太極拳選集

Taijiquan Master Reference

An Anthology

Volume 2

Compiled by
Michael A. DeMarco, M.A.

VIA MEDIA PUBLISHING | Articles from the Journal of Asian Martial Arts

Disclaimer

Please note that the author and publisher of this book are not responsible in any manner whatsoever for any injury that may result from practicing the techniques and/or following the instructions given herein. Participation in martial arts activities can be dangerous and can lead to serious injury. The material presented in this book is intended for reference only, and the reader assumes all risks associated with attempting to perform any of the activities described herein. Before attempting any of the physical activities described in this book, the reader should consult a physician for advice regarding their individual suitability for performing such activity.

All Rights Reserved

No part of this publication, including illustrations, may be reproduced or utilized in any form or by any means, electronic or mechanical, including photocopying, recording, or by any information storage and retrieval system (beyond that copying permitted by sections 107 and 108 of the US Copyright Law and except by reviewers for the public press), without written permission from Via Media Publishing Company.

Warning: Any unauthorized act in relation to a copyright work may result in both a civil claim for damages and criminal prosecution.

Copyright © 2025
by Via Media Publishing Company
941 Calle Mejia #822
Santa Fe, NM 87501 USA

Book and cover design
by Via Media Publishing Company

ISBN 979-8-9922430-1-7

www.viamediapublishing.com

Dedication

To all those who have contributed to the
Journal of Asian Martial Arts (1992–2016)
providing articles of high academic standards
that will continue to inspire research and practice.

Table of Contents

Preface — vii

- Going Beyond the Norm: An Interview with Chen Taiji Stylist Wang Xi'an — 481
  Asr Cordes

- To Bend or Not to Bend: A Look at Spinal Movement in Taijiquan and Other Martial Arts — 497
  Michael A. DeMarco, M.A.

- Comments on Selections from Chen Xin's *Illustrated Explanations of Chen Taijiquan* with Commentary from Chen Xiaowang, — 527
  Stephan Berwick, M.A., and translations by Dannie Butler, M.A.

- Dripping Oil Onto Parchment: Traditional Taijiquan Form Training in Chen Village — 542
  David Gaffney, B.A.

- Taiji Solo Form: The Benefits of Group Versus Individual Practice — 556
  John Loupos, B.S.

- From a Small Village to the Capital: The Li Family's Early Taijiquan Curriculum — 560
  Wong Yuen Ming

- Overlapping Steps: Traditional Training Methods in Chen Village Taijiquan — 569
  David Gaffney, B.A.

- In Memory of Wu Daxin: Wu Family Taiji Boxing Gatekeeper — 585
  Cai Naibiao; Y.L. Yip and Leroy Clark, Trans.

- Fear of Falling: Taijiquan as a Form of Graded in Vivo Exposure Therapy — 595
  Shane Kachur, B.M.R. (P.T), R. Nicholas Carleton, M.A., and Gordon Asmundson, Ph.D.

- Sanshou: Understanding Taijiquan as a Martial Art — 605
  Greg Wolfson, B.A.

- Ge Hong: Famous Daoist Thinker and Practical Martial Artist — 617
  Stanley E. Henning, M.A.

- Benefits of Non-Competitive Push-Hands Practice — 620
  Herman P. Kauz

- Taijiquan and Daoism: From Religion to Martial Art and Martial Art to Religion — 625
  Douglas Wile, Ph.D.

- Taiji Ruler: Legacy of the Sleeping Immortal — 671
  Kenneth S. Cohen, M.A., M.S.Th.

- Chenjiagou: The History of the Taiji Village — 695
  David Gaffney, B.A

- Zheng Manqing: The Memorial Hall and Legacy of the Master of Five Excellences in Taiwan — 711
  Russ Mason, M.A.

▶ A Comprehensive Introduction to Sun Family Taiji Boxing   733
   Theory and Applications
   Jake Burroughs, B.A.

▶ Xiong Style Taiji in Taiwan: Historical Development and   752
   a Photographic Exposé Featuring Master Lin Jianhong
   Michael A. DeMarco, M.A.

▶ Throwing Techniques in the Internal Martial Arts: 777
   An Elucidation of the Guiding Principle of 'Sticking and Following'
   Tim Cartmill, B.A.

▶ Liu Xiheng: Memories of a Taiji Sage   797
   Benjamin Lo, Xu Yizhong, Yuan Weiming, Xu Zhengmei, and Danny Emerick.
   Compiled by Russ Mason, M.A.

▶ Tensegrity: 828
   Development of Dynamic Balance and Internal Power in Taijiquan
   Michael Rosario Graycar and Rachel Tomlinson, M.Ed.

▶ Form and Function: 843
   Why Push-Hands is Essential to the Practice of Taijiquan
   Hal Mosher, B.A.

▶ Multiple Intelligences in the Process of Learning Martial Arts   855
   Using Taijiquan as an Example
   S. Dale Brown, M.A.

▶ Three Techniques of Dantian Rotation in Chen Taiji: Internal Energy   865
   Techniques and Their Relationship with the Body's Meridians
   Bosco Seung-Chul Baek (白承哲), B.S.

▶ Taiji and Qigong Health Benefits: How and Why They Work   886
   C.J. Rhoads, D.Ed., M.Ed., Duane Crider, Ph.D., and Dina Hayduk, D.Ed., M.Ed.

▶ Yoga Alchemy in Taijiquan   907
   Greg Brodsky, B.A., Lic. Ac.

▶ Ward Off, Diagonal Flying from Zheng Style Taijiquan   925
   Russ Mason, M.A.

▶ Chen Taijiquan: A Master's Touch   929
   David Gaffney, B.A.

▶ The Yang Style Taiji Spear Lineage   933
   Zhang Yun, M.S.

Sources of Original Publication   938

Index   940

Preface

Via Media Publishing was founded in 1992 in order to produce the peer reviewed quarterly *Journal of Asian Martial Arts* (1992–2012)—the first publication of its kind to focus on martial traditions in an academic format. Many of the authors were scholar–practitioners, who utilized their unique talents to present articles from various specializations, such as Asian Studies, kinesiology, history, anthropology, philosophy, and physical education.

Those who were serious about this field subscribed to the journal to read articles noted for their high academic and aesthetic standards. Most were in the United States, Canada, and Europe, but also in other areas of the world. These naturally included martial art schools and individual practitioners. There was a strong base among university and public libraries too.

As founder of Via Media, I've decided to assemble this anthology of articles relating to taijiquan. There are over three hundred million taiji practitioners worldwide, drawn to the art mainly for health maintenance and it therapeutic value. Researchers can benefit from this handy anthology, particularly for the information and analyses presented, including the rich bibliographic listings. Taiji practitioners will also gain insights to benefit their own practice, be it for health and/or self-defense.

Note that page numbering is consecutive from Volume 1 through Volume 2. The index covers both volumes.

Included here are sixty-four articles, the same number of hexagrams in the *Book of Changes* (*Yijing*). In addition to 735 illustrations, there are glossaries, maps, charts, and bibliographies. *Taijiquan* is the term representing the general category of study, but taijiquan can be subdivided into its branches, from the original Chen Family Style to the highly popular Yang Family Style. Other lineages are presented, such as the Wu and Sun systems.

The variety of material in this anthology reflects in-depth scholarly research and the experience of master practitioners. It will be a valuable source taijiquan enthusiasts for future decades. By making this book available to individuals and libraries, we hope this rare material will greatly contribute to further research in this field and inspire many to learn taijiquan with aspirations to mastery.

Michael DeMarco, Publisher
Santa Fe, NM, December 2024

Going Beyond the Norm:
An Interview with Chen Taijiquan Stylist Wang Xi'an
by Asr Cordes*

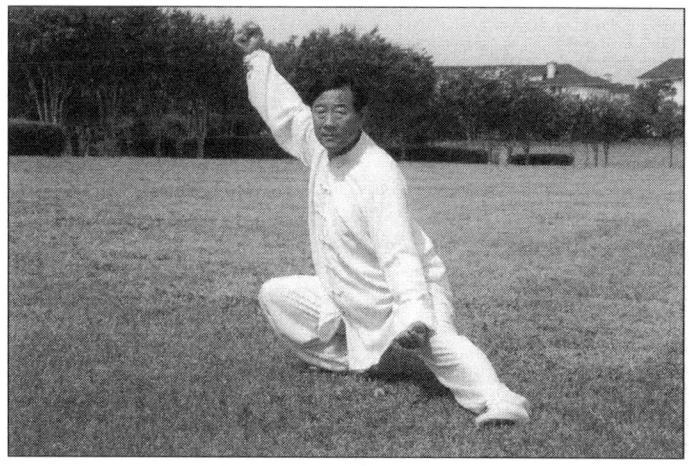

Chen Style Grandmaster Wang Xi'an.
All photographs courtesy of A. Cordes and Cheng Jincai.

Introduction

Wang Xi'an, a nineteenth-generation Chen Style taijiquan practitioner, is one of the leading representatives of the style. He is one of the celebrated Chen Style "Four Great Tigers," the others being Chen Xiaowang, Chen Zhenglei, and Zhu Tiancai. Mr. Wang has played a unique role in the preservation and proliferation of Chen taiji in Chen Village (Chenjiagou), where the style originated, and around the world.

Wang was born in 1944 in Xi'an, Shanxi Province, China. He and his family moved to Chen Village in 1945; Wang's parents were natives of Chen Village. About 120 years ago, Wang family ancestors moved to dynasty from Xingyang Village, which is south of the Yellow River.

Like most Chen villagers, Wang Xi'an began learning taiji when he was very young. However, his formal training did not begin until an eighteenth-generation successor of the style, Chen Zhaopei, retired from his civil service job and returned to Chen Village in 1958. He found that the level of taiji had diminished to the point that the standards of the next generation were uncertain. He subsequently opened the first formal classes. It was in these classes that Wang Xi'an and the other "Four Great Tigers" were taught. The "Four Great Tigers" subsequently studied with eighteenth-generation masters Chen Zhaokui and Feng Zhiqiang.

Wang Xi'an draws on his lifetime of Chen Style training to clearly communicate the mindset of Chen practice as well as vital keys to achieving success in Chen taijiquan training.

In May 2000, Wang made his first visit to the United States. To improve taiji here, two of Wang's students, Cheng Jincai (a lineage disciple and thirty-year student of Wang) and Li Shudong, sponsored Wang's visit. The following interview was conducted in Chinese Mandarin at Cheng Jincai's Chen Style Tai Chi Development Center in Houston, Texas.

INTERVIEW

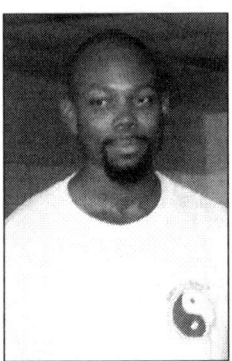

Asr Cordes, author and Chen Style practitioner.

■ *How did you came to study taiji?*

Well, it was the tradition and specialty of the area. Prior to the Cultural Revolution [1966–1976], everyone living in the village practiced. It was almost as if you couldn't live there without doing it. As a child living there you see everyone doing it, so naturally you try it too.

When I began learning taiji, all the people there were farmers. During the busy seasons, training was put on hold. When the farm work was done, training continued. At that time, taiji training was in the background of my life.

■ *At what point did you become serious about studying taiji?*

My serious training began when I was around eighteen years old, but my formal training didn't begin until I was twenty. At that time, Chen Zhaopei had returned to Chen Village and began teaching formal classes. Before Chen Zhaopei organized formal classes, everyone had their own small training groups and areas, usually at home. Family members of all different ages trained together. There were no big classes or anything like that.

I first studied small frame Chen Style and then large frame. I would like to note that the Chen small and large frames have a few differences between them. Based on my experience and observations, the old large frame of Chen Style yields a faster rate of development.

■ *We have heard that you have been instrumental in helping to preserve and promote Chen taiji. Could you tell us a little bit about that?*

Throughout the past, the popularity of taiji in Chen Village has had its ups and downs due to different events. The most recent down period was during the ten years of the Cultural Revolution. During the Cultural Revolution, I was in a unique position to help keep taiji going in the village as I held the position of *dui zhang*, which is like a vice mayor. Chen Zhaopei gave me the special responsibility of maintaining and promoting taiji development in the village. I knew I would need the help of the other teachers in the village. I invited Chen Zhaokui, an eighteenth-generation representative, back to the Chen Village to teach the new frame system of his father, Chen Fake.

I sought out the assistance of the local government leaders to help restore and promote the growth of taiji practice in and around the village. We organized all the small training groups into formal town classes. We put in place compulsory regulations that made it mandatory that these small groups form town classes. If a person trained well, they would receive special awards such as pay bonuses. If a person trained poorly, there might be pay deductions or overtime hours issued. These different groups also had small competitions in which people would receive special awards.

I also brought taiji training into the elementary and middle school curriculum. In addition to this, I opened school and public classes for advanced practitioners to bring them up to a higher level. After a few years, I opened a professional training school [*ti xiao*] with middle- and advanced-level classes. As a result, everyone in the village was into taiji training.

The Japanese began to develop a strong interest in taijiquan in 1981. After studying Yang taiji for a year, they learned that the major taiji styles had developed from Chen taiji and that the Chen Village was the source of taiji. In 1982, they approached the Henan Province Sports Committee about learning taiji in the Chen Village. I went as a representative to meet and interview the Japanese. In 1982, they brought a group of taiji enthusiasts from Japan to study at Chen Village. This was the first time the village had been opened to other countries.

This event drew such a large crowd that many police were needed to provide security. The event received lots of publicity from both the local and Japanese media. A well-known Japanese journalist, Shan Po Yinfu [Mandarin], was among this first group of visitors. He invited me to visit Japan in 1983. Japanese television and newspapers covered this visit extensively. I set up coaches for many cities in Japan and returned to China. About this time, taiji in general started to gain more popularity around the world.

Later, the Henan Sports Committee wanted me to go and teach in other areas. A few years later the other members of the "Four Great Tigers" moved from the village to teach in other places in China and around the world. Since nearly everyone was gone, and I knew someone needed to stay and keep up the level of practice in the village, I gave up the teaching post and returned to the hometown. Presently, my students are doing very well. I do not need to go see them compete anymore because I know how they will do.

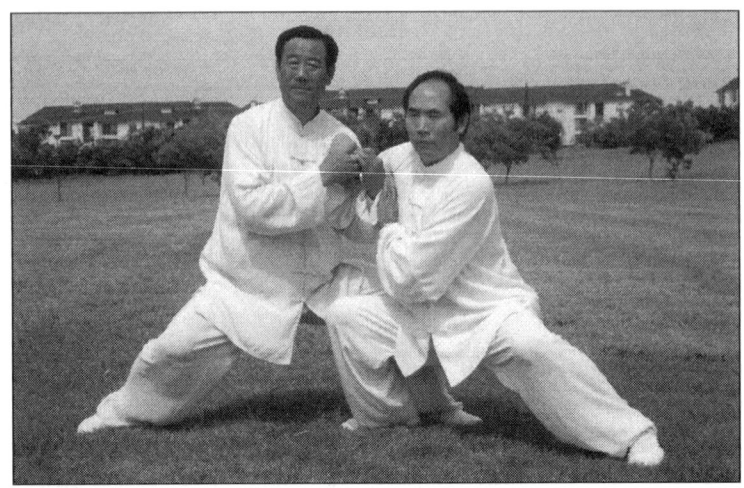

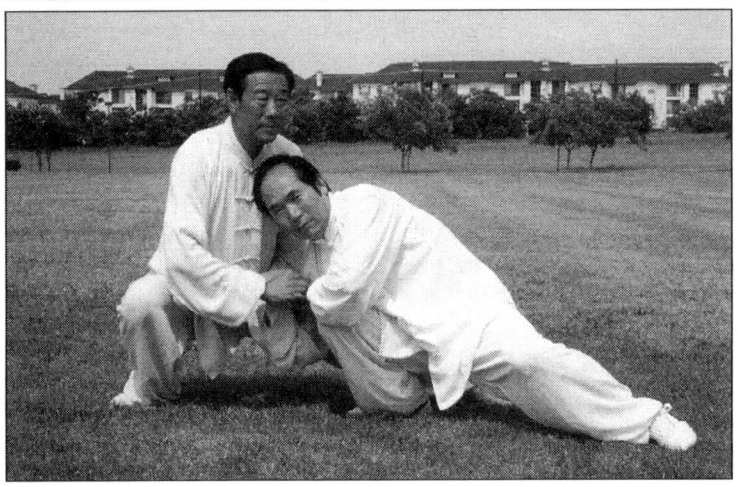

Wang Xi'an and Cheng Jincai practicing a counter to
a joint-locking application. (Plano, TX 5/2000)

■ *I have noticed that lots of martial artists acknowledge taiji as a good health exercise but not as an effective martial art. Could you explain a bit about taiji training to help us understand more clearly?*

Taiji training is very hard. You must train past your body's normal limits—many times past these normal limits. Normal training just will not do. You need to push. Back in Chen Village, all the people were farmers. The winter and spring were not busy times, so we had a lot of time to practice. So, I trained very hard through the summer heat and the winter cold. I had a large yard, and I don't know how many times a day I would train the routines. Too many to count. If you want to make real improvement, it is important that you work past your normal limits.

> Next page: Wang Xi'an practicing a movement from the
> Chen Style's first routine—shake foot and stretch down
> (Plano, TX, 5/2000); and from the second routine—
> wrap firecrackers (Paris, France 5/1994).

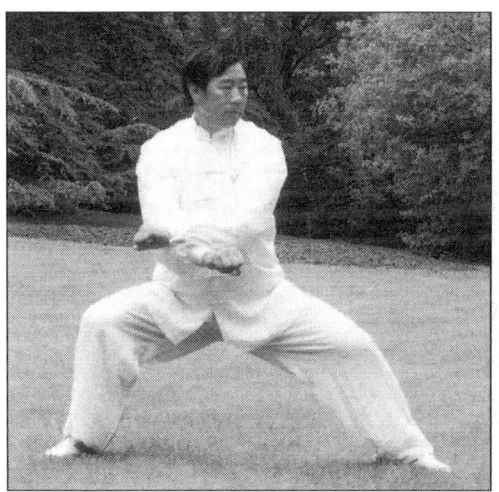
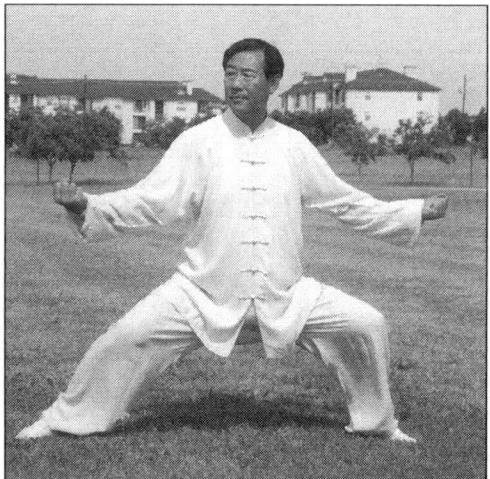

Even though we would have to lay off training to do the seasonal farm work, we could retain our gongfu or cultivation. Just a few days of warming up and you would be very good again.

Training internal energy it is like the rain. When it is raining very hard, the water comes down very strong and is abundant. When it is not raining, the water evaporates and dries up. When you are training internal energy very well, you need to keep it going and growing. Do not stop too long and allow your internal energy cultivation to evaporate or recede. It is not like an underground spring in where you dig until you hit water, and the water continues flowing forever. I used this analogy to clarify how you should train energy. If you want to build up very strong internal work, you must be consistent in practice, and I reiterate that you must train many times beyond your normal limits.

As far as the martial aspect is concerned, most martial arts have special and secret methods. Chen Style also has methods that are unique and are not taught to the public. Even I have methods that most taiji practitioners normally do not know.

The external martial styles are more straight in and straight out when it comes to punching and kicking. The internal styles emphasize more on breathing, mind control, and spiral movements. I feel that external styles are too demanding on the body. If practiced for too long, you will suffer when you get older. As the external martial artist ages, the bones and tendons start to show injury and then it is too late to really correct. If you only train "hard," the body is injured but you might not know it until it is too late.

Energy is generated from the inside and cultivated until it permeates the whole body from the most internal level to the surface of the skin. This makes you very healthy, but taiji is not just for that. It also builds very good fighting skills. External arts use explosive punching and kicking. The internal styles specialize in the use of spiral mechanics [*chansijing*], a unified way of delivering explosive power [*fajing*], as well as a way of dissipating power called *yin jin luo kong*. *Yin jin luo kong* means using your sensitivity to trick the opponent into attacking and then leading him into emptiness and then attacking him at his weakest moment. This is the internal arts usage of soft to fight hard. These are the high-level skills of taiji.

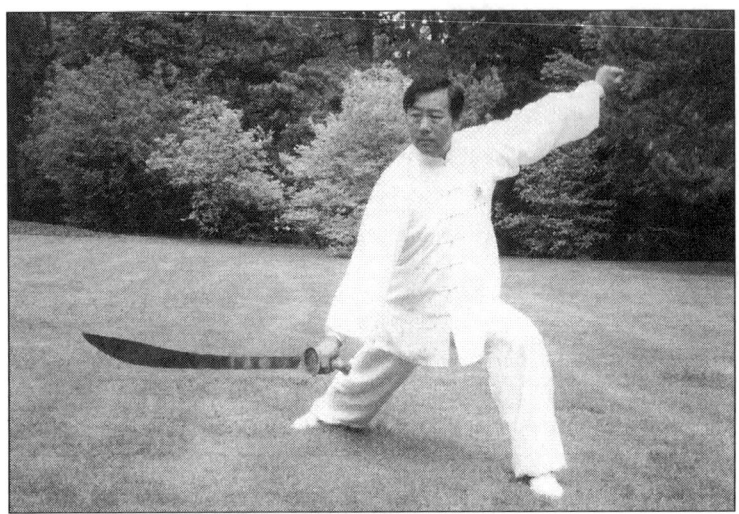

Wang Xi'an practicing a movement
from the Chen Style broadsword
rolling body chopping (Paris, France, 5/1994).

Normally people watch taiji and ask, "How can that be used for fighting?" At this level, people are not capable of understanding taiji's secrets. They only see the outside yet have no feeling to complete the picture. Once they start training and start developing to a higher level, they say, "Oh, now I understand a little." This process repeats itself until the many little breakthroughs lead to real skills. Progress comes by gradually building up. You can't push people and make them understand this kind of thing.

The internal arts include weapons practice, but they are not really used for self-defense. In the old days, people used them for protection, but since then things have cooled off. Now the martial uses have become more secret. In older times, people trained hard for protection. Now the emphasis has shifted more toward health. Currently, many people practice Yang taijiquan because it was the first to reach the public eye and is easier to learn. People are likely to do it when they are only looking for health.

Chen Style is not only soft, but also hard. It is not only slow, but also fast. Yang Style leans toward the soft side and the Chen Style sticks to perfectly balancing the two extremes and is easily adjusted to all ages and body types. Chen Style is very flexible but always maintains the internal training. The difference is who can improve faster. If you want to improve faster, you need to work harder to reach a high level. Yang Style has internal training, but soft training is not enough to reach high level or martial skill. If you want fighting skill, you will need special training.

First you build up internal energy from inside. You build up the whole body. The body becomes strong and internal energy can go through the whole body at the mind command. Then good fighting skill can be developed. Internal skills and health are developed at the same time. The special training for fighting skill requires in-depth knowledge of the applications of the Chen Style routines. Many people never reach this point in their training, so they never really understand about the fighting skills. That is the hard part of training.

■ *[Li Shudong]: I once had a traditional martial arts teacher. If he did not know a student well, he would teach them motions but not usage. He wanted to keep the tradition of transmitting to the right people. He needed to know who really wanted to train, if they had good character and manners. He made sure everything was correct and only then he taught the secrets. These teachings are not easily divulged to the public, right?*

No matter how much money people offer me, if they do not demonstrate the right character and I do not like teaching them, then no matter how much they pay, it won't matter. I would not teach them.

When it comes to martial skills, Chen Style has elements that the external styles have, such as numerous hitting, kicking, throwing, and joint locking techniques. Every style has those things. However, the spiral energy and short energy techniques, not everyone has those.

Taiji has five basic fighting skills: 1) feinting or dodging to trick an opponent, 2) grabbing techniques, 3) controlling, usually done with grabs and throws, 4) neutralizing attacks, and 5) hitting. These techniques are not isolated during usage. In fact, they are used together in various combinations according to the situation.

■ *[Wang stands up to demonstrate a movement called "lazy about tying a robe." He then asks me to grab both of his wrists with all my strength. Suddenly he circles his waist, generating a tremendous shaking power, which throws me away and frees him from the double-handed grab. The power generated was both soft and powerful, at once generating such an immense jolt that I was slightly disoriented.]*

I used this demonstration to show that not only do you have and use power, but you also use it very intelligently. You apply your power to just the right places that are the most vulnerable. Do not just hit the opponent. Sense the weakness in his power, then attack. In this case, the thumbs were the weak part of the hold, so they were attacked to neutralize the hold.

When executing the movements of the form, every small detail needs to be articulated. The attention to these subtleties in the forms will determine your success in developing real taiji combative skills.

■ *[Using the very beginning of the movement lazy about tying a coat, he circles both hands upward and does a small pressing action by extending and settling the wrists to the front.]*

This little pressing action at the top seems very small, but when it comes to martial technique, it is very important. You have this technique where the movement appears to be only neutralizing, but at the end there is a subtle attack hidden in the minute detail.

- *Could you please tell us of your experience with your teacher Chen Zhaopei?*

Chen Zhaopei was a very good person. He did not have a chance to receive a high education, but his memory was incredible. He committed to memory most of the important aspects of Chinese history. In his younger days, he worked for the civil service. When he returned to Chen Village, he used all his energy to help preserve Chen taiji. He would always try to answer every question a student had and watch their movements to try and understand what their problems were so that they could be corrected. He was extremely warmhearted. He would go way out of his way to teach and help people.

In 1972, the first competition was held in Dengfeng County, Henan Province. Chen Zhaopei was the head coach. By setting up formal classes and organizing competitions to promote development, he tried to build up Chen taiji from a secret family style to the level of a national art and sport.

I often had to attend meetings that would not end until late at night. After finishing my meetings, I would always stop by the school to find Chen Zhaopei inside with an oil lamp burning. So, I would go see him and he would teach me a lot. Chen Zhaopei was quite fond of singing. He often sang in a traditional free-style type of singing in which the singer sings whatever is in his mind. Chen Zhaopei would often sing these lines:

> When I hear the rooster crow, I awake and practice taiji.
> Right now, I am old, but I can still stick to the floor.
> I want someone who can be my successor.
> Even with sweat pouring out everywhere, I am quite happy.

- *What do you think about the level of taiji practice in the United States?*

I am pleased to see the popularity of taiji rising in the U.S., but presently the Japanese display a higher level. This is because they have been exposed to the top-level Chen masters for a longer time than the rest of the world outside of China. The higher-level Chen taiji has only been taught in the U.S. for a relatively short period. However, I am sure that the level will continue to rise in the next few years.

I am happy to see the rapid growth of taiji's popularity in such a short time. A lot of students are doing very well. However, I hope that they can practice more and for a longer time so that they can reach the deeper, more valuable aspects of taiji. I really appreciate the hospitality that everyone has shown me during this visit, and I hope everyone gets a chance to visit Chen Village.

I have done a lot of traveling and teaching around the world, and I have observed the constant rise in taiji's popularity. Right now, I am trying to build up Chen Village because, although it is the seat of Chen Style, it is a very poor village. It does not have a lot of the amenities that foreign visitors are accustomed to. Some serious students do not care about those kinds of things, but it would help things out greatly if the living arrangements were a little more comfortable during their stay. Also, I have made sure that there are higher-level teachers there so that more people can stay and get the desired training. With all this in mind, I am in the process of building a large professional training facility with dormitories. This also will serve to support Chen villagers who are really interested in training professionally: they can live there while training.

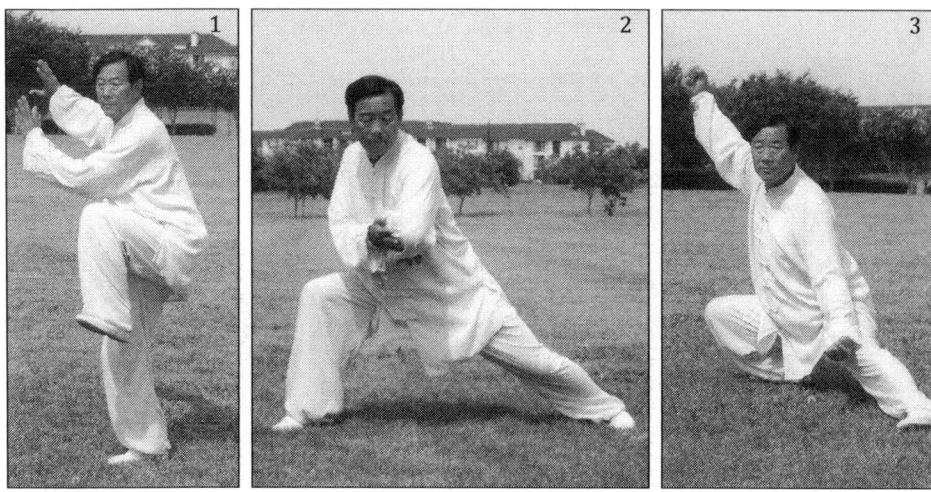

Wang Xi'an practicing. 1) a transitional movement from the Chen Style's first routine—Buddha's warrior attendant pounds mortar. 2) Chen Style's second routine—elbow hits the heart. 3) Chen Style's first routine—shake foot and stretch down (Plano, TX 5/2000).

TECHNICAL SECTION

Chen taijiquan is packed with highly effective martial techniques ranging from simple to profound. Practitioners become competent at the Chen Style's repertoire of high-level fighting skills through the practice of forms, push-hands, fighting drills, stepping drills, and body conditioning. The following applications present an introduction to Chen taijiquan's arsenal. These applications provide examples of how some of Chen Style's basic skills and methods are integrated in practical combative applications.

Strategically, Chen Style uses defense as its offense, yet it is very flexible and adapts to any situation as needed. Chen Style practitioners generally do not struggle with or seek to overpower the opponent. Instead, the Chen stylist uses sensitivity developed from push-hands practice to find the path of least resistance and uses the opponent's force against them, adding his own power and body weight to the opponent's power. Techniques are crisply executed in a swift and fluid manner with precise timing, attacking an opponent at the weakest place at the most vulnerable time.

It should be noted that all the essential concepts of Chen Style's numerous boxing skills are contained in the empty-hand and weapons forms. The applications featured in this article draw upon the following skills (Wallace, 1998: 58–89):

Eight boxing skills, also known as eight essential energies:
- ward off / resilient force
- rollback
- push
- press
- pluck
- split
- elbow strike, and
- leaning strike

The following technical section will illustrate the following:
- neutralization
- joint locking
- spiral energy or silk reeling
- return energy folding
- leading into emptiness
- striking
- stepping methods
- grabbing
- throwing
- kicking

Wallace, A. (1998). Internal training: The foundation for Chen Style Taijiquan's fighting skills and health promotion. *Journal of Asian Martial Arts, 7*(1): 58–89.

DEFENSE AGAINST A PUNCH

Skills Utilized: Neutralization of power, grab, and hit

1a The opponent punches at Cheng's face. He neutralizes the punch by sidestepping the attack while entering the opponent's space, blocking with his right hand without breaking the momentum of the punch.

1b Cheng quickly grabs the opponent's arm with his left hand then pulls the opponent into him, increasing the forward momentum of the punch. This literally sucks the opponent in and upsets his balance.

1c Cheng immediately punches to the side of the opponent's head. When applied at actual speed, the technique is executed in an instant and is very fluid utilizing sensitivity to fully capitalize upon the opponent's power.

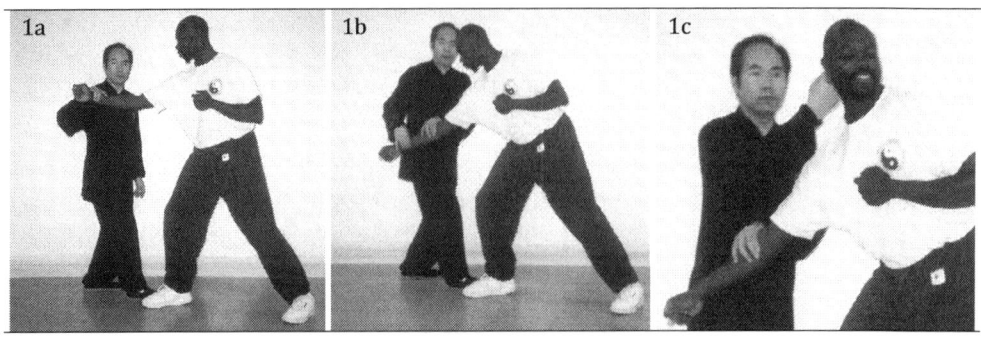

TAKE DOWN

Skills Utilized: Return/folding energy

2a The opponent grabs Cheng's arms as if to grapple with him.

2b Cheng relaxes his shoulders and chest to neutralize the grabbing of his arms. He then inserts his left hand outside of the opponent's right arm and his right hand inside the opponent's left. Using the points of contact as the controlling point, Cheng fakes a throw to the right causing the opponent to resist.

2c As soon as the reflex to resist arises in the opponent, Cheng uses his looseness and sensitivity to suddenly fold to the left.

2d Fully capitalizing on the opponent's returning energy, Cheng forcefully slams the opponent to the ground.

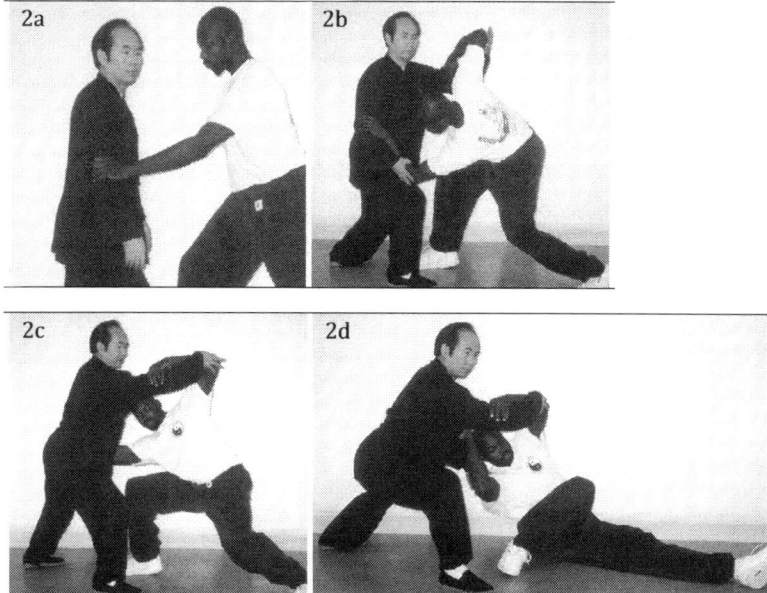

JOINT LOCK

Skills Utilized: Pluck

3a The opponent punches to Cheng's face. Using the rollback technique, Cheng intercepts and deflects the punch with his left hand.

3b Cheng catches the elbow from the bottom with his right hand hooking his fingers in the crease of the elbow he then applies the plucking technique, twisting and folding the joints.

3c After he manipulates the opponent into a very awkward position, he applies pressure to the locked joints generating great pain possibly dislocating the shoulder and seriously injuring the spine.

**See following page
for 3a, 3b and 3c.**

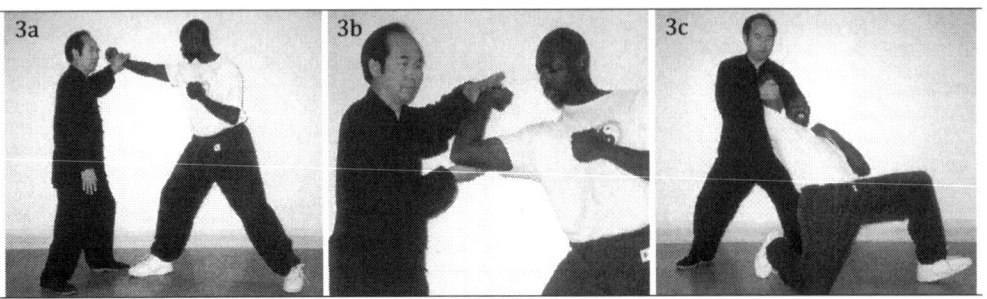

THROWING TECHNIQUE

Skills Utilized: Push (also translated as crowding or squeezing)

4a The opponent suddenly pushes Cheng's chest. Cheng immediately sinks down to stabilize his body.

4b He grabs the opponent's elbows and changes the angle of the elbow joints by rotating them outward. Cheng simultaneously expands his chest toward the opponent and pulls him in, generating the push or squeezing energy making the opponents arms collapse locking his wrists and causing his body to overextend forward.

4c Cheng then explosively spirals his body and weight down to the right destroying the opponent's balance.

4d Cheng then forcefully flips the opponent over on to the ground.

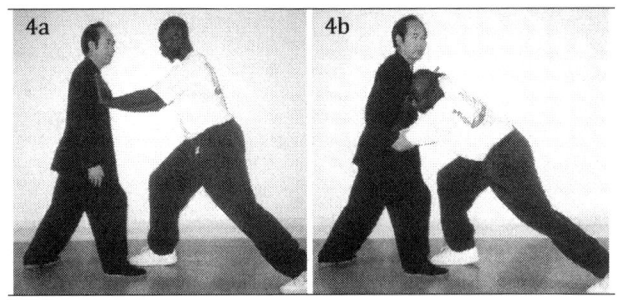

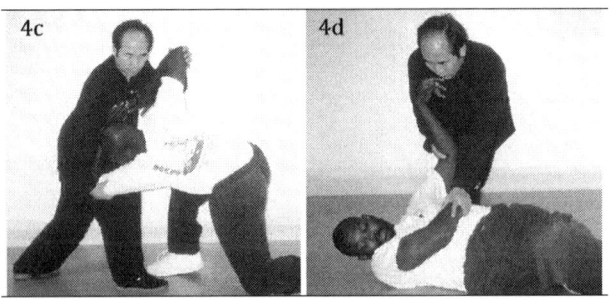

KICK NEUTRALIZATION

Skills Utilized: Kicking technique, neutralization of power

5a Cheng and the opponent square off.
5b The opponent delivers a front kick. Cheng rotates his body to the right, neutralizing the kick. He then catches the kick from the bottom.
5c-d Cheng completes the catching of the kick with his left hand locking the knee. He then delivers a side heel kick to the inside of the knee, which takes the opponent down, possibly dislocating or breaking the knee.

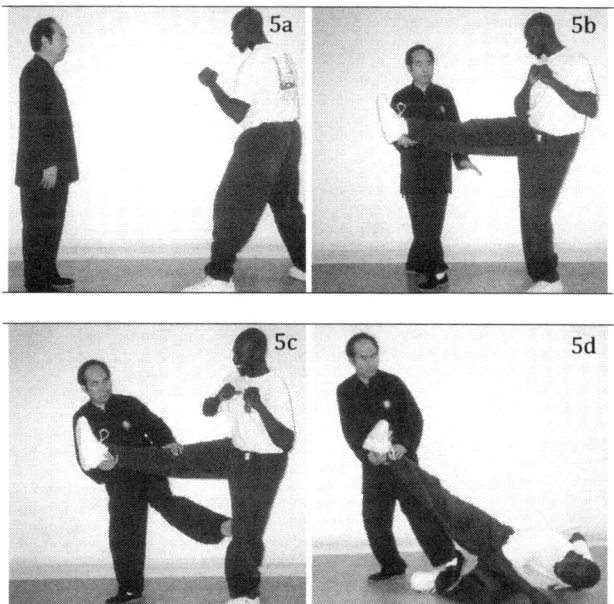

JOINT LOCK

Skills Utilized: Pluck

6a The opponent grabs Cheng's wrist.
6b Cheng rotates his arm clockwise exploiting the range of motion of the opponent's arm and then grabs the opponent's wrist before he can let go.
6c Cheng then sinks his body and opens his arm forward, generating immense pressure on the opponent's already locked wrist and forearm and setting him up to be hit in the face.

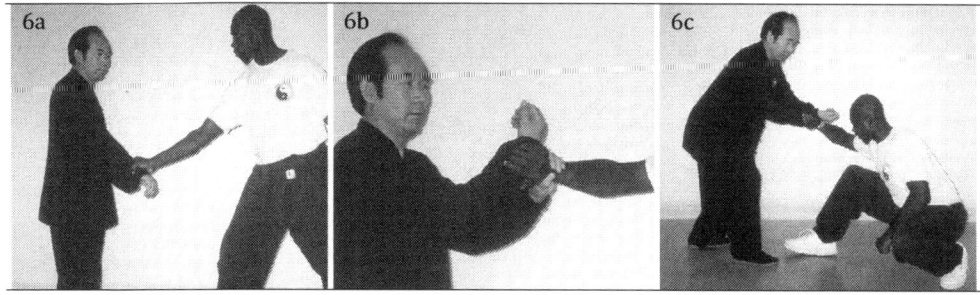

TAKE DOWN

Skills Utilized: Press, leading into emptiness

7a The opponent forcefully pushes Cheng's chest.
7b Cheng sinks his body and loosens his joints allowing the opponent's force to be conducted to the ground without toppling him. Cheng simultaneously places his hands on top of the opponent's forearms.
7c He then relaxes and hollows his chest while pressing downward on the opponent's incoming force. This causes the opponent to suddenly fall into emptiness.
7d As the opponent falls in, Cheng adds his own force pressing downward, slamming the opponent to the ground.

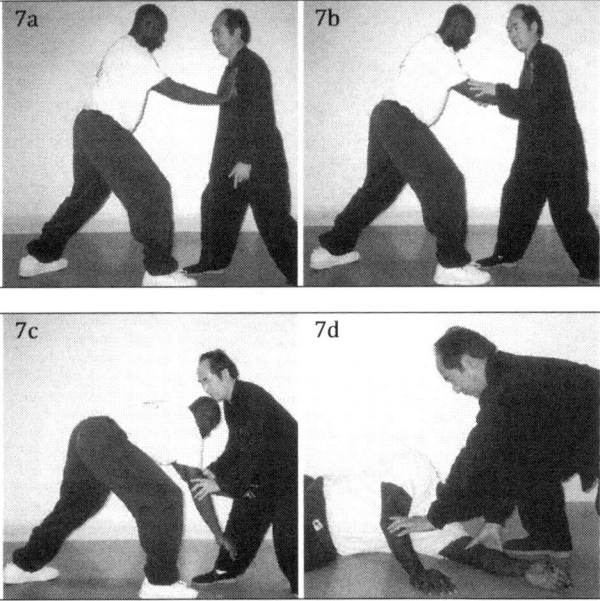

THROW

Skill Utilized: Joint locking

8a The opponent grabs Cheng's arms as if to grapple with him.
8b Cheng then grabs inside the opponent's right elbow with his left hand and outside the left elbow with his right hand. He twists the right elbow inside, locking the joints on the right while pressing the outside of the left elbow causing the opponent to fold to the right.
8c Cheng then drops his body weight while explosively spiraling the hips down to the left, forcefully slamming the opponent to the ground.

See following page for 8a, 8b and 8c.

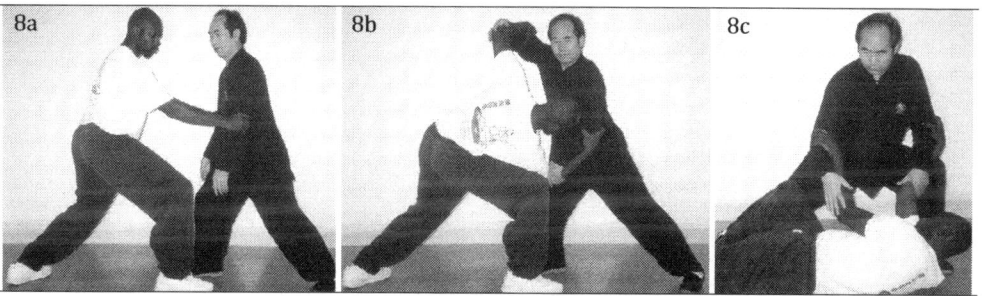

JOINT LOCK

Skills Utilized: Pluck

9a The opponent punches at Cheng's face. Cheng rotates his body out of the way and catches the opponent's wrist and elbow.

9b He then guides the opponent's elbow into the fold of his own elbow to stabilize the elbow while folding the wrist to create a very firm joint lock.

9c Cheng then applies pressure to the locked joints generating immense pain at the wrist allowing him to manipulate the opponent into a very vulnerable position and strike him or severely damage the tissues in the wrist.

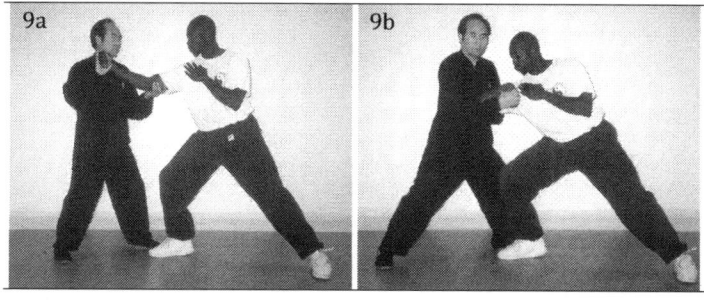

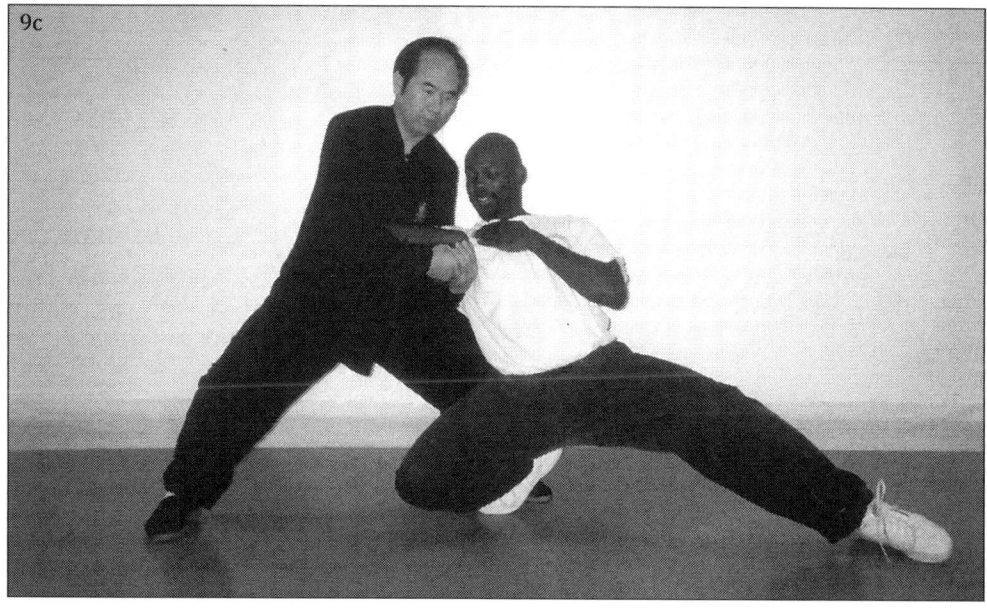

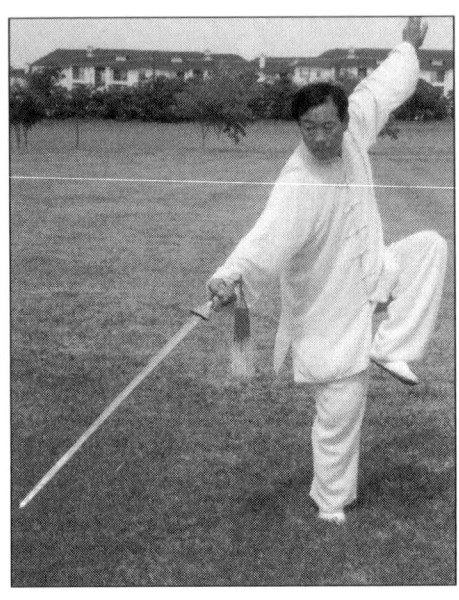

Wang Xi'an practicing a movement from
the Chen Style straight sword routine
called immortal points the way
(Plano, TX 5/2000).

* Special thanks goes to Li Shudong for helping with
the translation while conducting this interview.

NAMES OF PEOPLE

Chen Fake	陳發科
Chen Zhaokuai	陳照奎
Wang Xian	王西安
Chen Xiaowang	陳小旺
Chen Zhenglei	陳正雷
Zhu Tiancai	朱天才
Cheng Jincai	程進才
Li Shudong	李樹東

To Bend or Not to Bend: A Look at Spinal Movement in Taijiquan and Other Martial Arts

by Michael A. DeMarco, M.A.

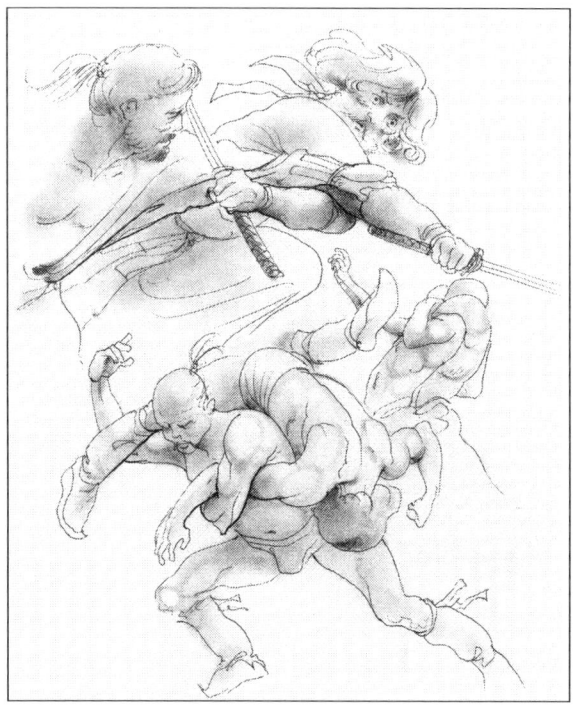

From artwork by Oscar Ratti.
© 2002 Via Media Publishing Co.

Abstract

Bending is one of the most contentious topics dealing with body mechanics found in the martial arts, and in taijiquan. In fighting traditions, "to bend or not to bend" is a matter of life or death and demands scrutiny. To offer a general picture of how the spine is viewed within these traditions, this article first gives an overview of the spinal structure, then looks to the relevant Asian martial arts literature and professional opinions on the subject. For a more practical approach, taijiquan was selected to help illustrate functional aspects of the spine under actual fighting conditions.

The purpose of this article is to present how the spine moves in the fighting arts, not just under ideal practice conditions, but also under more realistic combative situations. In so doing, there are many factors and variables to consider, such as form verses function, the dynamics of body mechanics, and the skill level of those involved. Because some skills are more difficult to obtain than others, it is expected that there are differences in theory and practice regarding this topic.

Introduction

There is a common admonition given to students by instructors of the various combative systems taught around the world: "keep your spine in proper alignment." This usually means straight, because an erect spinal column is considered a valuable key in maintaining balance and proper alignment for executing fighting techniques. However, upon close observation, we can see that the spine often flexes to extreme degrees during actual practice. Why? Is this a phenomenon associated more with beginning level practitioners than with advanced? Should the spine always remain straight, or are there exceptions to this rule? Do certain styles allow one to bend, while others forbid it? This article looks at how some noted martial art systems utilize the spine and asks readers to look within their own practice to discover for themselves the spine's role in their combative art.

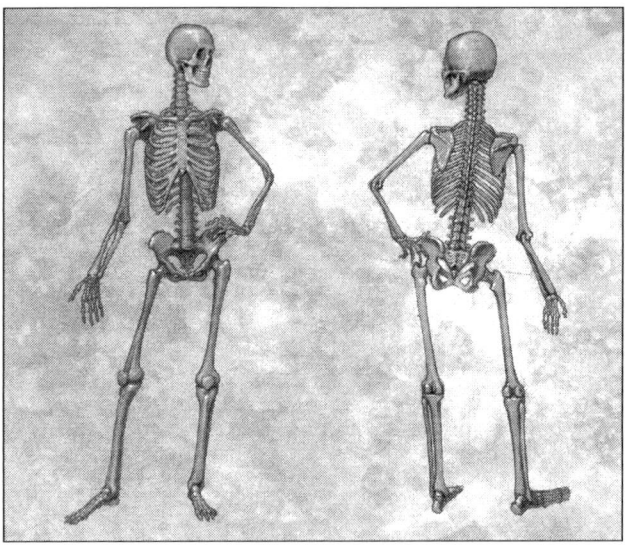

Structure of the Spine

All traditional martial arts, whether they practiced with or without weapons, build their systems upon an intimate understanding of human anatomy and related body mechanics. Before looking directly at the role the spine plays in the martial arts, we should look at the fundamentals of the skeletal system.

Made up of 206 bones in adults, the skeleton is the principal structure upon which all other bodily systems are arranged, such as the muscular and nervous systems. If we study a picture of a skeleton, it is soon apparent that the spine is the human body's biological axis. In the most simplistic terms, it functions as a conduit for all the vital organs. Whenever proper body posture is addressed, the spine ranks first in importance. The high value placed on proper spinal alignment is lauded by chiropractors and other medical specialists. Even analogies illustrate the vital importance of the spine, such as referring to a person as being the "backbone" of a team, or another as being "spineless" (one who is without strength or character). A spine even holds this journal together!

If we are concerned with martial arts and movement, then we should have a basic understanding of the spine and how it works. Medical books usually divide the spine into several sections to facilitate discussion. The bony segments that form the spinal column are called vertebrae, and these are demarcated according to their positions:

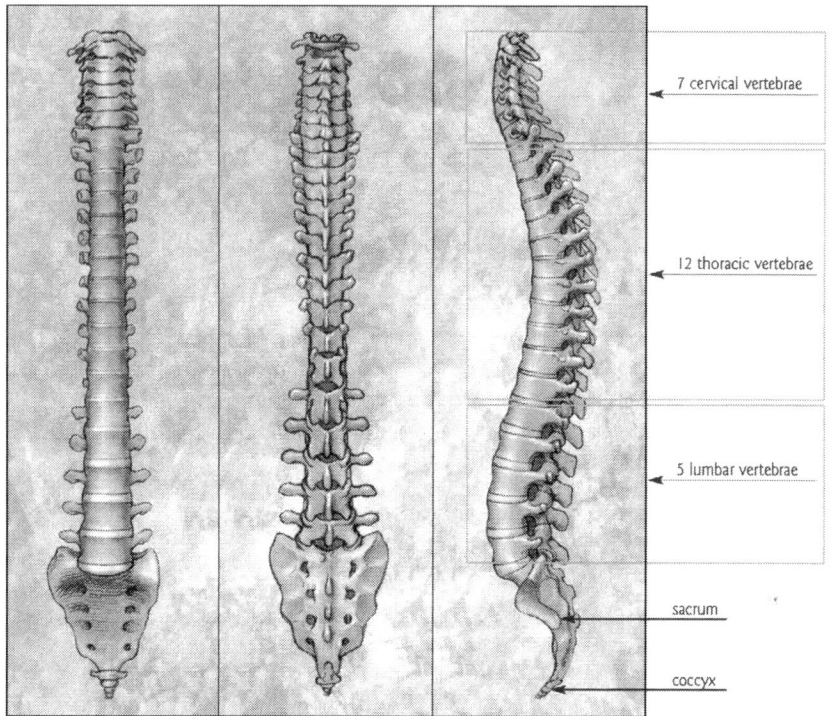

- cervical vertebrae (7): make up the neck
- thoracic vertebrae (12): make up the mid-back section where the ribs are attached
- lumbar vertebrae (5): located below the last thoracic bone and the top of the sacrum
- sacral vertebrae: caged within the bones of the pelvis
- coccyx: the terminal vertebrae.

Although the segments forming the spinal column give the body stability, they also allow it to be flexible. A healthy spine can bend easily and effortlessly under natural conditions. However, the vertebrae often become less mobile due to factors such as daily stress, disease, and injuries. Muscular tension probably plays the biggest part in this, often resulting from psychological responses that occur subconsciously. From infancy we are told to sit and stand up straight, lift with a straight back, and possibly are even scolded by a teacher or officer into "attention!" —with eyes front, heels together, and arms to the sides. Such conditioning has lasting effects. Similar conditioning is carried out in martial arts studios as well.

The Spine as Described in Selected Martial Traditions

From the brief discussion above, we can see that our regular daily lifestyles affect how we think about the spine, which manifests in our bodily movement. To further complicate matters, martial arts often follow the military tradition of strict "attention." There is commonly an oppressive atmosphere in martial art studios that molds individuals into a working order and forges students' forms into cookie-cutter images. The result may be a functional class and impressive forms, but the impetus is a forced one. Couple this with fears that arise out of facing sparring competitions or being judged by higher ranks, and we see an increase in tensions that can fuse one's spinal column. Bruce Lee had a miniature tombstone erected inside his studio that read: "In memory of a once fluid man crammed and distorted by the classical mess."

Lee was poking fun at the overbearing power of teachers and writings that dulled the human being's natural movement. One of the biggest causes of unnatural stiffening of the spine has been the concept of being "straight." For example, golf teachers and instructional books preach that all right-handed golfers should keep their left arms straight while addressing the ball. If this lesson is taken to heart without understanding the full meaning, the golfer is doomed to play as if his left arm were in a cast. "Straight" does not mean tense. Also, "straight" while addressing the ball does not mean that the arm should not flex while in movement. Likewise, we are often told by martial arts instructors and authors that we should keep our postures "straight." Perhaps we should maintain a straight posture that is without stiffness?

If we make a brief overview of references to the spine and posture in martial arts, there may be some common ground. For example, Dr. John Donohue (personal communication, August 18, 2002) writes: "In Shotokan karate, you don't bend. An upright spine is considered essential for proper balance and focus. When you're a beginner, a *sensei* [teacher] will place a *shinai* [bamboo practice sword] up against your spine to test whether it's straight enough. This is probably influenced by the erect spine in *zazen* [sitting meditation], with its associations of clear energy and breathing channels, etc. Same in kendo—we stand very erect, and a perfect strike is one where this posture is maintained. People bend while dodging strikes in sparring, but this is considered a cheap tournament trick and not classic technique."

In discussing another sword art, Dr. Deborah Klens-Bigman concurs with Dr. Donohue. She writes (personal communication, August 20, 2002): "Generally speaking, in Muso Shinden-ryu iaido, the back is kept straight, and the weight is centered. Movement comes from the *koshi* (lower back/hip region) while the upper back remains upright. The only exceptions occur when the iaidoka needs to transfer his/her weight onto the opponent's body to temporarily immobilize him, or in one case, when the iaido practitioner needs to clear an obstacle overhead to cut down an opponent."

Most martial arts discuss the spine in personal instruction, but often the topic is neglected in the written documents. Dr. Klens-Bigman points this out: "There is little 'major literature' in Muso Shinden-ryu iaido, though there are a couple of sources in Japanese. The posture aspect is part of the *okuden* (oral teaching) in every class I've taken in this style—a lot of emphasis is placed on maintaining an upright posture."

Most styles are known for keeping the spine plumb-line erect, i.e., perpendicular to the ground. Another idea is to align the spine with one of the legs. Dr. Karl Friday discusses the Japanese system he is most familiar with (personal communication, August 18, 2002) and points out this variation. He states: "While Kashima-Shinryu traditional literature contains no explicit discussions of the spine or upper body posture, these are very important matters in Kashima-Shinryu martial art, and receive a great deal of attention in direct instruction. All Kashima-Shinryu postures emphasize keeping the spine erect, without bending at the waist, and the upper body titled forward thirty to forty degrees, such that it forms a straight line with the back leg, which is also kept nearly straight. The elbows are flexed outward to form a circle, rolling the shoulders forward slightly, and smoothing out the curve of the spine. This position has numerous implications for control of range, for delivery of power, and for diffusion of incoming force or energy."

There are similar movements done with the sword that can be found in performances with other weapons as well, such as the staff or spear. Kim Taylor, states (personal communication, August 21, 2002): "In Iaido, Jodo and Niten Ichi-ryu, the back is straight; not only that but it remains as close to perpendicular to the floor as possible. There is very little twisting of the shoulders out of line with the hips, and the back is curved forward only in very special circumstances."

Mr. Taylor mentions one of the bigger problems associated with practicing with a "straight back": "In fact, one of the things I've noticed is that I can practice any of those arts for a couple of hours and at the end my lower back creaks from having frozen in place, as if I'd sat still in a chair for the same amount of time."

In these arts or any other stressing a 'straight back', the tensions may have the opposite effect of what we really desire. We desire freedom of movement to let our bodies respond instantaneously in any conflict. Too much tension and rigidity results in being "frozen." This can occur when one intentionally or unintentionally tries to make the spine straight, or when one eventually becomes too tense from over-practice.

THE SPINE IN IAIDO TECHNIQUES
Demonstrated by Kim Taylor

1) A normal draw and cut for iaido, with back straight and perpendicular to the floor throughout.
2) "Floating Clouds" (*uki gumo*) technique where the swordsman draws and cuts into the shoulder of a person who tried to gram the hilt. The sword must stay cut into the shoulder, so you have to bend over to do it.
3) A technique called "Under the porch" (*tana shita*) where one imagines he is under a veranda and slides forward out into the open to cut own the opponent. After the cut, the swordsman returns to the standard straight-back stance.

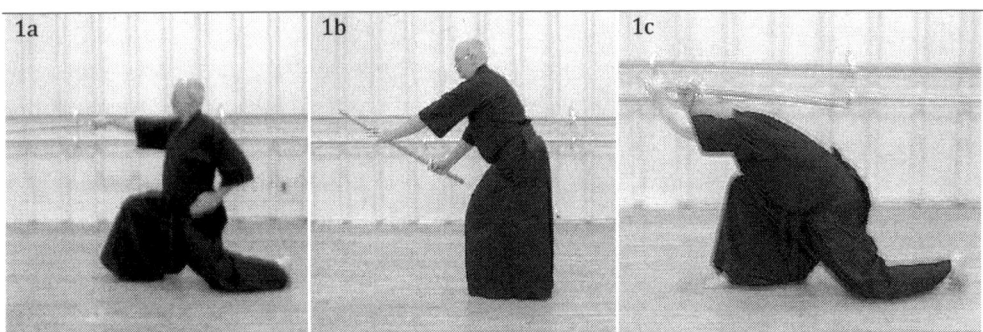

The ideas regarding the use of the spine in the sword arts are also found in other styles. Dr. Robert Dohrenwend (personal communication, August 18, 2002) points this out: "All those styles of karate and its derivative taekwondo, with which I am familiar, emphasize a straight back with low shoulders and level hips. The reason has to do with the efficient transfer of power from the hips to the point of impact. The only general exceptions are when the body leans to counterbalance a kick, but even then, the attitude of the back allows the karate-ka to recover his upright posture and solid balance as quickly as possible. In all the formal stances of karate and taekwondo, the back is kept straight and vertical. However, there is often a slight forward inclination from the hips when fighting or sparring, although the back is kept relatively straight . . . . The straight back is so basic to karate that it is often taken for granted, so few printed sources mention it explicitly. For Shotokan, Nakayama is as authoritative a source as exists."

> At all times, the upper part of the body must be kept perpendicular to the ground and the hips level. – Nakayama, 1977: 28

> The upper body must be firmly settled . . . and the back kept straight or perpendicular to the ground. – Nakayama, 1966: 23

For Okinawan karate, Uechi-ryu may be taken as representative, and George E. Mattson emphasizes a straight back in his book, *The Way of Karate* (1963: 55–56).

In referring to Korean styles, Marc Tedeschi states (personal communication, August 24, 2002): "Hapkido also has no particular philosophy about the back/spine being straight or vertical, or prescribing when and how it is bent. In some instances the spine is erect and over the hips; in others it is bent quite dramatically. It all depends on what creates the greatest technical efficiency, maintains balance, or contributes to one's energetic connection to one's opponent."

Mr. Tedeschi goes on to write that when compared to taekwondo, "Hapkido techniques (strikes, joint locks, throws) tend to make greater use of upper-body motions and pronounced leaning to increase power. The back/spine might be in any number of positions."

Just from the few samples above, it is apparent that the martial systems associated with Japan and Korea are noted for their uprightness. But there are exceptions. What we find in other cultures is very similar.

Dr. Phillip Zarrilli (personal communication, August 18, 2002) notes: "Given the foundation of kalarippayattu practice in Indian yoga, it is not surprising that practice is built around what I would describe as a 'lengthened' spine. Since Indian martial practice is concerned with awakening the internal energy (*kundalini sakti*) to be utilized in martial applications or health-giving therapies, the energy must be awakened and eventually travel along the line of the spine, i.e., from the base or 'root' of the navel through the top of the head. The sense of such a lengthened spine, with energy travelling along the spine-line, is gained through long-term practice of the basic exercises under the tutelage of a master teacher. One learns that support must always be kept in the region of the lower abdomen, with the awakened energy travelling from there downward into the earth, and up/outward through the upper torso/arms, and top of the head. For the practitioner who has 'actualized' an awakening of the internal energy, it is not necessary for the spine per se to always be literally 'lengthened,' i.e., as in the serpent pose of the CVN style,* the upper back might be tucked/rounded as the practitioner quickly turns under when executing the pose."

*NOTE: The CVN style referred to here is the style taught by Govindankutty Nair in Trivandrum, Kerala.

What we have found for the Asian traditions regarding references to the spine is found in other cultures as well, including the Western. For example, in European saber fencing: ". . . the trunk is held in an upright, or perpendicular position" (Crosnier, n.d.: 21). Alaux (1975: 128) writes that there is an "emphasis on keeping the body erect to facilitate greater mobility... The torso should be kept upright with the shoulders relaxed..."

Most of the fighting systems mentioned above are primarily striking arts. They focus on a standing position for defense and attack. However, other systems have a different approach, and their use of the spine offers a different perspective. These systems include the various styles of grappling, wrestling, judo, sambo, sumo, Brazilian jiujitsu, etc. Rather than having a focus on striking with hands and feet from a vertical position, these arts are often performed horizontally, on or near the ground. As a result, considerations for balance are different. Movements are performed with the expectation that gravity will act to assist in making throws, falls, and locks.

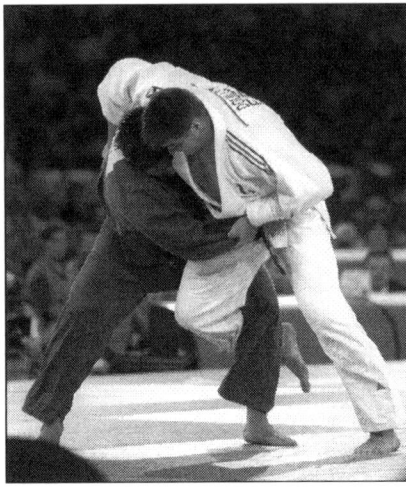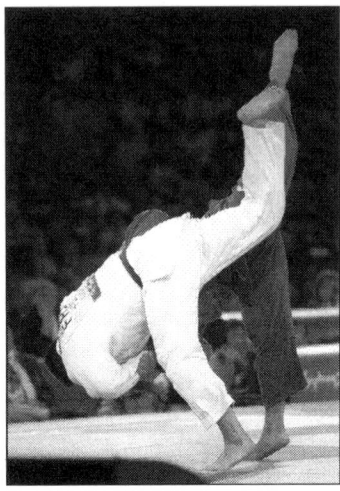

Beautiful technique shown by Douillet (white) in this 2000 Olympic judo bout with Shinohara. However, Douillet's sweep was not good enough to score as Shinohara's amazing dexterity allowed him to use uchimata-sukashi to win the match. Photos courtesy of David Finch.

Daniele Bolelli (personal communication, September 5, 2002) discusses some of the arts that often utilize movements that require the spine to bend and twist. He states that "some arts, particularly so the grappling ones, bend at the hips so that they look almost prone to the ground. Freestyle wrestling is a prime example of this. Whereas judo advocates always staying straight, freestyle wrestlers are closer to the ground in order to 'shoot' for the legs and to be ready to sprawl against a 'shooting' attack."

Also, another topic of interest may be the preparatory exercises used in some grappling arts. Mr. Bolelli gives the example of "bridging" (the bending of the back backwards and resting on one's forehead). He writes that bridging "is used by groundfighters to strengthen the neck muscles but also as an escape from the bottom position. Some people suggest that this may be harmful for the structural alignment of the neck, but most grapplers consider bridging one of the most important exercises of all."

From the previous material discussing the spine and its use in the various martial arts, most styles favor keeping the spine straight. The spine may align with gravity or be in alignment with the angle that favors one of the legs. The reasons given for this alignment involve the desire to maintain balance and to provide a solid anatomical structure for the execution of fighting techniques. Most martial traditions have solo routines that are practiced for perfecting their techniques. A straight spinal column allows the practitioner to experience movement in accord with the school's established tradition, providing a source of power and the kinetic beauty for which the martial arts are known.

The following section will focus on the spine as utilized within the taijiquan tradition, but represents similar views and practices found in other Chinese fighting systems.

TECHNIQUES FROM NORTHERN SHAOLIN BOXING
Demonstrated by Gao Fangxian
Photos courtesy of Robert W. Smith.

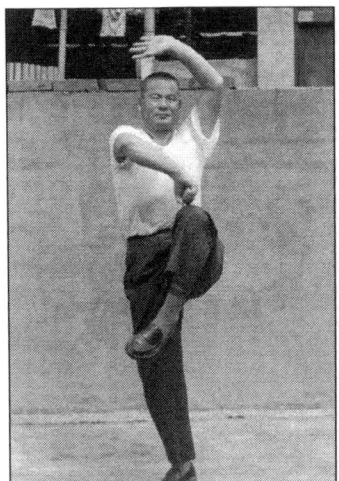
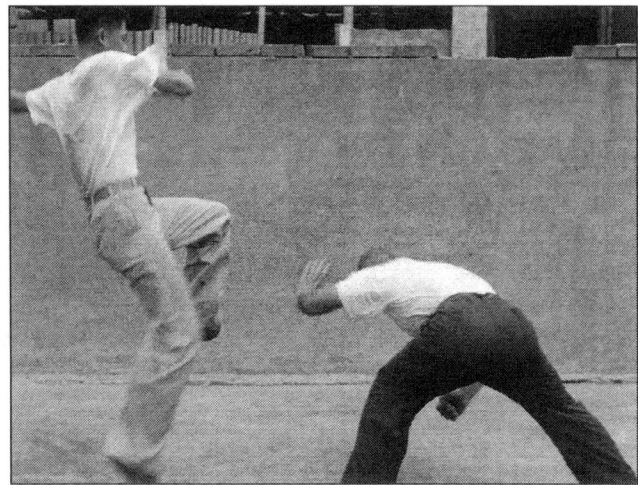

TECHNIQUES FROM DRAGON PALM BAGUA
Demonstrated by Mark Bow Sim
Photos courtesy of Shannon Phelps.

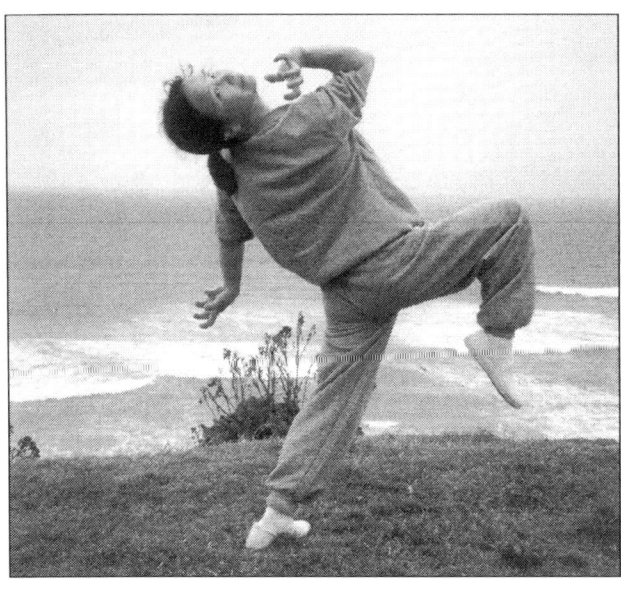

PEKING OPERA ACTORS PERFORMING A FIGHT SCENE.
Many fighting forms utilize bending backwards to evade attacks by spears, swords, and other weapons. Photos courtesy of the National Kuo-kuang Chinese Opera Company in Taiwan. Photograph by Lee Minghsun.

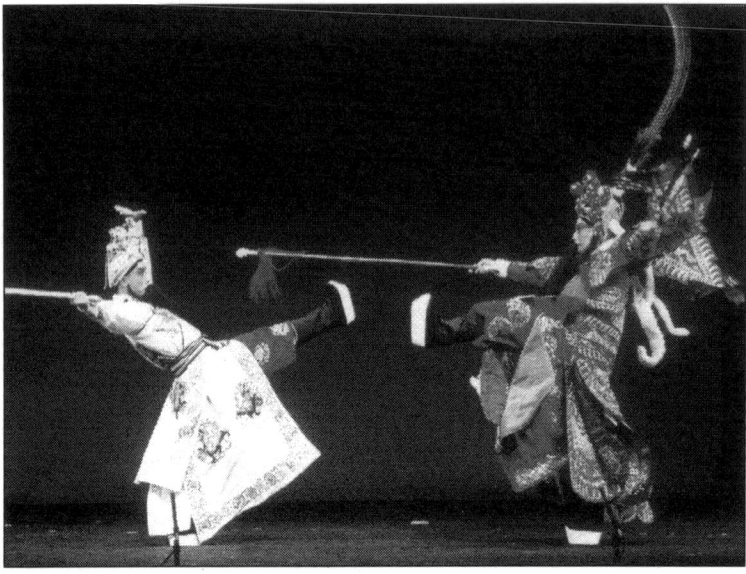

THE SPINE AS DESCRIBED IN THE TAIJIQUAN TRADITION

Regardless of taiji style (Chen, Yang, Wu, Hao, etc.), there is ample advice in the tome of taijiquan literature for the necessity of keeping one's posture erect during practice. The most common phrase is "to think of the head being suspended by a thread," thus straightening the backbone without tension. Since the "thread" does the work, there is no need for the muscles to make the back straight.

The importance of posture is noted by Sim and Gaffney, who have put great effort into bringing many of the Chen taiji teachings between the covers of a single volume:

> The mainstay of [taiji] movements and posture is the spine, as it links the head, the body and the limbs, facilitating whole-body movement. ... By keeping the spine straight, relaxed and strong, the gaps between the vertebrae will be opened naturally so that qi can pass through, up or down, very smoothly, facilitating ease of action. The spine should be like a flexible rope and not a stiff pole. If the spine is stiff, energy and power will not be transmitted from the feet to the hands.
> – Sim and Gaffney, 2002: 61

The above statement mentions keeping the spine straight, but also relaxed and flexible. This flexibility of the spine can be likened to the archer's bow. In taijiquan, there is an analogy depicting five main parts of the body that resemble "bows." They are the two arms, the two legs, and the body (Sim and Gaffney, 2002: 78–80). "Of the five bows, the body bow is primary, the arm and leg bows secondary" (Sim and Gaffney, 2002: 80). If the body bow is primary, then we know that the spine's movement plays a vital role in the Chen tradition.

But how flexible should the spine be? A clue can be found in a teaching formula that is presented by the leading representative of Chen family taiji, Chen Xiaowang. He details "five levels of skill" based on incorporating a proper mix of yin (soft) and yang (hard) into one's practice (Sim and Gaffney, 2002: 83–94). In the first level, there is "one yin, nine yang." At each successive level there is one more yin added, until the highest level is reached with "five yin and five yang— A True Master" (Sim and Gaffney, 2002: 93).

To balance hard and soft in one's movements means to let the spine have some flexibility. What remains unclear is the degree of flexibility allowed. If Chen Xiaowang said 50%, we would have to ask, "50% of what?!" We first need to know what the maximum is to know what such formulas mean. The maximum can only be felt through two-person practice, and push-hands is the favored method. Sim and Gaffney repeat an idea offered by many experts noted for their push-hands abilities: "If a person continues to yield when being pushed and does not know the boundary of the yield, balance will be lost. Yielding leads to neutralizing (*hua*)" (Sim and Gaffney, 2002: 151). If the above statement is correct and applied to the question of the spine's flexibility, then it seems that the ideal for the spine to bend would be 50% of the maximum, where one can maintain balance. One major problem in this equation is that the maximum differs for each practitioner.

We find much of the same throughout the *Taiji Classics*. In the Yang Style, which is often taught and practiced specifically for its health-nurturing benefits, we find solid rationale for keeping the spine straight. Zheng Manqing (Cheng Man-ch'ing), taiji master and Chinese medical doctor, writes that "the structure of the spine is not as important as its function which is the path and means of self-cultivation and preserving life" (Cheng, 1985: 41). He delves in more deeply in writing:

> If you are *cheng* (upright), there will be no cause for illness in the spine. Wei is the fear of not being upright and so courting illness. So, I advise [taijiquan] practitioners, "Make your spine upright." Upright is a string of pearls that does not lean. But being tense, holding oneself unnaturally erect, or over correcting are all real defects. You just must know that these are dangerous. – Cheng, 1985: 43

Dr. Douglas Wile (personal communication, August 21, 2002) says that "bending and double-weightedness must be two of the most contentious topics in taiji body mechanics. Pull-down, split, elbow-stroke, and shoulder-stroke are often described as compensation or recovery techniques for failures in timely ward off, roll-back, press, and push, and I think that bending is often compensation for failures in waist rotation and sinking. By sinking, here, I mean externally as well as internally, that is, literally dropping your center of gravity below the opponent's thrust. But enough of me. Qi Jiguang's *Quanjing* shows no bending. The Chen people are more tolerant of bending than the Yang, and Chen Xin specifically states that one should not be too dogmatic about it. The illustrations in some of the other early Chen books from the 1930s also show occasional departures from plumb erect. The Wu Jianquan style is kind of a special case, because they incline forward in many postures but deny that this compromises their internal vertical connection."

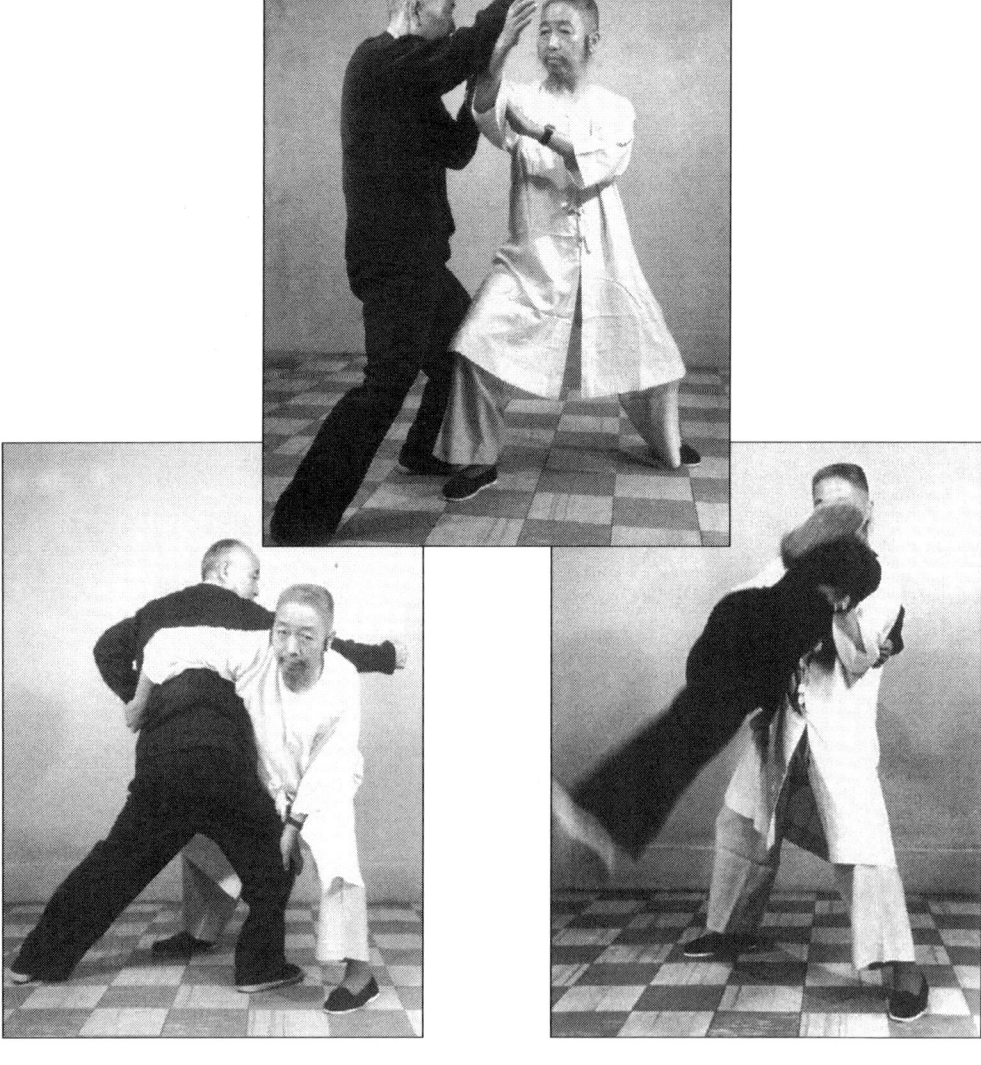

Above: Zheng Manqing in an exemplary classic taiji pose illustrating the ideals of upright spinal alignment. Right: Other photos of techniques showing bending while maintaining strenth and balance in movement. Photos courtesy of Robert W. Smith.

As we found in Dr. Karl Friday's description of Kashima-Shinryu, another example of holding the spine in alignment with a leg is found in Wu taiji. In some postures, such as forward press or push, the spine angles into a direct line with the back leg. This is one telltale trait of the Wu Style that makes it discernable from other taiji styles.

In contrast to the Chen Style, Yang practitioners seem to have a greater desire to have even more yin or softness in their form. Reasons for this are both health and self-defense related. Therefore, much of the real work in Yang Style is in teaching oneself the deeper aspects of relaxing and how it relates to body posture and movement. To become "soft," Zheng Manqing endorsed loosening the joints in the order of arms, legs, then back and that "Loosening the three joints of the back comes relatively late in training" (Lowenthal, 1991: 97). It is extremely important to note that most practitioners never reach the final stages in this practice. As Wolfe Lowenthal writes:

> You must be completely relaxed, without any resistance. If you are 99% correct you are 100% wrong. That is why [taiji] can be so frustrating: a practitioner can make a great deal of progress in subduing his ego but pay the price for a small residue of resistance in a split second of hardness that sabotages his best effort. – Lowenthal, 1991: 129

Wu Yuxiang (1812–1880), who created Wu taiji, states: "Power is emitted from the spine" (Yang, 2001: 5). The spine, as the primary bow, is used to lead attackers "into emptiness" and then provide a powerful counterforce. In the bows are stored power, which can be released like arrows. Again, the flexibility of the spine comes into question. Wu Yuxiang simply states: "Find the straight in the curved; accumulate, then emit" (Yang, 2001: 5). When martial arts texts refer to a "straight" spine, perhaps the dynamics of movement turn the "straight" into a "curve"?

A commentary Dr. Yang Jwing-ming makes on one of Wu Yuxiang's phrases is: "When you are pushing hands or sparring, you are exchanging techniques back and forth. You must be flexible and adaptable, folding and bending as appropriate" (Yang, 2001: 6). Push-hands practice was developed so martial applications could be learned in a realistic manner without the threat of severe injury or death. As such, proper push-hands practice offers insights into the art of taiji that is not easily found by only practicing the solo form. For this reason, the following technical section departs from the theories found in texts and attempts to see what happens in actual practice.

TECHNICAL SECTION

The following presentation attempts to show how the spine is affected in self-defense movements. We can do this in logical stages based on defensive theories that are common to many fighting systems.

STAGE #1: Stepping Away

"Self-defense" implies that someone is attacking somebody. The attack can manifest in numerous 1B ways, be it an attempt to strike, push, lock, or grab, etc. The simplest way to avoid injury when under attack is to move away from the attack. In these cases, the defender can move out of range of the attack by stepping backward, sideward, or diagonally.

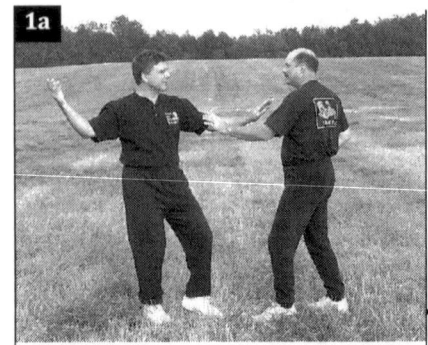

EXAMPLE 1A: Stepping Backward

The attacker steps in while throwing a round house strike. The defender uses "monkey-retreats," stepping backward to get outside the attack range, while catching the attacker's hand for a follow-up technique.

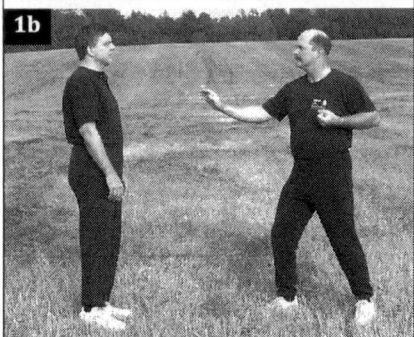

EXAMPLE 1B: Stepping Diagonally to the Right

The attacker steps in while throwing a left straight punch toward the chin. The defender uses "ward off," moving outside the attack range by stepping diagonally to the right and simultaneously blocking or catching the attacker's moving hand. A counter technique should immediately follow.

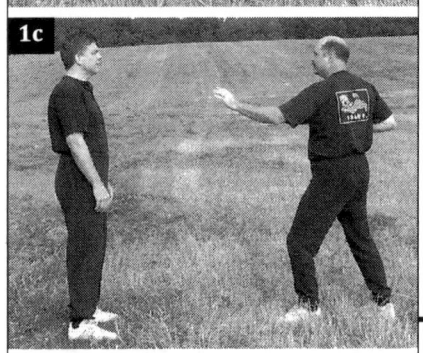

EXAMPLE 1C: Stepping Diagonally to the Left

The attacker steps in while throwing a right uppercut toward the chin. The defender uses "rising hands," moving outside the attack range by stepping diagonally to the left, blocking first with his left palm and then the back of his right forearm. A counter technique should immediately follow.

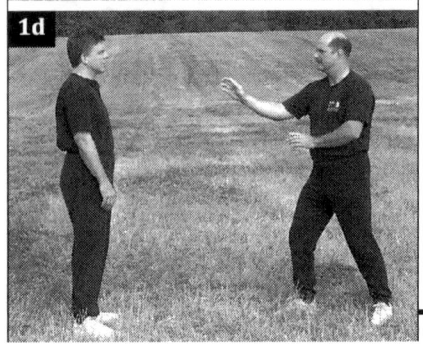

EXAMPLE 1D: Stepping to the Side

The attacker attempts a kick to the groin, but the defender uses "brush-knee," stepping directly to the side with his right leg, letting the left leg follow to keep it out of the kick's

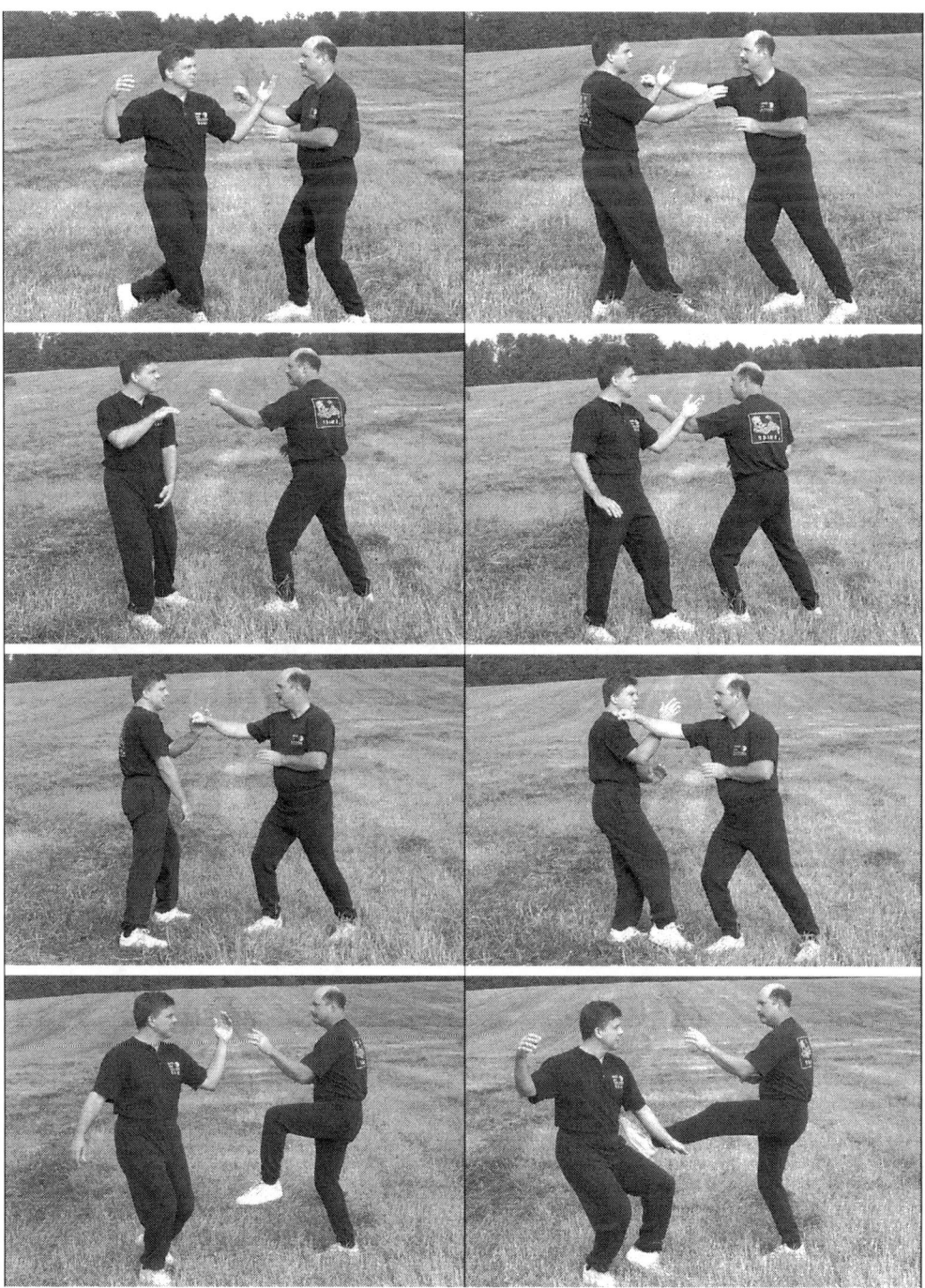

range. While stepping, the defender lets his left hand fall in a circular motion to catch the kick. A counter technique should immediately follow.

RESULT: In each case illustrated, the attacker is unable to make any contact, and the defender remains free from any outside stress. Therefore, his back can stay straight in all these cases.

STAGE #2: Stationary Feet — Stationary Spine

If the defender has room to move, it is possible to evade an attack and keep the spine straight. However, what happens when he cannot move his feet? There may be injured people buckled over next to him or somebody attacking from another side. Furniture or low ceilings may limit his moving in certain directions. For this reason, we look at basic attacks to a person who cannot move his feet but attempts to keep his spine straight. Once the defender finds himself locked in a stationary position, there is no doubt that pressures on his body will result from

EXAMPLE 2A: Forcing Backward

The attacker steps inward with a two-handed push to the chest. The defender tenses in an attempt to maintain his position, but is pushed off-balance backward. The pressure of the push to the upper body causes the front foot to lift. There is no time for a defensive technique to be employed.

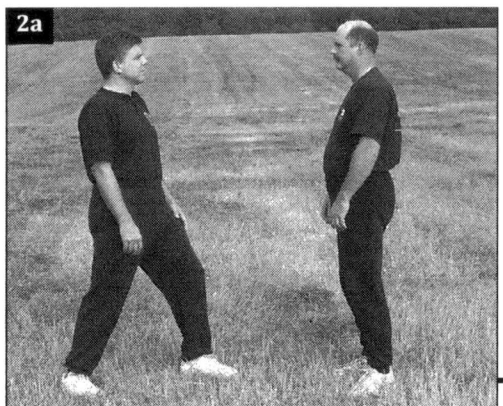

EXAMPLE 2B: Forcing Forward

The attacker grabs both wrists and pulls the defender forward. The defender tenses to maintain his position but is pulled off-balance forward. The effect of the pull on the upper body causes the back heel to lift or leave the ground if the technique is done to completion. There is no time for a defensive technique to be employed.

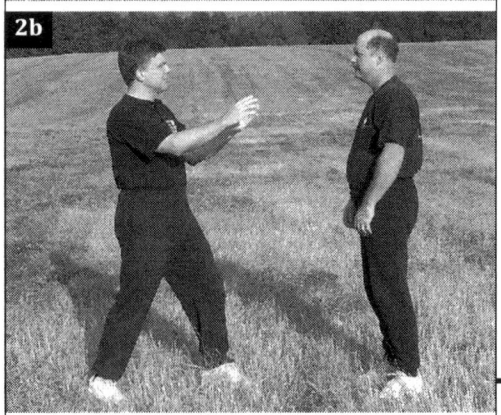

EXAMPLE 2C:
Forcing Sideways to the Left

The attacker grabs the right wrist and steps inward to use "ward off." The defender tenses in an attempt to maintain his position, but is thrown off-balance sideways. The effect of the arm across the chest area is that the defender's toes lift or leave the ground if the technique is done to completion. There is no time for a defensive technique to be employed.

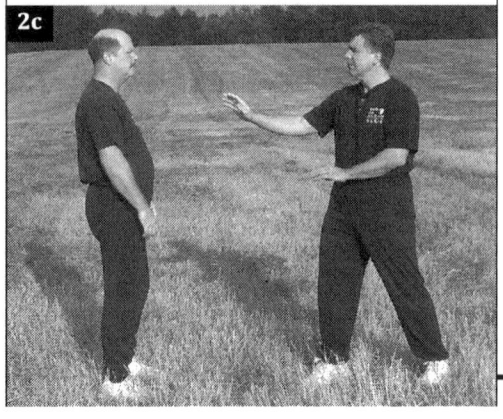

any attack. If he chooses to "hold his ground" or "freezes" from fear, a stationary posture held with tension affects any possible defensive maneuver.

In the following examples, we can see the results on the body of the defender who is attacked from the four cardinal directions. Here, we deliberately keep the spine in a locked position. Admittedly, this is an extreme case of rigidity, but it sometimes occurs in self-defense. The exaggerated examples are also attempting to show the effects of keeping the spine too tense.

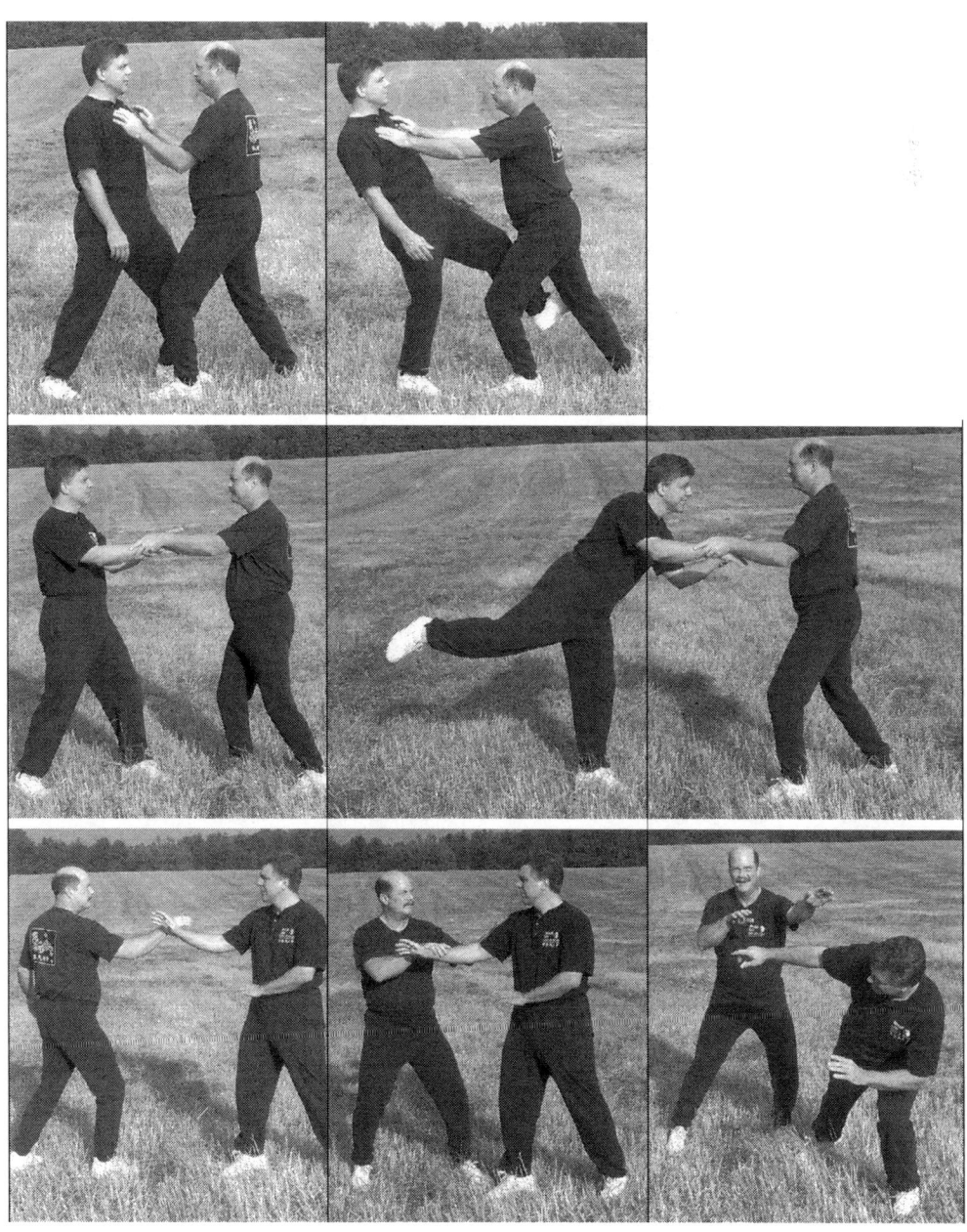

EXAMPLE 2D:
Forcing Sideways to the Right

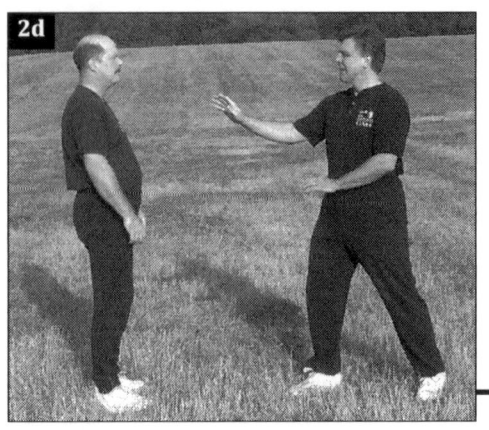

The attacker grabs the right wrist while stepping diagonally to use "rollback." The defender tenses in an attempt to maintain his position but is thrown off-balance sideways to the right. The effect of the force toward the shoulder area causes the defender's feet to lift or leave the ground if the technique is done to completion. There is no time for a defensive technique to be employed.

RESULT: In each case shown above, the defender finds himself in a dangerous predicament. By keeping the spine straight and stiff, the defender ties his bodily structure into one unit. Any pressure made above affects the stance below. Depending on the direction of the attacker's movement, the defender is easily set off-balance. You can see the effect in the feet with either the toes, heels, or sides of the feet first

---

STAGE #3: Stationary Feet — Shifting and Turning

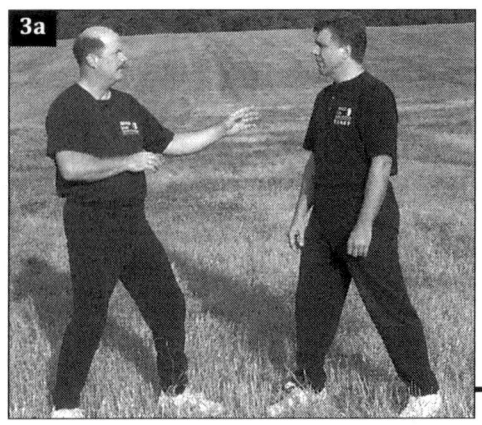

Try to defend yourself without moving your feet. You will quickly discover that some simple body movements aid in making defensive movements successful, such as: 1) shifting the weight from one leg to the other, 2) turning the spine to the left or right, or 3) a combination of shifting and turning.

EXAMPLE 3A: Turning

The attacker gives a strong single-hand push on the defender's shoulder. If the defender attempts to hold his position, the push would break his balance and cause his toes to lift. By relaxing and moving with the push by turning leftward, the attack is neutralized, and the defender can keep straight and balanced.

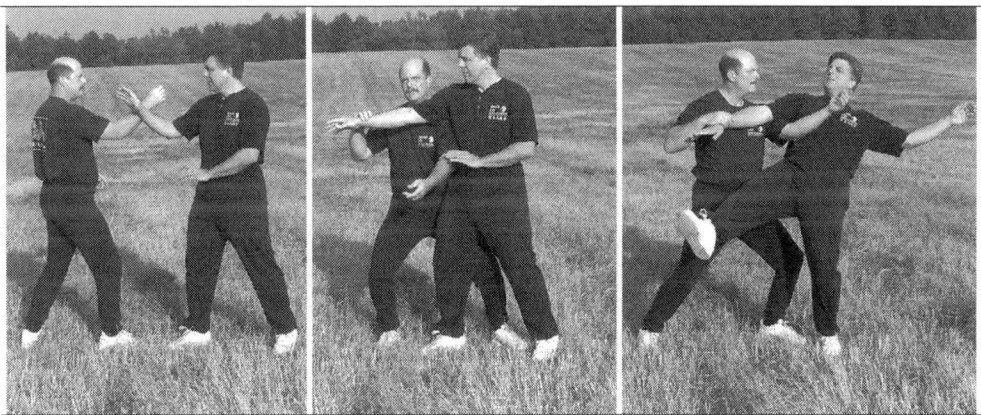

losing their root and oftentimes becoming airborne. Being off-balance makes counter-movements difficult to perform. Of course, the defender will try to use some technique for protection, but the result is usually the same. What may determine the result in this case is a matter of strength against strength. Since this rigid method does not work very well, we now look to further movement possibilities.

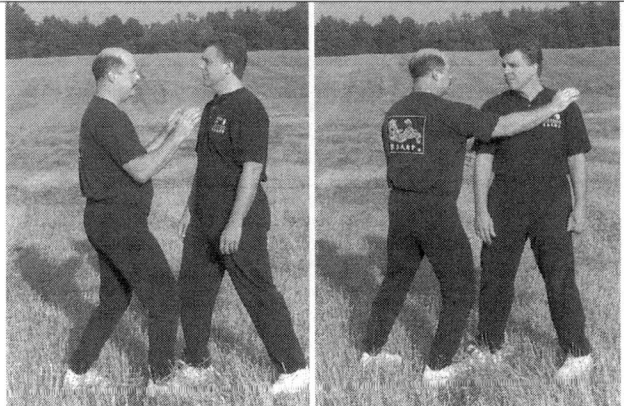

LIMITATION: The defender has successfully evaded the attack's main thrust, but another attack can immediately follow. If the defender attempts to 3B hold his position and the attacker is stronger, the defender can easily be pushed off-balance.

EXAMPLE 3B: Shifting Backward

The attacker gives a strong double-hand push on the defender's chest. If the defender attempts to hold his position and the attacker is stronger, the push would break his balance and cause his toes to lift. By relaxing and moving with the push, the attack is neutralized and the defender can keep straight and balanced.

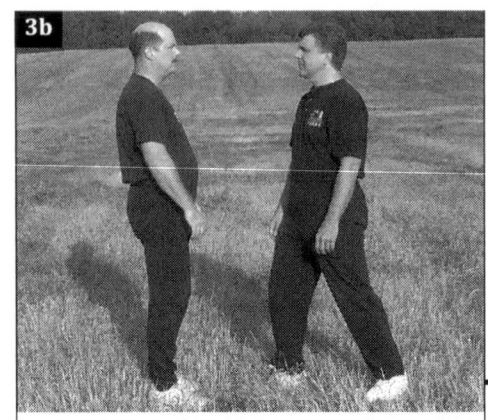

LIMITATION: If the attacker keeps his momentum going forward, the defender has already shifted to his limit and therefore will be pushed off-balance.

EXAMPLE 3C: Shifting Backwards and Turning

The attacker grabs the right wrist and steps inward to use "ward off." The defender starts to shift backward and turns his torso left while keeping his back straight. This maneuver can lessen, and slightly delay the attack's impact.

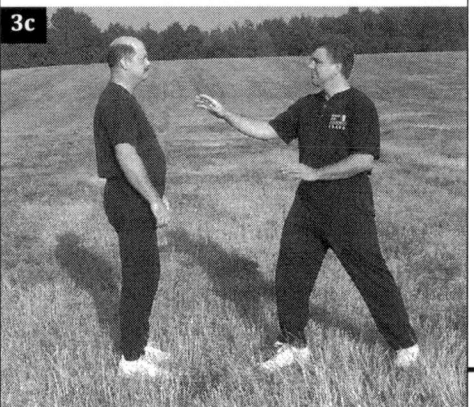

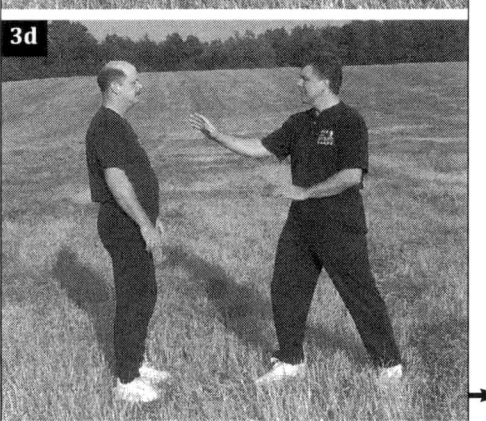

LIMITATION: Again, the stronger person will prevail. Thus, the defender can still be thrown off-balance sideways. The effect of the arm across the chest area causes the defender's toes to lift or leave the ground if the technique is done to completion. There is no time for a defensive technique to be employed.

EXAMPLE 3D: Shifting Backwards and Turning

The attacker grabs the right wrist while stepping diagonally to use "rollback." The defender attempts to shift backward and can pull his arm in and turn slightly to the right to protect the elbow joint. This maneuver can lessen and slightly delay the impact of the attack.

LIMITATION: Again, the stronger person will prevail. Thus, the defender can still be thrown off-balance sideways to the right. The effect of the attacker's left hand

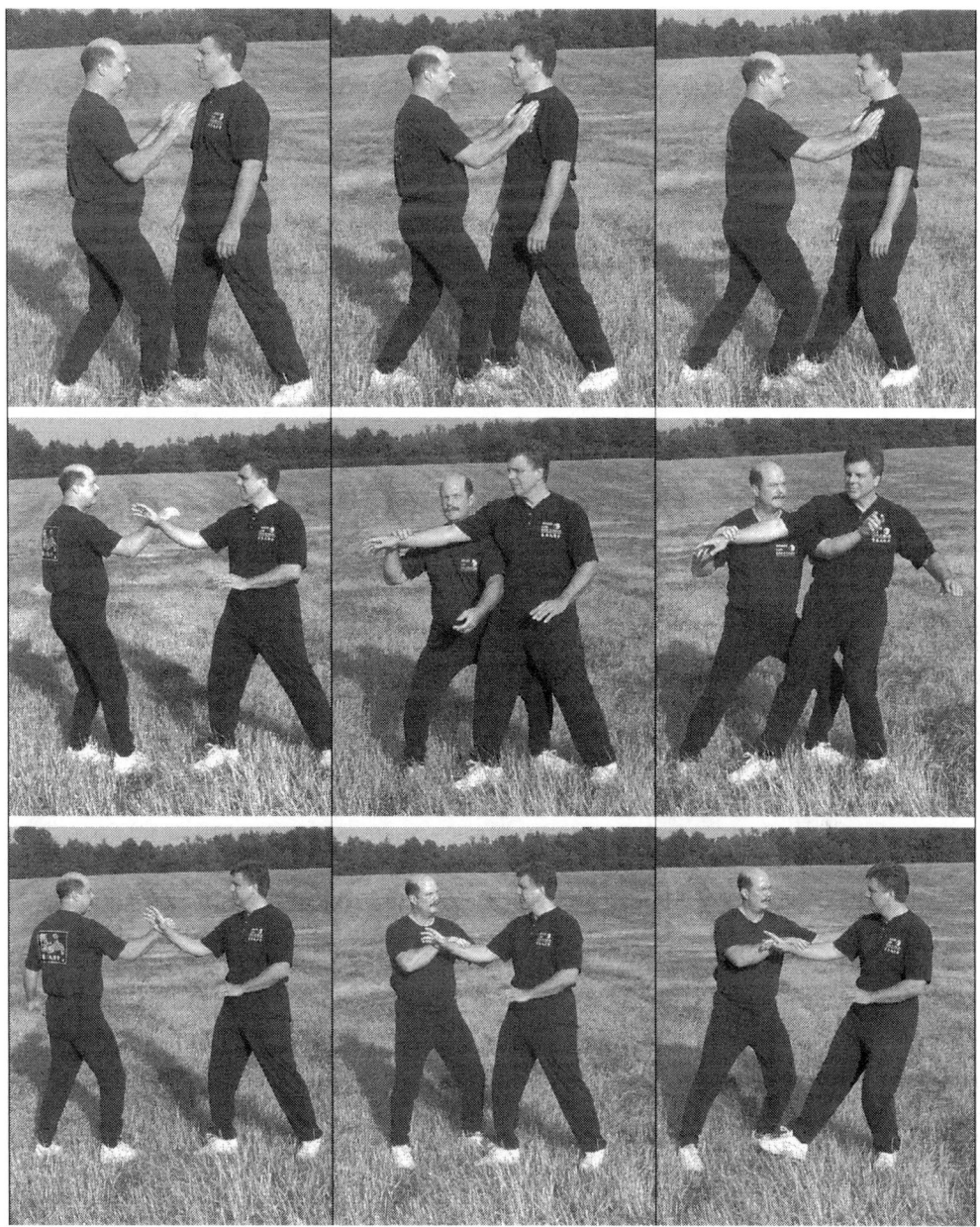

and forearm on the shoulder area causes the defender's toes to lift or leave the ground if the technique is done to completion. There is no time for a defensive technique to be employed.

RESULT: Shifting and turning make it much easier to move defensively than trying to defend in one position. However, even with the additional movement, if trying to keep the spine totally straight, the movements are limited and leave weaknesses in defense and offense. The result is pitting strength against strength where the stronger prevails.

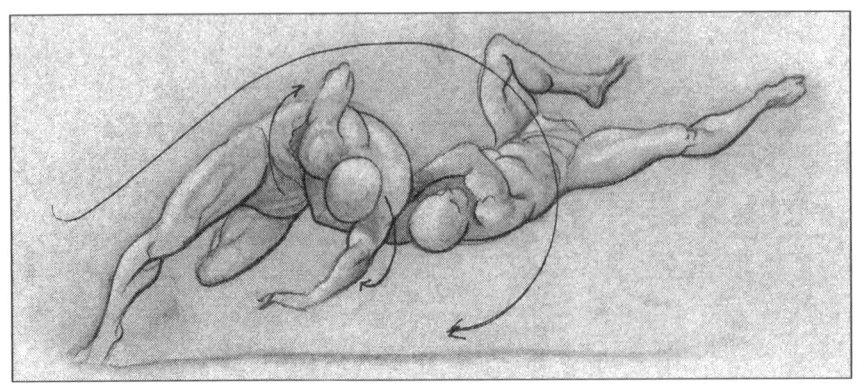

Above artwork by Oscar Ratti © 2002 Via Media Publishing Co.
Below artwork by Oscar Ratti © 2001 Via Media Publishing Co.

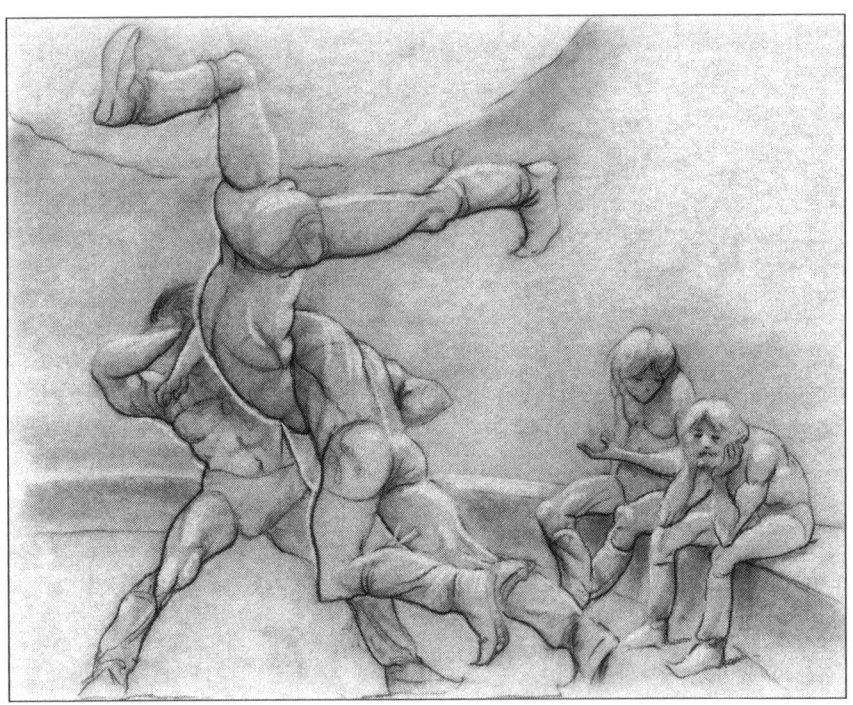

STAGE #4: Stationary Feet — Shifting, Turning, and Bending
So far in our experiment to see how the spine is affected in self-defense movements, we have seen that total freedom of movement makes self-defense relatively easy, allowing the spine to maintain an erect posture. When the feet are stationary, there is little time and distance to respond to an attack. Attempting to keep the spine perfectly straight without moving in any direction proves to be the most disadvantageous way to face an attacker. However, shifting and turning offers more time and distance, allowing for a greater range of defensive responses. Experimenting with an even greater flexibility in the spine, we find another possibility in self-defense movement.

EXAMPLE 4A: One-Hand Push to a Shoulder

The attacker gives a strong single-hand push to the defender's right shoulder. If the defender attempts to hold his position, the push will break his balance and cause his toes to lift (as in stage 2). While keeping a straight back, the defender can shift backward to obtain more time before the attacker closes the distance, but the defender soon reaches a limit where he cannot counter the push (as in stage 3). Therefore, since the feet are stationary, the defender can only move his upper torso away from the force by bending. Bending by itself is not a solution but must be done as part of an overall technique for neutralizing and countering. Note that in taiji, the defense is a natural outcome of the body movement, with the hands following the waist. A push can end the sequence.

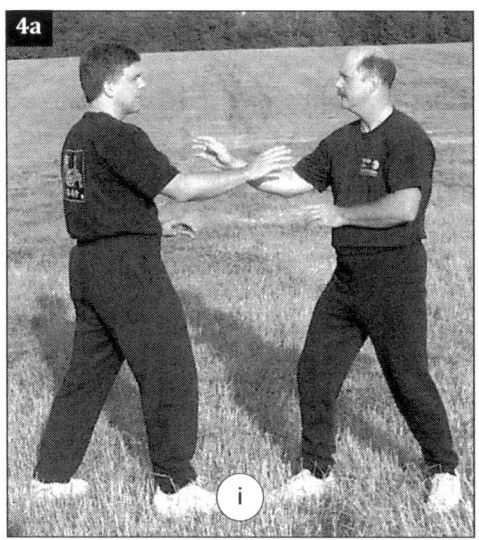
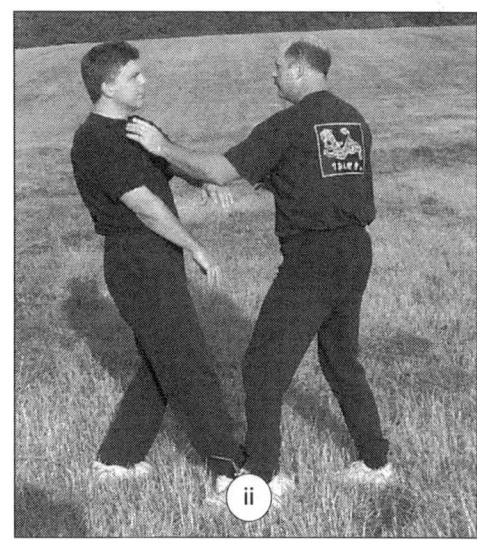
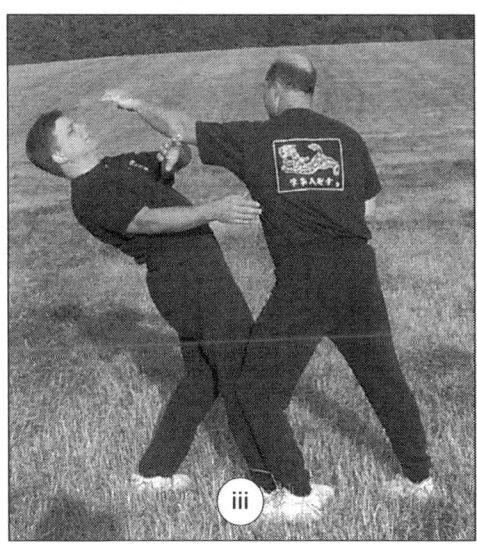
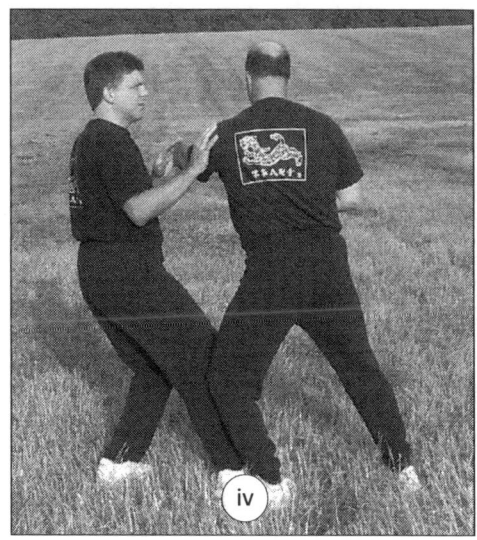

EXAMPLE 4B: Pulling the Lead Arm

The attacker grabs the defender's right wrist and starts to pull. If the defender attempts to hold his position, the pull will break his balance and cause his back heel to lift (as in stage 2). While keeping a straight back, the defender can shift forwards to obtain more time before the attacker closes the distance, but the defender soon reaches a limit where he cannot counter the pull (as in stage 3). Therefore, since the feet are stationary, the defender can only move his upper torso forward with the force by bending. Again, bending by itself is not a solution, but must be done as part of an overall technique for neutralizing and countering. In this case, the defender moves with the pull to a point where it becomes difficult for the attacker to keep pulling. In a continuous flow, the defender circles rightward with waist, upper torso and right arm. Because the attacker's grip is strong and he doesn't want to let go, the defender's smooth flow quickly brings the attacker into an awkward, off-balanced position. This usually leads to the attacker falling.

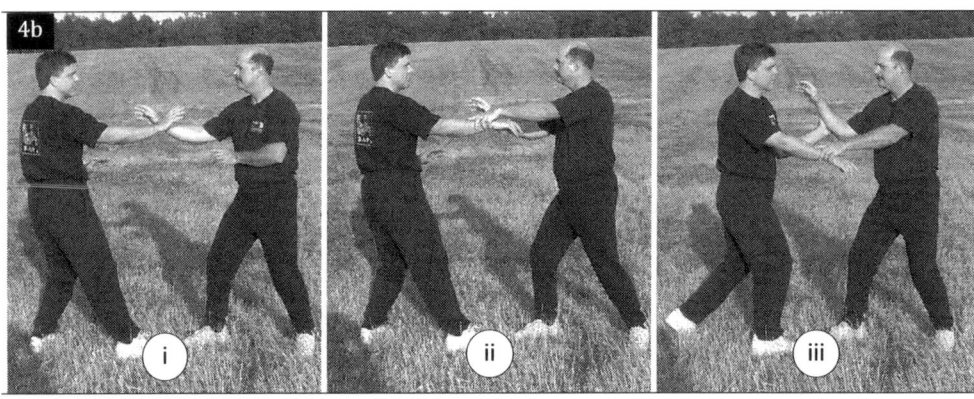

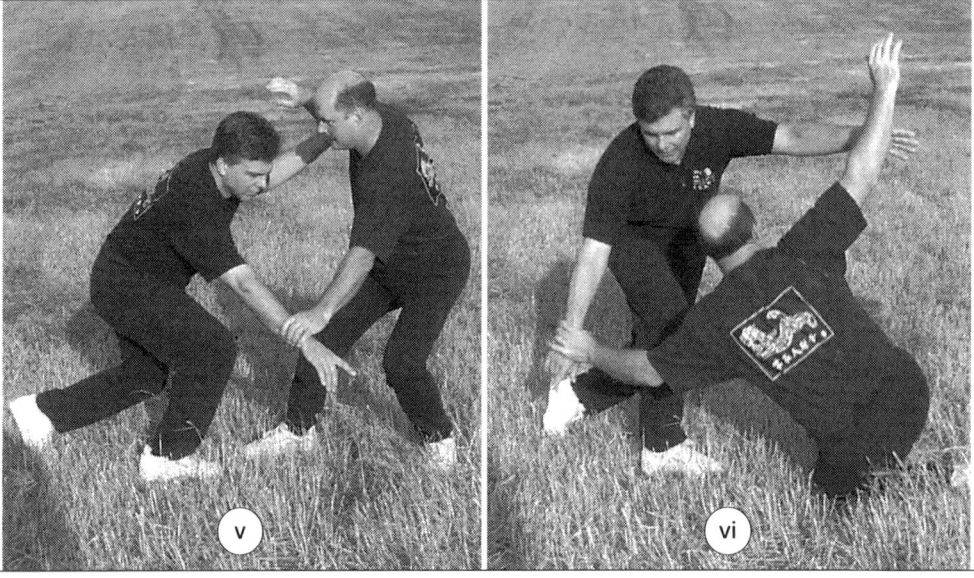

EXAMPLE 4C: Ward Off High

The attacker grabs the defender's right wrist and steps inward to use "ward off." If the defender attempted to hold his position, the ward off would off-balance him and cause his back toes to lift (as in stage 2). To distance himself from the main thrust of the ward off, the defender starts to shift backward while keeping his back straight, but the defender soon reaches a limit where he cannot counter (as in stage 3). Therefore, since the feet are stationary, the defender can only move his upper torso backward with the force by bending. Again, bending by itself is not a solution, but must be done as part of an overall technique for neutralizing and countering. In this case, the defender moves with the ward off arm. In a continuous flow, the defender circles his hands upward simultaneously with the upper torso's bending. Because the attacker's arm is aimed high, the defender has neutralized the attack by moving with the energy flow and then safely below the line of attack. This allows the defender to flow quickly into a counter using a double-hand push.

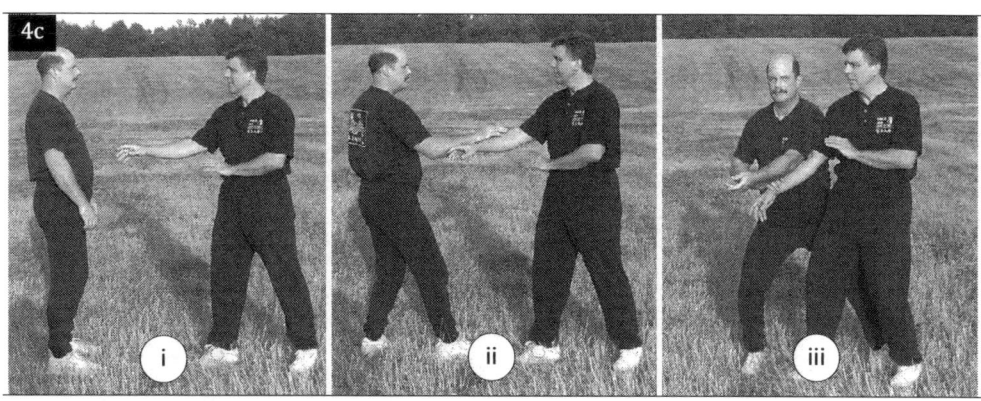

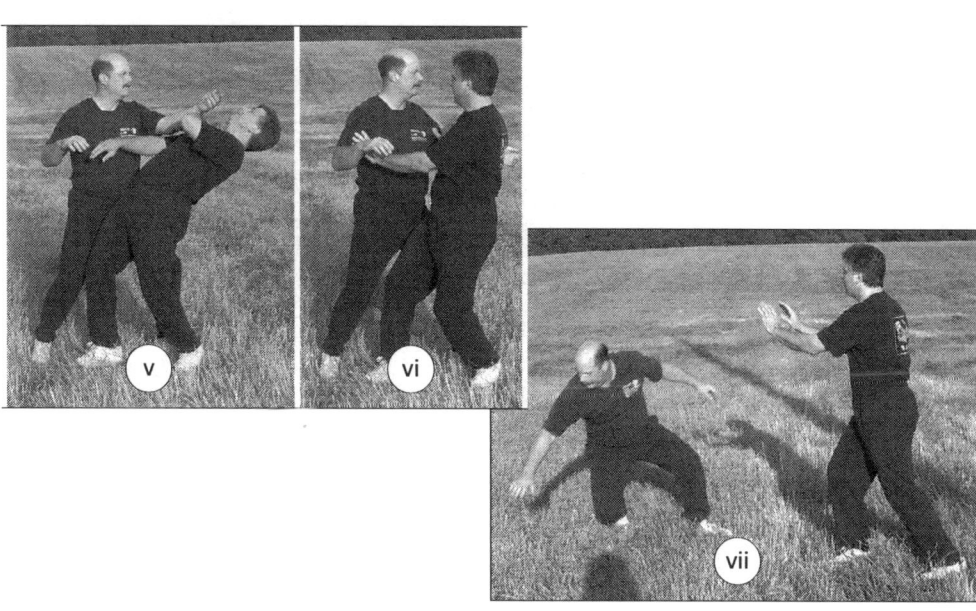

EXAMPLE 4D: Sideways Push

The attacker knocks the right arm away and steps in diagonally and attempts to push the defender over sideways. If the defender attempted to hold his position, the push would break his balance and cause his feet to lift (as in stage 2). To distance himself from the attacker, the defender may try shifting backward while keeping his back straight, but the defender would soon reach a limit where he could not counter (as in stage 3). Therefore, since the feet are stationary, the defender can only bend his upper torso forward, moving in the same direction as the attacking force.

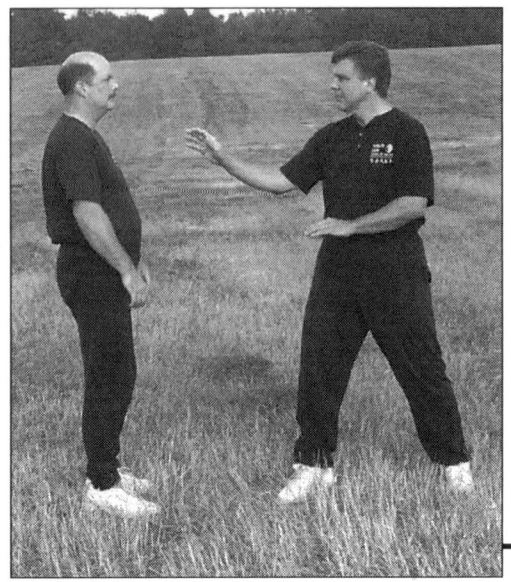

Again, bending by itself is not a solution, but must be done as part of an overall technique for neutralizing and countering. In this case, as the defender bends downwards, his right arm naturally circles downwards, then upwards to the back. Because the attacker's arm was targeted high on the back, the defender neutralized the attack by bending with the energy flow and then being safely below the line of attack. This natural movement is used to catch the movement of the attacker's pushing arm, which keeps the attacker's momentum going sideways. This defense also allows the defender to return to an erect position while simultaneously passing his left arm underneath his own right elbow to the attacker's left elbow, then letting it smoothly continue left while letting his right hand cross over to the right. This effectively pins the attacker's left arm and results in a double-hand push.

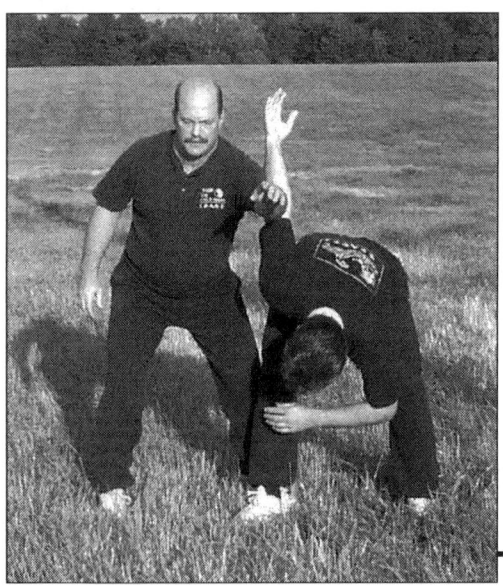

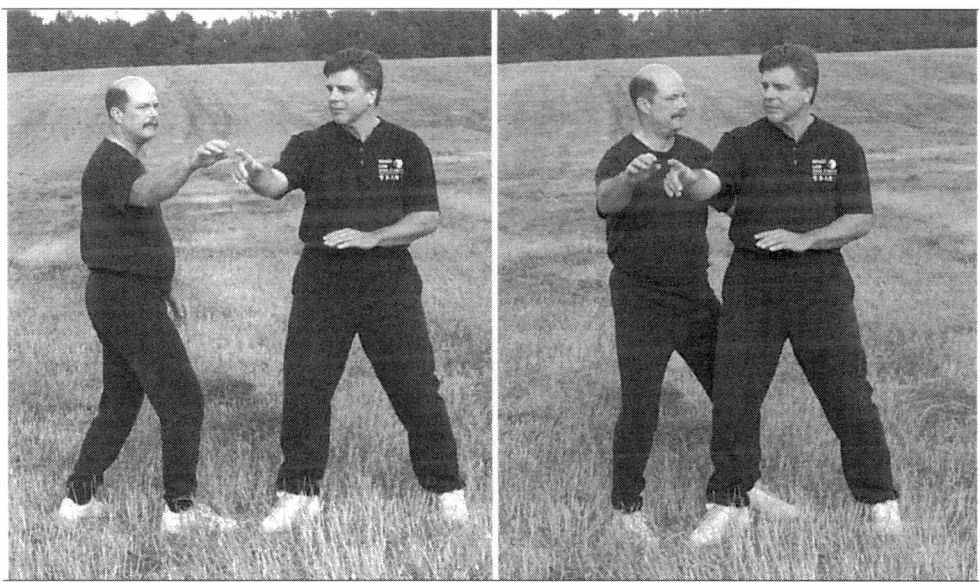

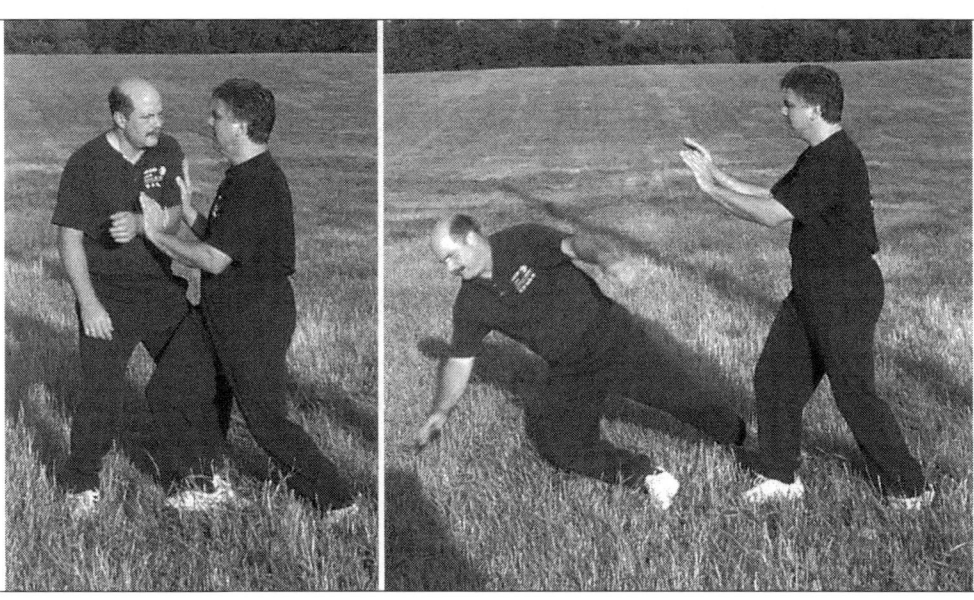

RESULT: We can see from the above examples that, when there is no alternative beyond shifting or turning, the bending of the spine adds another dimension to one's defensive capabilities. It does so by providing more time to move and distance oneself further from the attacker. In addition, it usually takes the target outside of the line of attack. This causes the attack to falter and gives the defender an advantage follow-up with his own technique.

THE SPINE IN FIGHTING MOVEMENTS: TO BEND OR NOT TO BEND?

Published literature and general instruction support this conclusion: all martial art practitioners should keep their spines plumb erect. Reasons given for this are many and the major points presented in this article are:

1) an upright spine maintains balance in all defensive and offensive movements
2) it provides the most efficient kinetics for powerful fighting techniques
3) the spine is the main conduit for all the vital organs, and is associated with the internal energy and breathing channels
4) an upright spine enhances the kinetic beauty of martial forms

All these reasons are legitimate. But does this only represent one side of the coin? Although there is overwhelming stress on keeping the spine plumb-erect, there are always hints that more should be considered before any conclusions are made.

In any substantial reference made to the necessity of keeping the spine upright and straight in martial practice, there are always exceptions noted. When practice is discussed, most say all should attempt to keep the spine erect. However, tiny red flags pop up when the exceptions show that the spine is much more flexible "in reality" or in "special circumstances." The spine bends when one wants "to dodge strikes," "escape from a hold," "transfer additional body weight onto an opponent," "clear an obstacle," etc. Plus, numerous books manage to show exceptions.

We need to ask ourselves why there is so much evidence in support of keeping the spine plumb-erect, and why there are relatively so few exceptions shown. It seems the answer is quite simple. Like "not seeing the forest for the trees," the reasons and practicality for bending the spine are hidden among the vast forest of basic instruction.

Most of the materials dealing with martial arts instruction are produced to teach beginners and semi-professionals. In so doing, there has been a focus on solo forms, such as kata, poomse, and other standardized routines. There really is no reason for bending the spine in most of these routines.

Even when two-person forms are shown or practiced, they are not realistic enough to call for much bending. For example, during self-defense practice, an attacker usually does not push or punch with enough speed or drive to force the defender to move "realistically." Why bend if the push stops short of pushing you off-balance?

Zheng Manqing wrote that loosening the joints comes relatively late in training. In the learning process, loosening is in the order of arms, legs, then back. Most never reach this final stage, and therefore such movements are seldom seen. Chen Xiaowang echoes this idea by stating that the highest level for a Chen Style practitioner to reach is manifesting "five yin, five yang" in his or her technical skills.

This mastery is a long way from "one yin, nine yang." Yang Jwing-ming comments on the Wu Style that one "must be flexible and adaptable, folding and bending as appropriate." Such ideas illustrate that practices utilizing the spine made flexible by loosening the vertebrae and adding the ointment of yin for pliability, should be a valid part of martial practice.

The key here seems to be: "bending as appropriate." In the great majority of cases, we never want to bend the spine, and we never need to. Generally, martial arts are practiced and viewed under ideal conditions, conditions where forms are a mainstay and sparring and other practices involving two or more people are governed by rules that keep such engagements on a safe level.

Conclusion

To see, analyze, and experience "how and why" the spine bends in the fighting arts, we need to consider factors we normally have no reason to encounter. For example, when we think of being balanced, we think of gravity and its effect on the body. Of course, when we stand on one foot, we need to align our whole body upright so as not to fall. This is a great test for balance! But this is under a static condition, the condition we are most familiar with. Laws of motion need to be applied and studied as they relate to martial movements. How do centrifugal and centripetal forces affect balance? What really happens to the whole body when making a truly committed attack? And what happens when all the complex dynamics of one person encounter another equally complex bundle of powerful human forces?

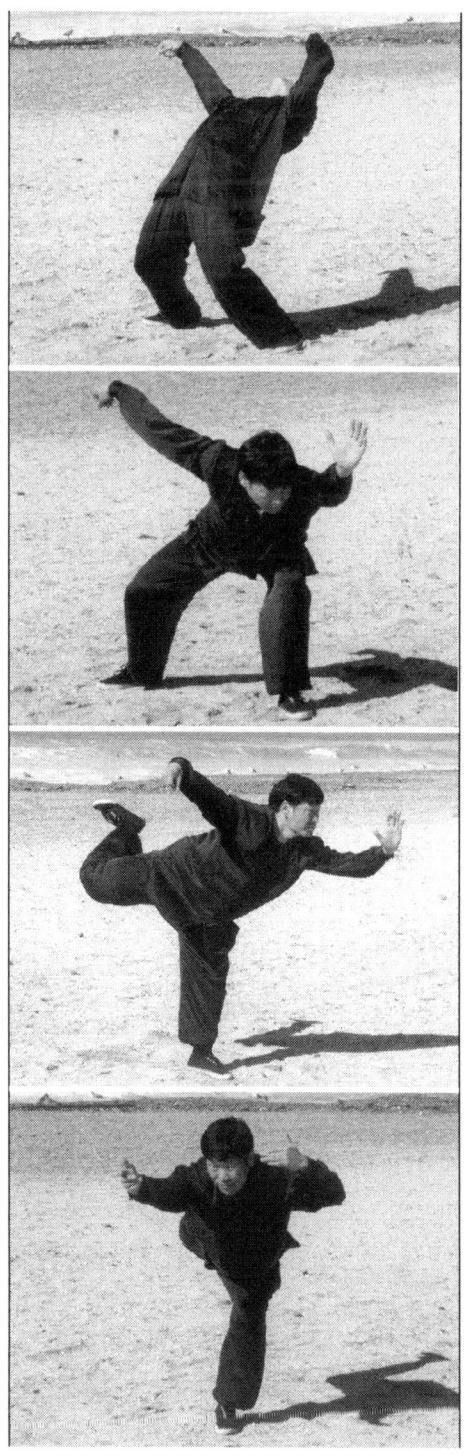

Victor Fu demonstrating *Sixiangquan* (found image boxing). This family style embodies essential elements from taiji, liangyi, xingyi, and bagua boxing systems. Photos courtesy of Shannon Phelps.

Jan Kauskas, who teaches taiji in Glasgow, Scotland, writes (personal communication, August 22, 2002): "I try to practice push-hands with a straight spine. My observation however is that, both in myself and others, when the going gets tough, the spine gets going. When we are under pressure from the other's advance, we often lose straightness and proceed from there."

In the end, we learn by doing. In the practice of push-hands, we can experiment with the dynamics of movement on many levels, starting with the elementary and moving up. As in any endeavor, however, change is difficult. If we train only in keeping the spine straight, it becomes impossible to bend even under conditions that call for such movement.

Many practice push-hands to intimately experience the possibilities of body movement, and to explore the vast number of variations possible in martial applications. They attempt to expand their skills, especially in sensing the bodies' energies and flow of movement. This requires a relaxed, flexible mind and body. Another reason some taiji practitioners practice seeking extreme spinal flexibility is to keep the vertebrae loose and healthy. Tensions in the spine limit one's self-defense capabilities as well as having an ill-effect on one's health.

Acknowledgments

My special thanks to the following people who have helped in some way with this article: Donna Bernardini, George Bernardini, Rhiannon Bernardini, Daniele Borelli, Barbara Davis, Robert Dohrenwend, John Donohue, Oscar Ratti, Richard Schmidt, Joe Svinth, Kim Taylor, Karl Friday, Jan Kauskas, Deborah Klens-Bigman, Marc Tedeschi, Douglas Wile, and Phillip Zarrilli.

Bibliography

Alau, M. (1975). *Modern fencing*. New York: Scribners.

Cheng, Man-ch'ing, (1985). *Cheng Tzu's thirteen treatises on t'ai chi ch'uan*. Berkeley, CA: North Atlantic Books.

Crosnier, R. (n.d.). *Fencing with the sabre*. New York: A.S. Barnes & Co.

Lowenthal, W. (1991). *There are no secrets: Professor Cheng Man-ch'ing and his tai chi chuan*. Berkeley, CA: North Atlantic Books.

Mattson, G. *The way of karate*. Rutland, VT: Tuttle.

Nakayama, M. (1966). *Dynamic karate*. Tokyo: Kodansha.

Nakayama, M. (1977). *Best karate-Comprehensive*. Tokyo: Kodansha.

Sim, D., and Gaffney, D. (2002). *Chen style taijiquan: The source of taiji boxing*. Berkeley, CA: North Atlantic Books.

Yang, J.M. (2001). *Tai chi secrets of the Wu and Li styles*. Boston: YMAA Publication Center.

Comments on Selections from Chen Xin's *Illustrated Explanations of Chen Taijiquan* with Commentary from Chen Xiaowang

by Stephan Berwick, M.A., and translations by Dannie Butler, M.A.

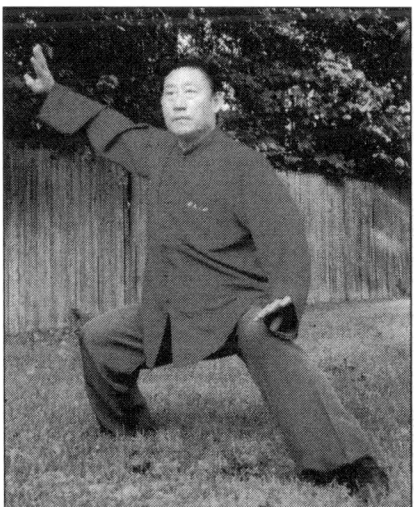 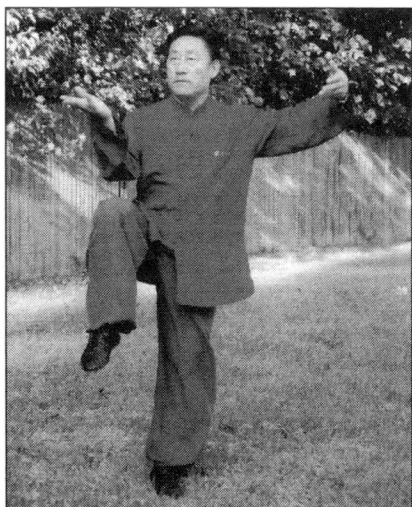

Leading representative of the Chen family system of taijiquan, Grandmaster Chen Xiaowang demonstrates a few classic postures. All photos courtesy of Chen Xiaowang.

Introduction

Historically, the level of boxing skill in Chenjiagou—the Chen family village from where taijiquan originated—always matched the times. During war and crises, skill levels dipped as compared to the high levels of skill exhibited during times of peace and prosperity. The 16th generation Chen family scholar, Chen Xin (1849–1929, also known as Chen Pinsan) divided his time between boxing practice and scholarly pursuits. When Chen Xin's highly influential classic, *Illustrated Explanations of Chen Taijiquan*, was published in 1933, the level of taiji in Chenjiagou was considered good, according to Chen Xiaowang. Chen Xin was a distant relative of today's acknowledged standard bearer of the 19th generation, Chen Xiaowang.

Regardless of the fluctuating quality in actual practice, taijiquan has always been subject to theoretical debate. The absence of any definitive publications emanating from Chenjiagou contributed to this, since Chen taijiquan theory was never recorded until the publication of Chen Xin's work. Handwritten in classical Chinese and published posthumously, it took Chen Xin over twelve years to write the book, from the 34th year of emperor Guangxu's reign (1908) until the 8th year after the formation of China's first republican government (1919). He produced four volumes containing hundreds of distinct classical Chinese characters. Of note, the well-known Chen taiji concept of silk reeling energy (*chansijing*) is a central theme throughout the book. Chen Xin successfully meshed the profound principles of the *Yijing* (Book of Changes), yin/yang theory, meridian theory, and practical technical descriptions, to produce a boxing manual of unprecedented comprehensiveness (Wu and Wu, 1976: 19).

The technical details of core Chen taiji technique contained in this seminal work have never been fully conveyed by and for contemporary practitioners. One must be able to read classical Chinese (a rarity even among most fluent Chinese readers) and have an intimate understanding of taiji to assimilate the book's contents. Thus, combining the language skills and taiji experience of the authors, this chapter provides the first-ever detailed English translations and analysis of some of the most complex technical sections from Chen Xin's work—along with commentary from Chen Xiaowang.

While Chen Xin's publication remains a masterwork on taijiquan, "the book itself is not enough to understand taiji," according to Chen Xiaowang. "Just language is not enough," he asserts. He insists that "Nobody, in any language, can write about taiji with true clarity and accuracy." He maintains that "hands-on corrections are more effective than any book."

Readers familiar with Chen family teaching methods, know that success in the art is largely based on a foundation of strict body structural skills that build the unique internal power (*jing*) characteristic of Chen taiji. Based on his insistence that skill development is based on "feeling," Chen Xiaowang has developed accessible teaching methods to instill the "feeling" of appropriate body structure, as Chen Xin sought to explain in his masterwork.

Chen Xiaowang teaches that "three languages are necessary to understand taiji":

The language of speaking and writing: To explain and theorize
The language of the body: To demonstrate and see
The language of corrections: To feel (the most important language)

The principles described by Chen Xin and as taught today by masters such as Chen Xiaowang apply to all versions of Chen taiji. Chen Xiaowang maintains that the principles described by Chen Xin permeate every variation of Chen taijiquan.

One of the principles expressed by Chen Xin in a particular chapter of his writings is a well-defined sense of purpose for practicing martial arts. While small portions of this chapter, "Essential Knowledge for the Study of Taijiquan," have been translated, the whole essay has not received a full translation and/or analysis of the context from which it was written. To that end, the authors include this essay in its entirety, with commentary, to enlighten and inspire readers' martial practice.

As an aid for readers, photos of Chen Xiaowang in the postures chosen for this article are presented along with Chen Xin's original hand drawn images. Also, Chen Xiaowang and Mr. Berwick's analysis is in regular type placed above the translated text which is emphasized by a gray line running parallel to the text, with a few comments in brackets from Mr. Butler and Mr. Berwick appearing throughout where applicable.

To help readers follow Chen Xin's diagrams and his highly detailed descriptions, he wrote:

> When doing taijiquan, it is not usually necessary to adhere to a specific direction. However, there is a certain standard for the pictures. The Big Dipper leads the heavens in the north, so it is appropriate that north is the primary direction. Therefore, to specify directions, the drawings all face north, with right corresponding to the east, left to the west, and the rear to the south.

The most influential technique of Chen taiji, single whip permeates all later forms of taiji and holds profound meaning for both internal development and combat usage. Single whip's practical applications depend on a sophisticated use of body skills and can be considered an "internal" interpretation of similar boxing techniques commonly seen in ancient Northern Chinese boxing forms. Chen taiji's silk reeling energy (*chansijing*) is highly refined when practicing single whip correctly. Thus, Chen Xin included supplementary diagrams to illustrate the silk reeling pathways that imbue single whip.

Chen Xiaowang expresses the principles described by Chen Xin as, "In the beginning, the outside (external) moves the inside (internal). When one's qi achieves a state of 60% qi "flowing," this feeling or sense of qi flow becomes more tangible and can then be controlled by the mind." And as described throughout Chen Xin's requirements for single whip, Chen Xiaowang's famed grandfather, Chen Fake, defined the internal energy of the crown of the head "as the essential qi from the heart" (Kohler, 1991: 14).

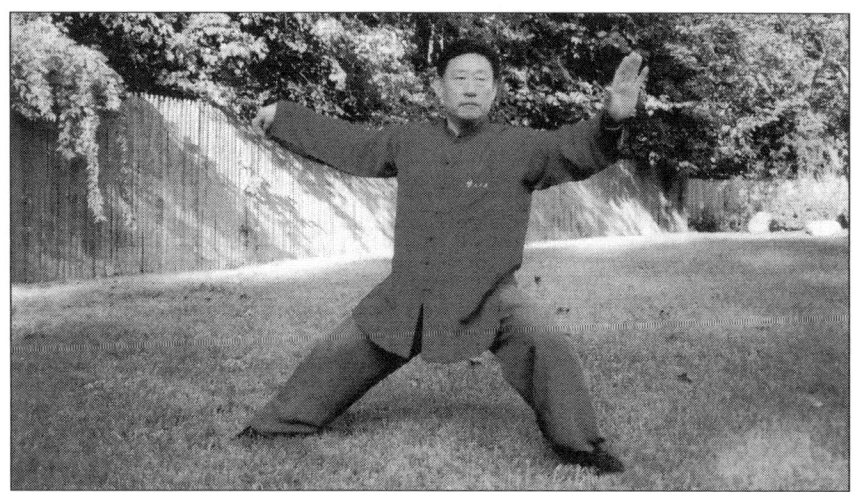

Single Whip

Single Whip

The central qi [or intrinsic energy] at the top of the head is the true qi. The intention of the mind leads it upward and it rises to the top of the head. The central qi is led up naturally; no object moves it. Thus is the intention.

When doing taijiquan, the mind is the ruler. The spine is key in moving the body left or right. The waist is key in moving the body up and down. The waist is raised by raising the qi. The waist is lowered by lowering the qi. Although it seems that there is a contention between raising and lowering, there is one qi throughout and raising and lowering are not at odds with each other. The left foot is led by the left hand. The right foot is led by the right hand. As for how the hands move at the top, and how the lower body and feet move at the bottom, everything rises and falls together. Top and bottom follow each other and naturally move in unison.

Moving the hands lies entirely in the palms and fingers leading the movements of the entire body. It is particularly important that the feet follow the hands. The central qi must move slowly through the forearms and upper arms. One must not become flustered and neglect to follow the natural principle. Moving naturally, do not favor one side. By means of the mind, the qi moves through both forearms. This is central qi. The back of the left hand faces north 10 to 20 percent. The back of the right hand faces the left hand 40 to 50 percent. The center qi moves to the fingers. This completely fulfills closure of the whole.

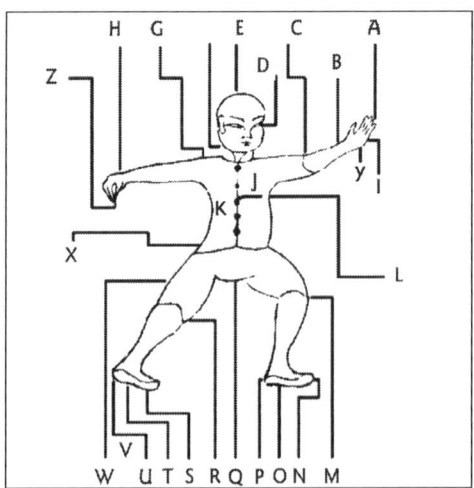

A: Force is used in the center of the fingers.
B: The left wrist must not be limp.
C: The inside of the elbow resembles the new moon or a bow, which is slightly bent.
D: The eyes focus on the middle finger of the left hand.
E: The energy of the top of the head leads upward. The top of the head is straight up.
G: The front and rear shoulders both collapse and must not rise.

H: The right wrist must not be limp. The fingers of the right hand
   all pinch together at one point. The front hand extends.
   The fingers of the rear hand restrain. This is the rear hand.
I: The front and edge of the palm use force.
   The back of the palm and the thumb use force.
J: Chest.
K: This space resembles the shape of the new moon.
L: The horizontal qi in the diaphragm is moved to the bottom of the feet.
   If one cannot do this, one should still move it to the *dantian* [lower abdomen].
M: The front knee bears the weight horizontally.
   The front knee sticks out fifty or sixty percent.
N: The toes of the left foot must grip the ground with force.
   The big toe especially must use force.
O: The left foot is slightly emptier than the right foot.
P: The heel first touches the ground, then the foot gradually
   comes forward until the left toes touch the ground.
Q: The groin is empty and round. Everything closes toward
   the center and naturally correlates.
R: The right knee sticks out twenty or thirty percent.
   It must not be limp but must bear weight.
S: The right foot faces north. It hooks slightly to the northwest.
T: There is a hollow in the yong quan.[1]
U: The heel must press on the ground with force. Only then will there be stability.
V: The right foot must be full. This is called "the front empty, the rear full."
W: The two thighs embrace inward from the outside.
X: The pelvis turns slightly upward and the lower abdomen closes.
   The groin is then rounded. A pulsing naturally occurs.
Y: The left hand? It closes with the right.
Z: The right hand should close with the left.

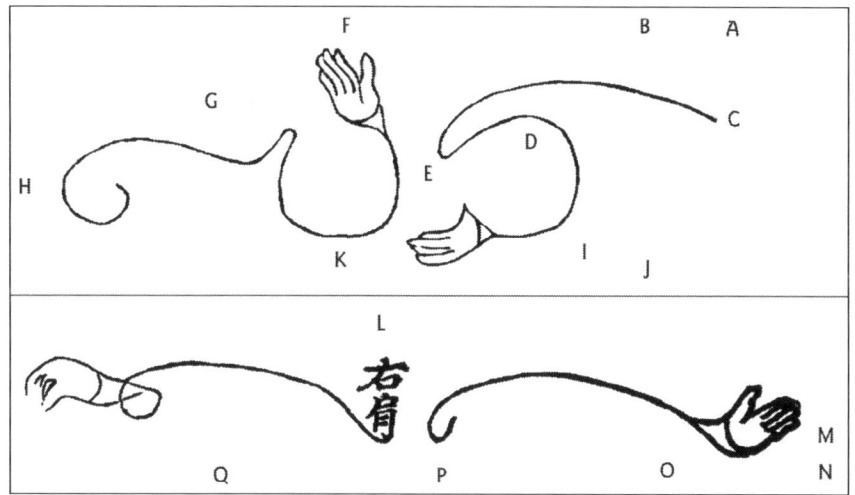

Hand Silk Reeling in Single Whip

A: This diagram goes with the diagram above. It faces north, and focuses on the right hand.

B: This is the closing of left and right. It is the transitional pulse between the previous posture and the next posture.

C: The left fingers are open and together. The forearm is relaxed. The left hand makes a circle and then moves west from below. The forearm is relaxed.

D: Starting point for the left hand.

E: Waist.

F: Hand starts.

G: The right hand moves thus.

H: The right hand stops.

I: The left hand leaves the waist and moves upward.

J: Before moving, the hand first makes a small circle and closes with the right.

K: This is *ge bo jin* [arm energy]. When the hand has turned enough, the back of the hand will be slightly forward.

L: Left shoulder.

M: The left hand stops. The left hand opens (unfolds).

N: Because this diagram also faces north, left and right are as above.

O: This is a diagram of the movement of the left hand. The left forearm bends to close with the right forearm.

P: The left hand begins. In the center, in the chest and abdomen, qi is exchanged from the *tiantu* acupoint to the lower abdomen. The qi hai, shi men, and guan yuan are like a *qing* [chime stone, made by hollowing out a hard sonorous stone], curved like a bow.[2] This is known as "hollowing the chest." It is closed. The energy must be insubstantial.

Q: The right forearm is turned backward and closes with the left hand.

R: The line in the circle is where the right hand originates. Before it originates, the right hand makes a small circle. The right hand restrains.

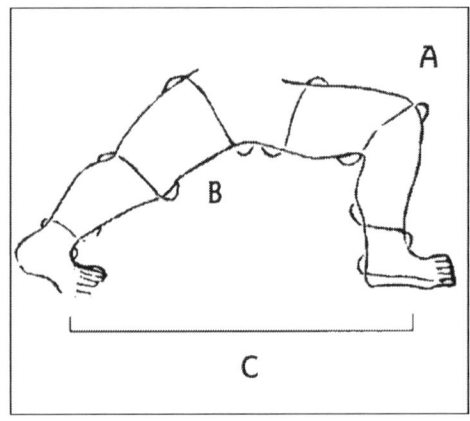

Lower Body Silk Reeling in Single Whip

The reeling is from the foot to the base formed at the top of the thighs. The energy reels from outside to inside. When it reels from the base and spirals back in the legs, hard qi is not used in the energy of the legs. When the knee closes inward, the five toes all close inwards. The leg naturally closes from top to bottom, and the groin is naturally rounded.

Method for Moving the Feet

The left foot first comes beside the right foot, with the toes touching the ground. It then steps out toward the west. The two feet are approximately one and a half feet apart.

    A: Left knee
    B: Right knee
    C: Diagram of correspondence between left and right energy

Method for Moving the Rear Heel

It need not be mentioned again that in single whip the left foot is first beside the right foot with the toes touching the ground, and then steps toward the west. As for the right foot, in the lazily tying coat [*lan ca yi*] posture, the toes are pointing toward the northeast. When the left foot takes a step to the left, the toes face northwest. Just prior to the left toes touching the ground, the right foot remains on the ground and the toes are facing northeast. The right heel twists on the ground toward the northwest, that is toward the west but slightly north. Therefore, it is said that the right toes and left toes touch the ground at the same time. The left foot touches the ground heel first then gradually comes down until the toes touch the ground. The left foot and right foot are closed. Only thus is the energy (jin) not dissipated.

    If one asks what is meant by "single whip," the answer would be that the two arms are not in front of the chest, but out to left and right sides of the body. When the left and right forearms extend, the motion seems weak, but it is as dangerous as a whip. The extension of the two forearms also resembles a whip. From this the posture gets its name. The left hand is primary. It moves upward until it is level with the navel, then makes a small circle from outside to inside. The right hand makes a small circle forward from the rear. The right and left close. As for the spirit, it should be as though two people were facing each other and talking.

    After this, from the closed position, the left hand leads the left side of the body from bottom to top toward the west. It then moves gradually toward the west, stopping at about 80 or 90 percent. While the left hand is extending, the eyes follow the left hand, and when the hand stops, the eyes remain focused on the middle finger of the left hand and do not look elsewhere.

    As for the central qi, the reeling method is the same as that for the right hand and right forearm in the lazily tying coat posture. When closing, the left foot is first pulled in beside the right foot with the toes touching the ground. This creates a posture for the next movement of the feet. When moving, the left foot moves toward the west together with the left hand. The left heel touches the ground as the left hand is about to stop. Movement continues until the left big toe touches the ground and the left hand stops at the same time. The form appears to stop, but the spirit does not stop. The left side of the body from top to bottom follows the extension of the left foot, which varies with the size of the person but is no less than approximately two feet.

As for the right hand, when closing it first makes a circle. When the left hand rises and moves toward the west, the right wrist is back. The right hand moves forward and then makes another circle. The arm slowly twists counterclockwise. This differs from the opening of the left hand. Not only is there energy in the right arm as it twists, but it also moves slightly toward the east and the back of the hand closes toward the front. Since the right hand moves toward the east while the left hand moves toward the west, it appears that there are two separate motions. They are the same in spirit. The reason the back of the right hand twists forward is to lower the pulse for the next move.

As for why the right fingers close together and remain closed, this is to prevent someone from grabbing the fingers from behind and bending them back, since the eyes are focused forward.

The silk reeling energy in the right arm spirals from the shoulder to the forearm, then to the right fingers. Although the right foot does not move, it twists based on the movement of the right hand. At first the toes are toward the northeast. Then as the right hand moves, the right heel remains on the ground while the toes twist toward the northwest. The right side of the body from top to bottom moves in this motion.

When the method is explained, it must necessarily be divided into parts. However, one must not take this to mean that it is divided. What is meant by "closed" is that the entire body closes together. Only then is there excellence.

As for the joints of the body, such as the left and right elbows and left and right shoulders, corresponding left and right joints must close and face each other. This needs no further explanation.

Those who do not understand may look at the illustration and copy the method once they have comprehended it. Everything goes back to keeping straight.

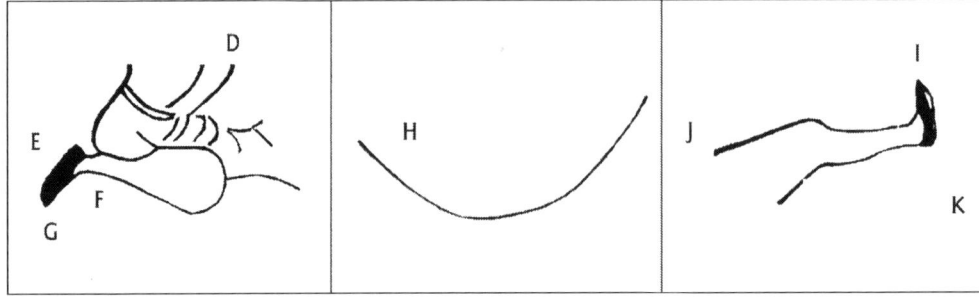

One must not lean to one side. The joints must be relaxed, and the arms must simply hang from the shoulders. The movements seem soft, but they are hard. The spirit is hidden within rather than revealed. This is great skill.

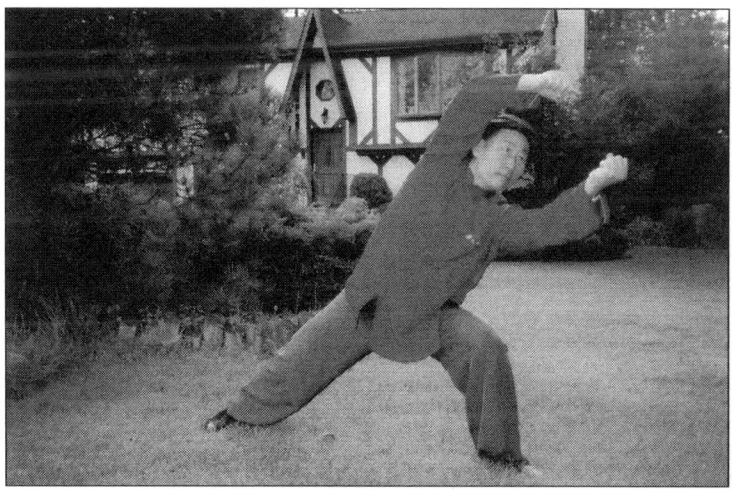

Overhead Cannon

The overhead cannon features Chen taiji's unique torque-like expression of explosive power releases (*fajing*). Usually seen at the end of the first form (*yilu*), this technique contains applications from striking to lesser-known throwing techniques. Chen Xin's description of overhead cannon's "pounding attack" (described below) does not just refer to pounding with the fists. He is likely referring to the defender using his body to pound the opponent at close range, from the side. Also, considering that Chen taiji can be considered a grappling art, his attentive descriptions of how the feet grip the ground, along with how the bodily joints "close" are like wrestling concepts taught globally.

The name of this posture describes its main movement, which is combined with a placement of the feet to form the posture. "Overhead cannon" refers to using a pounding attack against someone in front.

The left and right hands descend and move from the front to the right and back. From the right and back they rotate forward making a large circle, then seizing and pounding downward in front of the chest. The left hand [although the term "hand" is used, the forearm is also included] uses rotational energy, and the right hand uses counter-rotational energy. The left leg uses rotational energy and the right leg uses counter-rotational energy. The feet are placed as has been described. The right and left elbows face outward. The right and left pound with the arms and fingers facing upward. From top to bottom, the four limbs all use embracing energy. This is the energy in the center of the chest. It descends from the upper left, then rises and makes a circle from right to left. The chest closes toward the front. Groin energy is open, rounded, and closed. The toes of both feet face inward, and the energy is closed. Top of the head energy leads. The two shoulders, two knees, and two heels all turn in from the outside. The combined strength is concentrated in the pounding motion. The eyes look between the two hands. This move is called "protecting the heart" pounding motion. It is very similar to the first move, Jin Gang works the pestle. In both moves, Protecting the heart is paramount. If the heart is not shaken, the top, bottom, and all four sides can be handled without error.

Explanation of the Joints

All joints in the entire body face each other and the energy is closed. The qi is one from top to bottom and the energy is closed.

A: The energy of the waist descends. If it does not, there will be no strength at the bottom of the foot, and the groin cannot be closed.
B: The two elbows face outward, and the two fists face each other, one forward, one back. The energy is closed.
C: The two shoulders are relaxed and lowered. Do not raise them.
D: The energy of the top of the head leads. Downward extension of this energy is the key to a strong body.
E: The eyes focus on the left elbow and left fist.
F: The chest must face forward and be closed. It must be entirely empty. The countless forms all contain extreme emptiness.
G: The right foot hooks toward the inside. The inside of the heel kicks back. The toes close inward.
H: The right knee is slightly bent. With the knee bent, the groin opens.
I: The groin must be large. It must be empty. It must be round. It must be closed.
J: The big toe closes to the inside. The five toes and the heel all use force to grip the ground. The left knee is bent. Do not extend it beyond the toe.

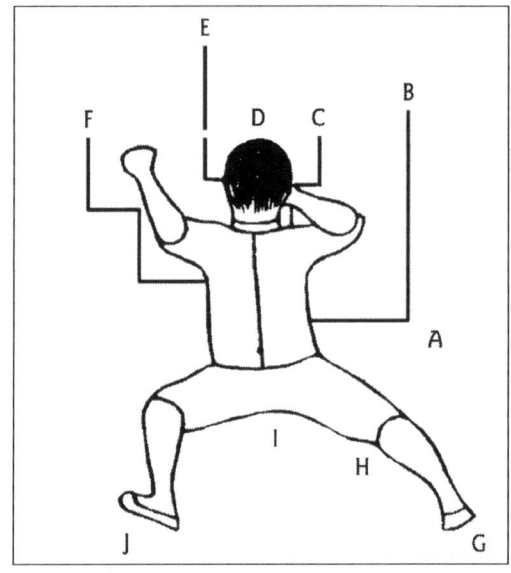

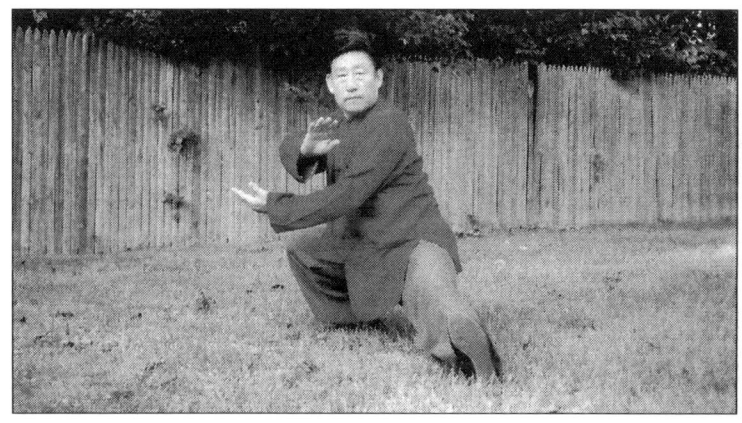

Falling Split
Grandmaster Chen Xiaowang in a variation of falling split.
The posture is low, but not touching the ground.

This is a signature movement from Chen taiji's first form (*yilu*), and Chen Xin's explication of this technique holds noteworthy historical details. It is the earliest written record documenting how this technique was practiced before the recent incarnations of this maneuver. All major schools of Chen taiji today practice this seminal movement in a sliding manner, usually with a stomp of the right foot to propel the left leg into a half-split. In Chen taiji's early history, the falling split (or "dragon creeps down") was practiced with a high vertical leap, falling into the half split position.

Leaping into leg splitting postures is common in many traditional Northern Chinese boxing systems. According to the commonly accepted history of Chen Taiji, Yang Luchan's teacher, Chen Changxing (of whom Chen Xiaowang is a direct descendant), is largely credited with removing the leaping motion when he standardized the original Chen family forms into the two highly dense, well-honed open-hand routines that survive to this day.

Of note, Chen Xin describes the seldom understood fighting application of falling split. His clear description of this movement's usage reveals that this classic Chen taiji maneuver boasts a simple combat utility that demands both high athletic and internal skills.

What is meant by falling split is that the body falls from the air and the legs form a split. The diagram shows the left leg extended out and the right leg bent. This is a single split. With a double split, it is impossible to rise again without a leap. This differs from the single split, in which the left heel is extended forward and closed, and the right knee is outward and open. One can fall or rise by turning the right heel with force. This is slightly easier, and most practitioners use this method nowadays.

The left hand extends out with the left leg as the right leg goes down so that it gradually goes forward. The right ear listens to the right side. The right arm extends, and the right hand looks as if it wants to move forward.

A: The eyes look at the left hand and left foot.
B: The top of the head energy must not be lost.
C: The left leg extends out and falls flat on the ground. The left foot kicks the enemy's shin. The left knee must not bend. The body must draw the qi and collapse forward. The right knee bends but must not rest fully on the ground. The hip bone is almost in a sitting posture, and there is an element of emptiness in its fullness. The top of the right foot faces down and the bottom of the shoe faces up. The Falling Split is reminiscent of the double rise. Whereas in the double rise one flies upward into the air, here one falls from mid-air and the two legs land on the ground. It is a natural correspondence rather than an artificial one. This adheres strictly to ancient precepts on devising routines. When the legs have been placed, the right arm is bent, and the left arm is extended. Both hands are to the left. Both hands then circle upward from the lower left to the right. The right arm unfolds, and the left arm is bent. Both hands extend. At this point, the right leg falls to the ground. As the right heel nears the ground, the left leg kicks out toward the southwest. The idea is for the movement of the left foot to resemble a crescent. The left hand moves as the left leg does; from the right waist it slowly arcs downward, then pushes out to the southwest simultaneously with the left foot. At first, finger strength is used, then palm strength is used. The right arm is back. Although the arm is extended, the hand still has the intention of moving downward and forward; it simply has not done so.
D: Diagram of the right leg.
E: In the Falling Split, the top of the head energy lifts, and the mind energy lifts the foot. The chest collapses to hold the energy. The hip bone is not completely seated. When the right foot comes down from mid-air, the bottom of the foot faces up.
F: The inside of the calf is empty rather than full.
G: This shows how the left foot kicks forward.
H: The left foot arcs slowly from the right and kicks forward. The heel uses force.

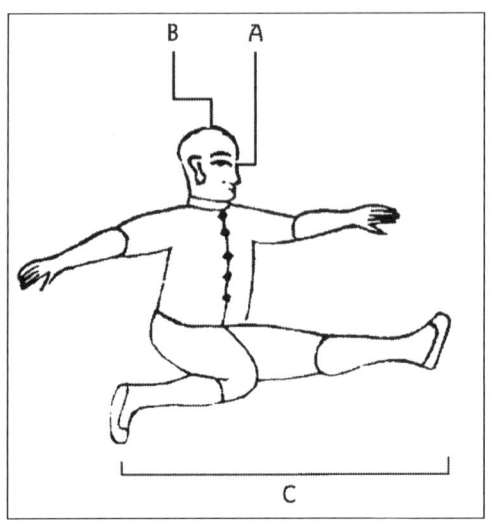

I: Illustration of the Left Leg Outward Kick.

J: When the left leg kicks out, the entire body's force is concentrated in the heel.

K: The main part of this move is the forward kick of the left leg. This kick is not empty. It is to kick the enemy. Therefore, the heel must use force. The forward push of the left hand is to help the left foot. The right hand is on the right side. This is also to help the left foot.

ESSENTIAL KNOWLEDGE FOR TAIJIQUAN STUDY

One of the hallmarks of the Chen family is their long-time connection to the military. Beginning with the General Chen Wangting, credited as the founder of taijiquan, and generations later, Chen Zhongshen, who was Chen Xin's father and a documented battalion leader against rebels during the Taiping Rebellion—the Chens appear to have always been a family of warriors. Consequently, the Chen clan exhibit an unusual sense of martial pride that imbues the ethos of their boxing art with a timeless and universal sense of purpose. Of this martial spirit, Chen Xin wrote the following:

When studying taijiquan, one must be respectful. Without respect, one will be careless with his teacher or friends without, and careless with his body within. When the mind has no restraint, how can one study an art?

When studying taijiquan, one must not be unruly. Unruliness will lead to trouble. One must not be unruly with his hands nor with his words. Outside, one must have the refined air of a scholar. If one is unruly outside, he will surely stray from the Mean.[3]

When studying taijiquan, one must not be complacent. Complacency will harm one's moves. As the saying goes, "Beyond the sky, there is more sky." If one can be humble, then he can accept teaching with an open mind. Who would not be willing to impart skill to him? When one's skill is the accumulated skill of many, it is great skill.

When studying taijiquan, one must carefully ponder each motion. If even a single motion is not pondered, this tendency will continue until one's reasoning is completely obscured. When something is being passed on and it is especially important to pay attention, if one does not pay attention at this point, the entire thread will become incorrect. The transitions will not be fluid, the motions will become disconnected, and it will be impossible to maintain the qi from beginning to end. If the qi cannot be maintained throughout, it will be difficult to even inquire about *tai he yuan qi* [great harmonious original qi].

When studying taijiquan, one should study books. Once the principles in books have been understood, the study of taijiquan will naturally become easier.

The study of taijiquan is the study of yin and yang, opening and closing. Yin and yang, opening and closing are already inherent in your own body. They cannot be increased or decreased through teaching. Once the inherent yin and yang, opening and closing are recovered, teaching stops. Teaching is instruction in the rule, that is, the principle of reaching perfection through the Great Mean.

Although taijiquan is not of great use, in this day many powers are contending with each other. Without martial arts, how can one survive? If this book is merely taken and practiced, it will be no small supplement to the marching drills of the army. If the people in our country practice it, then in hand-to-hand encounters with the enemy, even though the enemy may be strong, what can he do to us? This, too, then, is one way of protecting the country. Men of thought should not dismiss this as simply my humble remarks.

The study of taijiquan must not be used to rob or pillage. If one uses it to rob, then when Heaven seizes him, no supernatural spirits will help him, much less people. For whom in the world can tolerate it?

The study of taijiquan must not be used to bully and oppress people. One who bullies and oppresses people incurs the wrath of everyone and is chief among evildoers.

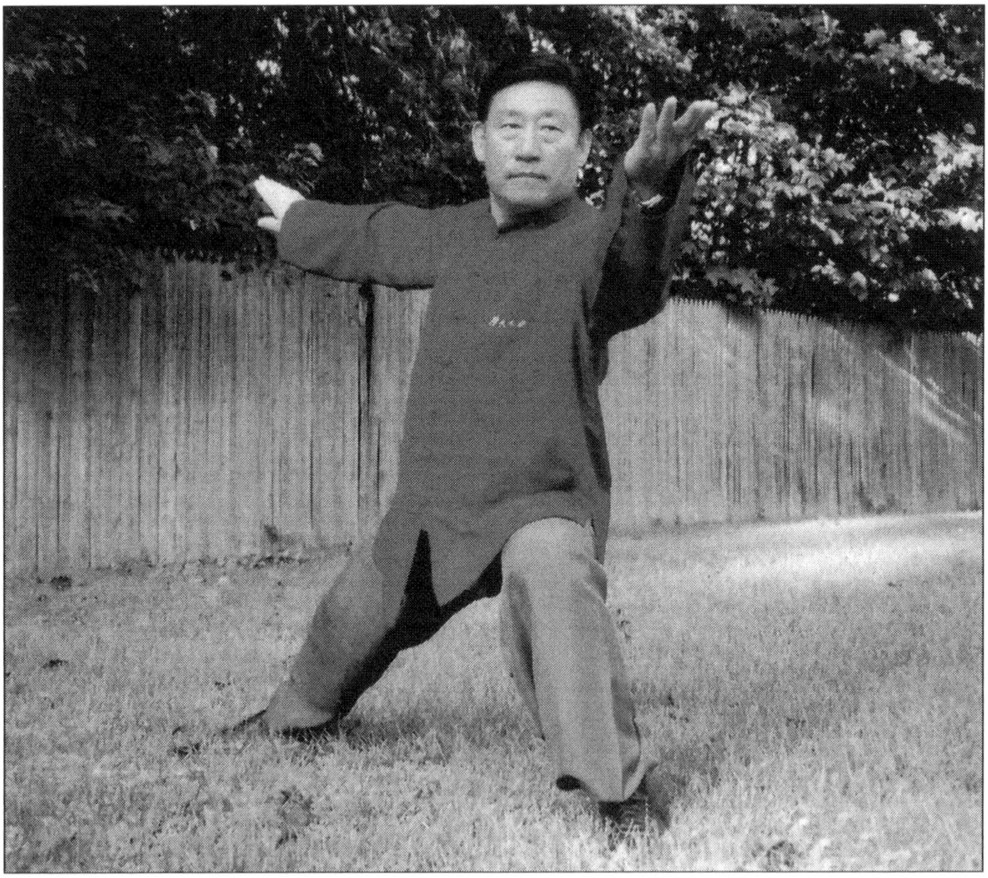

Grandmaster Chen Xiaowang finds
Chen Xin's theories in taiji practice.

Notes

[1] Reference to an acupoint (K17) in the center of the bottom of the foot.
[2] Reference to acupoints located in the lower abdomen, known as the *ming men* that lies vertically along the "conception" meridian.
[3] In the introduction to the Confucian classic, the *Doctrine of the Mean*, the character *chung*, rendered "mean" here, is defined as "being without inclination to either side." The Song dynasty philosopher Chu Xi states that it is "without inclination or deflection, [and] neither exceeds nor comes short" (Legge, 1971: 382).

Bibliography

Berwick, S. (2001). Chen Xiaowang on learning, practicing, and teaching Chen taiji. *Journal of Asian Martial Arts, 10*(2), 98–101.

Berwick, S. (2001). Chen Village under the influence of Chen Xiaoxing. *Journal of Asian Martial Arts, 10*(2), 88–97.

Chen, X. (September 30, 2002). Personal interview in New York.

Chen, X. (2000). *Illustrated explanations of Chen taijiquan* (Chen shi Taijiquan tushuo). Shanghai: Shanghai Bookshop Publishing Company. (Original work published in 1933).

Kohler, S. (Trans.) (1991). Internal energies of Chen and Yang styles. *Tai Chi, 15*(2), 14–19. (Original work published in 1975)

Legge, J. (1971). *Confucius: Confucian analects, The great learning, & doctrine of the mean*. New York: Dover Publications. (Original work published in 1893)

Liuxin, G. and Shen, J. (Eds.) (1963). *Chen shi taijiquan*. Beijing: People's Sports Publishing Company.

Wile, D. (1999). *Tai chi ancestors: The making of an internal martial art*. New City, NY: Sweet Chi Press.

Wu, T. and Wu, T. (1976). The yin and yang of tai chi chuan. *Self Defense World, 2*(2), 18–19.

Dripping Oil Onto Parchment:
Traditional Taijiquan Form Training in Chen Village
by David Gaffney, B.A.

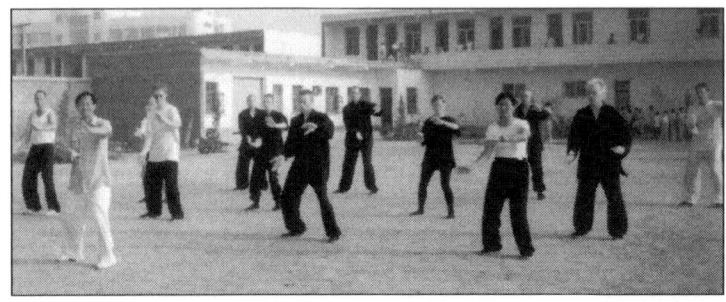

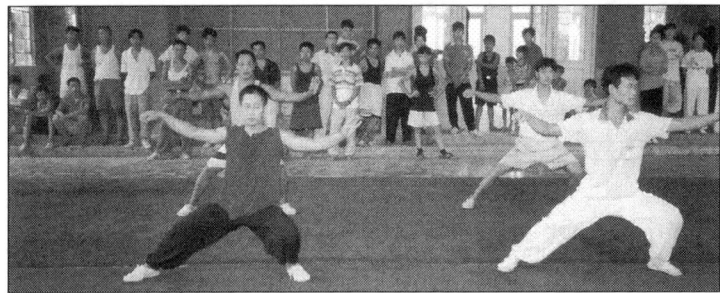

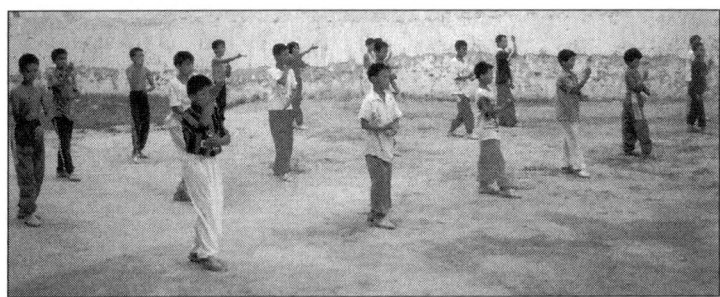

Top: Familiarity through repetition. Middle: Group demonstration in the main training hall in Chen Village. Bottom: From an early age form training is used to develop strong foundation skills. Children in Wenxian County (close to Chen Village) practice the old frame form during a physical education class. All photos courtesy of David Gaffney.

Introduction

Practicing taijiquan (often abbreviated as taiji) in its ancestral birthplace, Chen Village, allows one to cut through many misconceptions and to reach closer to the essence of the traditional manner of acquiring skill. The realization that you are tracing the footsteps of people like Chen Wangting (1600–1680), the creator of Chen taijiquan; Chen Changxing (1771–1853), formulator of the system as we know it today; and Chen Fake, who took taiji to the wider world, in effect, stepping on the same soil—gives one a great sense of continuity.

One area where East and West fully accord is in their belief that one should have a sense of the past to fully appreciate the present. That is why history is taught as a subject in school, and those of us who have been bored by it, and slept through the subject, are the poorer for it. With regards to taiji, perhaps even more important than recorded history is the method of acquiring skill that has been passed down orally from teacher to student for centuries.

Chen taiji has its own step-by-step comprehensive training method, of which, it soon becomes apparent, form training provides the foundation. Stories are handed down of the prodigious number of repetitions Chen Fake performed every day. Chen Xiaowang is said to have suspended building work on his house because it was interfering with his daily routine of thirty repetitions of the old frame first routine (*laojia yilu*). This tradition has survived with the current emerging masters from the village. Wang Haijun, three times overall champion in the Chinese National Taijiquan Tournament, recalled how his first eight years of training in Chen Village consisted solely of practicing the old frame first routine.

Form training is demanding. It requires the total attention and participation of mind and body. Elements such as patience, persistence, mind/intent (*yi*), strength, relaxation, and internal energy (*yi*) are crucial in honing one's taijiquan skills. In Chen Village, practitioners have for generations considered the hand form to be the base upon which all other taiji skills are built. Practicing the taiji form is not simply a matter of mindlessly repeating the sequences. Each routine has been carefully researched and meticulously arranged. The forms are the culmination of centuries of practical experience, each posture and maneuver having been tried, tested, and then assembled to construct the forms or routines we see today.

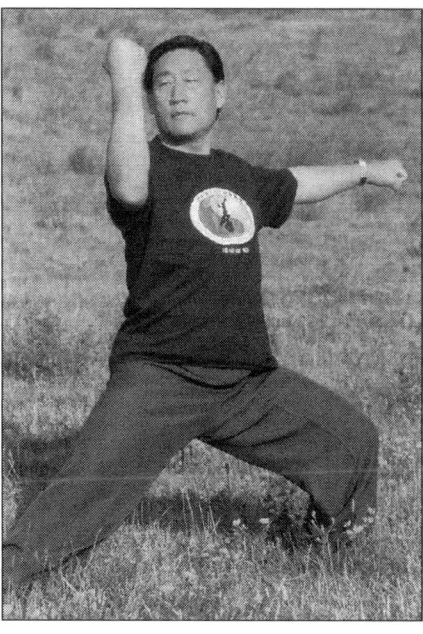

Chen Xiaowang performing the new frame (*xinjia*) routine.

Characteristics of the Traditional Hand Forms

While modern shortened versions of taiji are practiced as an introduction to the system, the main curriculum emphasizes two primary bare-hand routines. The first and more commonly practiced routine is the first routine (*yilu*), the second being the more dynamic cannon fist routine (*paochui*). The 14th-generation standard bearer Chen Changxing compiled these two routines, incorporating the more numerous ancient forms devised by systems founder Chen Wangting (Chen, 1993).

Compared to the cannon fist, the first routine's movements are comparatively simple, with more emphasis placed upon softness than hardness. The first routine focuses upon the development of silk reeling (*chansijing*) through the twining and coiling movements of the limbs and body, interspersed with issuing energy movements (*fajing*). In appearance, the form is relaxed, steady, and stable. The form, as the Chinese classics say, is "like a great river rolling on unceasingly." Throughout, the limbs are guided by the body in an uninterrupted sequence of opening and closing movements.

Great thought was given to the movements' features (hard or soft, difficult or easy, etc.) so that the art's complexities could be learned little by little over time. For instance, the first routine's beginning movements are relatively straightforward. The movements are comfortable and natural, with silk reeling as the most important principle. More softness and less hard movement make learning and practicing easier. This employment of coiling and twining movement is one of the major features of Chen taiji. Practicing the form while accurately following this method leads the student along the path to developing more effective issuing energy, and eventually gaining an understanding of how to apply and escape from joint-locking techniques (*qinna*). Conscientious training of the first form lays a strong base upon which more complex skills can subsequently be overlaid.

The second routine, cannon fist (*paochui*), is more difficult. Movements are more intricate, faster, and tighter, with shaking energy as the main principle. Through practice of this form comes an appreciation of the different requirements of each movement—for example, the positioning of hands and feet, bodily synchronization throughout the movement, and how to place the body most favorably for attack or defense.

High or Low Postures?

The optimum number of forms practiced, and the level of physical difficulty must be decided relative to the practitioner's strength, age, and vigor. For less-experienced students, it is preferable that actions be large, comfortable, and open. The expression of roundness, fullness, and continuous motion, as well as the alternation of opening and closing movements, can be more clearly seen when the spiraling silk reeling circles are larger.

Practicing in a high or low stance is left up to personal preference. In the early stages of training, low postures allow one to develop the lower body's foundation strength. In a lecture entitled "How to Practice Taijiquan" given during the First International Chen Style Training Camp in 1999, Chen Zhenglei stressed the vital importance of building up leg strength. He suggested that:

> When the legs are strong and can bear weight firmly, then the upper body can relax and sink down into them, making the top flexible. If the legs are not strong, the upper body is "afraid" of sinking down and remains top heavy and unrelaxed.

Low postures also allow the practitioner to see more clearly the folding movements of the waist and turning of the legs. As the skill level increases, it is normal for the postures to become higher. This higher stance is extremely agile, the practitioner being able to change naturally and easily between high and low positions. For the older beginner, a higher position may be more comfortable. Above all, in practicing the form, one should let naturalness be the guiding principle.

Training the Frame

The inhabitants of Chen Village refer to taiji practice as "training the frame of one's posture" (*lien panjia*). Great emphasis is placed on the quality of a student's position and fixing any deficiencies in his or her posture. The training syllabus requires the student to first learn the form's movements. Once familiarity with the form is reached, the process of correcting posture can begin. Correcting posture is a "hands on" process whereby the teacher adjusts the posture of a student until it eventually fulfills a set of requirements handed down over many generations. This is achieved in much the same way as a sculptor refining ever-greater details from a crude outline.

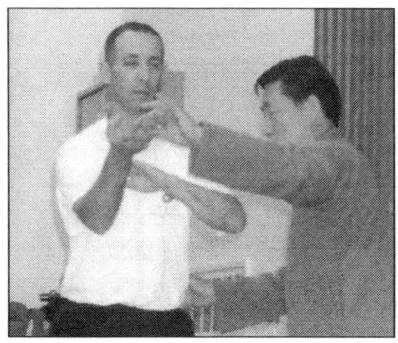

Correcting posture is a hands-on process.
Chen Xiaowang helping Mr. Gaffney.

Familiarity Through Repetition

Chen Zhenglei likens the process of achieving competence in the form to learning to write Chinese characters. In the early stages of practice, one should not look too far ahead to the more advanced requirements. Like learning the basic calligraphy strokes, the beginner should first concern himself with accurately learning the sequence. Concentration should be focused upon maintaining an upright position and performing the movements in a soft and balanced manner. Inexperienced practitioners often try to run before they can walk and would do well to heed the following advice:

> As for those errors that unavoidably crop up—like raising your shoulders or sticking out your elbows, filling your chest with unrestrained qi, panting when you breathe, your hands and feet trembling, etc.—it is not advisable to delve into these phenomena too deeply.
> – Chen, 1998

Different teachers from Chen Village often compare learning taijiquan to the wider educational system. Everybody accepts that they must go through primary education before they are ready to attend high school. Likewise, they must complete high school before they can attend a university. Those trying to acquire the more complex skills upon an inadequate foundation are destined to fail.

Repetitive practice of the form leads to familiarity with the movements. Certain optimum patterns of movement must be established, and these can only become set if they are repeated almost endlessly. Chen Zhenglei (1999) said that taijiquan movement's unique nature is designed to get rid of all body stiffness and rigidity. Through prolonged practice and training, the body's joints are loosened, the tendons are stretched and elongated, and all parts of the body are coordinated in motion. Every gap between the joints should eventually develop an elastic quality. This elasticity—the stretching of the tendons, plus developing whole body coordination—is what is known as taiji internal skill (*neigong*) (Si, 2000: 13).

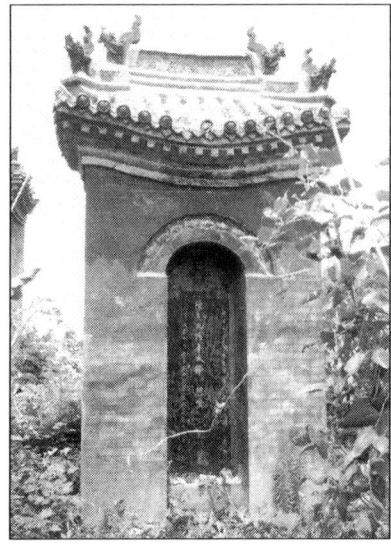

The tomb of Chen Zhoukui.

In time, coordination, flexibility, and relaxation are acquired throughout every movement within the form. The movement becomes fluid and unpredictable, changing instantly form slow to fast, from soft to hard, and from light to heavy. Relaxation provides the foundation of accumulating and releasing power (*fajing*). By seeking complete relaxation, the practitioner attempts to rid himself of stiff energy released en route during a movement. Speed and power are greatly increased by lessening the stiff resistance of muscles during movement (Si, 2000: 13).

In his discourse on fighting methods, *Training for Sparring*, Chen Zhaokui writes:

> Emphasis on slow movements alone leads to slow strikes which an opponent can counter easily. Emphasis on fast moves only makes it difficult to feel the path of your energy and makes it easy to strike along a longer path than necessary. Being fast refers to the speed generated through familiarity of the energy path. It is a speed without loss of quality.
> – Ma, 1998

Slowness as a Training Tool

When training the form, emphasis is placed upon slowness. Throughout each individual movement, the practitioner begins slowly, moves smoothly in transition, and gradually settles into the final posture. Using the slow approach allows one to fully concentrate upon each opening and closing, stretch and withdraw, and rising and lowering movement. Over time, slow practice enables postures to be developed exactly, to fulfill the martial applications contained within. Every form trains the body so that the practitioner becomes aware of the optimum position through all stages of each technique, and slowness enables the body to become fixed in its postures. Following this approach, when a movement is speeded up, it becomes natural and will not stray. Posture and movement developed in this way will grow to be habitual and can be utilized whenever an individual needs to move quickly and decisively—whether they are speeding up the movements of the form, practicing push-hands, or engaging in free-sparing (*san shou*).

Exponents of the external martial arts generally consider the development of direct force and superior speed and strength as the natural way by which an adversary can be defeated. From this perspective, taiji seems to be at odds with nature. At first glance, it seems obvious that, in combat, strength must be superior to softness and speed more successful than slowness. Taiji philosophy, however, holds that this assessment is invalid. Instead, taiji followers are asked to have confidence in the idea that softness can prevail over greater strength and that slowness can defeat speed. Performing movements quickly before the postures have become fixed and exact leads to a loss of detail and efficacy. Consequently, the use of slowness represents one of taiji's distinctive training methods rather than its ultimate objective.

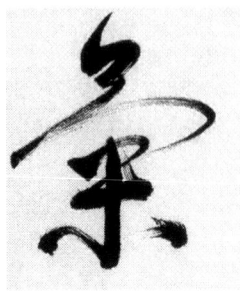 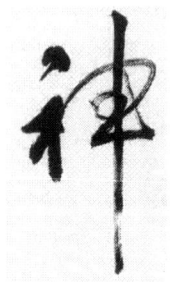 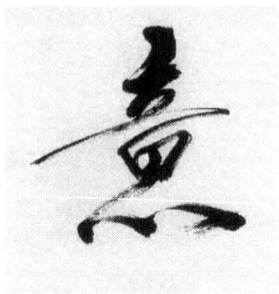

Vital energy (*qi*), spirit (*shen*), intention (*yi*). Calligraphy by Zhu Tiancai.

Fostering Mental Calmness and Its Roll Cultivating Qi, and the Development of Intention

Calmness of the mind is a fundamental requirement if the practitioner hopes to preserve the many finer points contained inside the forms. Impatience merely leads to hurriedness and a loss of detail. Composure of the mind enables vital energy to become quiet and subsequently to follow the intention. In this manner the intention can be fostered, facilitating the link between spirit (*shen*) and vital energy (*qi*). Chen Zhenglai (1998) suggests that:

> In practicing Chen Style taijiquan, you must keep your thoughts quiet, getting rid of all internal and external disturbances. Only in this way will you benefit by restraining your internal energy, and by guiding the rising and movement of internal energy.

In time, this approach allows the taiji practitioner to effect whole-body movement during the form, unifying internal spirit or consciousness with the external form, thereby uniting body and mind. Practicing slowly allows one to cultivate qi, increasing the health and vigor of the body. This provides the foundation from which martial stamina and skill can flourish.

Traditional taiji practice emphasizes the importance of the abdominal center of balance (*dantian*) and its rotation. When form training, the practitioner is required to focus on the dantian region. According to the study of meridians, the dantian is situated in the lower abdomen two to three fingers below the navel. In this area, there is a concentration of internal organs, mainly the reproductive and excretory ones. Concentrating one's mind intent on the dantian has several benefits: 1) it can lower the body's center of gravity making the lower plane (*xia pan*) very steady and balanced, 2) it enables massage of the internal organs, which increases the functions of those organs, 3) it can focus the mind-intent (*yi nien*) so that when you are practicing boxing you are actually resting your mind, and 4) it enables dantian breathing, namely abdominal breathing, which increases lung capacity (Si, 2000: 13).

In order not to hinder qi development, the forms should be practiced according to the principles, and one should not place a limit on each movement by focusing on one application. Every movement has many possible applications. Considering each as part of a circle, one realizes that all points on the circle can represent a particular application, depending on the situation. One should learn the method, not its manifestation (Chen, 1999). In other words, do not be concerned with individual applications but rather on how the body moves as a completely integrated system.

Fundamental to correct taiji practice is the constant involvement of the mind (*yi*) in all movements within the form arising from the mind's "intent." The mind moves the qi, which in turn moves the body. The taiji form requires the practitioner to develop a deep level of concentration upon the body's internal sensations, always focusing on the precise movement being performed. In terms of strictness and attention to detail, even the smallest detail must be clearly executed, with no brushing over a movement that is unclear. Each movement within the sequence should be carefully considered as to its function and characteristics: whether it is relaxed enough, where to open and close, whether to turn in the foot, if there is enough spiral movement, etc. The practitioner meticulously works out the requirements, slowly reducing the number of shortcomings and faults. With this mindset, each repetition of the form should lead to new discoveries and understandings, and ultimately mastery.

To develop *yi* and *qi*, the form must be practiced correctly for some time. Distinct stages must be passed through. First, the sequence must be mastered until it becomes very familiar. At this stage, emphasis is placed primarily upon attaining looseness in the joints and correct body structure. Initially, training should center on standardizing the movements of the form as closely as possible to fulfill the body requirements of Chen taijiquan. Each time the student comes to a fixed posture—for example, lazily tying coat (*lan zha yi*), single whip (*dan bian*), or preparing form (*taiji qi shi*)—he or she should focus strictly upon each part of the body, making sure that it conforms to the principles. This process requires considerable mental effort if the student is to avoid deviating from the correct path. Though many people can quote the taiji requirements and verses from the *Taiji Classics*, real understanding can only come through training these into one's body. For instance, it is not enough to know that the shoulders must be relaxed; the practitioner must discover how to relax them and to what degree. Or how to contain or store the chest (*han xiong*). At what point is it sufficiently stored? Too much, and the waist collapses; too little, and the shoulder tightens.

Once the form can be performed naturally, the internal energy can develop. With each completed posture, the vital energy sinks to the dantian and from there is distributed throughout the body. Through continual, diligent practice, more qi is accumulated and stored in the dantian. Chen Zhenglai (1999) likens the dantian to a large river, saying that if the water level is not sufficiently high, then water will not fill the smaller tributaries downstream. So, if the dantian has not filled with qi, qi cannot be pushed out to the extremities.

When the fixed postures have been standardized and the basic requirements fulfilled, the practitioner then must consider the movement principles: using the waist as the axis, moving sectionally, etc. At this stage, one must seek the correct route of each movement in the form, incorporating the basic requirements and movement principles. To understand one or two points is considered not bad, as it is not possible to understand every aspect at once. Improvement occurs in a step-by-step manner over time. For example, dividing the body into three sections, a requirement of all basic movements is that the outer sections (hands and feet) hold the energy, the two middle sections (elbows and knees) hold the position, and the two root sections (shoulders and upper thighs, *ku*) relax. To do all this simultaneously is very difficult, so it is better perhaps to concentrate on one point at a time (Si, 2000: 13). As the movement principles and body requirements are realized, the internal energy from the dantian can be accurately directed to the appropriate point, depending upon which movement is being performed.

The Hand Form as a Blueprint for Developing Martial Skill

The hand form provides the blueprint for developing the martial skills of Chen taijiquan. A multifaceted instructional tool, it incorporates many essentials that, when united, allow the practitioner to fully build up his fighting skills. There are no easy options if one seeks to acquire higher-level abilities. Inexperienced students often press the teacher as to the precise application and usage of movements early in their training. With the traditional Chen Village masters, answers sometimes seem ambiguous and vague. Instead of being shown some spectacular attack or countering technique, the student is told to look to the principle behind the movement. This can be very frustrating to those used to being spoon fed techniques, after all, it is argued, if you don't learn how to attack an opponent, how can this be a martial art? Impatient students may leave with the feeling that the real skill is being withheld or may gloomily conclude that their skill is not deemed sufficient to warrant an answer.

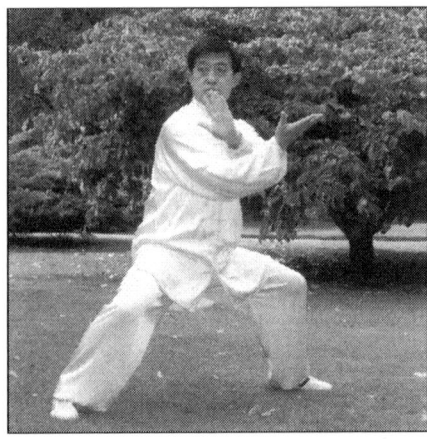

Chen Zhenglei in transition movement during the lazily tying coat posture.

During class one day, Chen Zhenglai likened taiji's martial application to Chinese medicine with its emphasis on cause rather than symptom. One should, he suggested, try to understand how a movement is generated rather than focusing upon its final expression. Approached in this manner, the form becomes a training method to ready the body for combat. In a treatise entitled "Training Method of Chen Taiji Routine and Push-Hands," Chen Zhaokui writes: "every position should be precise, and each destination should be clear" (Ma, 1998).

Taiji is a practical and no-nonsense martial art. Its proficient use rests upon an assimilation of its core principles if one is to grasp the internal substance and avoid the practice "flowery fists": nice to look at, but devoid of content. At all times, the practitioner must seek out the most difficult, the most challenging, and the most detailed aspects of the movements contained within the form. The temptation to cheat to circumvent demanding movements should be avoided. For instance, when performing the dragon on the ground posture, the practitioner drops into a low stance, and next, even more difficult, moves to the following position through arced movement.

Every movement and step in the form has been developed to prepare the student for a particular purpose, and all ought to be viewed as being important, not just those with immediately apparent martial applications.

Old Frame First Routine — Closing Sequence
1) crossed foot kick (*shi zhi jiao*)
2) punch to crotch (*zhi dang chui*)
3) white ape presents fruit (*bai yuan xian guo*)
4) six sealing and four closing (*liu feng si bi*)

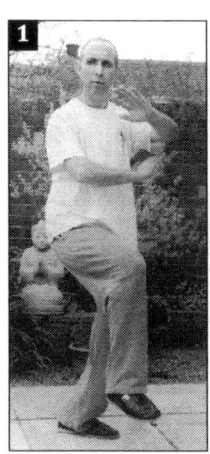
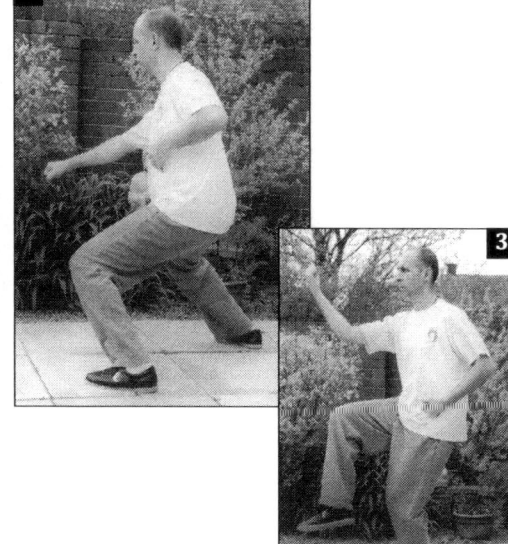
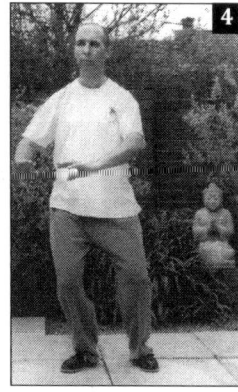

5) single whip (*dan bian*)
6) dragon on the ground (*que di long*)

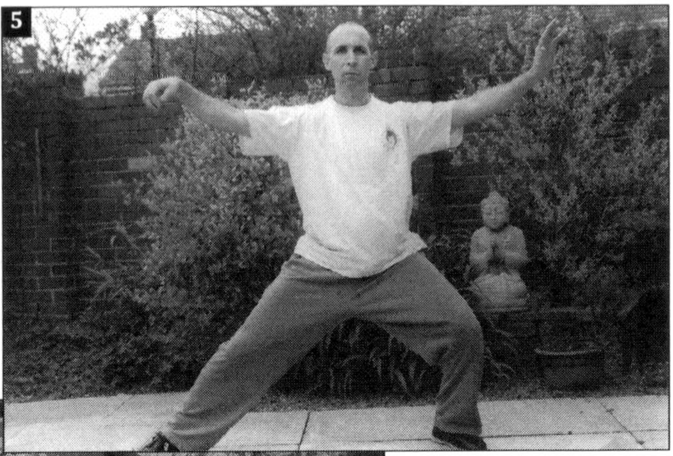

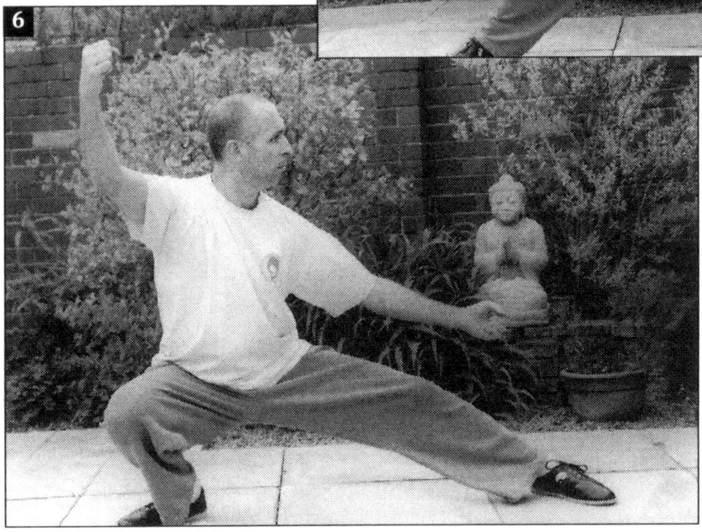

7) stepping forward with seven stars (*shang bu qi xing*)
8) step back to ride the tiger (*xia bu kua hu*)
9) head-on blow (*dang tou pao*)

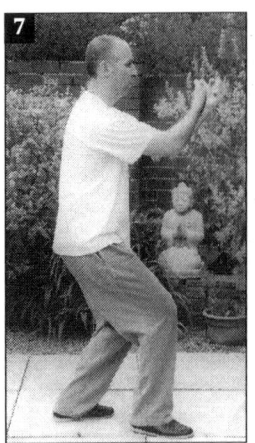 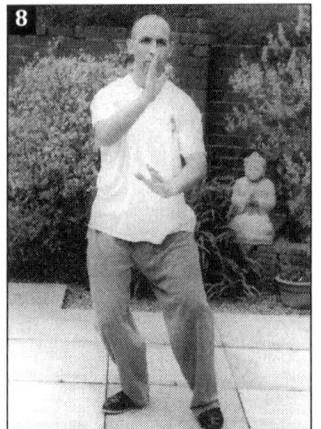 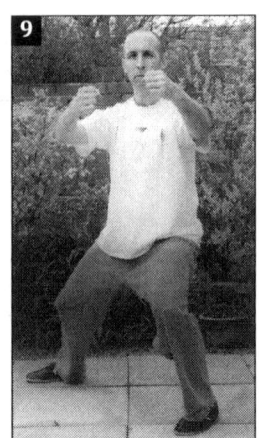

10) Buddha's warrior attendant pounds mortar (*jin gang dao dui*)
11) closing form (*taiji shou si*)

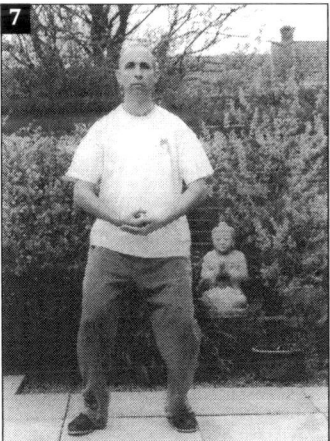 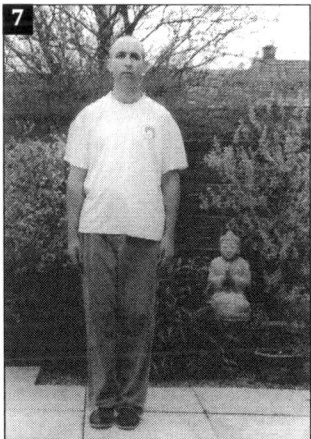

Requirements When Practicing the Form

In his book *Chen Style Taijiquan Method and Theory*, Ma Hong (1998), a disciple of Chen Zhaokui, lists sixteen requirements laid down by his teacher, which must be attended to during each posture:

1) eye movement (the direction of the eyes)
2) the shape of the hands, and how the hand changes as the movement is being performed
3) silk reeling (*shun-chan* and *ni-chan*) of the arms
4) footwork (how to execute changes when stepping)
5) silk reeling (*shun-chan* and *ni-chan*) of the legs
6) opening and closing of the chest and back
7) rising and falling of the buttocks
8) dantian rotation (waist and lower abdomen)
9) shifting weight (the relationship of substantial and insubstantial)
10) beginning and end points, as well as the transitional movements of the upper and lower limbs
11) how much strength to use, and where the strength should be concentrated (i.e., where is the attack point?)
12) position and direction of posture
13) the rise and fall of spiral movement (top and bottom coordination)
14) the change in tempo (alternating slow and fast)
15) breathing (coordination of breathing and movement)
16) listening (not just auditory, but with all senses)

The requirements are not rigid measurements but have got to be experienced and polished through continuous training. Their intricacy is reflected in an early taiji adage: "Only the gods know; impossible to transmit orally." To the inexperienced learner, Chen taijiquan's body requirements at times appear almost unbearably strict. Nevertheless, by following this route, an advanced level of ability can be reached in a step-by-step manner.

Over time, conscientious practice and study of the form allow the practitioner to identify and build into his arsenal both the attacking and defensive facets of the art. From a defensive perspective, the intention is to achieve the capacity to lure an adversary into emptiness. This requires training to a stage where one can stick, connect, adhere, and follow: neither losing contact with nor resisting the opponent. Offensive skills are acquired by refining taiji's eight energy methods (*ba fa*): *peng, lu, ji, an, cai, lei, zhou*, and *kou*. In time, the student tries to approach the level of skill often quoted in the *Taiji Classics* whereby "four ounces can overcome a thousand pounds."

To attain this level, the form must be honed until it becomes unbroken, with each movement flowing smoothly into the next, on the surface relaxed but inwardly strong. Where hard and soft elements are combined, the upper and lower body are coordinated, and the internal and external (*yi* and *li*) work closely together. Looking at accomplished practitioners, you see movement that is highly refined, devoid of all stiffness and clumsiness.

The development pace cannot be forced. Paradoxically, the more you try to hurry, the more difficult it is to progress. Highly regarded 20th generation practitioner Wang Haijun, an adopted student of Chen Zhenglai, cites an old Chen taiji saying that skill is acquired like dripping oil onto parchment until eventually the parchment is saturated. He says that the traditional way was to accept whatever the teacher was teaching at whatever pace, no matter how slowly. With prolonged practice, skill naturally develops. Those people who train daily for years reach levels of skill that seem impossible to achieve to those unable or unwilling to devote themselves as fully to training.

While individual goals dictate the level of intensity during practice, combat efficiency necessitates a high level of dedication in terms of time and exertion. The forms should not be approached as sequences of movements and techniques to be memorized and then repeated parrot-like. Rather, they are training tools with which one can hone the ability to move and react in a calm, natural, and potent way. Chen Xiaowang, in his critique "The Fajing of Chen Style Taijiquan" (n.d.), suggests that a fitting outlook when practicing the form is to train diligently, ignoring tiredness, and accepting the need to work hard. In the words of a well-known Chinese saying, if you hope to reach a high level of skill, you must be willing to "eat bitterness" (*chi ku*).

Bibliography

Chen, X. (n.d.). "The fajing of Chen Style Taijiquan," downloaded from Chen Zhenglei's official website: http://www.chenzhenglei-tj.com. In Chinese.

Chen, Z. (1993). *Wonderful taiji kungfu*. Zhengzhou: Zhengzhou Ancient Books.

Chen, Z. (1998). *Chinese taijiquan scriptures: Taijiquan Chen shi jia dushu*. Xi'an: Qu Ban Xian Gongsi.

Chen, Z. (1999). Notes taken during the First International Chen Taijiquan Training Camp, held in August 18th to the 28th in Handang, Hebei, China.

Ma, H. (1998). *Chen Style Taijiquan method and theory*. Beijing: Beijing Sports University Press.

Si, C. (2000). Demystifying taijiquan, *Shaolin and Taiji*, 11: 13. In Chinese.

• 40 •
Taiji Solo Form:
The Benefits of Group Versus Individual Practice
by John Loupos, B.S.

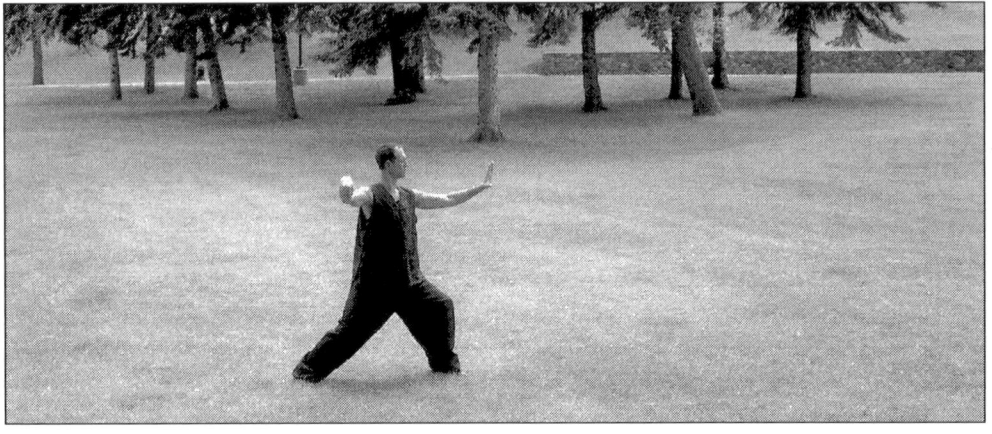

Photo courtesy of John Loupos.

> "Normally, taiji practice is a solo affair, hemmed in by the frenetic pace of daily life.... Though taiji is principally an individual journey, companionship along the road is to be treasured."
> – Dr. Jay Dunbar

As you might infer from the preceding quotation, there is no hard and fast consensus as to the relative merits of group practice versus solo practice. When you practice taiji on your own, you are the primary variable in the experience, there being no one else to take into consideration. Of course, other considerations, such as the conditions under which you practice (terrain, lighting, weather, your most recent meal, time of day, etc.), will have some effect on any given practice session, as can your own personal subjective aspects. But, if it's just you and your taiji, the potential for unanticipated influences from outside sources is about nil.

You are alone with yourself. It's a beautiful, brisk morning as you stroll out to your lawn, or the park, or the quiet confines of whatever personal sanctum you have available. As you stand in quiet preparation, prior to embarking on one more in an untold number of repetitions of your taiji form, you feel yourself rooting to the earth. Your body automatically enacts a multitude of minor adjustments, and your respiration softens and slows as the parasympathetic branch of your autonomic nervous system prevails, relaxing you down to a deeper level. With the first moves of your form, you feel any residual kinks in your body announcing their release and melting away. Soon your mind and spirit follow as internal energy (*qi*) starts to tingle through your body's energy pathways. In the whole universe, there is only you in your oneness with all, and the timelessness of the moment you are in.

Solo practice offers the opportunity to move at your own pace and with attention to your own agenda. If you have a notion to linger over this move or that for extra practice, that's your prerogative.

On the other hand, group practice offers the prospect of mingled energies, whether distractive or harmonious. When you practice your taiji with others, their presence can't not affect your experience. In fact, there are several reasons why practicing taiji in a neighborly way can yield benefits above and beyond what you might expect from solo training.

Whenever two or more people practice taiji together, the "energy" changes. As one member of a group, you may feel an aura of anticipation, a heightened sensitivity to the parameters of your physical space in proximity to those around you, or a peripheral awareness of timing your moves to the moves of others. Exactly how your energy changes may also depend on the specific group context. Practicing in your regular class, alongside familiar fellow students with your teacher at the helm will likely feel different from practicing with acquaintances at the park or with unknown peers at a tournament or taiji get together. Regardless of the context, group practice offers you an opportunity to learn how to engage the energy of your taiji with the energy of others who are on a similar path.

As a teacher, I have more than the usual opportunity, incentive, and responsibility to pay attention to the dynamics of group practice. Experience has taught me that any shift in energy can be used as an opportunity to learn something new and to increase one's perceptive abilities. For example, a feeling of enhanced sensitivity and refined perception are necessary precursors to synchronized timing. Synchronized timing implies your ability to match your moves exactly to the moves of others around you. Naturally, the whole issue of synchronized timing is moot if you are practicing alone. But when practicing alongside others, each person shares equally in the responsibility for keeping the group moving in unison. (Note: In actual practice, and depending on the size of the group, if novices or beginners are involved, more experienced students might be expected to shoulder a greater share of this responsibility to keep their practice within the ability range of the less experienced classmates.)

Synchronized timing may seem merely an aesthetic quality to casual observers, but it can take on added significance in any context in which you engage directly with others, whether in "verbal" negotiation, push-hands practice, or outright combat/self-defense. Reflect for a moment on whether you have ever engaged in a conversation or a negotiation, perhaps one that was a bit volatile, where there was a possibility of escalating conflict. Even in a relatively benign situation, short of out-and-out combat, the timing and nuances of your remarks, not to mention your body language, can influence how events play out. Poorly crafted or ill-timed verbal communication can inflame a situation, vice de-escalating it.

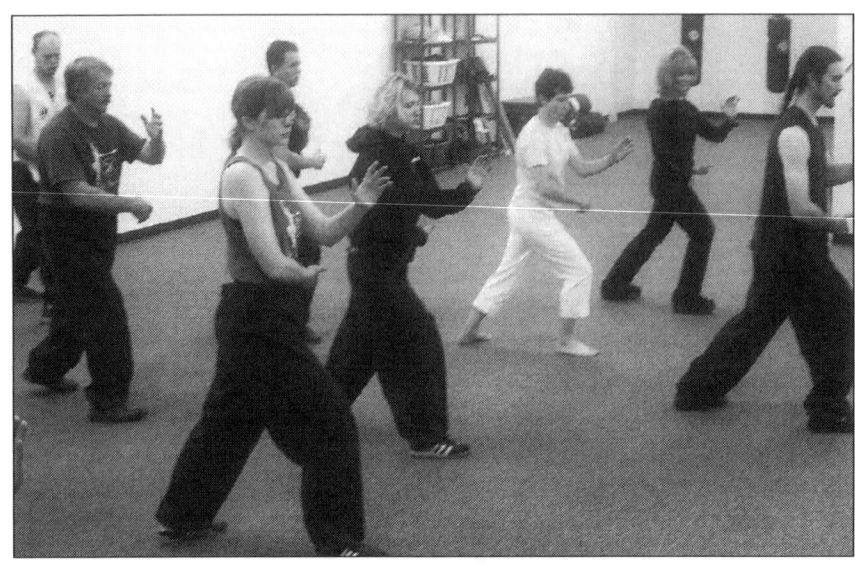

Seeking the benefits of group practice.
Photo courtesy of John Loupos.

The sensitivity that you develop toward others, often unconsciously, as one consequence of group practice can help you avoid misreads and respond more effectively in resolving conflict before it gets out of control. Group practice is clearly more conducive to the acquisition of enhanced sensitivity and refined perception, for the purposes of interaction with others, than is solo practice.

From a martial perspective, the issue of timing, or synchronizing your moves to the moves of others, is especially important. Taiji as a martial art necessarily entails interaction with others, whether for prearranged push-hands practice or during actual combat or self-defense.

Nowadays, taiji is often pursued as a personal development or fitness activity with rare thought given to its fighting application. People who study taiji are often motivated to do so by reasons that are quite different from those who study harder or more external martial arts styles. Nevertheless, taiji can be an effective fighting system for those who train with some regard for its martial aspects.

From a martial perspective, it is very important to know where your opponent is at all always to be able to sense instantly if your opponent closes his distance on you. This "knowing" can stem from visually observing your opponent, or it can stem from "sensing" his or her proximity. Practicing with others and developing an awareness of where they are at all times even in the absence of a direct visual line of contact, requires a certain peripheral awareness. This is most readily developed by practicing on a regular basis in close proximity to others. Of course, merely being able to sense an opponent's approach is useless if you lack the skills to respond accordingly, but that skill level requires preparation of a different sort.

Along these same lines, it can be instructive for any group to vary its practice speed. Learning how to keep your body properly adjusted while moving at variable speeds is essential from a martial perspective because, in a real situation, you may not be able to control the speed with which another person uses against you. Rather, you must be able to match your speed to that of your opponent. Varying the speed at which your group practices forces you to learn how to adapt to what could be a rapidly changing situation.

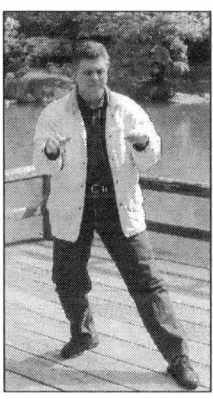

Seeking the benefits of individual practice.
Photo courtesy of Lin Shengxuan.

Another of the skills that group form practice teaches, even if inadvertently, is how to sense and maintain a fixed distance from those around you. Though you may have never thought of this skill as such, when you practice with others, for example in a crowded classroom, the likelihood is that you naturally become aware if someone encroaches on your space. At such times, you may automatically adjust the length or width of your step or stance, or perhaps the pace of your movements, to allow for a more manageable distance between yourself and those sharing your practice space. Taken to a more highly developed level, the same skill allows you to control and maintain a safe distance between yourself and someone who is posing a genuine threat.

Aside from the way group practice prepares you for engaging with others in push-hands or combat, there is simply the sheer joy of sharing your time and space with other people who are also committed to exploring the magic taiji has to offer. When you practice and train taiji, you are creating the potential to grow and evolve as a person. Such personal growth may not happen by quantum leaps, but every practice session will leave its mark in some way. Practicing *en masse* allows you and your fellow students the opportunity to learn from each other's mistakes and to share in each other's progress. Because there are few road maps outlining whatever route your personal taiji journey will take, group practice can offer solace in times of uncertainty and, in the words of Dr. Jay, "companionship along the way."

From a Small Village to the Capital:
The Li Family's Early Taijiquan Curriculum
by Wong Yuen Ming

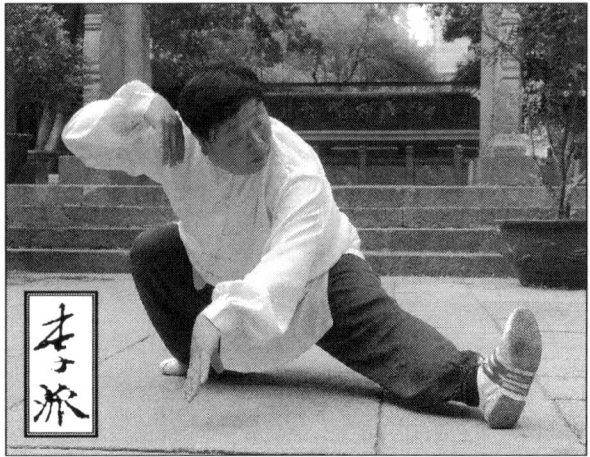
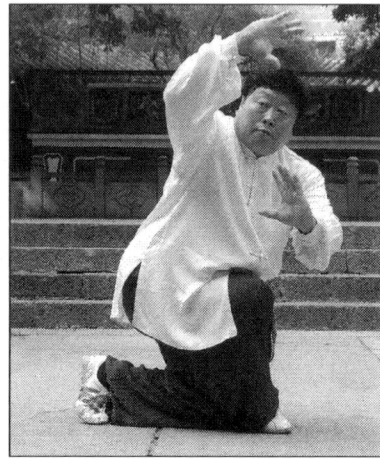

Zhang Shaotang (b. 1952), fourth generation Li Style master practicing.
Chinese characters for Li Family School.
All illustrations courtesy of Wong Yuen Ming.

Introduction

Hebei Province in northern China has been home to number of notable martial artists in the last couple hundred years. Placing their capital in Beijing, the Qing dynasty attracted many accomplished teachers who were looking for fortune, some found careers as escorts for the many rich merchants traveling across the country, and many others as martial arts teachers. The most influential taijiquan figure of that period was without doubt Yang Luchan (1799–c. 1875), who reached Beijing around 1850 with plenty of experience gained from numerous trips to Chen Village (birthplace of Chen Family Style Taiji). Later, he taught in his hometown of Yongnian. Modern taijiquan history basically started with Yang's arrival in the capital, and especially with his appointment to the court.

Yang Luchan Goes to Beijing

Yang Luchan went to Beijing with an introduction from Wu Ruqing[1] to teach at a rich family's compound. Wu Tunan (?–1988)[2] explains how Ruqing, who had passed the imperial examinations and was appointed to Beijing, had a friend called Mr. Zhang. Zhang's brother loved martial arts and having heard about Yang Luchan from Ruqing, invite Yang to the family estate to teach (Ma, 1984). In a short time, Yang and his two sons were working at the Zhang mansion training the young Zhang Fengqi.

According to Wu Tunan's account, the Zhangs had a successful preserved vegetable business and one of their outlets was in Xiang Shan, very close to where Prince Zaiyi[3] used to hunt. According to this story, Prince Zaiyi often stopped over at the Zhang's on the way back to the palace to purchase some of their famous preserved vegetables. On one of these visits, the prince happened to see Yang Luchan training Zhang Fengqi. Luchan's skills intrigued the prince, who invited him to his estate. This anecdote notes that the Zhangs were not happy with this at first, so an arrangement was made allowing Yang to teach at the prince's residence the first two weeks of the month and continue his teaching at the Zhang's the second half of each month.

However, the Li family has a slightly different story.[4] Wang Lanting (1829–?) wrote in 1874 that his introduction to the art of taijiquan was in the fourth year of the Tongzhi Era (1865) through his colleague Fu Zhongquan,[5] a military guard who worked at the Dun Prince Residence.[6] Three years later when Wang was promoted to chief officer (a third grade officer),[7] he had the chance to spend some time again with Fu Zhongquan. Realizing taijiquan's depth, Wang decided to follow Fu to Dongzhi Men, an area in Beijing where Yang Luchan was teaching. After encountering Yang, Wang asked to be accepted as disciple and later offered Yang a teaching position at the Dun Prince Residence.

Yang oversaw training the guards, who were mainly of Manchu heritage and already quite skilled in martial arts. The most famous of this group were the three comrades Wu Quanyou (1834–1902),[8] Ling Shan, and Wan Chun. All later studied under Yang Banhou (1837–1892, second son of Yang Luchan), and are therefore referred as third generation students in most Yang family writings. Contrary to common knowledge, Yang Luchan accepted a few disciples most of whom were only vaguely mentioned in later Yang literature, which focused mainly on his direct family successors. Some of these earlier students were completely written out of the Yang lineage by the second generation upon failing to accept the tutelage of Yang Banhou after Yang Luchan's death.

Wang Lanting's original name was Yongtai. He remained under Yang Luchan's tutelage for seven years, until Yang's death. This may sound odd to the general reader who believes Yang Luchan died in 1872. A brief explanation is necessary to put this information into perspective.

According to written and oral sources that Wang Lanting passed on to his disciple Li Ruidong (1851–1917), Yang Luchan died in Beijing between 1875 and 1880. Yang gave Wang a complete set of literature, which included classics (*jingpu*) from Yang Luchan's teacher Chen Changxing, manuals (*zongpu*), secret instructions (*koujue*), "heart transmissions" (*xinfa*), and various notes. Wang Lanting's manual preface dated 1874 specifies that Wang "was accepted as a disciple in the seventh year of the Tongzhi Era (1868) … and studied for seven years," not mentioning the death of Yang, thus confirming he was still alive when the preface was written. Later, Li Ruidong corroborates this assumption in his preface adding that "the old Master [Yang Luchan] died at the beginning of the Guangxu Era [starting 1875] …

[A]t the beginning of the Guangxu Era, I received the true transmission of taijiquan from my senior [*shixiong*] Wang Lanting . . .." This preface notes that, on behalf of Yang who had just died, Wang Lanting passed his knowledge to Li Ruidong. Since Wang and Li first met at the Li's residence in the fourth month of the sixth year of the Guangxu Era (1880), we are left with the first six years of Guangxu (1875 to 1880).

These manuals were then passed down to Li Ruidong, who added his insights along with manuals from his other teachers. The body of his transmission was originally called the Li Style martial system. It was later renamed Wuqing Taijiquan in respect of Master Li's birthplace and because of his emphasis on taiji. In the last 20 years or so, his descendants have started to refer to the school as Li Taijiquan to standardize its name with the common custom of naming family styles with the family name.

Great Master Li Ruidong

Li Ruidong (aka, Li Shuxun) was born in 1851 in Wuqing Prefecture (Tianjin) to a very rich and influential family. His father, Li Xiaoji, was a famous doctor and owned a medicine business. Their mansion had over eighty guestrooms, which people of skills in various arts visited all year round. The young Li Ruidong was attracted to martial arts since childhood, and his father, having seen his inclinations, arranged for various masters to teach his son and personally taught him traditional Chinese medicine.

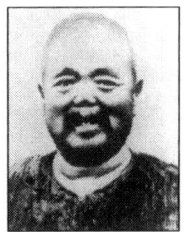 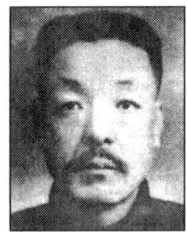

Left: Li Ruidong (b. 1851), founder of Li Style Taijiquan.
Right: Li Jiying, third son of Li Ruidong.

In 1880, the chief of the Dun Prince Palace guards, Wang Lanting, was passing by Wuqing and briefly visited his acquaintance, Li Xiaoji. The first night during dinner, Li Ruidong started to ask Wang about his favorite subject, martial arts. Lanting explained that he used to study Twelve Continuous Fists (*Shier Lianquan*, a branch of xinyiquan) but that he had switched to taijiquan after meeting Master Yang Luchan and had been learning from Dong Haichuan (1804–1880, founder of baguazhang) after his teacher passed away. Li Ruidong asked to continue the discussion in the library, were the two moved to drink some tea.

Having heard of the Yang family, Li asked Wang if he knew of Yang Banhou. Lanting replied, "He is not a stranger, of course. He is my junior classmate and son of my late teacher." In hearing this, Li got excited and asked if he could test his skills against Master Wang. With each of three attacks, Li Ruidong was sent to the floor. Impressed with such martial ability, Li immediately asked to be accepted as a disciple. Wang replied that, given his relationship with Li's father, he considered Li a junior of the same generation and was going to teach him on behalf of Master Yang. Wang Lanting proposed Li follow him to the capital, where he was first offered the position of officer of Garden Management (a fifth-grade officer), which was mainly a seasonal job where he could have plenty of time to practice with Wang.

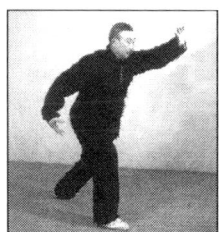 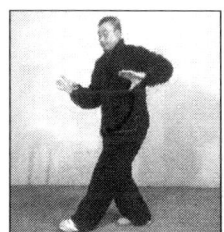

Zhang Wansheng, third generation Li Style master.

Early Curriculum and Learning Progression

In the preface by Li Ruidong dated 1881 of the family taijiquan manual, he recounts this learning progression:

> I first studied 13 postures, then I learned the 64 forms, and I was given a manual that was a must read for beginners. . . .. I studied eight positions, five steps, and eight techniques, all at the various levels of solo practice, partner practice, solo stepping, partner stepping, solo exercise, partner exercise, solo killing, partner killing. . . .

We can see here the original progression of study passed down to Li Ruidong. Later in the manual, the complete list of movements and description of those forms are recorded. Li was not a beginner, but we can establish from the same source that the above material was transmitted over three years. The 64 sequence is also referred to as the "Henan 64 Form," and it was possibly developed in Henan by the Chen family on the foundation of the earlier 13 postures, although its description and appearance do not entirely fit into modern Chen Style.

This material has been handed down from Yang Luchan to Wang Lanting, from Wang to Li, and is still part of Li curriculum. It is important to note the approach to training even more than the curriculum itself. Every movement is studied and performed alone many times. After many repetitions, the movement is held in a standing practice before going on with a new set. As for all other exercises, the progression for practice is from beginner practice to solo practice to partner practice.

Li Ruidong explains in his "Four Important Points of Solo Practice":

> Danlian is solo practice. While practicing alone, we do not have to strive [to subdue an opponent] but only try to get familiar [with the exercise]. We can choose one or two exercises and practice them—this is called learning appearance. We can take three or five exercises and perform them without rest—this is called learning breath. We can take a few simple moves and practice them at will—this is called learning the law. Or we can practice as per our imagination—this is called learning the secret wisdom. Taken together, these are the Four Important Points of Solo Practice....
>
> The law creates the appearance, the appearance moves the breath, borrowing the breath gives birth to the secret wisdom, acting the secret wisdom leads to the law....
>
> Without practicing the appearance, the appearance is not firm. Without practicing the breath, the breath is not smooth. Without practicing the secret wisdom, the secret wisdom is not active. Without practicing the law, the law does not break through. There is a progression and if one does not understand the law and wastes his time practicing the appearance, the appearance is not true. Trying to practice the secret wisdom without practicing the breath, the secret wisdom is not alive. Trying to practice the law without practicing the secret wisdom, the law is not round....

It was therefore the "eight doors" with the "five steps" that formed the curriculum's foundation. They were practiced first according to the beginner procedure (*chulian*), learning one movement at a time and holding it in the stillness of standing meditation and following the solo practice sequence. Only later were they linked to form the 13 postures and the 64 forms. The eight forms, with the foundation of five steps, then generate the eight techniques/ energies (*peng, lu, ji, an, cai, lie, zhou, kao*) that were performed at that time in both large and small frames.

After having progressed in solo practice, there was an intermediary phase in which the student receives from the teacher the oral explanations of the "five secrets" along with the practical "adjustment of hands and eyes." This is extremely important, but not easily covered within a few words and would be better addressed in a future writing.

The next step was partner practice, the door to practical employment of one's skill to combat. Li Ruidong passed down a "Three Important Points on Partner Practice":

> *Shuanglian* means practicing with a partner. When practicing with a partner, one should not follow a preset form, doing a preset form

becomes a dead system. Those who practice this way abandon their hearts and rush with their spirit, hands and feet execute false movements. They bend, but do not reach out, just like a theater performance showing an empty form, like a story without heart—only a nice-looking picture for the pleasure of those watching. Practicing like this for long does not only lead to no accomplishment, but it is also dangerous. If one wants to get benefit from partner practice, it is essential to receive constant instructions from a skilled teacher.

With a practice companion, one carries an attack, and one defends to train the distance and investigate each other's movement, thus understanding the principles of change. These are the two first important points. Then each partner chooses his favorite techniques and apply them full force in order to learn the importance of applications.

Taken altogether, these are the Three Important Points. Basically, within this framework of training, the introduction to actual fighting was a period of attack/response in which the apprentice was supposed to learn timing, distance, and the principles of change behind each movement. Once these points were understood, it was basically free fighting, where the students were expected to test their embodiment of the principles of the eight gates (*bamen*) and five steps (*wubu*) and react accordingly.

The reader may have noticed that no mention of "push-hands" was made. I believe push-hands was especially popular among descendants of Yang Luchan as a useful tool for friendly reciprocal test of skills when true fighting was not necessary. However, push-hands has gained much significance and broader acceptance since it was introduced, although seldom practiced, by the 2nd and 3rd generations of the Li family. They practice this mainly to meet the expectations of outsiders who are looking at a polite reciprocal test of skills. Most teachers in this lineage are quick to remind students that friendly and methodic exchanges like those in push hands easily get the practitioner to fall into a "dead system" that Li Ruidong warned about.

Li Ruidong had few equals during his time. His curriculum was immense, including training regimens he inherited from some of the most gifted martial artists at the turn of the century, which we will investigate later.

Useful Definitions
- **13 postures:** referred to as the early taijiquan routine based on the combination of the 8 doors and the 5 steps.
- **8 doors (*bamen*):** sometimes referred as the 8 techniques (see below).
- **8 techniques:** 8 expressions of fundamental taijiquan energies/movements—ward off (*peng*), rollback (*lu*), press (*ji*), push (*an*), pluck (*cai*), split (*lie*), elbow

(*zhou*), and bump (*kao*).
- **8 forms (*bashi*)**: set of exercises based on the 8 doors.
- **5 steps (*wubu*)**: 5 main spatial directions giving form to taijiquan footwork.
- **64 forms**: enlarged version of the earlier 13 postures, possibly created at the Chen Village and passed down to Yang Luchan.
- **Large and small frames**: the two main approaches to practice, in particular referring to their relative external appearance, being compact or expanded.

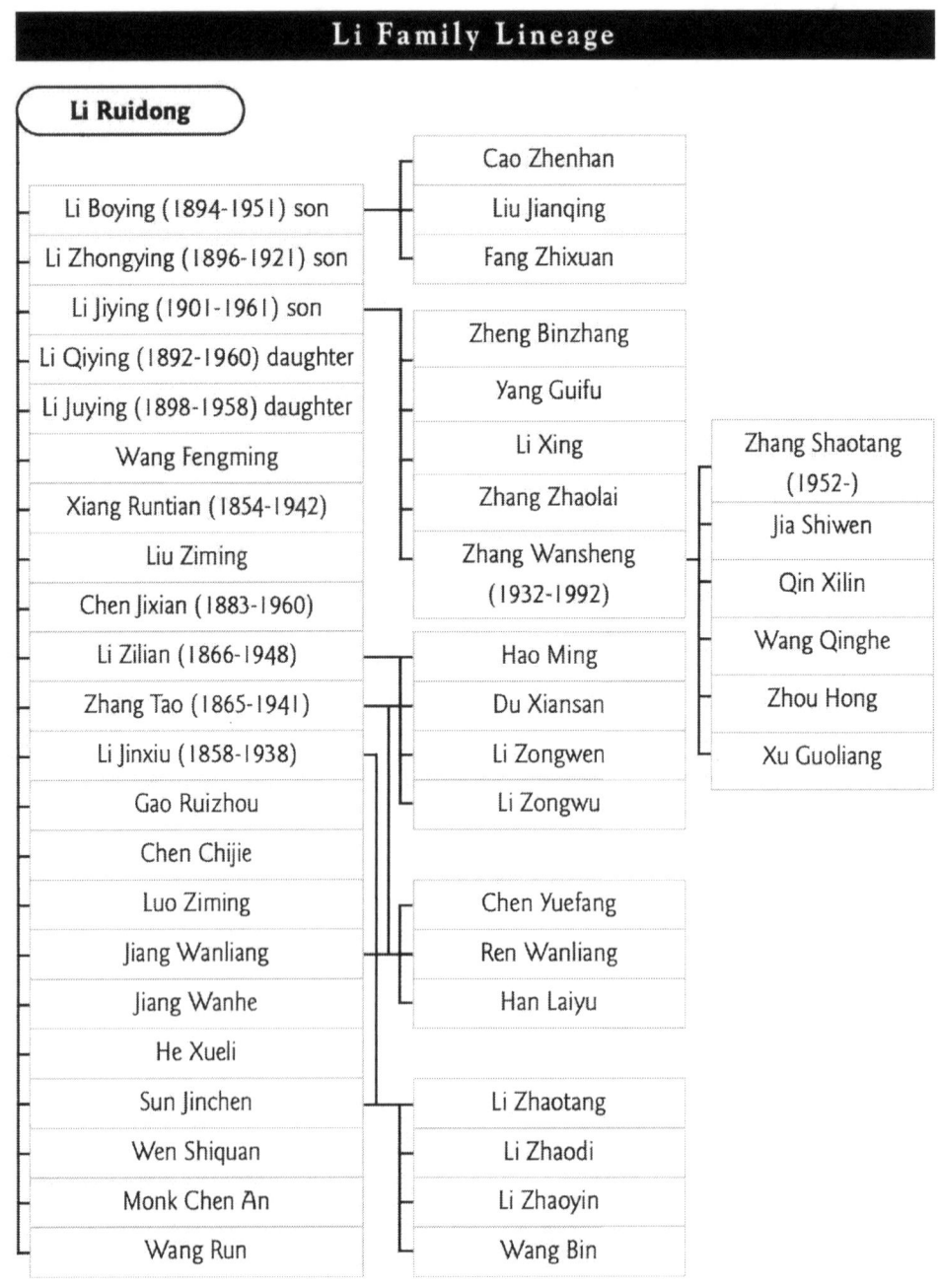

Glossary

Ba dashi	八大勢	Shidi	師弟
Ba xiaoshi	八小勢	Shier lianquan	十二連拳
Bafa	八法	Shijing	試勁
Baobiao	保標	Shixiong	師兄
Bashi	八勢	Shuangcao	雙操
Chenjiakou	陳家溝	Shuanglian	雙練
Chulian	初練	Shuanglian sanyao	雙練三要
Dancao	單操	Shuangsha	雙殺
Danlian	單練	Shuangxing	雙行
Danlian siyao	單練四要	Sifa	死法
Dansha	單殺	Taiji shisan shi	太極十三勢
Danxing	單行	Tianjin	天津
Dong Haichuan	董海川	Tongzhi (era)	同治
Dongzhi Men	東直門	Tuishou	推手
Fu Zhongquan	富仲權	Wan Chun	萬春
Guangxu (era)	光緒	Wang Lanting (Yongtai)	王蘭亭 (永泰)
Henan style 64 form	河北六十四勢	Wu Ruqing	武汝清
Ji	機	Wu Tunan	吳圖南
Jingpu	經譜	Wu Yuxiang	武禹襄
Koujue	口訣	Wubu	五步
Li	理	Wujing	武清
Li Ruidong (Shuxun)	李瑞東 (樹勛)	Wujue	五決
Li Xiaoqi	李小歧	Xiang Shan	香山
Ling Shan	凌善 (山)	Xinfa	心法
Lipai Quanfa	李派拳法	Xinyiquan	心意拳
Prince Duan	端王	Yang Banhou	楊班侯
Prince Dun	惇王	Yang Luchan	楊露蟬
Prince Zaiyi	載漪	Yongnian	永年
Qi	氣	Zhang Fengqi	張鳳岐
Quanpu	拳譜	Zhanzhuang	站樁
Quanyou (Wu)	全佑	Zongpu	宗譜
Shi	勢		

Notes

1. Elder brother of the more famous Wu Yuxiang, who was an early disciple of Yang Luchan in their hometown of Yongnian and whose descendants later originated the Wu/Hao Style.
2. Famous taijiquan teacher and scholar, disciple of Wu Jianquan (1870–1941).
3. Prince Zaiyi was the birth name of Prince Duan.
4. When Yang Luchan got to the prince's residence in 1868, Zaiyi was only thirteen. Zaiyi got married in 1885 and was ennobled as Prince Duan in 1889.
5. It is very probable that Fu Zhongquan was none other than Fu Zhou, whose descendants teach mainly in Baoding what they call "Inside the Palace Taijiquan" (Funei Pai Taijiquan).
6. Fifth son of the Daoguan Emperor (r. 1821–1850) and father of Prince Duan.
7. Officers were divided into nine grades with additional subcategories to create the so-called "Nine Grades, Eighteen Levels."
8. His son Wu Jianquan then used the surname Wu to create the name Wu Style Taijiquan.
9. In traditional Chinese society, family bonds and roles are quite strict. The same applies to martial arts families, two students from the same generation would refer to themselves as to "elder brother" and "younger brother." In certain schools, this refers to the amount of time in practice as opposed to actual age.

Bibliography

Li Family. (1874). Taijiquan family manual. Unpublished manuscript. Wang Lanting's preface dated 1874. Li Ruidong's preface dated 1881.

Ma, Y.Q. (Ed.). (1984). *Research on Taijiquan*. Hong Kong: Commercial Press.

Overlapping Steps:
Traditional Training Methods in Chen Village Taijiquan
by David Gaffney, B.A.

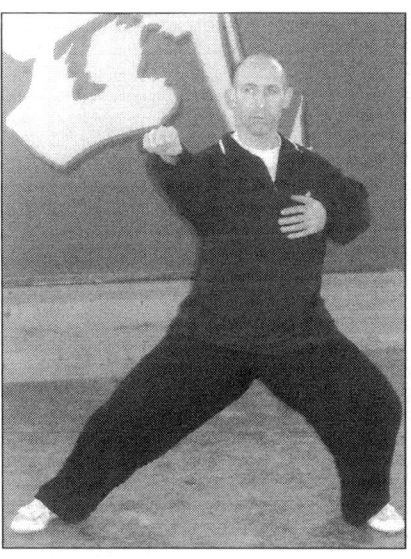

The author performing a Chen Style taijiquan movement called hidden fist. All photographs courtesy of David Gaffney.

Introduction

Though many people can quote the requirements of taijiquan and verses from the taijiquan classics, real understanding can only come through training. According to Chen Fake, the style's 17th-generation standard-bearer, those learning taijiquan must not only appreciate the theories intellectually, they must also train the methods into their body. Theoretical knowledge should be accompanied by practical action: "How much you accomplish depends entirely on how much effort you put in" (Ma Hong, 1988: 13). In his *Illustrated Explanation of Chen Family Taijiquan* (1986), Chen Xin goes further, suggesting that "all that idle talk does is to create a tide of black ink; actually putting it into practice is the real thing" (Gaffney and Sim, 2000: 94).

Chen taijiquan requires the body to be used in a unique, disciplined way and has a wide-ranging training curriculum encompassing standing exercises, single-movement exercises, bare-hand forms, push-hands, weapons, and supplementary equipment training. In common with other sports or martial arts, it is essential to begin with the basics. With time and conscientious practice, the body is strengthened, and one discovers a new way of moving. Each of the different training methods should be viewed within the framework of a larger system. Each facet of training, from the standing exercises to advanced push-hands drills, is interconnected and necessary. Considered in its entirety, the training process can be likened to a series of overlapping steps, each laid upon the underpinning foundation of the preceding one.

In Chenjiagou, it is commonly stated that all practice must be done "according to the principles" (Gu and Shen, 1998: 306). The principles start with the fundamental requirements and progress incrementally to the highest skill levels. Developing correct habits is a gradual process and the key to traditional training is to have patience en route to acquiring competence.

In the West, people often think of taijiquan as an easy option. Chenjia Villagers, however, have long understood that learning taijiquan is often painstaking and arduous. The Chen taijiquan student begins by seeking to understand and manage essential body requirements and execute basic body movements. Training is focused upon developing sufficient internal as well as external strength to carry out these actions rather than being impatient for the more complex techniques.

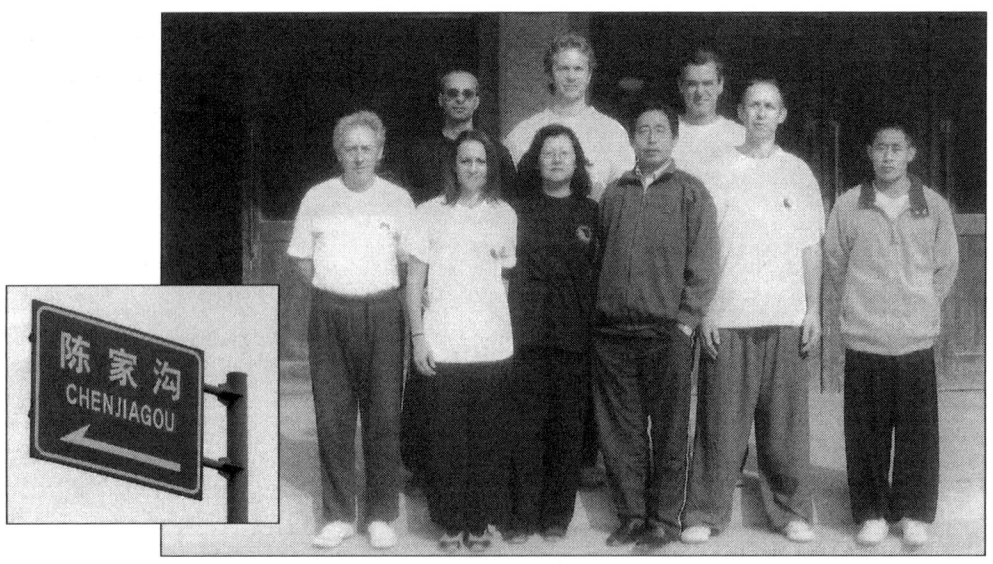

Left: Street sign showing the way to Chen Village. Right: November 2004 Intensive Training Camp organized by Chen Taiji Great Britain. Back row, left to right: Yaniv Morada (Israel), Neill Baker (UK), Fabrizio Cuminetti (Italy). Front: Riger Twigg (UK), Gabrilla Morgado (Portugal), Davidine Siaw-Voon Sim (UK), Chen Xiaoxing, David Gaffney (UK), and Chen Zhiqiang.

Standing Pole — Entering the Door

Chen Xin's *Illustrated Explanation of Chen Family Taijiquan* (1986) suggests that: "To train taiji, one must begin at *wuji*" (quiet, nothingness). This provides the guideline for entering the door of Chen taijiquan's traditional training curriculum. Standing pole (*zhanzhuang*) is the most basic taijiquan exercise and is common to many Chinese martial arts. Typically, the arms are held in front of the body as if holding a large ball as the practitioner stands and quietly observes the natural ebb and flow of the breath. The standing pole exercise, however, can be practiced using any of the end postures from the taiji form. During "standing practice, a static posture is maintained for a period, with emphasis upon developing awareness of and maintaining the most efficient and relaxed structural alignment necessary to hold the position.

To the casual observer, it may appear as if little is happening. The experienced practitioner, though, is intensely engaged in a variety of actions and sensations. Prolonged practice of this ostensibly uncomplicated exercise, along with enhancing postural awareness and calmness of mind, significantly increases leg strength. When the legs are strong and can bear weight securely, then the upper body can relax and sink down into them, making the top more flexible. If the legs do not have sufficient strength, the top is "afraid" to sink down, and the body remains top heavy and tense. All Chen taijiquan training methods look to develop extreme lightness and sensitivity in the upper body. Simultaneously, the lower body should exhibit a feeling of extreme heaviness and connection to the ground. At this stage, the practitioner can be said to be putting down roots. The importance of this is reflected in the verse "Cultivate the roots and the branches and leaves will be abundant" (Gaffney and Sim, 2000: 132).

Taijiquan is an internal martial art, entailing internal energy (*nei jing*) training in addition to external physical training. The power and strength of internal energy are manifested in external actions. To train internal skills, one must first train the body's intrinsic energy (*qi*). This includes cultivation, storage, and circulation of qi. Standing pole practice provides a means of increasing internal feeling and qi circulation. Regular standing for extended periods gives rise to acute body awareness as the practitioner learns to relax and sink their qi. By reducing the level of external stimulation, one can focus more closely upon sensations within the body. While the external body is still, internally the breath, blood, and qi are circulating. This represents a state of balance, or "motion in stillness."

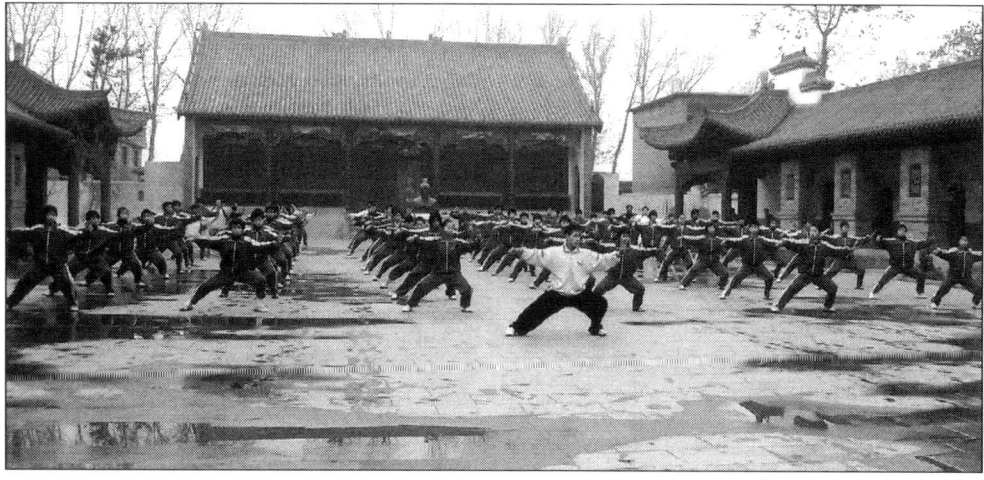

A demonstration by members of the Chen Village Taijiquan School
in the memorial ground of Chen Wangting.

Through prolonged training, qi becomes fuller and stronger, filling the energy center in the lower abdomen (*dantian*), breaking through blockages in the energy paths (*jingluo*), and then saturating the whole body. The body is like an inflated ball, full of elasticity and overflowing with a physical sensation of inward to outward expansion and strength (*peng jing*). With Chen taijiquan's spiraling silk reeling movement, this energy can be circulated throughout the body.

The standing pole training requirements are carried over to the taiji form: head erect, shoulders relaxed, elbows sunk down, chest relaxed, hips sunk, knees bent, etc. To correctly follow these basic and seemingly simple principles requires deep concentration. As one develops competence in the different aspects during standing, the feelings and sensations that arise can be transferred to the taiji form and push-hands.

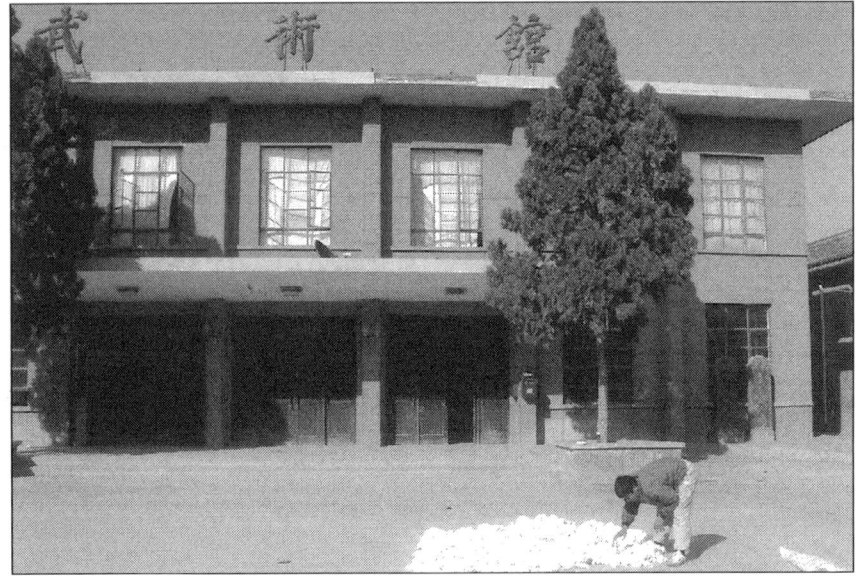

Above: The Chen Village Taijiquan School. Below, left: Statue of Chen Changxing.
Below right: Practicing the old frame first routine, golden rooster standing on one leg.

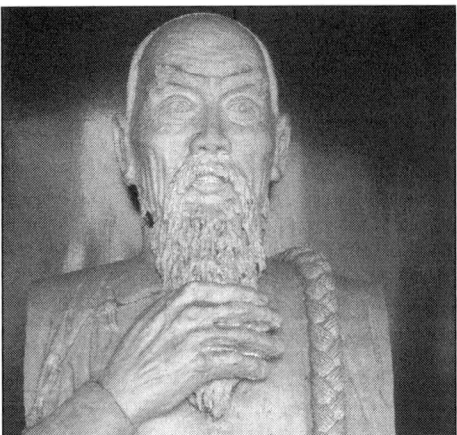
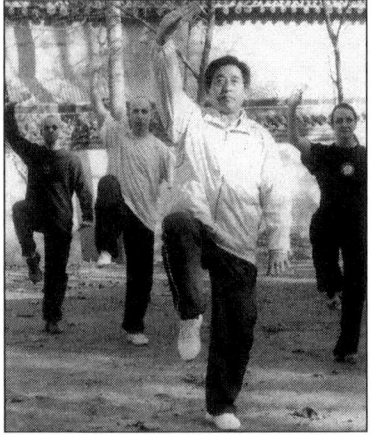

Empty-Hand Forms: The Foundation of Chen Taijiquan Skills

Form training has long provided the foundation of Chen taijiquan's step-by-step training method. Chen Wangting's original art was comprised of five empty-hand boxing routines that were passed down the next five generations. Chen Changxing (1771–1853), the 14th-generation standard bearer, refined the five routines into the two routines practiced today. These are the first routine (*yilu*) and the second routine (*erlu*, also known as the *paochui* or cannon fist form).

It has been suggested that some of Chen Wangting's unique art was lost. Chen Xiaoxing, principal of the Chenjiagou Taijiquan School, refutes this: "The synthesis of the five routines was not a matter of losing the old forms but of putting the five together, absorbing the essence of each. The first routine and the cannon fist contain the same essence as the original routines, preserving many of the movements and all the movement principles" (Chen Xiaoxing, 2004). Today, Chen Style taijiquan empty-hand forms consist of two main versions (frames): old and new (*laojia* and *xinjia*, respectively). The old frame has been handed down relatively unchanged since Chen Changxing's time, while 17th-generation master Chen Fake developed the new frame. The new frame incorporates more obvious silk reeling movement, more power releasing actions, and greater emphasis on joint-locking (*qinna*) techniques. Each consists of a first routine and cannon fist. Where the first routine is characterized by slow, soft movements, the second is predominantly fast and powerful.

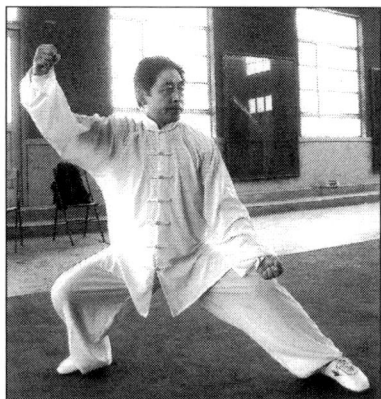

Chen Xiaoxing at practice—certain optimum patterns of movement must be established and these can only become set if they are repeated almost endlessly.

It is important to understand form training within the context of a larger system. Nowadays, people often equate knowing many forms with martial expertise. Adam Hsu (1998: 93) cautions that we should not confuse quantity with quality arguing: "Students who spend their time learning multitudes of forms are wasting their time. This kind of practice, void of a true foundation, is no more than folk dance" because "each form has its own purpose, and each form is one step in a clear progression of training."

In the beginning, the student should seek to standardize movement as far as possible in accordance with Chen taijiquan's basic requirements for each part of the body. Each of the requirements has practical implications for maintaining good health, for maximizing movement efficiency, for qi circulation, and for heightening martial effectiveness.

Primary emphasis is placed upon understanding the underlying movement principles and then progressing to standardized movement. Once this is accomplished, the next goal is to search for further realization of the internal circulation of energy. When you first come to the fixed postures, for example, lazily tying coat or single whip, in your mind you must very stringently adjust yourself according to the requirements for each part of the body. Everyone knows the requirements as they have been widely written about, it is the degree that is hard to realize. For instance, all experienced taijiquan practitioners are familiar with the requirement to "store the chest" (*han xiong*), but how do you store? If you store too much, the waist collapses, but what is too much? It is not like carpentry where someone just gives you the measurements and you can do it accordingly.

> Only through persistent practice and strict adherence to correct principles can one achieve a stage where one is able to produce just the right amount of *jing* [internal force], change at will, and rotate with ease. One must train hard in form practice so that the body becomes one single unit, which enables one movement activating all movements.
> – Chen Xiaowang, 1990: 29

In this context, we can understand the logic behind Chen taijiquan's traditional emphasis upon the first routine as the foundation form. The form's slower nature permits the practitioner to pay attention to details, to make certain that postures are precise, to test stability and balance during movement, to enhance lower body strength, and to become conscious of the circulation of qi throughout the body.

Herman Kauz (1989: 80) succinctly sums up the benefits of this intense attention to detail during form practice:

> Individual training of this nature enables the student to grow accustomed to the body mechanics involved in the performance of his techniques. He is not distracted by an opponent's shifting about evasively or attempting to counterattack. He has time in which to work on problems concerned with correct foot placement, body position or pulling direction. In an actual match, the opportunity to perform a throw appears only briefly, allowing insufficient time to give attention to the many factors involved. Certain optimum patterns of movement must be established, and these can only become set if they are repeated almost endlessly.

As the practitioner's skill increases, they may begin training in the cannon fist routine to develop the explosive release of strength (*bao fali*) as well as their endurance and stamina (*nai li*). Taijiquan is built upon the model of hardness and softness complementing and alternating with each other. Consequently, the two forms represent a complete balanced system of hardness and softness. The cannon fist routine is physically very demanding with many instances of energy release (*fajing*), fast movements, sweeps, elbow and shoulder techniques, and sudden changes of attack and defense. Where the first routine provides the means of developing internal energy, the second is said to consolidate and express this energy (Chen Xiaoxing, 2004).

Push-Hands: To Know One's Opponent
Chen Wangting created the two-person training drill called push-hands, the objective of which is to attain sensitivity to the movement and intention of an adversary while masking one's own intention and energy. Attaining this heightened level of sensitivity has long been the goal of Chen Taiji exponents. In the "Song of the Canon of Boxing," Chen Wangting states that one should seek to accomplish a level of ability where: "Nobody knows me, while I know everybody" (Chen Zhenglei, 1992, Vol. 3: 1).

Harmonizing with an opponent's movements, the practitioner works toward eliminating all tension and resistance within his own responses. In contrast to most external martial arts, the intention is not just to block an incoming force with greater force, but to "listen" to and "borrow" the opponent's energy to defend oneself.

This listening skill is not solely dependent upon the sense of touch but of whole-body awareness. Many people make the mistake of turning their heads to one side or closing their eyes while pushing hands. In fact, there must be a combination and coordination of sight, hearing, and touch; and one is not exclusive of the others.

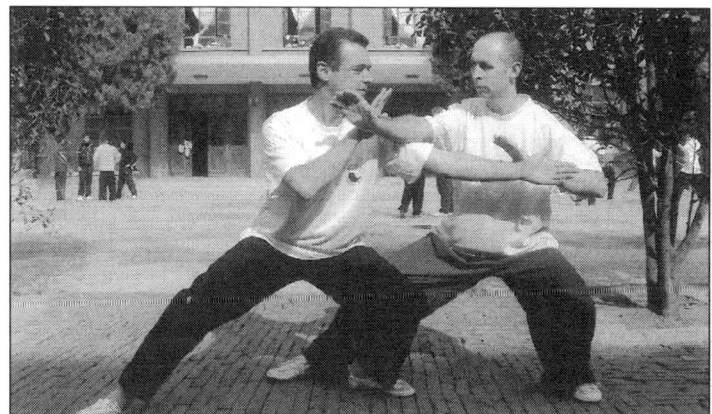

Fabrizio Cuminetti (left) and David Gaffney pushing hands —
single forward and back step.

According to Chen Xiaowang (1990: 29), push hands and form practice are inseparable:

> Whatever shortcomings one has in the form will certainly show up as weaknesses during push hands, giving an opponent the opportunity to take advantage. To this end, one needs to practice push hands; check on the forms; understand the internal force (*jing*); and learn how to express the force (*fajing*) as well as how to neutralize the force (*hua ing*). If one can withstand confrontational push hands, then it is an indication that one has understood the underlying taiji principles. Continuous training will lead to increased confidence. At this point one can step up one's training and bring in supplementary training such as shaking the long pole; practicing with weapons such as the sabre, spear, sword, and staff; and doing single-posture training such as fajing.

Understanding the trained energies of the body (*jing*) lies at the heart of push-hands practice. Fundamental to achieving this is a careful study of taijiquan's eight methods or *bafa*. From these eight methods or energies all skills and techniques are generated. The eight energies comprise four frontal methods (*si zheng*), which are quite familiar to most taiji practitioners: warding (*peng*); diverting (*lu*); squeezing (*ji*) and pressing down (*an*).

The next four skills, also known as the four diagonal methods (*si yu*), are less familiar: plucking (*cai*), splitting (*lie*), elbowing (*zhou*), and bumping (*kao*). Mastering these four is important if one is to acquire a true understanding of the throwing and striking that Chen taijiquan is famous for. Unlike the first four methods, *cai, lie, zhou*, and *kao* are typically instilled when the student begins practicing at higher speeds and with more force (Berwick, 2000: 191–2).

Taiji push-hands is built upon the foundation of forms practice. At this stage, the practitioner should have a good understanding of how to use their body in accordance with taijiquan's strict movement principles. Training centers on the interchange of energies between the two participants. For example, when a partner uses press down, you ward off. When he uses squeeze in, you divert away. Chen Changxing stressed the importance of painstakingly studying the different energy methods in his "Song of Pushing Hands": "Be conscientious about *peng, lu, ji*, and *an*. Following each other above and below, difficult for people to enter" (Zhu, 1994: 281).

For generations, Chen taiji boxers have sought to fulfill the push-hands principles of "connecting, joining, sticking, and following," "neither letting go nor resisting" (Wang, 1998: 10). Push-hands allows the practitioner to put to the test the body postures trained in the forms. Correct body alignment enables one to control others and yet prevent them from entering one's boundary.

Chen Style taijiquan traditionally uses five methods of push-hands:

- *Wuan hua*: fixed step, single- and double-handed exercises
- *Ding bu*: fixed step, double-handed
- *Huang bu* (*jin yi tui yi*): single backward/forward step, double-handed
- *Da lu*: moving step, low stance, double-handed
- *Luang cai hua*: free steps, double-handed

Beyond these is the practice of free pushing or *san tui*.

Lafcadio Hearn (1850–1904), former chair of English literature at the Imperial University of Tokyo, eloquently expressed his fascination of the Asian martial arts ideal of using sensitivity to overcome superior strength. Although he had probably never seen taiji push hands, his description of the approach to training he saw in late 18th-century Japan could have been written with it in mind:

> What Western brain could have elaborated this strange teaching— never to oppose force to force, but only to direct and utilize the power of attack; to overthrow the enemy solely by his own effort? Surely none! The occidental mind appears to work in straight lines; the oriental in wonderful curves and circles. Yet how fine a symbolism of intelligence as a means to foil brute force! – Hearn, 1989: 57–58

Single-Posture Training

For generations, Chen taijiquan practitioners in Chenjiagou have followed an integrated system designed to increase martial ability. The process involves form, push-hands and single-posture training and each has its unique part to play. While trained separately, the three are closely interconnected: "push-hands is the means by which the accuracy of the form can be tested; form training is the foundation upon which effective push-hands skills are built; single-posture training is the means by which martial skill is brought out" (Gaffney and Sim, 2000: 136).

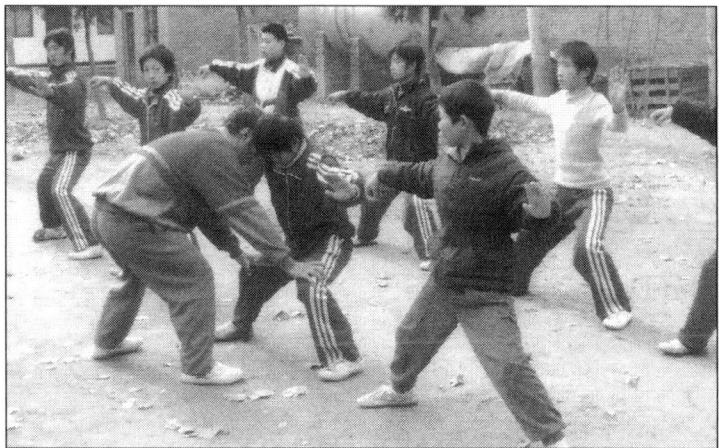

"Fixing the frame" — a young coach making sure that students' postures are precise.

Chen Zhaokui outlined some of the reasons single-posture practice must be included alongside the more widely seen form and push-hands training:

> Some applications of the movement cannot be used in push-hands. For example, elbow strikes, leg methods and also attacking vital points of an opponent, or qinna. Also, some very fast fajing movements in the form cannot be done successively, as it would be too exhausting.
> – Ma Hong, 1998: 21

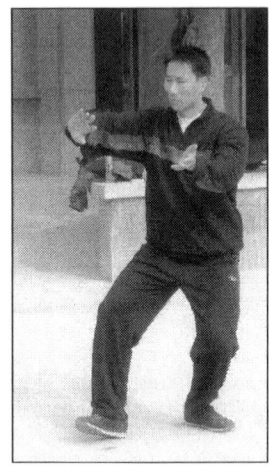
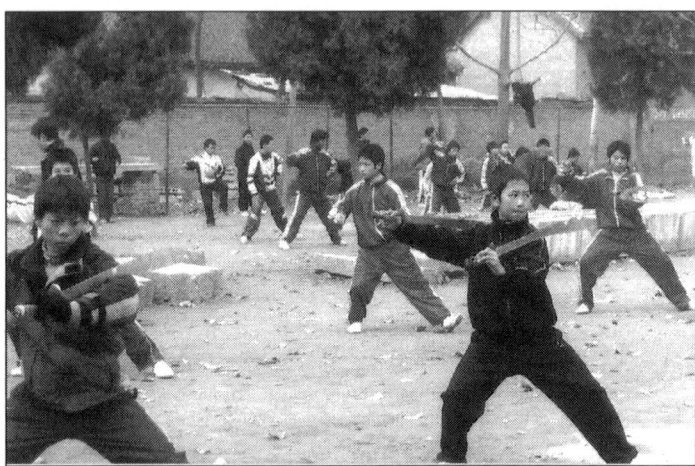

Training the empty hand form lays the foundation upon which all other skills are built. Children in the foreground practicing double saber. Many of the weapon forms have changed little since they were formulated, providing a window on taijiquan origins.

At first sight, single-posture training may seem tiresome and repetitive. Nonetheless, going over individual movements many times significantly increases the capacity to use them practically. Single-posture practice often focuses on building effective fajing ability. Even so, there should be no departure from taijiquan's core principles. Any movement where force is emitted must be characterized by looseness, pliability, and elasticity, rather than rigidity and stiffness. Just because a movement is fast and powerful, does not mean the practitioner should lose sight of the need to follow the silk reeling spiral path rather than straight-line movement (Ma Hong, 1998: 400).

Single-movement practice can be divided into several different groups, beginning with those actions performed while stationary. Examples in the old frame first routine include the stamping movement that concludes the Buddha's warrior attendant pounds mortar, the hidden thrust punch, and the green dragon Out of the Water. Other single movements embrace those that entail stepping, for instance, stepping forward using fajing while training the energy methods of taijiquan (e.g. *cai, lie, zhou, kao*), and retreating movements, as in the posture step back and whirl arms.

Short Weapons Training

Weapons training has always played an important part in the Chen curriculum. At the time of its creation, Chen taijiquan was practiced essentially to develop the Chenjiagou villagers' martial and military skills. Without a doubt, the training would have greatly enhanced the taiji boxers' health, but this was not the main reason for practicing the art. In Chen Wangting's day, guns had yet to appear, traditional weapons were still being carried onto the battlefield and used in combat.

Today, most people consider the weapon routines of the assorted Chinese martial arts only from the perspective of demonstrating or exercising in the park. Viewing the Chen weapon forms in this way shows a superficial appreciation of their fundamental nature. Preserved within each of the Chen weapons routines is a complex martial training manual. As well as the flexible sinuous movements, the forms include numerous dynamic actions; swift changes in tempo; and fierce chopping, slicing, or thrusting movements.

Viewed in the light of the whole system, weapons training adds to the empty-hand training by magnifying certain requirements. For instance, the mind and intention must be extended all the way through the weapon's length; movements must stay relaxed, agile, and efficient at the same time as one controls a weighted object; and footwork must be lively and responsive to permit rapid changes in the fighting sequence. Within the Chen training curriculum, numerous weapons are still practiced, including sword (*jian*), broadsword (*dao*), spear (*qiang*), halberd (*guandao*, often rendered *quandao* or *kwando*), pole, double sword, double broadsword, and double iron mace.

The sword is one of the oldest weapons in Chinese martial arts history. Archaeologists have uncovered swords from as far back as the Bronze Age. When the terracotta army was unearthed in the early Chinese capital Xi'an, a find dating back to the Qin dynasty more than two thousand years ago, the statues of officers were carrying swords (Tian and Zhen, 2004: 102).

The Chen taijiquan sword is generally light in weight, with a flexible blade. For the Chen taiji swordsman, success on the battlefield depended upon skill, precision, and speed. Chen taijiquan contains one single straight sword form consisting of forty-nine postures. In his book *Chen Family Taiji*, Chen Zhenglei (1997: 217) explains:

> The forty-nine postures can be sub-divided into thirteen basic techniques: thrusting downward (*zha*), level or upward thrust (*ci*), pointing by flicking the wrist (*dian*), chopping (*pi*), slicing levelly or obliquely upward (*mo*), sweeping (*sao*), neutralizing in a circular path (*hua*), circular deflection with point uppermost (*liao*), hanging (*gua*), pushing up (*tuo*), pushing (*tui*), intercepting (*jie*), and raising the opponent's weapon overhead (*jia*).

The sword's flexibility allows the proficient swordsman to inflict injury from a great range of angles utilizing many diverse techniques. Its great versatility has led to the saying that there is "no gap the sword cannot enter, and no gap that another can enter" (Chen Zhenglei, 1992, Vol. 1: 180).

The different weapons help to train the many diverse qualities essential in honing a "taijiquan physique." Practicing the Chen sword form allows an exponent to develop the ability to project energy in a relaxed manner to the sword tip. It also helps to create an efficient taiji body, with repeated practice loosening the large joints such as the hips and shoulders, as well as helping to increase the suppleness of the wrists and hands.

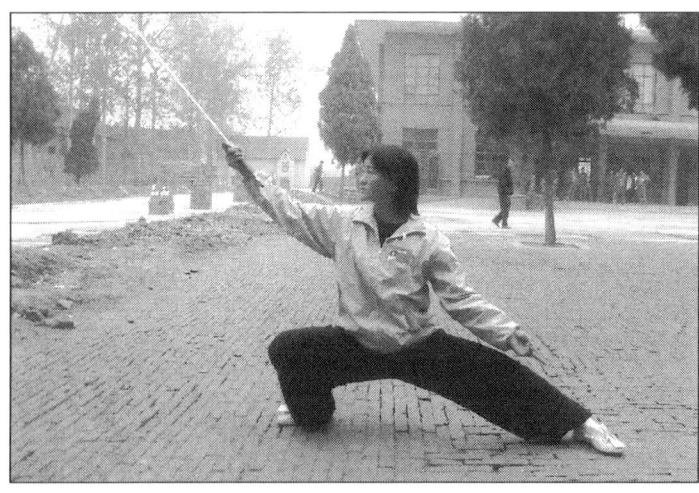

In Chen taijiquan, the sword used is generally light in weight, with a flexible blade.

Easily distinguishable from the sword, which is double edged and light, the broadsword is single edged and heavy. The broadsword's strength led to cutting movements that are large, expansive, and powerful. In appearance, using the broadsword is said to be "like splitting a mountain." In character, the broadsword is traditionally compared to a ferocious tiger, with each movement being more direct and easily understandable than the straight sword. This is reflected in the Chinese martial arts saying "*Dao*—like a fierce tiger; *jian*—like a swimming dragon" (Chen Zhenglei, 1997, Vol. 1: 217).

The Chen broadsword form is short and dynamic. Although classified as a short weapon, the broadsword can cover a surprisingly long distance by utilizing explosive leaping and jumping movements. Movements can be performed in different ways depending upon the ultimate objective of practice. Often the routine is executed with long, low stances as a way of conditioning the body, increasing one's power and speed.

As a means of overall body training, the explosive leaping and jumping movements have much in common with modern plyometric exercises used by many of today's elite sports performers. Simply put, the combination of speed and strength is power. For many years, coaches and athletes have sought to improve power to enhance performance. Throughout the last century and no doubt long before, jumping, bounding, and hopping exercises have been used in various ways to enhance athletic performance. In recent years, this distinct method of training for power or explosiveness has been termed plyometrics (Flach, 2005: 14). In Chenjiagou, taijiquan exponents have long understood this method of training to enhance the individual's explosive actions.

Using very low stances, however, prevents the dexterity and fleetness of footwork required in a real conflict. The taiji boxer focusing on training the applications within the broadsword routine would usually practice in a higher posture to enhance mobility. Consequently, to achieve both martial and conditioning benefits, Chenjiagou practitioners have traditionally trained over a range of heights.

Long Weapons

Chen taijiquan also has several weapons for long-range combat, including the halberd, long pole, and the "king of weapons" — the spear. An often-cited phrase—"one hundred days to practice broadsword, one thousand days to practice spear"—reflects the form's intricacy and difficulty level (Chen Zhenglei, 1992, Vol. 2: 52).

Also known as the "pear flower spear" and "white ape staff," the Chen taijiquan spear form includes the functions of both spear and staff. The routine dates to Chen Wangting, making it one of the earliest taiji forms. In his comprehensive review of taijiquan, *The Origin, Evolution, and Development of Shadow Boxing*, Gu Liuxin cites the evidence gathered by historian Tang Hao, who concluded that the texts of famous Ming dynasty (C.E. 1368–1644) General Qi Jiguang had a profound influence on Chen Wangting's creation of taijiquan. Qi's military training text documented the spear techniques of the Yang Family 24-movement spear form. The Yang family in question refers to a renowned Song Dynasty (C.E. 960–1279) (female warrior who used the form to avenge the slaying of her male relatives, so should not be confused with the Yang taijiquan family (Gu, 1996).

The Chen taiji spear form's earliest version followed the sequence of the Yang 24-movement form in both posture and name. Its uniqueness came because of the application of taiji movement principles to the existing method. In the ensuing years, the Chen spear form has increased from 24 to 72 movements, adding a variety of staff movements.

Watching a skilled exponent performing with the staff, its martial roots are immediately apparent. The overall tempo is forceful, direct and rapid, with few movements being done slowly. Although it is highly unlikely that anyone would need to use the spear for combat today, the Chen family spear form remains a highly practical training tool. Spear practice enhances empty-hand skills by improving balance with intricate and rapid-stepping movements as well as developing upper body strength and overall flexibility.

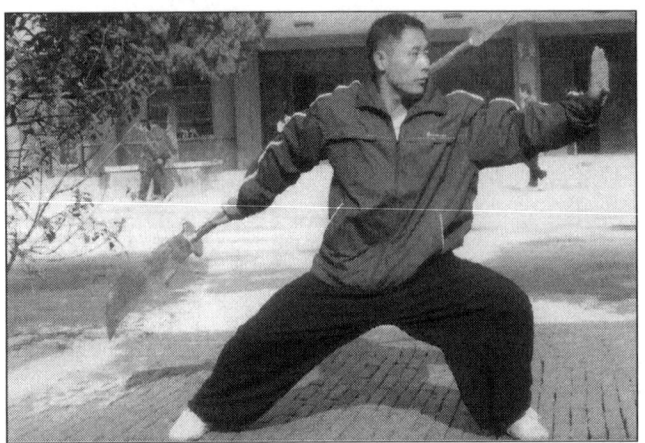

Training with the guandao: the favored weapon of Chen taijiquan creator Chen Wangting.

Variously known as the spring and autumn broadsword, the green dragon crescent moon broadsword, or simply the "big knife," the halberd (*ji*) is one of the system's oldest weapons forms. Characterized by strong and powerful movements, the halberd is a large and heavy weapon requiring a high degree of upper body strength and a stable root to manipulate it freely. The Chen taijiquan halberd trains the practitioner to move and be responsive in every direction. The favored weapon of Chen Wangting, it is recorded in the genealogy of the Chen Family (Chen Zhenglei, 1999: 4), that:

> Wangting, alias Zhouting, was a knight at the end of the Ming dynasty [C.E. 1368–1644] and a scholar in the early years of the Qing dynasty [C.E. 1644–1912]. He was known in Shandong Province as a martial arts master, once defeating more than a thousand bandits. He was the originator of the barehanded and armed combat boxing of the Chen school. He was a born warrior, as can be proved by the broadsword he used in combat.

While the individual names of the weapon or empty-hand forms describe the movements, the halberd form is unique. Each of its thirty movements is given a seven-character song or poem. When taken in their entirety, they recount the story of General Guan, a famous warrior from the turbulent Three Kingdoms Period (C.E. 25–220). Consequently, every time the form is practiced, his exploits are re-enacted (Gaffney and Sim, 2000: 188).

Contemporary practitioners should not overlook the importance of the weapons routines as they offer a tangible link to past generations.

The forms are at once practical and aesthetic. Artistically pleasing to watch, the weapons routines are physically complex and demanding to complete. Many of the weapon forms have changed little since the time of Chen Wangting. Consequently, they provide a window to the origins of taijiquan and represent an important legacy to today's taijiquan practitioner. – Gaffney and Sim, 2000: 172

Supplementary Equipment Training

Standing pole, forms practice, silk reeling exercises, push-hands, etc., all lead to an increase in internal strength. As the practitioner reaches a more accomplished level, the use of supplementary exercises with a variety of training equipment can further amplify this energy. Skills such as neutralizing, yielding, grappling (*qinna*), and fajing are more efficient when backed by greater physical strength.

Past masters placed great emphasis on supplementary power training methods (*xing gong*). In Chenjiagou, in the garden where Yang Luchan, the progenitor of Yang taijiquan, is said to have learned from Chen Changxing, there is still a stone weight weighing about eighty kilograms that the two are reputed to have trained with to increase their hand strength.

Also popular to this day is the exercise of shaking a long pole as a means of increasing the power that can be transmitted from the dantian out to the extremities. Cut from the baila tree, the pole is typically about four yards long and roughly an inch and a half in diameter. This type of wood is flexible and springy, allowing the practitioner to transmit force through it. It is said that Chen Fake performed three hundred repetitions of this exercise daily, as well as at least thirty repetitions of the empty-hand form.

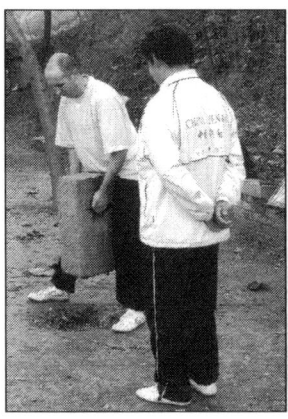 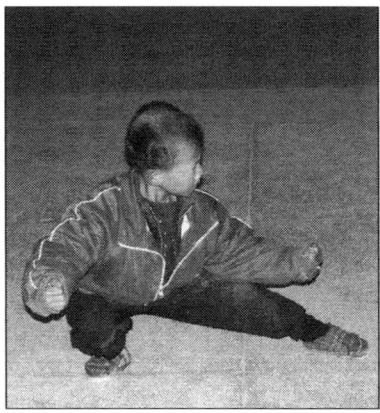

Left: Supplementary equipment training. Chen Xiaoxing watches the author lifting a stone weight to increase hand strength. Right: Training starts at a young age in Chenjiagou. A three-year-old child going through his form.

Conclusion

Chen Village taijiquan is a unique example of Chinese martial culture, providing a tangible link to past generations of taiji practitioners. Changed little through the passing generations, this art today draws increasing numbers of practitioners attracted by its characteristics of power, grace, and agility. To succeed, modern practitioners would be well advised to look to the appropriate method for their stage of development and not to be in a hurry to learn new things. Above all, practice must be patient, systematic, and persistent if advanced ability is to be attained. To quote an old Chinese proverb: "One day's chill does not result in three feet of ice" (Gaffney and Sim, 2000: 148).

Bibliography

Berwick, S. (2000). The five stages of Chen taiji combat training. In *Ultimate guide to Tai Chi: The best of Inside Kung Fu*. Chicago: McGraw-Hill/Contemporary Books.

Chen, X. (1990). *Chen Style Taijiquan transmitted through generations*. Beijing: People's Sports Publishing.

Chen, X. (2004). CTGB Interview, Nov. 2004 Chenjiagou Training Camp.

Chen, Z. (1992). *A compendium of taijiquan boxing and weapons (Volume 1)*. Beijing: Higher Education Press.

Chen, Z. (1992). *A compendium of taijiquan boxing and weapons (Volume 2)*. Beijing: Higher Education Press.

Chen, Z. (1992). *A compendium of taijiquan boxing and weapons (Volume 3)*. Beijing: Higher Education Press.

Chen, Z. (1999). *The art of Chen family taijiquan*. Shanxi: Technical Sports Publications.

Chen, Z. (1997). *Chen family taiji: Master's insights*. Xi'an: World Books.

Flach, A. (2005). The complete book of isometrics. Long Island City, NY: Hatherleigh Press.

Gu, L. (1996). The origin, evolution and development of shadow boxing. In *Chen Style Taijiquan* (Feng Zhiqiang and Feng Dabiao, Eds.). Beijing: People's Sports Publishing.

Gu, L. and Shen J. (1998). *Chen Style Taijiquan*. Beijing: People's Sports Publishing.

Hearn, L. (1989). *Jiujutsu. In Martial arts reader: Classic writings on philosophy and technique*. New York: Overlook Press.

Hsu, A. (1998). *The sword polisher's record: The way of kung-fu*. Boston: Tuttle Publishing.

Kauz, H. (1989). The aim of individual form practice. In *Martial arts reader: Classic writings on philosophy and technique*. New York: Overlook Press.

Ma, H. (1998). *Chen Style Taijiquan method and theory*. Beijing: Sports University Press.

Tian, Y. and Zhen, Q. (2004). *Wondrous wushu*. Guangxi: People's Publications.

Wang, X. (1998). *Push hands skills and methods*. Henan Sports Publications.

Zhu, T. (1994). *Authentic Chenjiagou taijiquan*. Percetaken Turbo Sdn. Bhd., Malaysia.

In Memory of Wu Daxin: Wu Family Taiji Boxing Gatekeeper
by Cai Naibiao; Translated by Y. L. Yip and Leroy Clark

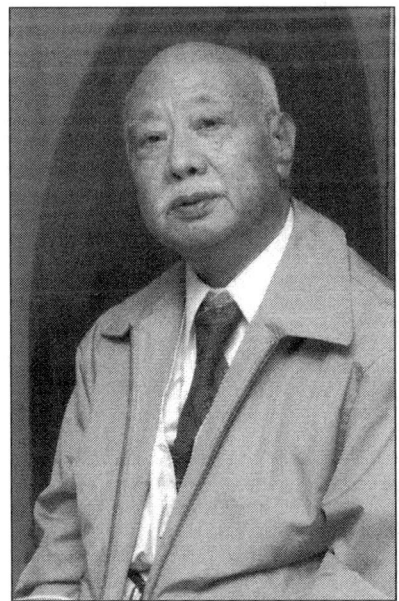
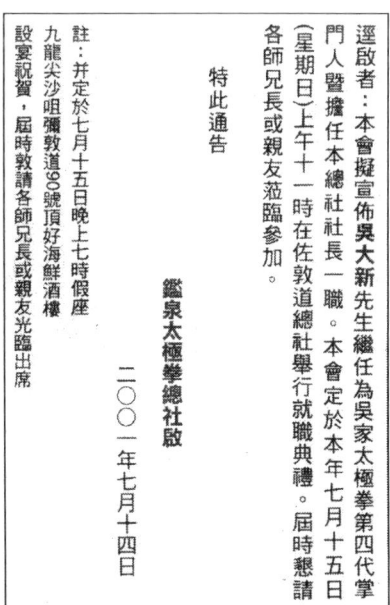

Wu Daxin on his birthday in 2005.
Newspaper advertisement dated July 14, 2001: an announcement stating that
Wu Daxin formally takes up post of gatekeeper of the Wu Style lineage.

On January 16, 2005, Wu Daxin (Wu Tai-sin; cant. Ng Dai Sun) passed away quietly at the Hong Kong Sanatorium Hospital. Wu was the latest in the bloodline of Wu Family Style taijiquan adepts, representing the 4th generation and selected as "gatekeeper" of the family boxing art. The gatekeeper is the main person who represents, guards, and monitors the family art. This person is selected and appointed by the previous gatekeeper, usually a blood relative. The person selected must have attained a respectable skill level, appropriate knowledge, and a suitable personality to represent the family system.

Wu Daxin was born in Mainland China on November 26th, 1933, only 22 years after the fall of the Qing Dynasty (1644–1911). It was an era of warlords, civil strife, and war. It was also the period immediately preceding the invasion and horrific occupation by Japan. Wu Daxin's father was Wu Gongzao (1903–1983), the second son of Wu Jianquan (1870–1942), and younger brother of Wu Gongyi (1900–1970). He was the brother of Wu Daxin.

In the mid-1930's, the Wu family was forced to move from Shanghai to avoid the unrest and warfare in China. In doing so, the family passed through Guangzhou, Macao, and finally settled in Hong Kong. Their sole means of support was their family heritage, i.e., the martial art of taiji boxing.

The family managed to survive and eventually thrive in such a poor, small island town because it had already secured fame in taiji boxing throughout China. By the time the Wu's had settled in Hong Kong, there were many rich celebrities, traveled and educated merchants, and societal movers and shakers in Hong Kong and Macao who knew of the Wu's boxing art. The family established a foothold on Hennessy Road in Wanchai, a Hong Kong suburb.

This Hong Kong neighborhood was home to the red-light bar district described famously in the 1960 movie, "The World of Suzie Wong." The area later became the proving grounds for Wu Dakui's (1923–1972) taiji skills. He was the eldest son of Gongyi and eldest grandson of Wu Jianquan. Dakui fought and defeated dozens of porters and workers on the rough waterfront. He was undefeated in Wanchai and before that on the Pearl River Delta, where Hong Kong, Macao, Guangzhou, Fo Shan, and Shun De are found. The area was a virtual gold mine of martial artists. This was the home of the famous Huang Feihong (cant. Wong Fei Hung, 1847–1924) and Ye Wen (cant. Yip Man, 1893–1972); and also, the home of Li Haiquan (cant. Lee Hoi Chuen, 1901–1965, father of Bruce Lee).

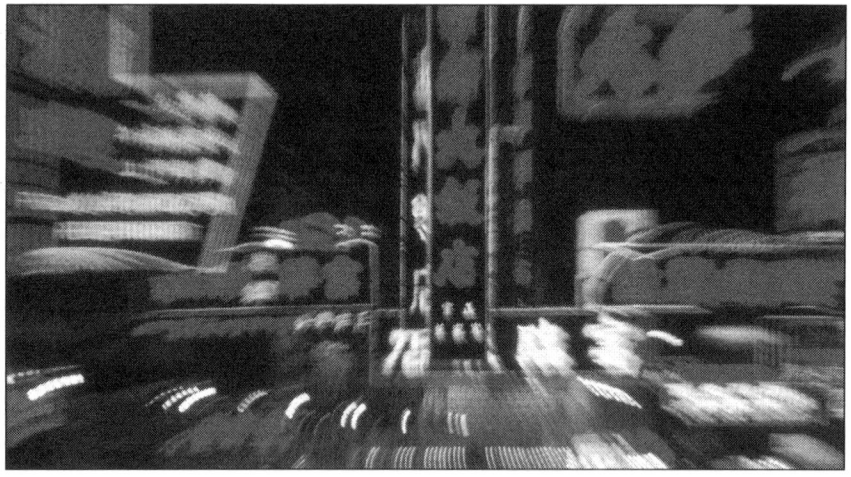

Wanchai District at night.

The Wu family was later invited to teach taiji for the Hong Kong Jin Wu Sports Association, South China Sports Association, and the Hong Kong YMCA. These teaching endeavors, however, lasted only a few years. By 1941, Hong Kong had fallen to the Japanese military. Refusing to be exploited by the invaders, the patriotic Wu family fled in several small groups back to Shanghai. Not until 1945, with Japan's surrender, did the Wu family return to Hong Kong.

This author was also born on Mainland China. By 1932, my mother brought my family to Hong Kong to avoid the war, civil strife, and the debilitating famine. I remember suffering through the infamous, meager food rationing of that war period. After the war, I entered the Jianquan Taiji Association on Lockhart Road in Wanchai and studied Wu's boxing method.

In the beginning, Zhong Yueping[1] taught me. He later became my "gongfu elder brother" (*shixiong*). It was at that time that I met the young Daxin. I knew immediately that he had suffered nearly the same fate as I had. His parents were far away on Mainland China because of the war. The only difference was that I was an orphan by that time. We became the closest of friends. On weekends, we used to go to Shatin in the New Territories to Shen Xianglin's villa. Shen was a senior disciple of Gongyi. Daxin and I slept in the same room. In fact, this was where Shen and his sons, Shen Dongqiang and Shen Dongfu, and Shen's godson, "Rock" Wu Guotai, studied under Gongyi on weekends.

Even as late as 1997, during the handover of the British Colony, I was asked by then gatekeeper Wu Yanxia (1930–2001) to share the teaching load a few nights a week with Daxin in the Jordan School. Sometimes he would arrive early in the afternoon. He would then plead with me to accompany him to various places in the city, sometimes as far away as Yuan Lang, near the Chinese border. We visited restaurants to snack on to pass away the time. Daxin shared some of his food with me while waiting there.

Master Wu Daxin followed his uncle Wu Gongyi in taiji boxing up to his uncle's 1972 death. Daxin was always at his master's side throughout the day as well as when the master taught boxing. He was like a son to him. Gongyi said that Daxin was the one who had learned the most from him and the one who received most of his art. "As for how much he eventually achieves," Gongyi also said, "it depends strictly on his diligence."

This was quite unlike Gongyi's own two sons. Wu Jianquan raised and taught taiji to Gongyi's oldest son, Dakui. Wu Gongyi's younger son, Daqi (1926–1993), was absent for many years while his father was still alive, having gone to Southeast Asia to teach taiji.

During the mid-1950's, after I had finished assisting Zhong Yueping teach on the top floor of the Lockhart Road school, we would go down one flight of stairs to the fourth floor where the main school was located.[2] Shortly after that, Wu Gongyi began to teach advanced material to Daxin, Zhong Yueping, and Guo Shaojiong, husband of Wu Yanxia. As a junior, I was only allowed to observe from the sideline. After those sessions, we would invite Gongyi to a restaurant for a late-night snack. Those were memorable days indeed. This was also how Daxin received so much personal coaching from Wu Gongyi.

There are some very special events about Daxin I remember with fondness and with awe. Around 1954 or 1955, one night after the annual celebration of the birthday of Daoist Grandmaster Zhang Sanfeng, we were in the Kam Ling (man. *Jinling*) Restaurant. The dinner party had finished. We left the restaurant and walked down the street only to find that gang members had punctured Wu Dakui's car tires. The street thugs were standing brazenly nearby. A brawl broke out and Daxin was grabbed from behind and attacked by three of the hoodlums. In one single motion, he punched the two in front and freed himself from the bear hug. All three fell. They immediately scrambled up and ran away.

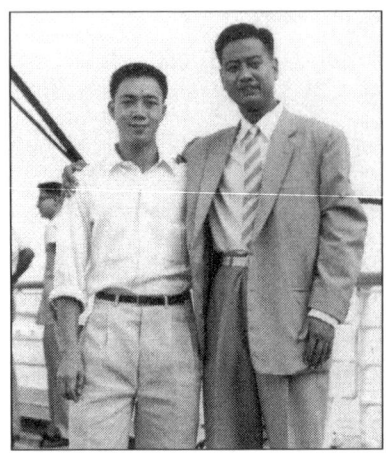 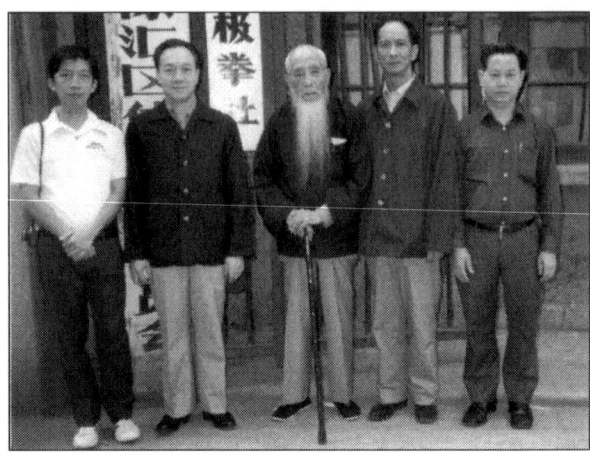

Left: The author and Wu Daxin (r.) on a liner heading for Singapore on June 29, 1956. Right: left to right: Liao Xiangsang (cant. Lau Heung Sang), Cai Naibiao, Wu Gongzao (1903–1983), Wu Dazhun, and Wu Kangnian (cant. Ng Hong Nin). Photograph taken in Shanghai, outside the Jianquan Taiji Association's Main School, June 12, 1981.

I remember well the date January 17th, 1954, when twenty-year old Daxin along with Zhong Yueping were the two personal assistants to Wu Gongyi for the famous Wu-Chan fight.[3] They assisted in the ring as well as on the trip from Hong Kong to Macao and back again.

On June 29th, 1956, Daxin took the Liner Carthage to Singapore to take the reins of the Jianquan Taiji Association there. This was really a milestone in Wu Family Taiji development because of the influence he would have there.

In 1979, Wu Gongzao, Daxin's father and the younger son of Jianquan, came to Hong Kong. The family was at last reunited after a separation of many years. Wu Gongzao mostly taught the most senior students such as Zhong Yueping and Lu Botang.

The book *Wu Family Taijiquan* (known as the Gold Book; Wu, 1984), based on Gongzao's taijiquan (known as the Green Book, 1933) was published in Hong Kong. Many observed that Gongzao's leg had been traumatized.[4] After some time, Gongzao gradually recovered. His fundamentals were still very impressive. He was much better than us even at his advanced age and in his poor physical condition. We could push and attack with all our might, yet he did not shift his step even one bit. His style looked like that of his nephew, Wu Dakui. But then, they had both learned from father and grandfather Wu Jianquan. In 1982, he returned to Hunan to visit old friends. Unfortunately, he died there.

During his stay in Hong Kong, Gongzao tried to arrange a marriage for Daxin. He wrote me about it. He told us his old injury, caused by the decades of confinement and torture, had been cured by a lady with excellent acupuncture skills. I had been present during some of those treatment sessions. It really was quite remarkable. After some massage and the removal of the inserted acupuncture needle, some old dark blood was extracted. Gongzao then felt much better. He was eventually cured. Gongzao was very grateful. He felt that the acupuncturist was an especially good person. He tried to arrange a marriage between her and his forty-year-old son Daxin. It was unsuccessful and Daxin remained single. I have treasured this letter from Gongzao all these years because it is in Gongzao's valuable, personal handwriting. It is also a piece of Wu family history. In addition, it is a record of certain wonderful and amazing traditional medicine.

In October 1988, the building holding the Lockhart Road School was to be demolished. Daxin purchased property on Moreton Terrace in Causeway Bay with his own funds.

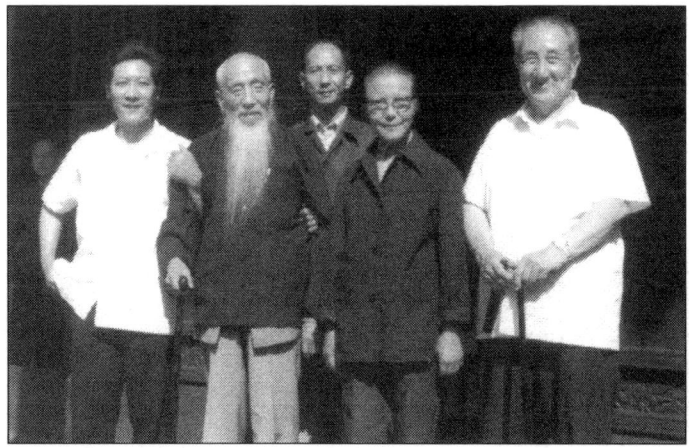

Left to right: Ma Jiangxiong (son of Ma Yueliang), Wu Gongzao (1903–1983), Wu Daizhung (cant. Ng TaiJing, elder brother of Wu Daxin), Wu Yinghua (1907–1997), and Ma Yueliang (1902–1998). Photograph taken in Jade Buddha Temple, Shanghai, 1981. Below: Handwritten letter from Wu Gongzao to Cai Naibiao which discusses introducing Wu Daxin to an acupuncturist who cured him. Dated 1982.

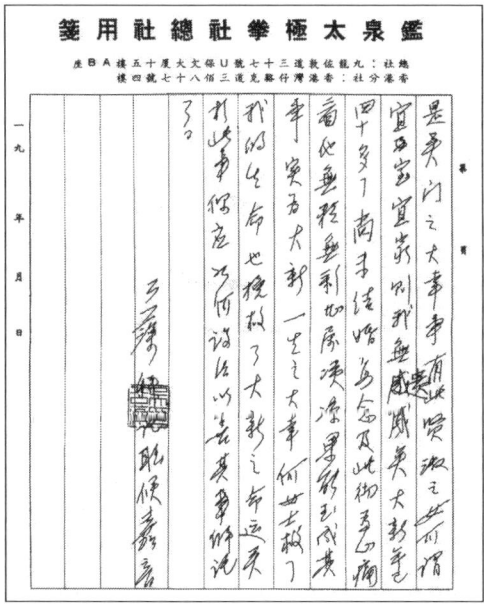
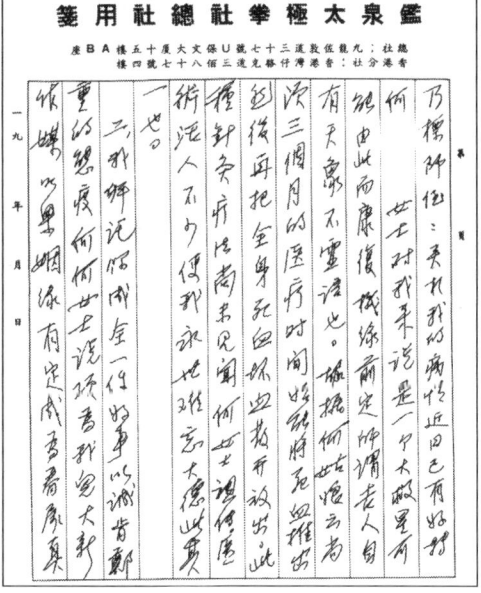

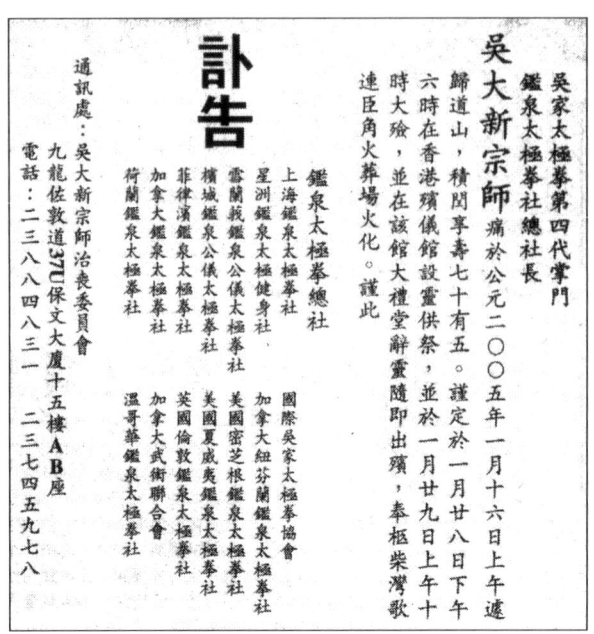

Newspaper obituary for Wu Daxin dated January 16, 2005.

After the 14 July 2001 death of Wu Yanxia, Daxin became the Wu family gatekeeper. The ceremony was held the next day in the Jordan Main School. A dinner party was held in the Best Seafood Restaurant (Ting Ho Restaurant) in the Tsim Sha Tsui section of Kowloon.

The first Wu family gatekeeper was Wu Quanyou, followed by his son, Wu Jianquan, then his son Wu Gongyi. After Gongyi's death, his son Wu Dakui became the gatekeeper in Hong Kong and outside China. Dakui died in 1972. His younger brother, Daqi, was then appointed gatekeeper. When Daqi passed away, the younger sister of Dakui and Daqi, Wu Yanxia, took over. She died in 2001. The above were all descendents of the Wu Gongyi line. Wu Daxin, on the other hand, was the son of Wu Jianquan's other son, Gongzao.

Master Daxin adopted ten batches of disciples; many are overseas. Among them are Wu Wenbiao, now chief coach in the Jordan Main School; Wu Kangnian, Wu Chaojie, Deng Huijian, and Kelvin Steel. Daxin and Wu Gongzao were famed for their taiji saber. Wu Gongyi, Wu Dakui, and Wu Yanxia were all very good with the double-edged sword. It is noteworthy that all of Wu's sword experts came from the Gongyi lineage. This had a direct effect on the disciples and was seen in their respective emphasis.

Daxin used to perform the saber routine during the annual Zhang Sanfeng Birthday Festival. In recent times, however, during Yanxia's term as gatekeeper, he also demonstrated push-hand exercises. Sometimes he would have his disciples demonstrate and then he would come out and teach them how they might improve. Occasionally he would demonstrate his simple, concise, and elegant solution to a particular situation. His skills were documented on video.

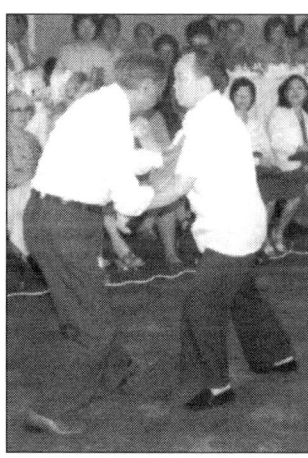 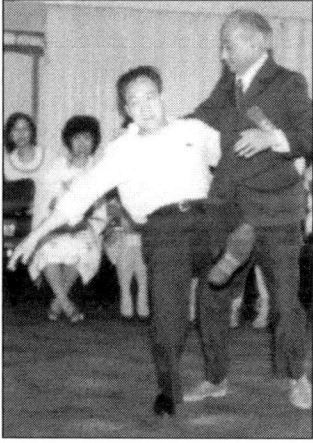 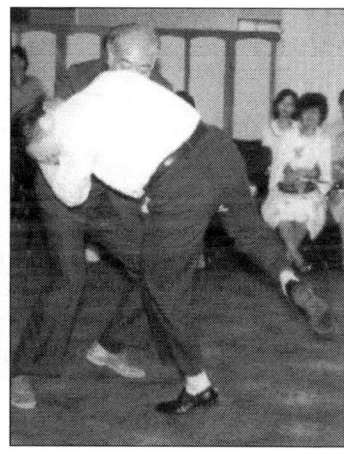

Wu Daxin and the author push-hands during celebrations for the annual Zheng Sanfeng (legendary founder of taijiquan) Birthday festival. Photographs taken in the Pearl City Restaurant, 1983 and 1984.

Daxin's push-hands skill was quite unique. More than any other, he really had the feel for Wu Gongyi's method. Seldom did he do push-hands in the school. Rather, he would just sit and observe. We frequently commented that Daxin seldom even moved his hands. Even when he did the exercise, he usually finished it off quickly with minimal moves.

Whenever I did push-hands with him, I would usually advance my hand and he would nearly simultaneously, directly strike back. It appeared he was attacking an attack. In fact, it was the advice of the ancients to wait until the other moves, but you arrive first. He did this in one simple coordinated movement. In fact, just his initial, interceptive position already nullified part of my attack. The strike on contact used a certain rotation and countered my offense. Thus, he could just spiral back and nullify and borrow my energy. Outwardly, that movement looked plain and simple. However, it was anything but plain and simple. Those who tasted it were filled with awe and respect. The higher their level, the more appreciation students voiced. For this reason, many followed him for years hoping just to see him show the movement. It was beautiful in its simplicity, yet few could do it.

During a meeting of our generation with Master Daxin, sitting next to him were Lu Botang, my gongfu older brother (*shidai*) who used to be the "demonstration dummy" for Wu Gongyi, and who had written extensively about Wu Gongyi in the newspapers; and Ye Shuliang, the chief coach of the now-closed Wu Dakui Mongkok School. Ye used to collect the special tuition fee for Daxin when he taught saber in Dakui's school. Thus, they were quite friendly with each other.

Lu Botang asked about the progress Daxin had made over the years. Daxin just let the seated Lu grasp his wrist. Quite quickly, he made a slight imperceptible movement. Involuntarily, Lu stood up gently. Lu was totally bewildered as to how Daxin had done that. Daxin told them, "This is ward off [*peng*]!" After this, Lu was completely convinced Daxin had indeed acquired Gongyi's art.

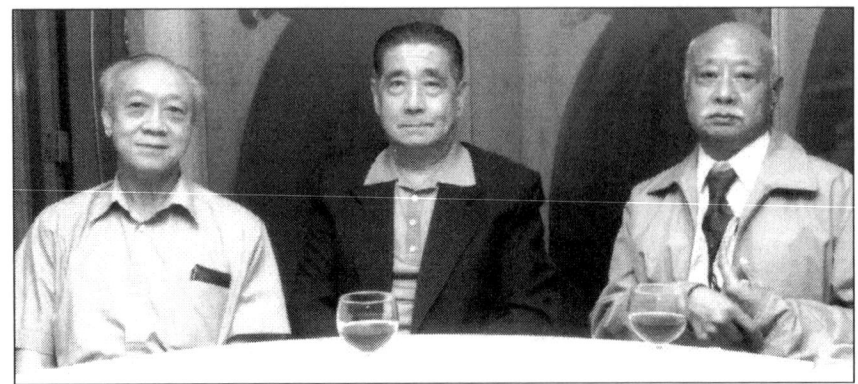

Left to right: Cai Naibiao with Xiao Huilong (cant. Siu Wai Lung) and Wu Daxin. Photograph taken in a Hong Kong restaurant on November 16, 2001, during a gathering to celebrate Wu Daxin's birthday. Mr. Xiao is the last surviving disciple who studied directly under Wu Jianquan.

After this demonstration, Ye Shuliang asked Daxin for any special gems he might give them to further their practice. Daxin then uttered, "jing"—meaning silence, serenity. This was probably the last gem of wisdom he left us.

South China Morning Post newspaper reporter Ravina Shamdasani interviewed Daxin for an article when he was sixty-eight years old. It was the commemoration on becoming gatekeeper. Commenting on that and on his and his cousins' practice, Daxin said, "I was lazy practicing taiji when I was growing up." Others, however, remember him practicing very diligently and that he understood the family tradition had continued for generations. He said, "It is my duty and honor to carry the tradition forward." Daxin explained, "It is a heavy burden, but we have been prepared from early childhood. In fact," he continued, "since I was in my mother's tummy." Wu Daxin was a superb master and gatekeeper.

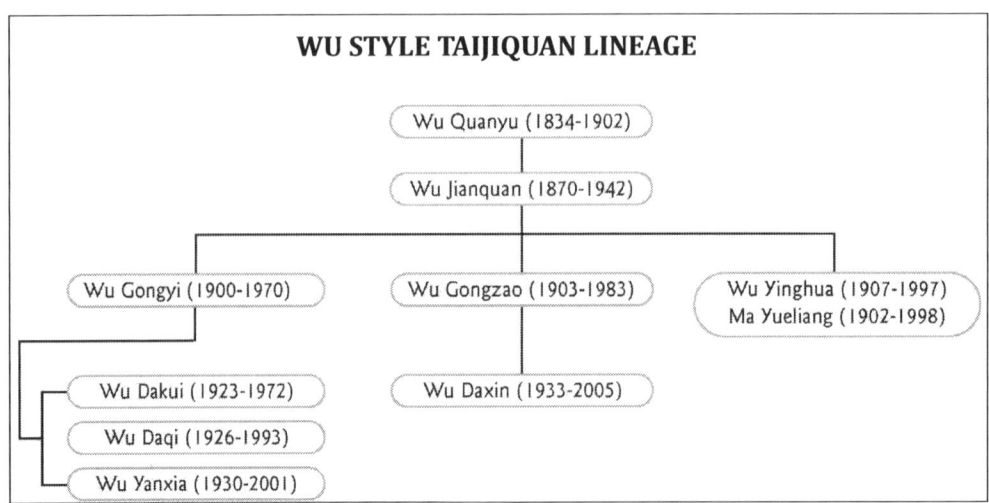

GLOSSARY

Pinyin		*Cantonese (Hong Kong)*
Cai Naibiao	蔡乃標	Tsoi Nie Biu
Deng Huijian	鄧惠堅	Dang Wai Gin
Fo Shan	佛山	Faat Shan
Guo Shaojiong	郭少炯	Kwok Siu Gwing
Huang Feihong	黃飛鴻	Wong Fei Hung
Jing	靜	Jing
Jian Quan	鑑泉	Kam Chuen
Taijiquan Association	太極拳社	Tai Chi Chuan Association
Li Haiquan	李海泉	Lee Hoi Chuen
Lu Botang	盧柏堂	Lo Pak Tong
Ma Yueliang	馬岳樑	Ma Ngok Leung
Shen Dongfu	沈東福	Shum Tung Fuk
Shen Dongqiang	沈東強	Shum Tung Keung
Shen Xianglin	沈香林	Shum Heung Lam
Shi Bo	師伯	Si Pak
Shi Di	師第	Si Tai
Shi Shu	師叔	Si Suk
Shi Xiong	師兄	Si Hing
Shun De	順德	Shun Tak
Wu Chaojie	吳超杰	Ng Chiu Kit
Wu Dakui	吳大揆	Ng Tai Kwai
Wu Daqi	吳大齊	Ng Tai Chai
Wu Daxin	吳大新	Ng Dai Sun
Wu Dazhun	吳大諄	Ng Tai Jeun
Wu Gongyi	吳公儀	Ng Kung Yee
Wu Gongzao	吳公藻	Ng Kung Cho
Wu Guotai	吳國泰	Ng Kwok Tai
Wu Jianquan	吳鑑泉	Ng Kam Chuen
Wu Kangnian	吳康年	Ng Hong Lin
Wu Wenbiao	吳文表	Ng Man Piu
Wu Yanxia	吳雁霞	Ng Ngan Ha
Wu Yinghua	吳英華	Ng Ying Wa
Wu Quanyu	吳全祐	Ng Chyun Yau
Ye Ruli	葉汝立	Yip Y.L.
Ye Shuliang	葉樹良	Yip Sue Leong
Ye Wen	葉問	Yip Man
Yuan Lang	元朗	Yuen Long
Zheng Tianxiong	鄭天熊	Cheng Tin Hung
Zheng Yongguang	鄭榮光	Cheng Wing Kwong
Zhong Yueping	鍾岳平	Chung Ngok Ping

Notes

[1] Zhong Yueping also taught Zheng Tianxiong, the nephew of Zheng Yongguang (a disciple of Wu Jianquan). Zheng Tianxiong had a very successful school in Mongkok. He won open championships and taught generations of students who also performed well in tournaments against a variety of martial art stylists. He was responsible for training and assessing taiji coaches in the Hong Kong Public Parks. He founded the largest taiji organization in Hong Kong at that time: the Hong Kong Taiji Main Association.

[2] Years later, a group of disciples combined resources to purchase the flat on the top floor of Po Man Building, near King George V. Garden, Jordan Road, for the Jianquan Association. This became the main school while the Wanchai school became a branch. Wu Dakui ran the Mongkok school.

[3] Note by Leroy Clark: After enduring decades of torture and imprisonment, Gongzao had nearly forgotten how to do the form. His leg injury would not allow him to do the form properly. His students report that Communist government officials had known that he was an adept in martial arts and, therefore, he had been deliberately tortured on his legs. Gongzao while imprisoned was only able to practice a qigong that did not require body movement. The guards were unable to keep him from doing at least that. During this politically charged period, torture methods for martial masters were selected to damage the masters' specialties, i.e., those who excelled in the use of the upper body limbs would be tortured on the upper limbs; those who excelled in leg work received trauma to the legs.

[4] January 1954 saw the much-publicized challenge of taijiquan's Wu Gongyi by White Crane stylist Chan Hak Fu. In Asia this was the fight of the century. It brought to the ring for the world to see for the first time the mysterious internal art against the widely accepted and understood external fighting art. The young, externalist Chan Hak Fu challenged taijiquan's senior, internalist Wu Gongyi, son of the widely known and respected Wu Jianquan. For an in-depth view of the challenge and impact, Yip and Clark (2002) Yip Y. and Clark, L. (2002). "Pivot." *Qi, the Journal of Traditional Eastern Health and Fitness*, (12) 3.

References

Wu, G.Z. (1933). *Taijiquan*. Hong Kong: Published by the Wu Family.
Wu, G.Z. (1984). *Wu family taijiquan*. Hong Kong: Published by the Wu Family.
Wu Family. (1995). *Wu style taijiquan and sabre*. Hong Kong: Published by the Wu Family.

Fear of Falling:
Taijiquan as a Form of Graded in Vivo Exposure Therapy
by Shane Kachur, B.M.R. (P.T), R. Nicholas Carleton, M.A.
and Gordon Asmundson, Ph.D.

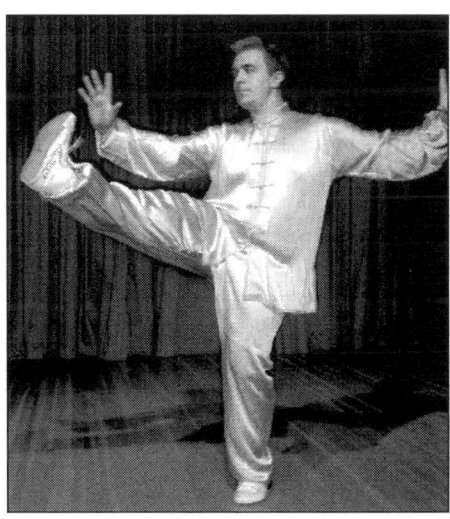

All photographs courtesy of S. Kachur.

Introduction

Falls in the elderly have enormous personal and logistical costs (Tinetti and Williams, 1997), often leading to permanent loss of function and independence. Preventative efforts for reducing falls focus on the causes of falling: both extrinsic and intrinsic to the individual (Lajoie and Gallagher, 2003). Extrinsic factors include improper footwear, unstable living conditions, and weather-related complications. Intrinsic factors include neurological complications caused by medications, syncope, vision impairment, and frailty. Defined as a reduction in physiological reserves and behavioral capacities (Wolf et al., 1996), frailty has long been believed the most common cause for falling in elderly populations; conversely, empirical investigations have identified loss of postural sway, poor balance, and fear of falling as the three key factors associated with predicting falls in elderly populations (Lajoie and Gallagher, 2003). Accordingly, traditional treatment to reduce falls has been exercise programs focused on reducing frailty and increasing strength, flexibility, and balance (Shumway-Cook, Gruber, Baldwin, and Liao, 1997; Tideiksaar, 1997).

Measures of postural sway and balance have been used to determine fall risk by evaluating how elderly people control their center of mass over their base of support. However, a cognitive construct—fear of falling—may also affect physical performance, reducing balance and increasing postural sway (Tinetti, Medes de

Leon, Doucette, and Baker, 1994). Indeed, measures of fear of falling may help identify individuals that are at risk for falling. One of the first attempts to identify a relationship between balance performance and fear of falling indicated that those who reported being afraid to fall also demonstrated significantly poorer results on postural sway with balance tests (Maki, Holiday, and Topper, 1991). Since then, fear of falling has been shown to be a stronger predictor of falls relative to postural sway and balance (Delbaere, Crombez, Vanderstraeten, Willems, and Cambier, 2004; Lajoie and Gallagher, 2003); therefore, it is now garnering additional attention from researchers and clinicians. Furthermore, the relationship between fear of falling and actual falls suggests treatments including fear-reduction techniques are likely to have a greater efficacy than treatments using exercise in isolation.

Fear of Falling – Research

Research has demonstrated that 30% of people over 65 years of age report a substantial fear of falling, despite never having fallen (Hadjistavropolous and Carpenter, 2006). In an attempt to understand how psychological indicators such as fear of falling are related to balance, Myers et al. (1996) assessed a sample of 60 community-dwelling seniors aged 65–95 (71.2% women; Mage = 74.6; SD = 7.5; see Table 1 for statistical definitions). Two yes/no self-report questionnaires were used to measure fear of falling and activity avoidance—the Falls Efficacy Scale (FES; Tinetti, Richman, and Powell, 1990) and the Activities-specific Balance Confidence Scale (ABC; Powell and Myers, 1995). These questionnaires, along with posturographical measures of balance, were examined to identify the relationships between various psychological indicators of balance confidence. The groups were separated based on their answers on the FES and then compared based on their ABC scores. The fear of falling and activity avoidance groups scored significantly lower than the non-fearful group on the ABC ($t = 3.91$, $p < .001$ and $t = 7.19$, $p < .001$, respectively). The ABC was also positively correlated with measures of mobility ($r = .56$, $p < .01$). Subsequently, Delbaere and colleagues (2004) demonstrated statistically significant negative correlations ($r = -.49$, $p < .01$) between biomechanical (i.e., physical strength and postural control) and psychological measures (i.e., fear and avoidance).

Similar analysis of the relationship between fear of falling and gait (Chamberlin, Fulwider, Sanders, and Medeiros, 2005) has demonstrated that fearful elderly have significantly different gait characteristics—such as slower speed, wider stride width, and a longer double limb support phase—than age-matched non-fearful controls. The marked changes in gait and the associations with fear of falling, avoidance behavior, and physical performance further support fear of falling as an important factor of physical performance. Fear and avoidance appear to have some influence on biological mechanisms that control ambulation and balance. Strong fears may have immediate influences, such as a startling fear that results in a fall; subtle fears may, over time, result in physiological adaptations that contribute to increases in frailty.

Somatic complaints driven (or exacerbated) by fear-avoidance have also been identified as a significant component in the development of chronic musculoskeletal pain (Asmundson, Norton, and Crombez, 2004). Briefly, fear of pain or physical harm leads to pain-related anxiety that results in avoidance behavior and subsequent disuse and deconditioning (see Figure 1). The feedback loops presented in Figure 1 show a reinforcement of fearful beliefs that serves to maintain activity avoidance and disability. Based on the fear of pain model, a model for the role of fear of falling on activity avoidance and falls can be proposed (Figure 2).

TABLE 1: Statistical Terminology
- M = mean, or average
- SD = standard deviation, represents roughly the average of individuals differs from the group average.
- n = the number of people in the sample
- p = the probability that the result is due to chance. A p = .05 would indicate that there is a 1/20 chance that the result occurred due to chance.
- t = the t score derived from doing a t-test, the t-test is one way to compare the mean scores between two groups to see if the groups differ significantly.
- r = represents the strength of a correlation between two groups. It can range from -1 to +1, a score of +1 would indicate that the two groups are maximally correlated and a change in one would cause the same increase in the other, whereas a -1 would indicate that increasing one group would cause the same magnitude decrease in the other.

FIGURE 1: The Fear–Anxiety–Avoidance Model of Chronic Pain
Redrawn and adapted from: Asmundson, Vlaeyen, and Crombez (2004). Understanding and treating fear of pain, p. 15. Used with kind permission from Oxford University Press.

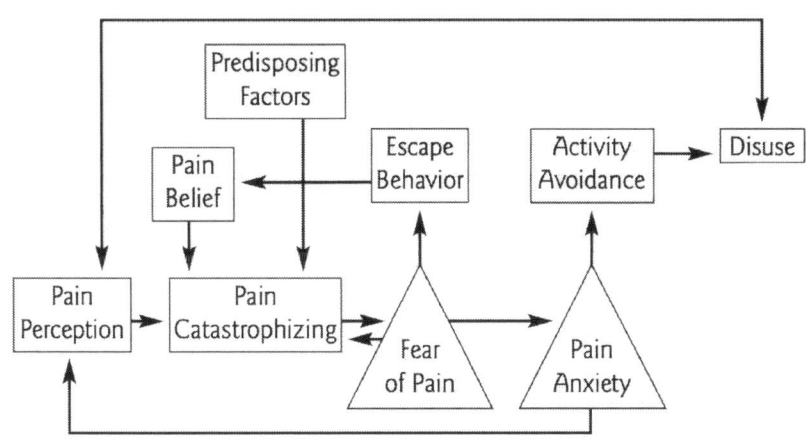

The Role of Fear of Falling

Existing research suggests fear of falling promotes falls via one of two pathways (Figure 2). First, fear and the resulting trepidation may result in an actual change in physiological gait mechanics and postural control (Chamberlin, et al., 2005). These changes constitute measurable increases in postural rigidity. The second pathway seems mediated by avoiding certain activities. Activity avoidance leads to losses in strength, range of motion, and promotes frailty, all of which increases the risk of falling (Delbaere, et al., 2004). Through these pathways, fear of falling may act as a pervasive vulnerability for frailty and falling. The feedback loops involving postural rigidity and activity avoidance maintain fear of falling, enabling a vicious cycle similar to the fear-avoidance models of chronic pain (Asmundson, et al., 2004). For example, after experiencing a fall, a person is more likely to be fearful of falling, which leads to avoidance, which can lead to disuse, postural rigidity, and an increased risk of falling.

FIGURE 2: Fear of Falling as an Antecedent of Falls

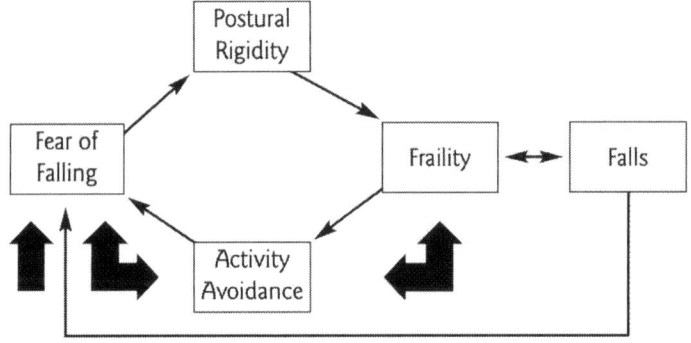

Current Treatment for Fear of Falling

Growing recognition of the role fear and avoidance plays in somatic conditions has resulted in specialized psychologically-focused treatments, particularly for chronic pain sufferers. The effective treatment of fear and avoidance related to chronic pain often revolves around a concept called graded *in vivo* (in life) exposure (Vlaeyen, de Jong, Leeuw, and Crombez, 2004). Graded in vivo exposure involves the systematic desensitization to fear-inducing stimuli through gradual exposure to feared activities in a safe environment. It has been succinctly described as "a keystone treatment method, [in which] individuals progress through an incremental series of anxiety provoking encounters with phobic stimuli, while utilizing relaxation as a reciprocal inhibitor of increasing anxiety" (Vlaeyen et al., 2004: 327). It is most likely that confrontation of fearful stimuli, not the relaxation component, is primarily responsible for fear reductions. By disconfirming the belief that harm will occur from the feared activity, graded in vivo exposure has been shown to result in reductions in fear, pain, and perceived disability, leading to increases in function (Boersma, et al., 2004; Vlaeyen, de Jong, Leeuw, and Crombez, 2004).

Taijiquan

Taijiquan is an ancient Chinese martial art that has evolved into an exercise regimen for health, resulting in improvements of range of motion, cardio-respiratory function, balance, and posture (Wolf, Coogler, and Xu, 1997). Taijiquan could be seen as a form of graded in vivo exposure. Taijiquan slowly, but progressively, exposes its practitioners to increasingly difficult postures that simulate situations that may also provoke fear of falling. Classically, taijiquan routines can have up to 108 movements; however, most research uses some modified form of taijiquan containing only 10–20 movements (Wayne, et al., 2004). Taijiquan also promotes a calm, relaxed attitude and atmosphere during each of the postural movements. Thus, it comprises both the graduated exposure and relaxation components of graded in vivo exposure. As a possible form of graded in vivo exposure, taijiquan reduces fear of falling as it improves balance (Taggart, 2002; Wolf, et al., 1996).

Taijiquan has received increasing scientific attention as a method for fall prevention in the elderly. Thus far the focus of these studies has been on taijiquan's effects on physical/neurological control systems of posture and balance (Haas, et al., 2004; McGibbon, et al., 2005; Tsang, Wong, Fu, and Hui-Chan, 2004; Wayne, et al., 2004; Wolf, Coogler, and Xu, 1997). These studies of balance and posture demonstrated that, as a treatment strategy, taijiquan improves postural control and balance (Hass, et al., 2004); moreover, taijiquan appears effective in improving balance and posture even for persons suffering from peripheral vestibular disease (McGibbon, et al., 2005; Wayne, et al., 2004).

Taijiquan may contribute to preventing the development of frailty. A sample of 20 taijiquan practitioners (50% women; Mage = 70.7; SD = 5.1) with a mean of 7.2 years (SD = 7.2) of practice were compared to 20 age-matched controls (60% women; Mage = 67.8; SD = 4.5) and a group of 20 healthy university students (40% women; Mage = 21.5; SD = 1.6) (Tsang, et al., 2004). The taijiquan and university student groups performed significantly better on computerized tests of balance than the aged-matched non-practitioner controls. This suggests that taijiquan practitioners (between 65.6 and 75.8 years of age) had the same balance control as younger, healthy individuals. This study and the vestibular-postural studies suggest that taijiquan improves balance as governed by the neuromuscular systems.

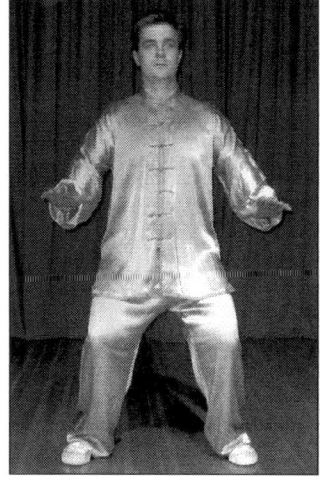

Picture 1: Commencing Form

This posture, with its large base of support, would have a low threat factor and can easily be made more difficult by adding different weight shifts and perturbations.

Picture 2: Functional Commencing Form
This posture resembles key functional activities such as getting off a bed or out of a chair.

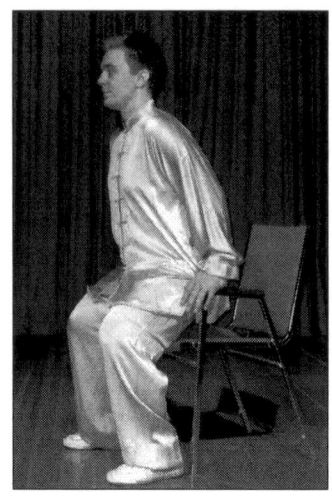

Taijiquan has also been compared to more traditional or 'Western' methods for balance improvement. A randomized controlled clinical trial compared taijiquan, computerized balance therapy, and education (Wolf, et al., 1996). Biomedical variables (strength, balance, and flexibility), functional variables (activities of daily living), and psychological variables (depression and fear of falling) were measured from a sample of 200 community dwelling seniors [81.0% women aged over 70 years (M = 76.2)]. The participants were randomized into three groups: taiji (n = 72), computerized balance training (n = 64), and education classes (n = 64). The taijiquan group practiced for 15 weeks. Repeated measurement analyses revealed that those participants practicing taijiquan outperformed both the computerized balance group and the educational group by way of a statistically significant reduction in fear of falling (p < .05). No statistically significant differences were found between the taijiquan group and the computerized balance therapy on measures of balance. In addition, after a four month follow up the taijiquan group had 29 falls, the computerized balance group had 44, and the education group had 37 falls. Taijiquan was found to reduce the risk of multiple falls by 47% in falls during this four-month period. It is noteworthy that the cost per participant associated with group taijiquan classes was lower than one-on-one computerized balance training with a physical therapist. Taggart (2002) replicated Wolf's findings, finding a similar effect of taijiquan practice on balance, functional mobility, and fear of falling in older women over the age of 65. After 3 months of normal activity the participants underwent taijiquan classes twice per week for 3 months. Following the taijiquan training, improvements were found in balance, functional mobility and fear of falling. Relative to alternative interventions, taijiquan may be more cost-effective and better at reducing fear of falling, improving balance, decreasing the rate of falls, and attenuating the development of frailty (Tsang, et al., 2005).

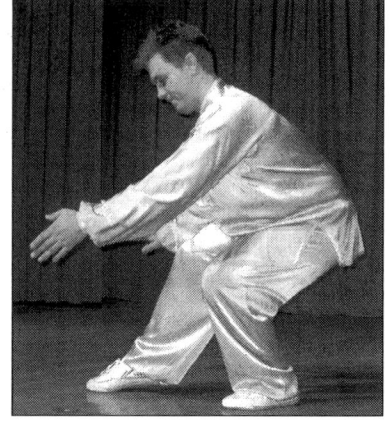

Picture 3: Needle at the Bottom of the Sea
This posture is more challenging than commencing form as there is more weight on one leg, forward inclination of the torso towards the ground, and forward reaching.

Picture 4: Functional Needle at the Bottom of the Sea
This posture can easily be made to simulate grasping objects from the floor.

Picture 5: Stand on One Leg
Progressing in difficulty, standing on one leg, presents a higher level of threat as balance requirements are increased. It is important to confront fears of falling. This can be done by acknowledging any attempts of the activity and reward gains to reduce fear and build confidence. Distraction, by focusing on the relaxation associated with taijiquan, can also be beneficial.

Picture 6: Functional Stand on One Leg
There are many functional applications that can be relayed with this particular posture, such as walking, stepping into the bathtub, or ascending stairs.

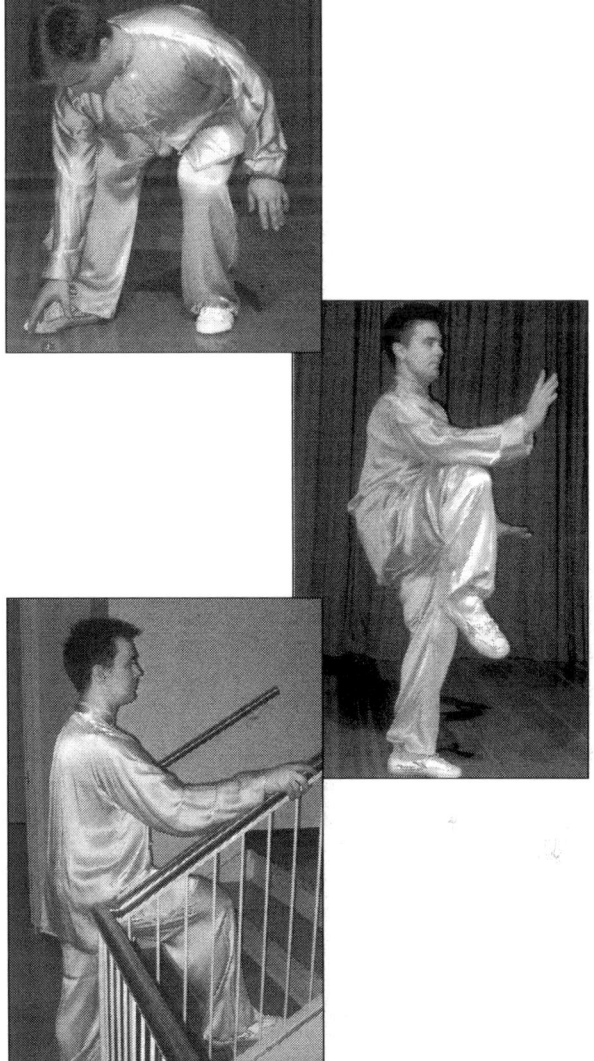

Picture 7: Progressions
As fear subsides and confidence is gained the fearful taijiquan practitioner should practice more efficiently and gain strength and balance associated with taijiquan practice. This then can be progressed into more difficult movements, such as kick with right heel.

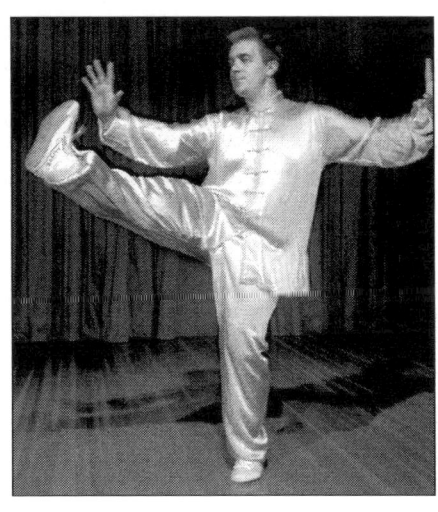

Beyond the aforementioned benefits of taijiquan, it can also facilitate a positive socially-reinforced exercise regime. If taijiquan therapy is engaged prior to a fall—or better yet, prior to the development of any disabling fear of falling—most falls may be prevented. The concept of taijiquan as a form of graded in vivo exposure therapy seems reasonable and peripherally supported by empirical investigations. Research is still needed to evaluate this possibility; however, there are some challenges to be addressed.

Specific research issues involve deciding which form and perspective of taijiquan should be applied. There is no standardized form of taijiquan and, moreover, large variability in instructor experience. These methodological limitations may make generalizability of research findings to community instruction settings difficult. There is also debate within taijiquan instructor circles as to the role student intentions play in obtaining health improvements. That is, some taijiquan schools suggest that maximal health benefits can only be acquired if the student learns the movement as a martial art, rather than exercise or therapy. There may be substantial resistance from instructors to adjusting their pedagogy for treatment purposes; however, there are already schools of taijiquan that use a dance model, rather than a martial arts model, focusing on choreography and repetition without any concern of the movement's combative purposes (Hong, 2006).

Despite the challenges, taijiquan seems to have tremendous potential for reducing falls. Four concepts, based on the principles of graded in vivo exposure, should be incorporated into teaching/practicing taijiquan when teaching/practicing to maximize the effects of exposure:

- First, ensure students understand that taijiquan is not harmful. This should be done verbally and through instructor demonstrations of movements prior to student attempts or practice.
- Second, wherever possible, relate the taijiquan movements to activities of daily living (see pictures 1 to 6); focus should be on any movements related to activities the student has indicated fear of performing. There should also be a progression starting with activities that are less fearful with a gradual increase to those that are more fearful.
- Third, movements should be progressive, starting with those that are least fearful and gradually introducing those that are more fearful as confidence and success is achieved (see picture 7).
- Fourth, and finally, confront student statements that convey beliefs that he or she is incapable of, or in danger, while performing any given daily activity. This might be accomplished (after appropriate taijiquan training and practice) by pointing out that the student is already performing the daily activity during taijiquan practice.

The benefits of taijiquan, applied as a form of graded in vivo exposure, need to be evaluated to ensure potential health benefits, particularly reductions in falling, are documented and communicated to health professionals interested in frailty and illness prevention. Hopefully this paper will influence health researchers to investigate taijiquan as a viable, cost-effective, and attractive method of fall prevention therapy.

▼●▼

Bibliography

Asmundson, G., Norton, P., and Vlaeyen, J. (2004). Fear-avoidance models of chronic pain: An overview. In G. Asmundson, J. Vlaeyen, and G. Crombez (Eds.), *Understanding and treating fear of pain*. New York: Oxford University Press.

Boersma, K., Linton, S., Overmeer, T., Jansson, M., Vlaeyen, J., and de Jong, J. (2002). Lowering fear-avoidance and enhancing function through exposure in vivo: A multiple baseline study across six patients with back pain. *Pain*, 108, 8–16.

Chamberlin, M., Fulwider, B., Sanders, S., and Medeiros, J. (2005). Does fear of falling influence spatial and temporal gait parameters in elderly persons. *The Journals of Gerontology*. Series A, Biological sciences and medical sciences, 60, 1163–1167.

Delbaere, K., Crombez, G., Vanderstraeten, G., Willems, T., and Cambier, D. (2004). Fear-related avoidance of activities, falls, and physical frailty. A prospective community-based cohort study. *Age and Aging*, 33, 368–373.

Haas, C., Gregor, R., Waddell, D., Oliver, A. Smith, D., Flemming, R., and Wolf, S. (2004). The influence of tai chi training on the centre of pressure trajectory during gait initiation in older adults. *Archives of Physical Medicine and Rehabilitation*, 85, 1593–1598.

Hadjistavropolous, T., and Carpenter, M. (2006). Fear of pain and fear of falling in the elderly. Presentation at the Canadian Pain Society 2006 Annual Conference, Edmonton, June 14–15. Edmonton, AB.

Hong, J. (2006). *Chen style taijiquan practical method* (Z. H. Chen, Trans.). Edmonton, Canada: Hunyuantaiji press.

Lajoie, Y., and Galagher, S. (2003). Predicting falls within the elderly community: of postural sway, reaction time, the Berg balance scale, and the Activities-specific Balance Confidence Scale for comparing fallers and non-fallers. *Archives of Physical Medicine and Rehabilitation*, 85, 1593–1598.

Maki, B., Holliday, P., and Topper, A. (1991). Fear of falling and postural performance in the elderly. *Journal of Gerontology*, 46, 123–131.

McGibbon, C., Krebs, D., Parker, S., Scarborough, D., Wayne, P., and Wolf, S. (2005). Tai chi and vestibular rehabilitation improve vestibulopathic gait via different neuromuscular mechanisms: preliminary report. BMC *Neurology*, 5, 1471–1483.

Meyers, A., Powell, L., Maki, B., Holliday, P., Brawley, L., and Sherk, W. (1996). Psychological indicators of balance confidence: Relationship to actual and perceived abilities. *Journal of Gerontology*, 51, 37–43.

Powell, L., and Myers, A. (1995). The activities-specific balance confidence (ABC) scale. *Journal of Gerontology*, 50, 28–34.

Shumway-Cook, A., Gruber, W., Baldwin M., and Liao, S. (1997). The effect of multidimensional exercises and balance, mobility and fall risk in community-dwelling older adults. *Physical Therapy*, 77, 46–57.

Taggert, H. (2002). Effects of tai chi exercise on balance, functional mobility, and fear of falling among older women. *Applied Nursing Research*, 15, 235–242.

Tideiksaar, R. (1997). Falling in the old age: Its prevention and management (2nd Ed). New York: Springer.

Tinetti, M., Medes de Leon, C., Doucette, J., and Baker, D. (1994). Fear of falling and fall-related efficacy in relationship to functioning among community-living elders. *Journal of Gerontological Medical Science*, 49, 140–147.

Tinetti, M., Richman, D., and Powell, L. (1990). Falls efficacy as a measure of fear of falling. *Journal of Gerontological Psychologial Science*, 48, 239–243.

Tinetti, M., and Williams, C. (1997). Falls, injuries due to falls, and the risk of admission to a nursing home. *The New England Journal of Medicine*, 337, 1279–1284.

Tsang, W., Wong, V., Fu, S., and Hui-Chan, C. (2004). Tai chi improves standing balance control under reduced or conflicting sensory conditions. *Archives of Physical Medicine*, 85, 129–137.

Vlaeyen, J., de Jong, J., Leeuw, M., and Crombez, G. (2004). Fear reduction in chronic pain: Graded exposure in vivo with behavioral experiments. In G. Asmundson, J. Vlaeyen, and G. Crombez (Eds.), *Understanding and treating fear of pain*. New York: Oxford University Press.

Wayne, P., Krebs, D., Wolf, S., Gill-Body, K., Scarborough, D., McGibbon, C., and Kaptchuk, T. (2004). Can tai chi improve vestibular postural control? *Archives of Physical Medicine and Rehabilitation*, 85, 142–152.

Wolf, S., Barnhart, H., Kutner, N., McNeely, E., Coogler, C., and Xu, T. (1996). Reducing frailty and falls in older persons: An investigation of Tai Chi and computerized balance training. *Journal of the American Geriatric Society*, 44, 889–903.

Wolf, S., Coogler, C., and Xu, T. (1997). Exploring the basis for tai chi chuan as a therapeutic exercise approach. *Archives of Physical Medicine and Rehabilitation*, 85, 886-892.

Note

This work was supported in part by New Emerging Team Grant PTS—63186 from the Canadian Institutes of Health Research (CIHR) Institute of Neurosciences, Mental Health and Addiction. Dr. Asmundson is supported by a CIHR Investigator Award and R. N. Carleton by a CIHR Canada Graduate Scholarship Doctoral Research Award. S. S. Kachur would like to acknowledge his taijiquan teacher, Master Nick Gracenin for his support and guidance. Correspondence concerning this article should be addressed to Gordon J. G. Asmundson Ph.D., Anxiety and Illness Behaviours Laboratory, University of Regina, Regina, Saskatchewan, S4S 0A2.

Sanshou: Understanding Taijiquan as a Martial Art
by Greg Wolfson, B.A.

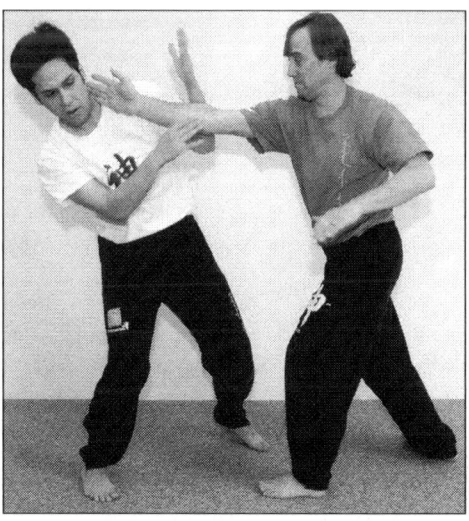

The author (left) playing push-hands (*tuishou*) with his teacher,
Scott M. Rodell. All photographs courtesy of Great River Taoist Center.

Introduction

The martial art taijiquan is popularly associated with the slow, graceful movements of the empty-hand form. Those with some exposure to the art might be familiar with the "push-hands" exercises (*tuishou*). In these partnered drills, each side tries to push the other off-balance using the art's eight basic techniques while maintaining physical contact. Their intent is to develop "listening energy" (*ting jin*) by feeling the strength and direction of their partner's pushes. With *tuishou*, the taiji player can practice redirecting incoming energy (in this case, pushes) without being thrust immediately into a more realistic combat environment. Few students, however, have applied these acquired skills in the "free hands" stage of training (*sanshou*), where they are tested in a full-contact, full-power environment. This is a major omission for any student wishing to learn the complete taijiquan system.

Traditionally, *sanshou* practice begins with taking individual techniques out of the empty-hand form and practicing them slowly in response to a variety of attacks. This is done repeatedly until the movement becomes natural and precise at full speed and power. From there, the student practices putting techniques together in combination. His goal here is to move freely and spontaneously from one move to the next, keeping his partner unbalanced. Eventually, the students practice full-contact play, where they must use this continuous freedom of movement to deal with whatever offense their partners bring.

This method of *sanshou* training should be differentiated from the choreographed two-person sanshou sets often practiced today. In these two-person forms, each player learns a set sequence of movements and then practices then in tandem with a partner, like a dance. The earliest recorded evidence of such sets within the Yang system is Chen Gong's 1932 book, *Combined Taijiquan, Broadsword, Double-edged Sword, Staff, and Sparring* (Taijiquan Dao Jian Gan Sanshou Hebian). By comparison, writings of the first three generations of Yang family masters, including transmitted instructional writings and Yang Chengfu's two books, *Complete Form and Practice of Taijiquan* (Taijiquan Tiyong Quanshu) and *Taijiquan Practical Methods* (Taijiquan Shiyongfa), contain no mention of such a form. The latter two books do contain descriptions of the other forms practiced by the Yang family, including their empty-hand, pushing-hands, saber, double-edge straight sword (*jian*), and staff forms. The existence of a two-person sanshou set dating back to Yang Chengfu's time would imply a glaring omission in the writings of the third-generation master.

One reason for the lack of *sanshou* training is the vast difference between the objectives of taijiquan's founders and many of today's adherents. Most students of Yang Style taijiquan are unaware that the art's founder, Yang Luchan, made his living not as a taiji teacher in the contemporary sense but as a military instructor. Both he and his sons, Banhou and Jianhou, taught provincial militia and then at the military garrisons in Beijing, enjoying the patronage of Manchu princes (Wile, 1983: xi–xii). They trained soldiers at a time of great civil unrest in China; the Qing rulers had to contend with the Taiping Rebellion in the east as well as minority uprisings in the north and west. That Yang Style taijiquan flourished in the military during such a period leaves little doubt as to its martial effectiveness.

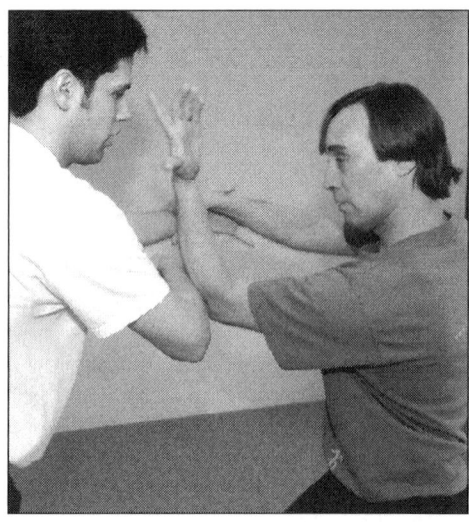

Scott M. Rodell (right) and the author developing
the "hands on" feel of taijiquan that can only
be obtained by practicing with others.

Yet today, many people take up this proven art not to achieve martial excellence, as its founders intended, but to improve their health or to exercise. They want taijiquan's ability to relieve stress, revitalize their bodies, and foster a strong, calm spirit. These students wonder what participation in "violent" sanshou training has to do with cultivating health and calmness. They do not understand that they must practice taijiquan as a martial art to achieve their goals. As the taiji master Zheng Manqing said, "[Taiji] form practice that ignores functional application bestows health benefits that are artificial at best" (Cheng, 1999: 6). Without an in-depth knowledge of martial technique gained from sanshou training, the student will not realize the vibrant health that taijiquan can produce. To understand why this is, we must explore the nature and components of the Yang family's art.

The Taijiquan System

To cultivate martial skill, taijiquan's creators developed a method of training that in many ways resembles the scientific method. Consider that in science, the scientist begins by theorizing some general principle or formula about the world. He conducts extensive research and formulates hypotheses. This is akin to the taiji player practicing the hand form. Through the form's slow, mindful movements, the player visualizes each technique's application, at the same time refining the body mechanics and internal energy (*qi*) circulation required to execute that technique.

For each technique, the practitioner imagines a training partner feeding him an idealized, slow-motion attack. The Chinese term for this partner (either real or imaginary) is *duifang*, literally "opposite direction," a term that has none of the adversarial connotations of its usual English translation, "opponent." The practitioner's responses to their duifang using the form postures are taiji "hypotheses." Master Zheng referred to this method when he instructed his students to "do the form as if someone is there" (Lowenthal, 1991: 109).

The next step for the scientist, once his theories are sound on paper, is to conduct laboratory experiments. He controls all aspects of the test environment, including the qualities of the test subjects and how much freedom of action they have. These procedures clarify the scientist's grasp of the principles underlying his theories.

Tuishou or "push-hands" exercises are one of the taiji player's laboratories. In these paired exercises, each partner attempts to unbalance and topple his now real duifang by redirecting his pushes, thereby creating openings for a counter-technique. By practicing the movements with a real person, one experiences first-hand how important precise timing and point of application are to a movement's effectiveness. The practitioner must develop a tactile sensitivity to the movements of his duifang, a "listening" skill that he uses to sense an incoming technique; he then responds with the appropriate counter at the appropriate time and place. Having gained this awareness of timing and distance in tuishou, the student can now recalibrate the actions of his imaginary duifang during form practice. This increases the accuracy of his responses.

The final test of the scientist is in the wild, where laboratory-tested theories are exposed to the real world's countless variations and uncertainties. As in the laboratory, the scientist analyzes this feedback and further refines his theories. For the taiji player, realizing this "real world" application is difficult (short of picking a fight). The sanshou or "free hands" stage of training described above closely simulates real combat with only those handicaps necessary for relative safety.

The greater distances and more precise timing of a sparring environment make sanshou a more difficult arena than tuishou. Circularizing a punch or kick from a charging duifang is much more challenging that redirecting pushes while in constant physical contact (as in tuishou). Any deficiency in one's practice, be it in body mechanics, understanding of technique, or inadequate listening skills, will greatly impair one's effectiveness. The more challenging setting forces the student to refine his understanding of distance, timing, and each of the form's martial applications.

Taijiquan and Good Health Revisited

With this broader understanding of the taijiquan system, we now have the vocabulary for linking this martial practice to the good health it promotes. When a taiji student practices the solo routine, he moves his body and circulates his internal energy (*qi*) with the express purpose of performing martial applications. The student must rigorously test his knowledge of application and principle in tuishou and sanshou; otherwise, his understanding of martial technique will be shallow, improper, or even absent. Lack of focus in the solo routine will, in turn, result in a low level of internal energy development. Master T.T. Liang said that taijiquan "is a combination of civil and martial aspects," and that "neglecting either [aspect] is not a real [taijiquan]" (Liang, 1974: 54). To shun taijiquan's martial tradition (the martial aspect) is to throw away the very method of internal cultivation (the civil aspect) devised by its creators. The taijiquan practitioner obtains the desired health benefits of the art only by focusing his physical and internal development on specific martial application.

Using this training paradigm, we now turn to exploring how sanshou broadens the practice of taijiquan.

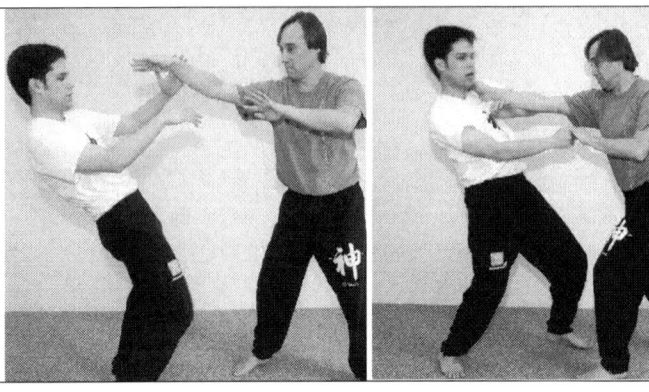

Push-hands is the first step in training the spontaneous use of taijiquan's principles.

Softness and Steel

The Yang family writings, a collection of texts expounding the principles of taijiquan, describe the advanced practitioner's body as "iron concealed in cotton" (Wile, 1983: 12). Although the player's exterior muscles are softened, they mask an inner structure of bones and sinews that is incredibly hard and powerful. This steel-like strength can be expressed at any moment to send the *duifang* flying. Many students, seeking to emulate the cotton "softness" in form practice without first improving their body mechanics, achieve only a spaghetti-like state that lacks strength and will collapse under pressure.

The Chinese term *fangsong*, which is loosely translated as "to relax" but more accurately means "to unclench the muscles," contains the proper method for cultivating this body state. First, the practitioner puts his body in order through stretching and solo routine practice, using the structure of his bones and sinews to support his body instead of external muscular tension. Stretching the waist and lower back are essential to making proper knee and spine alignment possible. Without alignment, the body will collapse and lack strength when trying to execute techniques in tuishou or sanshou.

Only with this framework in place can the practitioner proceed to step two: using the mind to consciously let go of remaining muscular tension, tension accrued from a lifetime of misalignment. The student constantly monitors his body during solo routine practice and while holding postures, letting go of any unnecessary tension (for example, unshrugging the shoulders and letting the elbows hang naturally). One must be clear that the inner "iron" structure is the first requirement; only then can outer "cotton" be achieved.

This new body state increases martial skill in a variety of ways. With less obstructing muscular tension, the taiji player can more easily direct the body's movements and receive its signals. He will be able to use his waist and his internal structure to freely direct his body as one coordinated unit. This will make his steps and attacks more fluid, efficient and effortless.

As his muscles unclench further and further, the advanced practitioner will become increasingly sensitive to tactile information. If, for example, he crosses

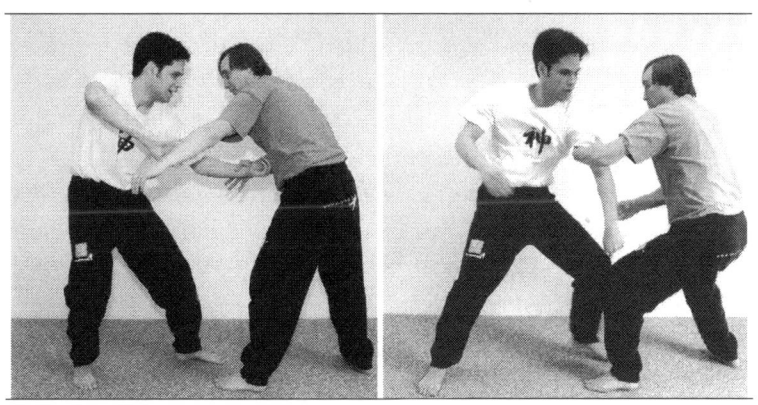

arms with a duifang who tries to give him a two-handed push, the taiji player's *fangsong* allows him to interpret the length and direction of this energy and begin the appropriate deflection. Less and less tension clarifies these signals until the smallest action by the other person triggers the correct response. In this way, the advanced player seems to have foreknowledge of his duifang's intentions. Hence the Yang family saying: "At the opponent's slightest stir, you have already anticipated it and moved beforehand" (Liang, 1974: 29).

Just as a high level of *fangsong* will increase the practitioner's effectiveness in sanshou, understanding the fault of stiff muscle tension will increase his ability to control his duifang. Consider an opposite that sticks his arm out stiffly to punch. This arm functions like a handle or lever connected directly to the duifang's spine. Executing a basic "splitting" technique (*lie*) along the line of this "lever" will disrupt the duifang's spine and, therefore, his entire body structure. During that moment, he becomes completely ineffective and easy to topple.

Stiffness during sanshou practice is not only caused by improper body mechanics; it also occurs when over-extending while "releasing energy" (*fajin*), as in a push. If one pushes to the point where the arms are fully locked, the arms tense and become handles to the spine as described above. Thus, the Yang family taijiquan writings caution that "energy should be preserved slightly [by bending the limbs somewhat] so that there is a surplus in order to avoid exhaustion" (Liang, 1974: 28). While this fault also occurs during tuishou practice, it is more common during sanshou. In the latter, the distance between players is more variable, and practitioners tend to "reach" to connect with their duifang instead of moving their body within range.

Staying Centered: Achieving Calm in Combat

Sanshou practice tests the taiji player's ability to stay calm as much as his ability to execute techniques. Cultivating this skill can pay big dividends, as Scott M. Rodell explains: "Learning not to follow thought when stung in sanshou, it is easier to let go in the everyday" (Rodell, 2005: 49). Conversely, if a student cannot maintain his cool and adhere to the principles during sanshou, he is not prepared to face a truly aggressive duifang or to use his practice in dealing with everyday confrontations.

How a student practices the solo routine has a dramatic effect on how well he will be prepared for tense situations. Improper solo routine practice—tensed from improper body mechanics and without martial intent—prevents students from settling and focusing either their minds, breath, or internal energy (*qi*). During tuishou and sanshou, these same practitioners tense up when pressed by their duifangs, anxiously resisting or dodging blows instead of calmly using their waist to direct the body and deflect the attacks.

Proper form practice cultivates the inner calm needed in the sanshou arena. Master T.T. Liang describes this method for moving towards calmness in his book, *T'ai Chi Ch'uan For Health and Self-Defense* (1974: 74):

Because the movement is slow, it is tranquil; because it is tranquil, the (qi) can sink deeply into the dantian and abide there; when the (qi) can sink deeply and abide in the dantian, then one can maintain oneself firmly. This is called the central equilibrium of mind and (qi). When the mind can be maintained firmly, then a calm unperturbedness can be attained . . .

The taiji player begins this process by placing his mind firmly on the meridian point called the dantian, located three finger-widths beneath the navel. As he learns to execute the form with less tension, the player's breath and qi will sink naturally to the dantian, and he obtains this state of "central equilibrium." With the breath and qi concentrated, the mind will come to rest in the waist where it can consciously direct the entire body. It will then become easier and easier to maintain this cultivated mind-body state during the rigors of sanshou.

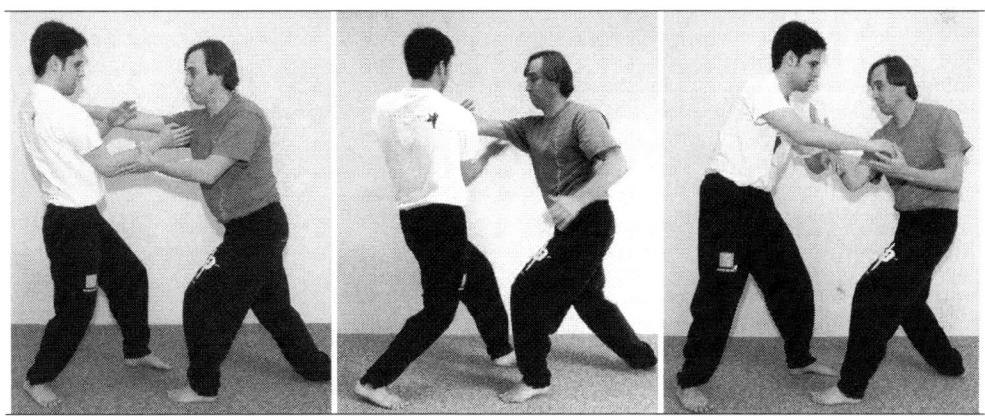

The author and his teacher Scott M. Rodell practicing freeform push-hands.
Quick and soft, concealing internal power, techniques from taijiquan's
repertoire manifest by themselves with proper training.

Victory is Achieved from the Side

Sanshou provides an opportunity to investigate techniques not easily understood through tuishou and form practice alone. For instance, consider the application of the movement "step forward, parry down, punch" from Zheng Manqing's simplified form. This technique illustrates the Yang family saying, "the bull's-eye is reached by attacking from the side" (Wile, 1983: 79). When the duifang attempts a right cross to the face, the taiji player intercepts it with his left hand and deflects it downward, redirecting his opposite's force to the right. The deflected arm becomes a lever that turns the duifang's body, presenting his right floating rib or "soft flank" for attack. The parry has manipulated the opposite's body and exposed his side, a position from which he cannot quickly recover or easily counterattack. In sanshou, the student practices a variety of similar deflections that create openings in the duifang's position.

Separation and Stepping

When practicing the solo routine, the taiji player pays special attention to how he distributes or separates his weight. Each step he takes is empty, with 100% of the body's weight resting on the opposite leg. In this way, the empty or insubstantial leg is free to kick or stomp as well as step. Additionally, good separation sends the mass of the body and spine directly through the weighted leg into the ground, as if you had rammed an upright spear deep into the earth. This rooted, vertical feeling provides a proper axle around which the waist can rotate freely and direct the body.

The taiji boxer can maintain this axle if most of the body's weight is on one leg; he loses the axle when he becomes "double-weighted," meaning each leg holds 50% of the body's weight. In this situation, equal distribution of weight means the spine is equally connected in each leg. The waist now has two competing axles around which it could rotate. Just as a wheel cannot rotate around two axles, double weighting binds the waist, restricting its freedom of motion. Consequently, the taiji player can no longer turn effectively, and all his movements will be slow and clumsy. He will not be able to adapt quickly and freely to his duifang's movements. While this ineffectiveness is visible in tuishou, it is exaggerated in sanshou, where the distance between combatants is greater and the timing of deflections and counters is more precise.

In addition to separation, successful stepping in sanshou requires a deeper understanding of another cardinal taijiquan principle, "the waist is the commander." In his *Mental Elucidation of the Thirteen Postures*, taijiquan Master Wang Zongyue states "when advancing and retreating, it is necessary to turn the body and change the steps" (Liang, 1974: 27). Master T.T. Liang explains this proper method for using the body in his commentary on this classic:

> **"When advancing**
> **and retreating,**
> **it is necessary**
> **to turn the body and**
> **change the steps."**
> – Liang, 1974: 27

Turning the body to regulate the distance between oneself and the duifang is impossible without first having proper separation to give the waist a definite axle to turn around. To compensate for double-weightedness and not using the waist, beginning sanshou students often blindly thrust their legs forward or backward when opportunity or necessity requires it. Instead of using the waist to position themselves for deflections and counters, they simply leap backwards to dodge blows or jump recklessly into perceived openings. This is an extremely imprecise and difficult way for finding a "superior position" from which they can perform techniques.

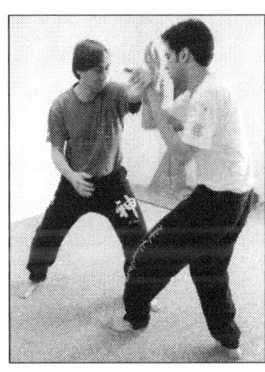
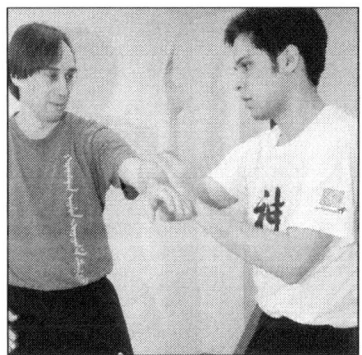
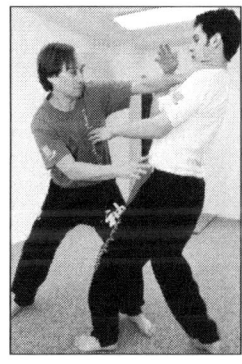

When your opponent strikes the left side of your body so fast that he gives you no chance to counterattack, you must yield and turn your body slightly to the left, while stepping back with your left foot to regain a favorable and superior position. After you have regained a superior position, you must turn your body slightly to the right if you want to counterattack with your left hand.

Listening Skills: Linking Tuishou and Sanshou

The taijiquan student is first introduced to the concept of "listening" (*ting jin*) during fixed-step single-hand tuishou. In this exercise, the two players face each other in opposing bow stances and touch forearms on the same side as their leading foot. The exercise begins when one side initiates a push anywhere above the belt and below the collar, such as pushing through their duifang's arm towards the right side of their body. It is then the other player's job to listen to the push through their tactile contact, deflect the incoming force and, if possible, counter.

It is important to note that tuishou matches aren't about swatting pushes aside and lunging at the duifang. The taiji player practices "sticking and following," two terms which he must understand to gain this tactile "listening" ability. "Sticking" means that the practitioner neither loses contact with nor offers resistance against the movements of the duifang. In this way, one can maintain constant awareness of the duifang's intentions through touch.

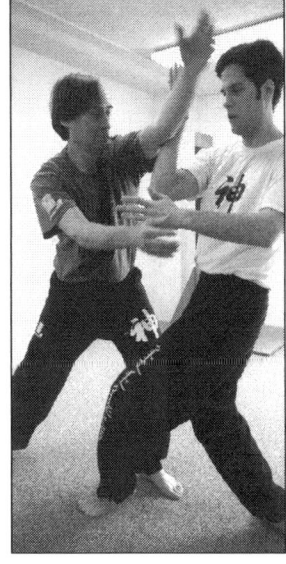

Knowing the duifang's intentions alone is not enough; one must also know the proper response. "Following" means not initiating a set offense of your own but allowing your opposite's actions to determine the appropriate response. As a simple example, consider a duifang that strikes the taiji boxer with his left hand. One appropriate response is to execute the basic technique "split" (*lie*). Turning his waist to the right, the boxer deflects the strike to his right arm. The turning of his waist simultaneously causes the left hand to shoot out in a counterattack. Before the duifang attacked, there was no intent to strike from the left. The boxer simply listened to his opposite's intent and allowed the offered attack to determine his response. The duifang has defeated himself; the taiji boxer is simply the means to that end.

In sanshou, one applies the listening skills developed in tuishou across the greater distances of free sparring. The student must use the techniques of sticking and following, even though he is not always in physical contact with the duifang. The Yang family secret transcripts describe this increased ability to "interpret energy":

> Only when one understands
> the visual awareness of looking far,
> near, left and right; the aural awareness
> of rising, falling, slowness, and haste;
> the kinesthetic awareness of dodge,
> return, provoke and finish;
> and the movement awareness of turn, exchange,
> advance, and retreat, can one truly be said
> to have mastered interpreting energy.
> – Wile (Trans.), 1983: 92

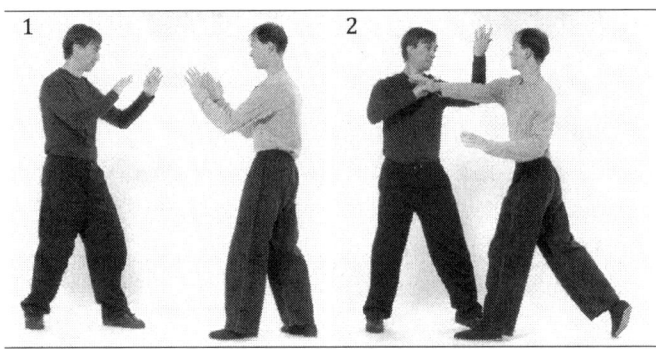

Here, Rauno Gordon attempts to strike Rodell, who uses
the deflection rollback into "brush knee and strike."

This full awareness of the duifang cannot be understood through form practice and tuishou alone. They simply do not provide the speed or variety of attacks that will properly season a student's understanding of how to execute taijiquan techniques. He will not learn how to stick to and follow his opponent in a manner not bounded by tactile contact.

In tuishou, the student must stick to his duifang continuously, always ready to respond appropriately to an attack or retreat. In sanshou, the situation is no different. Usually, the beginner will stick and adapt until he takes the offensive, at which point the greater distances of sanshou will force him to overreach and lock his arms (as described in the section on *fangsong*). Tensing up in this fashion makes it difficult for the student to remain calm and aware of his duifang, and he cannot respond appropriately if his opposite deflects and counters. The Yang family writings were aware of this possibility and cautioned that "the energy may be broken off [i.e. discharged], but the mind-intent remains" (Liang, 1974: 30). Even when the taiji player discharges into his duifang, he must remain mentally connected to him, aware of his position and intent and ready to continue adapting.

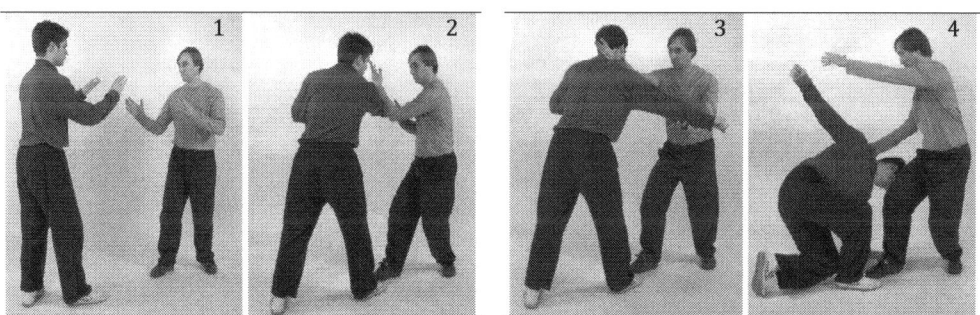

Rodell intercepts the attack with this left elbow and swings
his left forearm downward, creating an opening on the neck for his right hand.
A circular movement right ward off off-balances the attacker into an effortless throw.

Sticking continuously also allows the taiji player to maintain the initiative when on the offensive. The reality is that in sanshou, the sparring is almost never ended with only one strike; a combination of counters that act as one is necessary to subdue the duifang. If the sanshou player is always aware of his duifang's position and intent, he can keep constant pressure on his opposite and maintain the upper hand. A focused series of attacks based on continuously sticking to and following the duifang will be increasingly difficult to neutralize. The taiji player's listening skills allow him to be a step ahead of his partner's deflections, forcing the latter to deal with a new attack before he has even recovered from the previous one. Yang Luchan, the founder of Yang Style taijiquan, called this "movement like a mighty river" (Wile, 1983: 109), bowling over the hapless duifang. With such skill, victory is a matter of discerning opportunity.

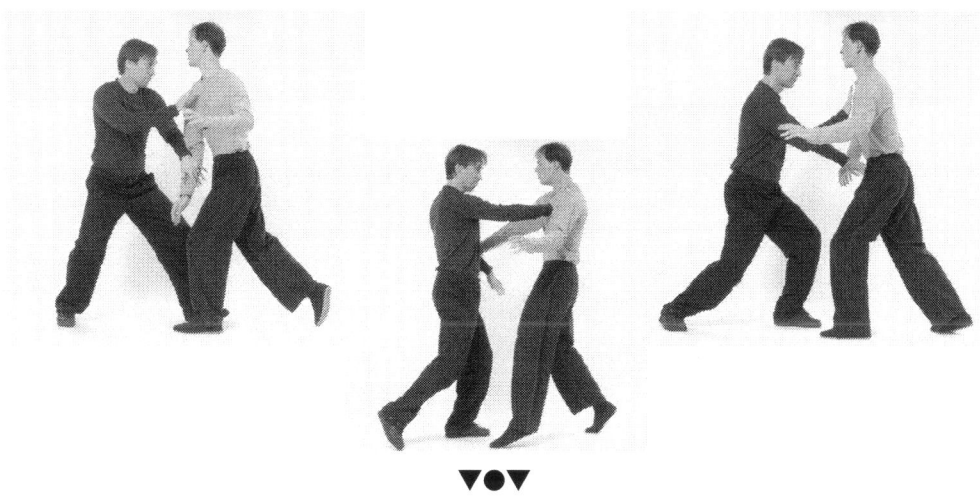

▼●▼

Chinese	**Terms**
dantian	丹田
duifang	對方
fajin	發勁
fangsong	鬆
lie	挒
qi	氣
sanshou	散手
taijiquan	太極拳
ting jin	聽勁
tuishou	推手

Acknowledgment

Special thanks to Great River Taoist Center and teacher Scott M. Rodell for all the training, editorial input, and inspiration. All push-hands photographs courtesy of Tim Fenoglio.

Bibliography

Chen, Gong (1943). *Taijiquan dao jian gan sanshou hebian* (Combined taijiquan, broadsword, double-edged sword, staff, and sparring). n.p.

Cheng, Man-ching (1999). *Master Cheng's new method of t'ai chi self-cultivation.* Trans. Mark Hennessy. Berkeley, CA: North Atlantic Books.

Liang, T. (1974). *T'ai chi ch'uan for health and self-defense.* New York: Vintage Books.

Lowenthal, W. (1991). *There are no secrets: Professor Cheng Man-Ch'ing and his tai chi chuan.* Berkeley, CA: North Atlantic Books.

Rodell, S. (2005). *Taiji notebook for martial artists.* Annandale, VA: Seven Stars Books and Video.

Wile, D. (Trans.). (1983). *T'ai-chi touchstones: Yang family secret transmissions.* Brooklyn, NY: Sweet Ch'i Press.

Yang, Chengfu (1931). *Taijiquan shiyongfa* (Taijiquan practical methods). n.p. Reprinted as Taijiquan Yongfa Tujie. Taipei: Wuzhou Chu-banshi, 1996.

Yang, Chengfu (1934). *Taijiquan tiyong quanshu* (Complete form and practice of taijiquan). Hong Kong, n.p. Reprinted, Taipei: Wu Xue guan (Lion Books), 2001.

Ge Hong: Famous Daoist Thinker and Practical Martial Artist
by Stanley E. Henning, M.A.

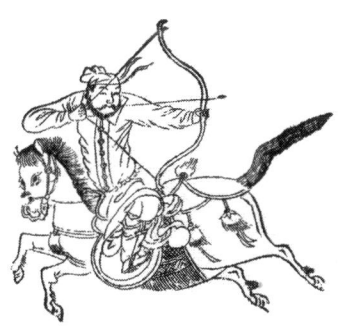

While in the military, Ge Hong killed two pursuers and a horse with archery from horseback. The illustration is from a 1609 edition of *Comprehensive Illustrated Encyclopedia* (*Sancai Tuhui*). Courtesy of the University of Hawaii, Hamilton Library.

Ge Hong, also named Zhichuan (Youthful River) and Baopuzi (One Who Embraces Simplicity) (283–363 CE), known primarily for his Daoist pursuits, was not only an important intellectual figure of his time, but also a military officer versed in martial arts. Although he only offers a few short lines on the subject in all his writings, they reveal valuable insights into the place of martial arts in society and aspects of their practice through the ages to modern times.

Ge Hong was a fascinating individual: a combination Confucian, Legalist, and Daoist intellectual, military officer, and official who had practiced martial arts and experienced combat, and a Daoist recluse and alchemist. In sum, his philosophy was to cultivate the inner saint and perfect the outer prince; to seek immortality through good works, other Daoist practices including alchemy, and improve the world by implementing the moral and legal way.

In the "Outer Chapters" of his *Baopuzi*, Ge Hong discusses success and failure in human affairs and what is permissible in matters belonging to the realm of Confucianism. It is no accident that he mentions martial arts in his postscript to this section as opposed to the "Inner Chapters," which he dedicates to Daoist pursuits. Ge Hong may actually be reflecting satire within his self-effacing tone that contrasts his own postscript to the "Outer Chapters" with that of Three Kingdom's Emperor Wei Wendi's (a.k.a. Cao Pi, 187–226 CE) postscript to *Discussing the Classics* (*Dian Lun*).[1] He notes that the Emperor's purpose was to speak of things he knew, such as archery, chess and fencing in which he was adept, while Ge Hong, on the contrary, claims to speak of things that he is not good at, including martial arts.

The Emperor boasts about his archery skills in hunting and his demonstration at a feast with a stick of sugar cane as a sword to thrice defeat General Deng Zhan's famed bare-hand-against-weapons fighting skills.[2] Ge Hong, on the other hand, merely notes in passing that he is not as skilled as young boys in throwing tiles and boxing (basic martial arts skills) and that, although he was not particularly strong in drawing a bow, he once had to use his mounted archery to kill two men and a horse to save his skin. He notes that archery was one of the Six Arts (Confucian disciplines including rites, music, mathematics, writing, charioteering and archery) that could also be used to defend against bandits or for hunting. He then notes that he had studied broadsword and shield, single-handed broadsword and double halberds and, later in life, seven-foot staff with which one could counter the blade of the large halberd. Finally, he explains that all the martial arts have secret formulas to describe important techniques and secret, mysterious methods to overcome an opponent. If an opponent was unaware of these, one could defeat him every time. In other words, Ge Hong was no mere novice.

When pieced together, Ge Hong's comments in his postscript to the *Baopuzi Outer Chapters* along with Emperor Wei Wendi's postscript to *Discussing the Classics*, which Ge Hong references, provide a panoramic view of the martial arts in Chinese society of his time. To begin with, we can see that the martial arts were widely practiced in one form or another at all levels and by all elements of society, from leaders to the commoners who formed militias. Even the literati were familiar with archery, one of the Six Arts they were expected to learn. Among various forms of play, many young males practiced boxing and the martial arts related sport of tile/stone tossing (for accuracy and distance).[3] These arts were practiced as worldly, not religious or spiritual activities, as Ge Hong clearly reflects. Later sources reveal that martial arts were practiced in Buddhist monasteries as well, after all, monks also came from society at large, and monastic property needed to be protected, especially in times of famine and political unrest. In any case, Ge Hong lived over 100 years prior to the founding of Shaolin Monastery, most well-known for its later association with the martial arts.

As for the incident between Emperor Wei Wendi and General Deng Zhan, the latter's touted ability to defeat an armed opponent using his bare hands is an example of what boxing was really all about in those days—basic training for use of weapons, to assist in the use of weapons in some cases, and to use as a last resort when one was weaponless.[4]

Finally, Ge Hong refers to the role of oral formulas (*kojue*) and secret methods (*mifa*) to support martial arts practices. These were mnemonic devices (common to the Chinese learning process of memorization) that provided insights on proper technique in practice. Ge Hong emphasizes that the techniques described in these oral formulas and/or secret methods can be effective if the opponent does not know them (they describe fighting tactics and techniques). They were often unintelligible or unclear to those outside the group that used them in training. They were brought to life by the hands-on instruction of one's teacher.

Ge Hong's concise, matter of fact comments on martial arts practices in his time provide us one of the best descriptions ever written. This description is, in turn, a key to our understanding of the role of the martial arts in Chinese society over the centuries. As for Ge Hong himself, he spent his final years in seclusion, seeking the path to immortality through alchemy at Mount Luofu outside Guangzhou.

Notes

1. It seems plausible that Ge Hong's reference to Cao Pi's postscript to the *Dian Lun* is meant to be a rejoinder to the condescending way citizens of the northern Kingdom of Wei viewed their counterparts, such as Ge Hong, from the southern Kingdom of Wu—barbarians who fastened their garments from the left side.
2. Deng Zhan is described as good at boxing/grappling (*shoubi*) and use of the five weapons (*wubing/wurong*), listed in the *Li Ji* (*Record of Rites*) as, bow and arrow, lance, spear, pike, and halberd. Also see Green, Vol. 1 (2001: 67).
3. The Former Han History (77 CE) notes that the military officer, Gan Yanshou, was exceptionally strong and practiced boxing and stone tossing.
4. The Cefu Yuangui (1013 CE) describes a three-day battle that took place in 582 between Chinese troops and a Turkic Tujue army. The Chinese fended off the Tujue force, but not before losing over 80 percent of their men and, with their weapons reduced, fighting the Tujue off with their bare fists to the point that one could reportedly see the bones in their hands. Chapter 395 cont. p. 4694. Also see Green, Vol. 1 (2001: 67).

Bibliography – English

Green, T. (Ed.) (2001). *Martial arts of the world: An encyclopedia*. 2 Volumes. Santa Barbara, CA: ABC-CLIO.

Knapp, K. Ge Hong [*Internet Encyclopedia of Philosophy*]. A summary of Ge Hong's life and thought. <http://www.iep.utm.edu/g/gehong.htm>

Bibliography – Romanized Chinese

Ban Gu (1936). *Former Han history*. Shanghai: Zhonghua Press.

Chen Feilong (2002). *Baopuzi outer chapters, modern notes and translation*. Taiwan Commercial Press.

Critique of Literature. <http://ef.cdpa.nsysu.edu.tw/ccw/03/dl.htm>

Li Gang. Ge Hong and his humanistic philosophy. <http://www.siwen.org/xxlr1.asp?id=299>

Wang Liqo (1974). *Discussion of Ge Hong*. Taibei: Wunan Press.

Wang Mengou (1997). *Record of rites—Modern notes and translation. Vol. 1.* Taiwan Commercial Press.

Wang Ming (1985). *An explanation of the Baopuzi internal chapters*. Beijing: Zhonghua Press.

Wang Qinruo (1960). *Library of the grand tortoise* (1013). Hong Kong: Zhonghua Press.

Benefits of Non-Competitive Push-Hands Practice
by Herman P. Kauz

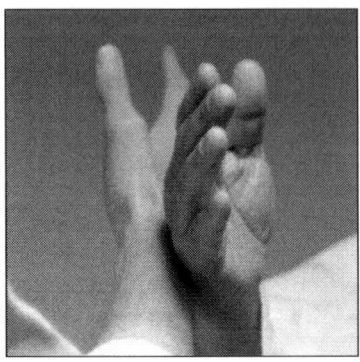

Photograph courtesy of Akiko O. Dykhuizen.

Introduction

In recent years we have learned about the health benefits of taijiquan (usually shortened to taiji). *Taiji* means to most of us a slow-motion set of connected movements resembling boxing, performed solo. It is widely practiced in China, especially by older people. Chinese city parks are filled early each morning with people doing various forms of exercise, a strong contingent of taiji practitioners among them. This practice strengthens legs, improves balance, calms the mind and spirit, and generally improves mental and physical health.

Related to this solo form exercise is a practice called push-hands. Here two persons face one another and attempt to break one another's balance using only a minimum of strength. It is generally done slowly from a fixed foot position. That is, if you are losing your balance, stepping in any direction to regain it is incorrect. The couple then breaks off and returns to a few moves of a simple form which precedes a freer style of attack and counterattack.

The reason we generally practice with a fixed foot position is that our response in both attack and defense comes primarily from a change in our body position and not through a foot movement. We must react to an attack by shifting our center and by yielding to the slightest pressure. The "center" is that point on the body where our opponent can control us. This point is constantly shifting as the opponent attempts to break our balance and as we try to evade.

As an attack is mounted, the defender not only neutralizes it but attempts simultaneously to counterattack. The attacker is somewhat vulnerable to a counter as he gets to that point in his forward movement where his weight is equally distributed between his feet. This is termed "double weighting" and results in a temporarily weakened position. If the defender counterattacks at this point, the attacker must neutralize it and continue the attack. We say that attacking is yang and defending is yin. But as we see in the taiji circle, yang has a small circle of yin in it, and yin a small circle of yang. Thus, while the defender mainly yields (*yin*) he also at the right moment counters (*yang*). The attacker is mostly yang, but he yields (*yin*) to the defender's countermove.

These attacks and counters often occur in split seconds. Though we attempt to practice slowly, our opponent may suddenly speed up, and we must keep pace. Another complication lies in our attempt to use only a minimum of strength to attack or to counter. Often, we use more than a few ounces of pressure in whatever we do, allowing a more skillful opponent to use this overdoing against us. We try then to be rooted in our feet and to be relaxed and flexible from the ankles up. We might think of the body as a piece of hanging cloth which absorbs and neutralizes an incoming force without harm. The attacker might then overextend and lose balance, expecting a solid surface and meeting no resistance.

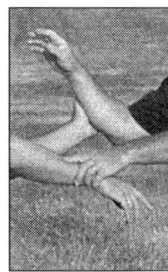 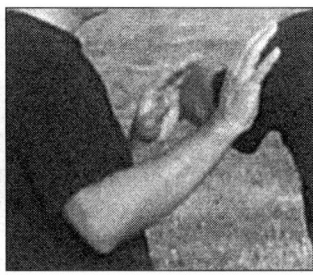 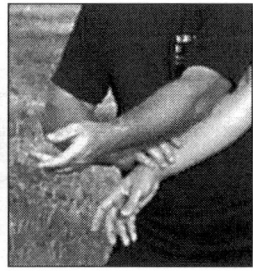

Photographs by Donna Bernardini.

The relaxed alertness and calmness gained from solo form practice is clearly going to be more difficult to maintain when your partner is trying to upset your balance. If we sense aggressiveness from our partner or an unwillingness to yield, we may become angry. All the difficulties we may have in dealing with others in daily life will gradually make an appearance. If we are open to it, we can learn a great deal about ourselves in push-hands. Most of us, as nothing we do works to our satisfaction, will experience some degree of frustration. We will try to follow our teacher's suggestion to avoid both resisting a push and pushing into hardness. Our teacher will show many times that resisting a push to maintain our balance will cause the opponent to instantly attack from a different direction and the game will be over. Also, attacking a point that seems unyielding with more strength gives the opponent a chance to suddenly yield, causing our overextension and loss of balance.

When a problem comes up in our daily life, we try to think of a solution. Logical, linear thought might be of some use in trying to figure out what is going on in push-hands. But in the moment the action occurs any advance planning or strategy will probably fail because you can't predict the opponent's response. Moreover, trying to think in push-hands will cause one's body to tense while figuring things out. More importantly, as beginners, we are limited in awareness and are often too hard, too tense, or our timing is faulty. So even if we do our best to follow our teacher's directions, we are incapable of doing what is required. To begin to get a sense of what is going on, our awareness and sensitivity must grow and sharpen. This is a never-ending process. Continuing to make progress in this direction requires almost daily push-hands practice. But, if we practice incorrectly, by using strength, for example, our progress will be slow or nonexistent. What is ultimately required is an internalization by our physical and mental systems of an instant thought-free response to the slightest stimulus. Moreover, to be successful, our response must consist of an optimum mix of softness, sensitivity, and timing, to name just a few qualities.

The process resembles that experienced by the Zen archery student, who must practice endlessly to lose a shot which he does not let go consciously. Instead, in a particular moment the archer, the bow, the arrow, and the target become one. To cite another example, the solution to a Zen koan cannot be rationally arrived at but must come in some other way. In both archery and Zen, the student does all he can to get a hoped-for result. This means he will use his mental and physical ability to do what seems to be required, only to have his efforts rejected or deemed unsuccessful. This sad situation may last a few years, but his efforts, or non-efforts, may one day bear fruit, only to be followed by a further period of failure.

Focusing again on push-hands, common student errors are failing to find the opponent's center, using too much strength, resisting an attack and trying to think their way through the pushing process. If our opponent is more skillful than we, every pushing encounter will result in failure. This outcome can be quite frustrating, unless the student comes to the training with no expectations or preconceived ideas and is willing to be open to what unfolds as he attempts to follow taiji principles. There is no final goal—it is an endless refining process.

It is only an illusion that the sought for result in push-hands is to push the opponent or to avoid a push. Instead, we should be trying to react in a thought-free way to what our system senses in the moment. This pattern stops the stream of thought having to do with past or future and puts us, if even for a little while, fully in the present. Halting our incessant mind chatter is a marvelous method for opening us to a sense of the spirit (or whatever one wants to call it) that permeates or suffuses us and everything around us. This aspect of push-hands may seem a bit too extreme or esoteric for some, but it is there for those who are ready for it. The benefits for our lives with this emphasis far outweigh those which accrue from limiting ourselves to just the physical.

Push-hands training then can be regarded as learning to become more responsive and more sensitive. To help us in this direction, all our attacking and defending moves should be limited to a mere few ounces of pressure. If we employ even a little too much force, a skillful opponent will use our overdoing against us. Also, all we need do is to unbalance our opponent. The instant this occurs, were it a self-defense situation, we could deliver a further attack to a vulnerable point. Pushing someone 10 or 20 feet away is regarded, from a practical standpoint, as losing your opponent. Unless he is at the edge of a cliff, he has a chance to regroup or to avail himself of a weapon and then return to the fray.

If our reason for doing push-hands is to develop improved fighting ability, we could well retard our development of the more important responsiveness and sensitivity we seek. It is true that push-hands practice can lay a superb foundation for fighting arts, but too great an emphasis on fighting techniques as we do push-hands will make us harder. I taught a kind of self-defense to taiji students for over twenty years, to familiarize them with attacks from punches, strikes, and kicks. I don't think this training helped much to improve students' abilities in push-hands, though it gave them some measure of self-defense ability.

At any rate, we are far better served, in terms of positive benefits, by developing our sensitivity. Even for martially oriented individuals, gaining additional awareness and acting in a timely way to defuse a situation is far superior to having to physically engage an opponent.

As our push-hands develops over the years, we may be fortunate enough to encounter a highly developed practitioner who offers no resistance and whose center is unavailable. While we are searching for some slight degree of solidity, we find we have overextended and somehow have lost our balance. If we use more strength and speed, the result is worse. Everyone who does push-hands seems to approve of softness and yielding and even to believe that is how they are pushing. An actual experience with someone who is skilled may open our eyes to the vast possibilities for development in the physical aspects of push-hands. Of course, we will want to know how we can reach this higher level. The answer is to give up strength, and to "invest in loss," as Zheng Manqing (1902–1975) put it. By this he meant avoid all resistance and try to learn from each push.

We are also faced with another problem. Language is inadequate to express what goes on in push-hands. This statement sounds like nonsense but try as we might we really can't put into words what is happening in a particular moment. We can talk about the moment before it occurs and after it has occurred, but in the instant, something happens our trained physical and mental system responds, either successfully or not. Many factors come together in a particular moment and thinking about what is happening will inhibit movement. We might well become frozen and fail to move at the right time. Essentially, we will have lost the flow.

A few hurdles, some rather high, stand in the way of our practicing to rise to a higher level. Among them are such handicaps as a strong body, skill in other martial arts, and a competitive turn of mind. One's system will respond to an emergency by doing what it has been trained to do. Changing a previous conditioning is the work of many years. Reverting to what our systems have previously learned will keep those connections alive and functioning. New connections must form in the brain and in our body if our response is going to change. These slowly form as we practice correctly over the years. If we can't give up what we have, we will fail to move in the direction we believe we want to go, no matter how long and hard we practice.

Our competitive culture has spawned push-hands contests. The Chinese also engage in such competition. Training to win such a contest will probably produce a different attitude toward push-hands than if "winning" in an encounter is of no consequence. We will tend to use strength, become ruthless, and generally ignore or give only lip service to the push-hands advice found in the *Taiji Classics*.

Push-hands styles range from a kind of Japanese sumo wrestling to the very sensitive. The classics state that if even a fly lights on your shoulder, your body should be set in motion. It takes many years of practice to develop the ability to perform in this lighter and more responsive way. But our impatience for results and craving for success will lead to our resisting pushes and to using too much strength. Possibilities for mental and spiritual growth are present in all martial arts. But when these arts are practiced as sport, the emphasis is on winning. Taijiquan practice is also vulnerable to this interpretation. There is no question in my mind that this approach, unfortunately, precludes the attainment of the kind of development we say we are seeking.

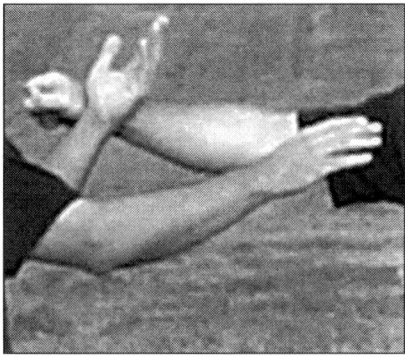

Photographs by Donna Bernardini.

My teacher, Zheng Manqing, among others, spoke of push-hands as a precious gem. He would teach everyone the taiji solo form because it would improve their health. But he refused to teach everyone push-hands. Those of us who practice correctly over the decades would probably also conclude that we have been given something of great value.

Taijiquan and Daoism:
From Religion to Martial Art and Martial Art to Religion
by Douglas Wile, Ph.D.

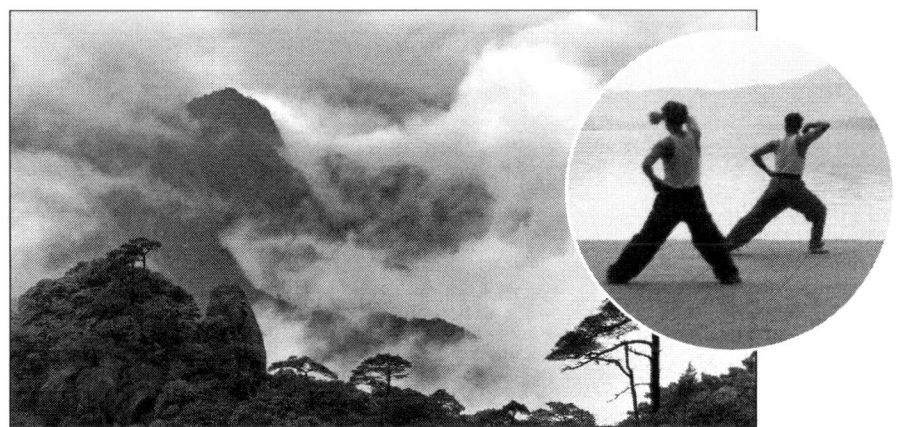

Misty scene over Wudang Mountains. Courtesy of www.photo2easy.com. Chen Style taiji practice along West Lake in Hangzhou city. Photograph by Michael DeMarco.

Introduction

The question of taijiquan's origins—and specifically whether they are Daoist or not—is no mere academic exercise but a major theater in China's culture wars for nearly a century. A recent mass-market book *Five Hundred Unsolved Mysteries in China's Cultural History* lists the origins of taijiquan as one of Chinese history's most contentious cases. In the 1930s, Tang Hao (1897–1959), China's first modern martial arts historian, was the target of an assassination plot for daring to unmask the myth of taiji's Daoist origins, and in 1999 a prominent martial arts journal, *Jingwu*, after ten years of extensive coverage, declared a moratorium on the topic. Why all the fuss?

From the middle of the 19th century to the beginning of the 21st, taijiquan has played a very public role in China's cultural life. Exponents of taijiquan were active in the self-strengthening campaigns of the late Qing Reform Movement and Nationalist Revolution; taijiquan played a leading role in the national and provincial martial arts academies of the Republican period; it was standardized and popularized for the masses during the Mao era (1949–1976); and today, taijiquan is still the site of hostile clashes between modernizers and traditionalists, even as it increasingly becomes a leading cultural export and tourist attraction. What began in the 17th century with Huang Zongxi's (1610–1695) wrapping a martial art in religion has come down in the 21st century to Neo-Zhang Sanfeng cultists wrapping religion in a martial art. This chapter will explore the ways in which the construction and deconstruction of a martial arts-Daoist connection has figured in political ideology, cultural identity, and commercial interest during the past century of Chinese history.

Defining taijiquan is at least as controversial as defining Daoism itself. If there are three Daoisms—philosophical, religious, and macrobiotic—there are also three taijis—martial, meditative, and medical. Similarly, there are three stereotypes of taiji masters: recluses who perfect their art with the help of nature or supernatural forces, secret masters living in the world who reveal their art only when pressed or for righteous causes, and public masters who defend the honor of their lineage and accept all challenges. We can trace taijiquan as a philosophy or a lineage, a generic or a brand. All styles claim Daoist philosophical content, and most claim to be successors to a transmission originating with a famous Daoist immortal. The terms "Daoist" and "Confucian" function in Chinese society with roughly the same degree of precision as do liberal and conservative in the West. A Daoist is someone who gathers herbs on misty mountains and meditates in a cave; by contrast, a Confucian sits on a throne or adjudicates stacks of lawsuits. A Daoist seeks seclusion, whereas a Confucian is asked to leave. All the arts and sciences are automatically ceded to Daoism by default because of Confucianism's "amateur ideal" and its distain for instrumental knowledge and individualism. Hence, painting, calligraphy, and poetry are considered Daoist arts; medicine is considered a Daoist science; and even military strategy has a Daoist mystique. The rise of taijiquan represents the attempt to assimilate martial arts into high culture, and for this purpose, only Daoism will do. Methodologically, the history of taijiquan has been told by materialists and idealists. The materialist, or humanist, says that trial and error, or practice, precedes theory, and that knowledge is cumulative, synthetic, and cross-disciplinary; the idealist believes in a transcendent realm of laws or principles accessible only to divine beings or great men. Essentially, the debate in taijiquan historiography has been between creationism and evolution. Of the three kinds of masters in the *Zhuangzi*—sages, craftsmen, and freaks—the creationists side with the sages, the humanists with the craftsmen, and the freaks we will save for the end of our story.

What are the role, status, identity, and image of the martial artist in traditional Chinese society? Bodyguards, bandits, family feudists, militiamen, assassins, knights-errant, rebels, opera singers, and market place performers. The army had no use for martial artists, either because their skills were flowery and impractical, or because solo virtuosos did not function well in battlefield formation. The subordination of military to civilian authority in politics and the elevation of the civil (*wen*) and military (*wu*) to virtual cosmological categories has allowed the scholar to maintain superiority over the warrior.

The best-known association of martial arts with religion in China is the Shaolin monks. As early as the Northern Wei (220–265), they had alternately been persecuted for participating in rebellions but at other times were enlisted by emperors to put down rebellion, piracy, and invasion. Martial arts were most likely to be officially banned during foreign dynasties, such as Mongol and Manchu, and martial arts training, together with quasi-religious doctrines and rituals, were often part of the lure and threat of secret societies. Martial dance for religious ritual and pure esthetics goes back to our earliest written records in China, but the marriage of qigong energetics with a martial art is not attested in detail until Chang Naizhou in the 18th century, a development that reaches its peak with taijiquan in the 19th and 20th centuries.

Whether we define Daoism as an institution with card-carrying members or a certain band on a perennial philosophical spectrum, there is no escaping the heroic efforts to associate or disassociate taijiquan with Daoism. Chinese thinking is often characterized as "correlative" to distinguish it from Western notions of linear causality. Analyzing states and changes based on yin and yang, the five phases, and stems and branches is indeed one mode of Chinese thinking. However, when direct causality is employed, say to assert that the immortal Zhang Sanfeng created taijiquan, we must decide whether this is ignorance, deception, or a discursive practice that places the Wudang Mountains, Zhang Sanfeng, the Internal School, Laozi, the *Yijing*, and taijiquan in a single narrative for the same reason that traditional medicine includes the kidney, "gate of life," foot *shao-yin* channel, ears, brain, hair, nails, anus, the color black, water, and winter, in the "kidney orb." Is it religious faith, the mythic mind, or simply another kind of rational thought? Is building up layer upon layer of Daoist associations for this martial art a form of magical protection against predatory appropriation? This chapter will explore both the ways in which taijiquan partakes of Daoist theory and the efforts to align taijiquan with Daoism. The continued outpouring of fictional accounts of taiji history in the 21st century may appear to be transparently political or commercial, but sometimes it can only be explained as the persistence of a cultural practice that refuses to conform to modern notions of "fact" and the search for a Chinese style of spirituality that retains faith in psychosomatic self-perfection and the possibility of embodied immortality.

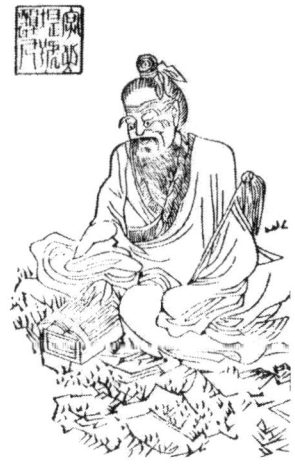

Illustration of Zhang Sanfeng taken from the *Collected Works of Zhang Sanfeng* (1844). Illustration courtesy of Douglas Wile.

Zhang Sanfeng and the Internal School

In the 1650s, after years of resistance to Manchu consolidation in the South, philosopher Huang Zongxi (1610–1695) gave up armed struggle and retired to his native Yuyao in Zhejiang Province, where he undertook a comprehensive reassessment of the philosophical and political roots of China's weakness. Among his prolific writings is the *Epitaph for Wang Zhengnan*, written for a former comrade-in-arms, whom Huang praises as a great martial artist, fierce patriot, and righteous knight-errant. He describes Wang as the only living successor to a martial arts lineage called the Internal School (*neijia*) and names Zhang Sanfeng as its founder. He locates Zhang in the Song dynasty, calls him a "Daoist alchemist," and says that Zhang invented the art by reversing Shaolin's reliance on hardness and emphasizing the defensive and offensive advantages of softness.

Huang Zongxi's son, Huang Baijia, himself a student of Wang Zhengnan, wrote a manual of the Internal School art, attributing Zhang Sanfeng's inspiration to a visitation by Xuanwu (God of War) in a dream. As set forth in Baijia's *Internal School's Boxing Methods*, the form bears little resemblance to taijiquan as we know it, contains no reference to internal training, and apart from its soft-style strategy is chiefly distinguished by its pressure point techniques. Moreover, Baijia says that as Wang's only student, the transmission will die with him. The reader is left to ponder whether the Huangs uncritically recorded Wang's account of the Internal School's origins or used biography to encrypt a political allegory for China's survival strategy under Manchu rule.

Contradictions abound: Huang Zongxi was one of the most sober rationalists in Chinese intellectual history and not given to myth making; he was personally opposed to alchemy and the self-delusion of immortality; there is no record of a "Zhang Sanfeng" in the Song dynasty (960–1279); and there is no mention in the Ming (1368–1644) histories or hagiographies of Zhang Sanfeng of any connection between the immortal and the martial arts, just as there are none between Bodhidharma and Shaolin gongfu in the Buddhist literature. The 19th century *Complete Works of Zhang Sanfeng* and 20th century *Zhang Sanfeng's Secret Transmissions on Taiji Elixir Cultivation* do not contain a single credible text, let alone one on martial arts. In other words, Zhang Sanfeng, the immortal martial artist and his Internal School, appear out of nowhere in the Huangs' *Epitath for Wang Zhengnan* and *Internal School's Boxing Methods* and disappear without a trace until the turn of the 20th century, when the first generation of mass market taiji publications begin to name Zhang Sanfeng as the father of taijiquan and the Internal School of Wudang as its precursor.

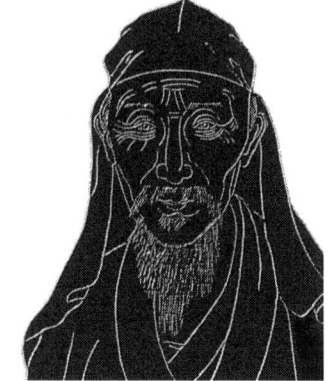

Drawing of Huang Zongxi dated 1873.

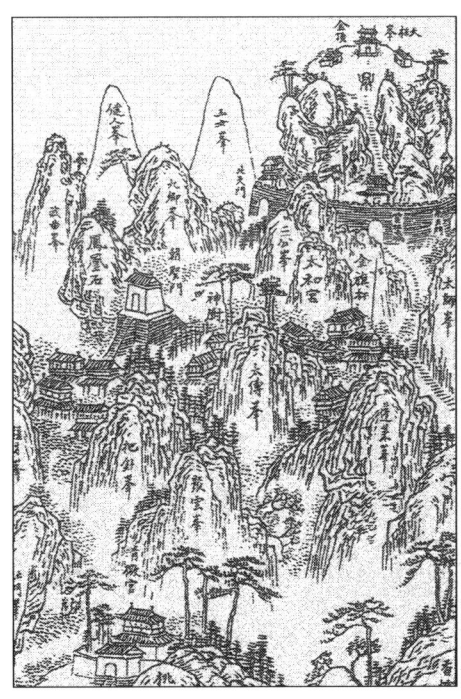

Illustration of Wudang from *Dayue Taiheshan Gazetteer* dated 1922.

Lineage and Legitimacy

Lineage has been an important means of establishing political legitimacy in China from at least the time of the Shang aristocracy, and it is no less important in the arts. In the Asian martial arts, status devolves from style founder to sons of style founders to "indoor students" of style founders or their sons, and finally to public students, ranked by successive removes. The most prestigious credentials in taijiquan are personal study with members of the Chen, Yang, Wu/Hao, Wu, or Sun families. More esoteric transmissions, usually claiming Daoist origins, are traced from master to disciple, without resort to kinship ties. Lineage establishes personal credentials, but styles often invoke historical, semi-historical, or supernatural founders as totemistic figureheads for the transmission as a whole. Perhaps the only exception in the taiji world is the Chen family, who have simply mythologized their own genealogy. Rather than be left out in the cold, most styles have followed the Yang family lead and adopted Zhang Sanfeng as the patron saint of taijiquan. In keeping with the hard-soft taxonomy established by the Huangs, the terms "Wudang" and "Internal School" became generic designations for martial arts based on yielding and qi cultivation, thus allowing xingyi and bagua to be grafted onto the Internal School tree as sharing the same principles, though lacking a direct line to a Daoist immortal. Where the seams begin to show is in the inconsistency of legendary narratives and in the splicing of the legendary onto the historical period.

For the sake of convenience, and to some degree coherence, let us trace the fathering of taijiquan onto a Daoist lineage through the various styles, style founders, and authors. The first published work introducing taijiquan to the world was Sun Lutang's (1861–1932) 1919 *The Study of Taijiquan*. Sun, student of Hao Weizhen (1842–1920) and founder of the Sun Style, credits Zhang Sanfeng as the founder of taijiquan but gives no biographical details. He weaves the various creation myths of three martial arts into a chronology, starting with Bodhidharma and Shaolin, followed by Yue Fei and xingyi, and culminating with Zhang Sanfeng "of the Yuan" with taijiquan. Omitting bagua from his narrative, he specifies that Zhang created taiji as a corrective to the harmful hard-style exercises practiced by his fellow immortality seekers. Although the Sun Style continues to be practiced, there are no other major books in this transmission. Hao Weizhen's teacher Li Yiyu (1832–1892) says in his *Short Introduction to Taijiquan* that, "the origins of the art are unknown" (Gu, 1982: 376), and since the Zhang Sanfeng of the *Epitath for Wang Zhengnan* is Song, the source of Sun's attribution seems to be some vague body of martial arts lore. Moving from the mythic to the legendary to the historical, he names Wang Zongyue as author of the classics and Wu Yuxiang (1812–1880) as the link to Chen Qingping (1795–1868) in Zhaobao. This geneology is remarkable for completely leaving Chen Changxing (1771–1853) and Yang Luchan (1799–1871) out of the picture. In fact, the Yang transmission, by far the most influential in the development and dissemination of the art in the last century, is never mentioned.

The second book of the modern era is Xu Yusheng's (1879–1945) 1921 *Illustrated Introduction to the Taijiquan Form*. Xu presents a two-part genealogy, tracing the theoretical origins to Fuxi, Yu, the Yellow Emperor, and Hua Tuo, and the practical martial applications to a series of obscure and largely unattested figures, beginning with Xu Xuanping of the Tang, and including Li Daoshan, Cheng Lingxi, Hu Jingzi, and Song Zhongshu. The second phase begins with Zhang Sanfeng, a name which Xu concedes is shared by more than ten figures, none of whom are recorded to have studied martial arts. Xu also gives an alternative version of Zhang's career, making him a Song figure, who single-handedly kills 500 Khitan invaders and transmits his art to hundreds of disciples in Shaanxi. Continuing, he says that during the Yuan, Wang Zongyue revived Zhang's transmission and wrote the classics. Later it was transmitted to Eastern Zhejiang, then to Zhang Songxi and Ningbo, where it was learned by Wang Zhengnan. After many more years it reached early Qing anti-Manchu rebel and folklore hero Gan Fengchi. This is the southern branch. The northern branch continued from Wang Zongyue to Jiang Fa to Chen Changxing and then Yang Luchan. Xu cites the *Prefectural Gazetteer of Ningbo* and *Lost Tales of Knight-Errantry* as his sources but was also clearly influenced by Song Shuming's early Republican *Treatise on the Origins and Branches of Taijiquan* (Dong, 1948: 108; Wu Zhiqing, n.d.: 268–271). He calls Zhang a "Confucian" and makes no special attempt to hang a Daoist label on his lineage. Xu was an un-aligned martial arts promoter, who did not name his personal teachers in the book but acknowledges the consultation of Yang Shaohou and Wu Jianquan at the Beijing Physical Education Research Institute that he headed. The book has no pretensions to critical scholarship, but Xu's work is unique in citing sources for his historical account and in offering multiple versions of taiji's origins. Although Xu's *Illustrated Introduction to the Taijiquan Form* created the formal template for future taiji instructional manuals, this aspect had no imitators.

Sun and Xu established the two prototypical origin myths that came to be adopted by virtually all subsequent writers: Zhang Sanfeng as sole creator of taijiquan, or Zhang as transmitter of an art with earlier antecedents. Exceptions are the Chen family, who had much to lose by myth and everything to gain by keeping creation under their own roof, and the Hao family, representing the Wu Yuxiang style, who did not produce their first book until 1963. The remaining and most prolific styles and writers hail from the Yang and Wu family transmissions. The first publication written on behalf of the Yang family art is that of Yang Chengfu's (1883–1936) student Chen Weiming, who in 1925 published the *Art of Taijiquan*. His very first chapter consists of a fanciful biography of Zhang Sanfeng, complete with all the standard miraculous flourishes. The text makes no reference to martial arts, except for the last sentence, which says that what is known as taijiquan began with him. His second chapter gives a general survey of the evolution of the martial arts, again naming Zhang Sanfeng as founder of the Internal School. Rather than confusing Wang Zong of the *Epitaph for Wang Zhengnan* with Wang Zongyue, however, it simply places Wang Zong a century after Zhang, but in direct line of transmission, and places Wang Zongyue in the Qing as author of the classics and teacher of Chen Changxing. He makes no special pleading for Daoism, but the last chapter consists of a series of quotations from the *Laozi*, together with parallel principles in the *Taiji Classics*. The next book in the Yang transmission is third generation Chengfu's 1931 *Self-defense Applications of Taijiquan*. Probably ghostwritten by Dong Yingjie, it begins with a photo gallery of Chengfu and chief disciples and a detailed genealogy from Zhang Sanfeng to Wang Zongyue. He mentions an "Eastern Branch" in Zhejiang, which "regrettably has died out," probably following Baijia's statement that Wang Zhengnan had no successors. However, the Henan Branch continues with the Chen's and Yang's. This is followed by a hagiography of the immortal Zhang, and at the end of the book a highly romantic tale of Zhang's cultivation practices. In a fantastic episode, Zhang Sanfeng is led by a display of heavenly lights to a mysterious cave deep in the mountains. Here he encounters two golden snakes and the source of the celestial emanations: two miraculous spears. Nearby he also discovers a manual called the *Taiji Sticky Thirteen Spear* from whose principles he distills the techniques and sparring form reproduced in the *Self-defense Applications of Taijiquan*. This is perhaps the first example of the genre of pure martial arts fantasy, lacking any antecedents in the Huangs' writings or *History of the Ming* biography of Zhang Sanfeng, to be found in a taiji publication. Chengfu's 1934 *Complete Principles and Practices of Taijiquan*, probably ghostwritten by Zheng Manqing, shows a bit more restraint. It contains no genealogy chart, but cites Zhang Sanfeng several times in the prefatory matter as creator of the art. Its narrative genealogy makes no distinction between northern, southern, or eastern branches, and streamlining the transmission, follows Xu Yusheng's introduction of Jiang Fa to deliver the art to Changxing. Departing from Chen Weiming, however, it does not place Changxing and Jiang Fa in a master-disciple relationship. It has no special pleading for Daoism as such.

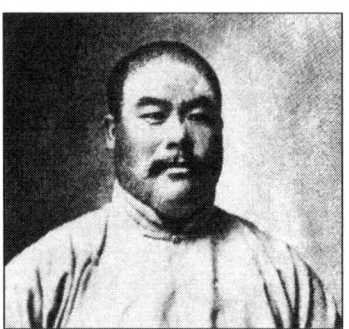

Yang Chengfu (1883–1936).

Writing in their own names, Zheng Manqing's 1946 (published 1952) *Thirteen Chapters on Taijiquan* contains no genealogy chart, no biography of Zhang, and only two passing references to Zhang as the creator of the Internal School of Wudang, whereas fellow Chengfu disciple Dong Yingjie's 1948 *Principles of Taijiquan* contains not only genealogy chart and biography of Zhang, but reproduces Song Shuming's *Treatise on the Origins and Branches of Taijiquan*, with Dong's personal endorsement of the view that taijiquan predated Sanfeng under different names. Three decades later, undoubtedly provoked by Cultural Revolution anti-feudalism, Zheng felt obliged to defend taiji's lineage against modern-minded scholars in his *New Method of Self-Study in Taijiquan*: "Some people have indulged in wild slander, claiming that taijiquan was not created by the immortal Zhang Sanfeng. I do not know what their motives are." He goes on to recite a number of principles from the *Laozi* shared by taijiquan, concluding, "Who but Sanfeng could have attained this…. Sanfeng took the principles of the Yellow Emperor and Laozi and applied them to the martial arts. Therefore, we call it the internal system. The Buddha was from India, that is, from a foreign country. Bodhidharma was a Buddhist and, therefore, his art is called external" (Zheng, n.d.: 20). Although accepting folklore as fact cannot endear him to historians, nevertheless, Zheng's message as a cultural ideologue is unmistakable: taijiquan's status as the Chinese martial art is inseparable from its special relationship with Daoism. Passing these genes to the next generation, Zheng's Chongqing era student Zhang Qixian in his 1969 *The Essential Principles and Practice of Taijiquan* gives a highly imaginative account of Zhang Sanfeng, complete with precise birth information (nineth day, fourth month, 1247 CE, following mother, nee Lin's, dream of a great stork coming from the sea). According to Zhang Qixian, Sanfeng created the art from observation of a snake's successful defense against a bird, *Yijing* cosmology, and the methods of past martial artists such as Xu Xuanping. Zheng Manqing's Taiwan era student Song Zhijian in his 1970 five-hundred-page magnum opus *The Study of Taijiquan*, not only accepts the Song Shuming genealogy, but offers complete biographies of all its unattested figures, and even a biography of Song Shuming himself. The trend among Yang lineage authors to magnify the mythological and Daoist trappings over time may be a deliberate counter-discourse to modernist movements on the mainland, but also thumbs its nose at deconstructionist practices in progressive Western scholarship. The scientific backgrounds of many of these authors and the amount of space devoted to legitimizing the art through appeal to Western science is also in stark contrast to their willingness to recapitulate and even embellish the most fabulous origination myths.

The next most widely practiced style is that founded by Wu Jianquan (1870–1942), whose father Quanyu (1834–1902) was a student of second-generation Yang family scion, Yang Banhou (1837–1892). As with the Yang transmission, the first published book was by a non-family member, in this case Wu Tunan's 1928 *Taijiquan*, which following on his 1926 *Brief Introduction to Chinese Martial Arts* presents formal biographies of all the unattested figures in Song Shuming's genealogy. Wu's background as an archeologist did not prevent him from exceeding all others in fabricating the minutiae of Zhang's travels and contacts, but there is no mention of how he came by martial skills. Zhang Sanfeng's life is a caricature of the Daoist immortal, but there is no special pleading for Daoism itself. Contradicting the *Epitath for Wang Zhengnan*, he places Wang Zongyue next in line after Zhang and makes Gan Fengchi the end of the southern branch. Jiang Fa of the northern branch brings the art to Chen Village. In his 1984 *Studies on Taijiquan*, Wu, nearing centenarian status, reaffirms his faith in the Xu Xuanping origination myth. In 1935, two other Wu Jianquan students, Ma Yueliang and Chen Zhenmin, published a manual with photos of Wu Jianquan, entitled *Wu Style Taijiquan*. This work takes an unusual approach to lineage. Truncating the Wu Tunan chart, it eliminates the southern branch and all pre-Zhang figures. Moreover, using an evolutionary analysis, it insists that self-defense is a natural ability of man, systematized by Bodhidharma, and refined by Zhang Sanfeng. This Darwinian analysis allows them to simultaneously acknowledge mythological origins, pay homage to the Yang family, and leave room for their own superiority as a further development on Yang. In the same year, Wu Jianquan's second son, Gongzao, published *Commentaries on Taijiquan*, which continues to prune the family tree, eliminating all charts, biographies, and any mention of Zhang Sanfeng. He pays homage only to his own father and close disciples, but this does not mean that he is turning his back on Daoism. On the contrary, he says that taiji's principles, "coincide perfectly with Daoist meditation and really constitute a Daoist practice" (Wu, 1935: 13).

With the phenomenal success of the Yang family in the 20s and 30s, Chen family standard bearer Chen Xin sought to reassert proprietorship of the family art and to buttress in the literary realm what Chen Fake (1887–1957) had accomplished for the family honor in the gymnasia and arenas. To this end, he began in 1919 and published in 1933 the monumental *Introduction to Chen Family Taijiquan*, presenting the Chen family form together with many pages of theoretical essays. By contrast, the traditional Chen family manuscripts discovered by Tang Hao in the village consisted of little more than lists of forms with posture names and a handful of terse training songs. Needing an ancestral progenitor, Chen Xin names Chen Bu, the first to relocate the family from Shanxi to Wen County in Henan, as creator of taijiquan. To compete with the Yang mystique, however, he still needed to establish Daoist credentials. This he accomplished in two ways: first, his book is a tour de force in cosmology and medicine, and second, he introduces a poem attributed to ancestor Chen Wangting in which the latter mentions his devotion to the *Scripture of the Yellow Court*, a famous Daoist cultivation work. He thus attempts to demonstrate, strictly within the parameters of family lineage, that it is possible to create a martial art with Daoist content and inspiration without a Daoist first cause. As we shall see later, rivals in neighboring Zhaobao effectively abandon family lineage and hitch their wagons directly to Zhang Sanfeng.

Positing historical lineages preceded by remote mythological progenitors and ancestors is a common cultural pattern among many peoples. The folkloric process may have been at work with Wang Zhengnan, but it was literati Huang Zongxi and Huang Baijia who presented it to the world. In the case of the Chen's and Yang's, the Chen's had no tradition of Zhang Sanfeng, and Yang Luchan would not have heard this in Chen Village. Even if he had been aware of the *Epitaph for Wang Zhengnan* and *Internal School's Boxing Methods*, unlikely for an illiterate peasant, he probably would not have associated this with the art he was taught in Henan so far from Zhejiang. The Huang documents are the *locus classici* for the Zhang Sanfeng creation myth, and derivative versions were carried in the *Ningbo Prefectural Gazetteer, Strange Tales from the Studio of Idleness* and *Complete works of Zhang Sanfeng*. We do not know who made the first link between Zhang Sanfeng and taijiquan, and no two versions are the same, but we do know that the promoters of this lineage were among the educated elite, including many with Western scientific knowledge, and could hardly be considered part of a folk process. Their motivations, then, must have been conscious and deserve further exploration.

The first generation of taijiquan books were written against the background of an unstable republic, warlordism, and the Northern Expedition, but not yet a strong communist movement or imminent Japanese invasion. What is interesting at the present juncture is that in spite of Tang Hao, Xu Zhen, Gu Liuxin and many other's attempts to deconstruct these invented traditions, we now enter the 21st century with claims on behalf of the Yangs more fantastic than anything these pioneering martial arts historians were obliged to explode. Although the first three generations of Yang family masters have been the object of extreme veneration and no small amount of apocrypha, they are still derivative of the Chen art, which in turn is viewed by some as a rustic retention of the exalted art of the immortal Zhang. If Yang Luchan could be linked directly with a Daoist source, this would reduce the Chen role to kindergarten and turn Luchan, whom Tang Hao determined to be a peasant bondservant, into a Daoist initiate.

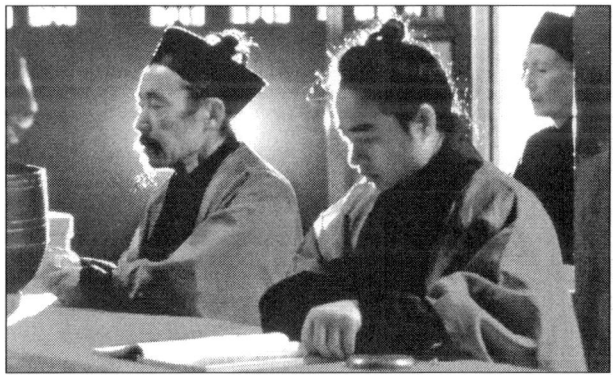

Daoist monks inside a temple. Photograph by Kipling Swehla (www.kiplingphoto.com) and courtesy of the Taoist Restoration Society (www.taoarts.com).

Although Luchan lived in the 19th century and is the founder of taijiquan's most widely disseminated style, there is not a shred of reliable biographical information about him, in fact, while arguably the most famous son of Yongnian County, his name does not appear in the local gazetteer, either as a degree holder, or even as a martial artist. Firsthand impressions of Luchan by grandson Chengfu are seriously undermined by the fact that Chengfu was born twelve years after Luchan's death. Controversies have centered on Luchan's background (was he a peasant or literatus?), his martial arts education (did he learn in Chen Village from boyhood, or did he make the fabled "three pilgrimages?"), and more recently, was he really a tutor to the Manchu princes in Beijing? Questions that might trouble sober scholars have not restrained He Hongming, a student of Li Yaxuan (himself a student of Luchan's grandson Yang Chengfu), who reports that Li told him that on his "third trip" to Chen Village, Yang was given the "classics" written by Zhang Sanfeng and then set out to the Wudang Mountains to learn inner alchemy from reclusive adepts. This led him to eliminate the jumps, stamps, hard kicks and strikes, and uneven tempo found in the Chen form and to give taijiquan the distinctive "internal" characteristics we now associate with it (He, 1999: 34-35). Zhao Youbin, Lu Dimin, Feng Fuming, and Yong Yangren are also in agreement that Yang Luchan received the classics from Chen Changxing (Zhao, Lu, and Feng, 1989: 22-24; Yong, 89, 26-31). Although this contradicts many firsthand accounts describing the gradual softening of the form through the first three generations of Yang masters and its adaptation to the urban intelligentsia, He Hongming's tale forges a much closer connection between the Yang's and Daoism, making Zhang Sanfeng the author of the *Taiji Classics*, putting them into Yang's hands in Chen Village, and sending Luchan himself to the Wudang Mountains to study with "Daoists." This version also minimizes the role of the Chen family and effectively erases the Wu's and Li's. A similar assertion is made in a recent article by Li

Shirong, "revealing" that Luchan received the classics from his teacher Chen Changxing, who preserved the Wang Zongyue manuscript of Zhang Sanfeng's writings (Li, 2000: 26–27). Again, this flies in the face of Tang Hao's finding no writings or oral tradition of Zhang Sanfeng in Chen Village and the absence of same in Chen Xin's *Introduction to Chen Family Taijiquan*. While making no attempt to refute, or even acknowledge, the findings of responsible scholars, He and Li seem willing to trade in Yang Luchan's historical role as a humble but gifted lineage founder for an invented role in the Zhang Sanfeng transmission and a Daoist initiate.

A few scholars have managed to avoid being kidnapped in either the Wudang Mountains or Chen Village. Bian Renjie (Bian, 1936: 5–9), Hu Puan (Wu, n.d.: 194), and Zhuang Shen (Zeng, 1960: 223–228) review the many mutually contradictory claims, concluding that the evidence advanced by partisans on all sides is false and credible records still unavailable. Wu Zhiqing, a 1917 student of Yang Chengfu, can steer clear of sectarianism and mystification, coming to the enlightened and elegant conclusion that:

> Taijiquan is not a mysterious and bizarre magical art; neither is it the shallow skill of bodyguards and street performers. Rather, it is a natural self-defense, exercise, and health system that arises from the natural world.
> – Wu, n.d.: 1

Similarly, Zhao Ximin (Zhao, 1979: 85–105), Wang Juexin (Wang, 1976: 5), and Zhou Jiannan (Zhou, 1976: 77–99), writing in Taiwan in the wake of the mainland's Cultural Revolution, nevertheless were able to free themselves from Cold War bias to mete out praise and blame on strictly scholarly criteria. However, their writings were not available in mainland China, where they could have served to correct some of the blind spots in Tang Hao's official view, and they were likewise ignored by overseas anticommunist cultural conservatives, just as they are today by the Neo-Zhang Sanfeng taiji religionists. In the end, these voices of reason were not able to carry the day, and one set of narrow views prevailed as the official version on the mainland, while the other became the self-appointed opposition and exclusive export model.

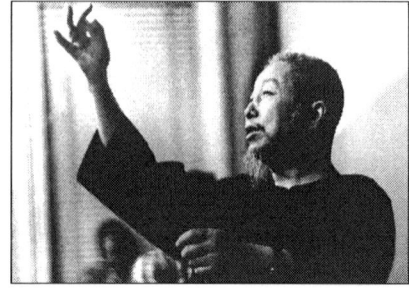

Zheng Manqing lectured on taijiquan, traditional Chinese medicine, and Chinese philosophy.
Photo courtesy of Kenneth Van Sickle. www.sinobarr.com

Consonance with Daoist Philosophy

Fabricating a lineage from a famous immortal in Chinese folklore is one approach to linking taijiquan to Daoism, but taiji's claim to being the thinking man's martial art rests more securely on its theoretical consonance with Daoist philosophy. Ironically, although the "*Taiji Classics*" have many embedded quotations from the *Yijing, Great Learning, Book of History, Records of the Grand Historian*, Zhu Xi, Zhou Dunyi, and Mencius, there are none from the *Laozi* and *Zhuangzi*. The first generation of modern taiji books, those of Sun Lutang, Chen Weiming, Xu Yushseng, and Chen Xin, are similarly eclectic in their use of philosophical sources. Sun Lutang credits the *Yijing* with inspiring Zhang to soften the qigong regimen of immortality seekers, and though he himself does not cite the *Laozi* directly, the Wu Xingu and Chen Zengze prefaces are devoted chiefly to establishing the Daoist connection. Xu Yusheng says that "Zhang Sanfeng based his art on the *Confucian* [author ital.] principle of taiji" (Xu, 1921: 2) and mentions Zhuangzi's "from skill we approach the Dao," but makes no special appeal to Daoism as taiji's official philosophy. In fact, in a preface to Xu's work, Yang Chang says despairingly, "In the midst of the current difficulties, most of our educated men escape into Buddhism and Daoism" (Xu, 1921: 4). In Zhang Yiling's preface to Xu's book, he credits Japan's victory over Russia to the former's promotion of judo, which he hastens to point out is borrowed from China (Xu, 1921: 1). Like everyone else, Xu uses *Yijing* cosmology to explain the principles of taijiquan, but says, "Today, science has reached an advanced stage, where it can be anticipated that in the future, geometry and mechanics will be used to explain the principles of taijiquan, without resorting to the *Yijing*" (Xu, 1921; 3). Xu then proceeds to a detailed exposition of Zhou Dunyi and Shao Yong's *Yijing*-based cosmologies and how they relate to taiji.

Representing the Wu Jianquan transmission, Wu Tunan's 1928 *Taijiquan* adopts the Song Shuming genealogy but uses no cosmological language or references to any philosophical school. Instead, it praises taijiquan as scientifically superior to both hard Chinese styles and Western calisthenics. Similarly, Chen Zhenmin and Ma Yueliang's *Wu* [Jianquan] *Style Taijiquan* says, "Because taijiquan appears relatively late and its history is fairly short, its system is more clearly delineated . . .. In all branches of learning or skill, later creations are superior to earlier . . . and martial arts are no exception to this rule" (Chen and Ma, 1935: 1, 3). This work also emphasizes taiji's consonance with modern science, downplaying cosmological language and debts to traditional philosophy. Representing the Yang transmission, Chen Weiming is sparing with cosmological jargon but concludes his *The Art of Taijiquan* with a lengthy series of parallel quotations from the *Laozi* and the *Taiji Classics*. Fellow Yang Chengfu disciple Dong Yingjie provides a biography of Zhang, but no separate section of parallel quotations. Zheng Manqing, another Chengfu disciple, in his *New Method of Self-study in Taijiquan* gives no biography but provides relevant quotations from the *Yijing, Laozi,* and *Neijing*. Yang Chengfu's 1931 *Taijiquan shiyong fa* begins with a biography of Zhang Sanfeng but has no extended cosmological expositions. His 1934 *Taijiquan tiyong quanshu*, however, does contain an introductory discussion on philosophical roots, and in Zheng Manqing's preface to the work, he specifically addresses the question of philosophical affinity, giving explicit priority to Daoism. Reviewing other traditional texts that countenance hardness as the natural complement of softness, Zheng finds in *Laozi* the only consistently soft-sided philosophy:

> Only the greatest hardness can overcome the greatest softness; only the greatest softness can overcome the greatest hardness. The *Yijing* says, "Hard and soft rub against each other, and the eight trigrams knock together." The *Book of History* says, "The thoughtful and imperturbable conquer by hardness; the wise and skillful conquer by softness." The *Book of Odes* says, "He would not eat the hard or spit out the soft." But when it comes to the application of hard and soft, there cannot be two approaches. Why is it that Laozi alone says, "The highest softness overcomes the highest hardness," and "The soft and weak triumph over the hard and strong?"
> – Yang, 1934: 3

For Zheng, the principle of uncompromising softness goes beyond self-cultivation and self-defense, and in national policy constitutes "the means for strengthening the nation and alleviating the people's suffering" (Yang, 1934: 4). Zheng expresses taiji's relationship with Daoism in this simple equation: "Taijiquan enables us to reach the stage of undifferentiated pure yang, which is the same as Laozi's 'concentrating the qi and developing softness'" (Zheng, 1952: 6). To achieve this level, however, Zheng struggles with the line in the *Taiji Classics*, "Those with qi have no strength." Parsing the distinction between strength, qi, and mind, Zheng combines Laozi's "Concentrate the qi and develop softness" with the inner elixir formula, "Refine the essence into qi and the qi into spirit" to explicate the classics' "The mind must be on the spirit and not on the qi; if it is on the qi, there will be blocks, and where there is qi, there is no strength; without qi there is pure hardness" (Zheng, 1952: 8). Zheng looks to Laozi for the highest expression of spiritual attainment and that practice without enlightenment and faith in softness can never lead to "essential hardness" (*chungang*) or "spiritual power" (*shenli*). Zheng's student Song Jianzhi continues this theme, "We cannot be certain who first created taijiquan, but judging from its name and principles, there is no doubt it was a Daoist. . . Daoism begins with Laozi . . . and his principles are precisely those governing the practice of stillness and action in taijiquan as well as inner elixir cultivation" (Song, 1959: 11). For Zheng and his disciples, the efficacy of softness could only be demonstrated after a considerable period of "*xue chikui*" (investing in loss), as only "supreme softness" will cause hardness to defeat itself.

It would be difficult to find any martial arts style during the late Qing-early Republican period that did not use Daoist language to legitimize itself, appeal to intellectuals, and contribute to the construction of national identity. It goes without saying that taijiquan shares its movement principles and inner energetics with sister arts xingyi and bagua, but soft-style philosophy was adopted even by Shaolin during this period. The *Traditional Shaolin and Secret Transmissions of Shaolin Boxing*, judged by Tang Hao to be no earlier than late Qing, express Shaolin's principles in terms of hard and soft, full and empty, and the pseudonymous author consistently refers to Shaolin as "the art of softness" (Zunwozhai, n.d.: 1–2; Tang, 1986: 70). To further elide any essential philosophical distinction between Shaolin and Wudang, the traditional Shaolin insists that the terms "internal and external," refer not to training or tactics, but to Shaolin's Buddhist origins. Tang Hao, who studied in Japan, also points out that the language of the Shaolin manuals sounds reminiscent of Japanese judo literature. Thus, at a time when China was under siege by Japan, China's martial arts ideologues may well have been aware of the role of judo in Japan's martial arts revival and in building a sense of superiority to the West and thus adopted its soft-style stance. In fact, the *Secrets of Shaolin Boxing* even attempts to adopt Zhang Sanfeng himself, characterizing him as a Shaolin master who in his later years systematized the "72 pressure point techniques," which he learned from a Daoist named Feng Yiyuan (Zunwozhai, n.d.; 108; Tang, 1986: 79).

No martial art has expended as much effort to establish its philosophical pedigree as taijiquan. The persistence of this view can be seen in a recent article by Ma Yuannian, entitled "Taijiquan and Confucian Thought" (*"Taijiquan he rujia sixiang"*):

> It is well-known that taijquan is a Daoist art and that its symbol is the taiji diagram . . .. However, historically Daoism, Buddhism, and Confucianism have influenced and learned from each other, and therefore, although purely a product of Daoism, taijiquan has also absorbed some Buddhist and Confucian elements, especially Confucianism's philosophy of the "golden mean." – Ma, 1998: 32–33

Even in an article ostensibly devoted to exploring the Confucian contribution to taijiquan's development, the author has already conceded that taiji is a "Daoist art."

In the *Laozi*, softness overcoming hardness, or softness within hardness, are presented both as martial ethic and strategy. However, pacifist themes in the *Laozi*, such as, "Compassion allows us to be courageous," and "Weapon are not auspicious instruments," are not nearly as well developed in the taiji literature as in judo, aikido, or even Shaolin. Strategically, the *Laozi's*, "I do not dare to play the host, but play the guest. I would rather retreat a yard than advance a foot," "Courage in daring gets us killed; courage in not killing allows us to live," and "The sage does not contend, and therefore no one in the world can contend with him" become in taiji a defensive strategy of disarming the opponent by apparent yielding, while giving him enough rope to hang himself. Laozi's "nonaction" (*wuwei*) functions in taiji as letting others strike the first blow, neutralizing the incoming energy, sticking to it, borrowing it, and returning it. "Egolessness" (*wuwo*) in the *Laozi* corresponds to taiji's "emptying," so that the opponent's force "lands on nothing." Martial arts writers from Huang Zongxi and Huang Baijia to the present have appreciated the wider allegorical significance of martial arts' soft-style strategy. In a postscript to a 1980 reprint of Wu Gongzao's *Commentaries on Taijiquan* no less a figure than Jin Yong, China's most celebrated martial arts novelist, makes very explicit the relationship between taijiquan, Daoism, and international political strategy:

> Humility invites advantage; pride courts disaster—this is China's political and personal philosophy.... Legend has it that taijiquan was created by Zhang Sanfeng, and Zhang Sanfeng was a Daoist. Taijiquan perfectly expresses Daoist philosophy. However, Daoist philosophy does not advocate pure passivity. Rather, Laozi emphasized that if you want to get something, you must first give something, and thus he said, "Great nations remain humble," meaning that the powerful do not puff themselves up but conserve their strength, while their enemies exhaust themselves. This is the time to strike. – Wu, 1980: 135–37

It is important to remember that in all three of the dominant versions of the Zhang Sanfeng myth, he is not a Daoist quietist but a warrior who goes forth to slay bandits. In Chinese, of course, "bandits" (*fei, zei, kou*) can refer to domestic rebels or foreign invaders. What did "Daoism" mean to turn of the century martial arts ideologues? In the late 19th century, reformer Tan Sitong strove mightily to harmonize Confucianism, Buddhism, and Christianity, but banished Daoism as encouraging passivity, Legalism as too repressive, and Neo-Confucianism as too puritanical. The seminal works on taijiquan written during the 1920s and 30s obviously had a different understanding of "Daoism." For them, the philosophy of hardness within softness, as for Huang Zongxi, was consonant with the non-confrontational political policy of appeasement pursued by both the late Qing Manchu regime and early Republican KMT (Kuomintang, 1912–1924).

Hundreds of books and articles have been devoted to establishing that taiji practice derives from the *Yijing*'s principles of hard and soft, full and empty. The majority of these are based not only on the idealistic assumption that theory precedes practice but that the *Yijing* is a Daoist work. Since the time of the *Cantongqi* and *Neijing*, cosmological language has been used to describe the internal energetics of meditation and medicine. Its earliest recorded wholesale application to the martial arts is seen in Chang Naizhou and the *Taiji Classics*. Because Confucius is traditionally credited with editing the *Yijing* and because of its importance in Song Neo-Confucianism, even some taiji exponents are prepared to concede its Confucian origins. Others, however, fearing dilution of the Daoist association explain that although Zhou Dunyi, author of the *Taijitu shuo* was not a Daoist himself, he stole the taiji symbol and its theory from a Daoist, usually identified as the immortal Chen Xiyi. However, by far the majority of taiji writers simply adopt the *Yijing* as a Daoist work. In the Chinese popular imagination, anything expressing arcane principles in mysterious symbols is associated with Daoism.

Following the correlative logic of the Daoism-*Yijing*-taijiquan triangle, it becomes increasingly clear that during taiji's maturation period in the 19th and early 20th centuries, to say something was Daoist was simply to say that it was Chinese. Calling it Confucian or Buddhist during the late Qing would not do, as the Manchu rulers had successfully co-opted both. Ironically, it is during times of national emergency that the Confucian theme of service to the state seems to have no rallying power and heterodox faiths promising supernatural power and a vision of the sublime come to the fore. Like these millenarian communities and secret societies, the martial arts movement of the turn of the century was not simply escapist but provided a channel for repressed nationalism, religiosity, and masculinity. The promotion of Daoism in China, wedded to the knight-errant (*xia*) tradition, parallels the resurrection of the samurai spirit for Japan's modern army, whose officers carried swords as symbols of the Japanese soul.

Associating taijiquan with philosophy was intended to make it palatable to the intelligentsia at a time when it was imperative to overcome the "sick man of Asia" syndrome and for effete literati to put aside their disdain for physical culture. Most martial artists were not members of the gentry class, however, let alone Confucian or Daoist, and literati like Huang Baijia, Wu Yuxiang, and Zheng Manqing have only studied with and glorified them during periods of national emergency. Although 19th century reformers had pointed out that archery and charioteering were part of the classical Confucian curriculum, they could only sell the martial as an expedient for national salvation and could not turn it into something transcendent. If progressive 19th century reformers rejected Daoism as representing passivity and superstition, a subset of conservative intellectuals intuited that only Daoism could transform the martial arts into a Dao.

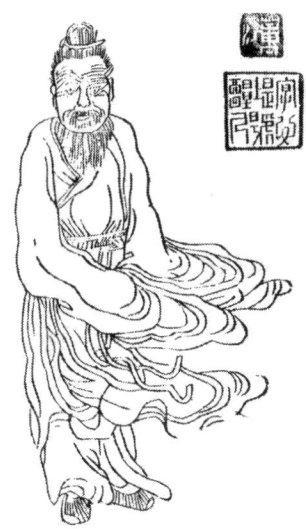

Illustration of Zhang Sanfeng taken from the *Collected Works of Zhang Sanfeng* (1844). Illustration courtesy of Douglas Wile.

Taijiquan and Daoist Cultivation

With a Daoist lineage and Daoist principles, taijiquan has its figurehead and its philosophy, but there are many paths to Daoist realization. The story of Zhang Sanfeng deriving the principles of a martial art from observing the battle of a snake and crane is like Fuxi abstracting the trigrams from gazing at heaven and earth. Shen Nong, the God of Agriculture, who "tasted a hundred herbs," and master butcher Pao Ding, whose knife met no resistance and so never dulled, are the prototypes of experimentation and induction, "approaching the Dao through skill." The shamanistic aspect of Daoism may be seen in the immortal Zhang's receiving the martial art in a dream from the god Xuanwu. The deductive approach to the Dao is seen in Zhang's reversal of Shaolin's principle of hardness and speed for softness and stillness. Another path is abstraction, or self-emptying and desirelessness, that allows the background consciousness, which is one with the Dao, to come to the fore. Finally, there is inner alchemy, a process that seeks to transform the body's intrinsic energies and achieve immortality through the triumph of the prenatal over the postnatal and yang over yin. It is the last of these that is chiefly the focus of self-cultivation in taiji theory. Self-cultivation, in turn, tends to be represented in two ways: cultivation as the servant of self-defense, or self-defense as a skill leading to enlightenment or the Dao. In the mythic, idealistic realm of Zhang Sanfeng, enlightenment precedes the creation of the martial art, but in the historical realm of human practice, cultivation leads to mastery of the art, and mastery of the art leads to realization of the Dao.

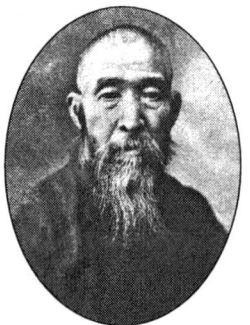

Sun Lutang (1861–1932).

Zhuangzi scoffed at yogic self-cultivation, as did Ge Hong, although for different reasons, and even *Complete Works of Zhang Sanfeng's* most frequently cited "*Da dao lun*" (Treatise on the Great Dao) says, "Some aspirants engage in massage and daoyin, breathing exercises, and herbs as methods of self-cultivation. Although these methods can temporarily relieve some illnesses, they cannot confer immortality and are considered laughable by true adepts" (Li, 1844: juan 3). Li Xiyue and his Sichuan circle, who forged the Zhang Sanfeng canon in the early 19th century, had no thought that this might prove to be an embarrassment to early 21st century revivers of Zhang Sanfeng as the patron saint of taijiquan. Despite attributing the Internal School to "a Daoist alchemist," there is nothing in the *Art of the Internal School's Boxing Methods* that relates to internal cultivation techniques. The Chen family material, likewise, contains no evidence of qigong importations prior to Chen Xin's early 20th century book. We find it full-blown, however, in Chang Naizhou's 18th century writings:

> The central qi is what the classics on immortality call the source yang or what medicine calls the source qi. Because it dwells in the center of the body, martial artists call it the central qi. This qi is the prenatal true monadal qi. Spiritual cultivation produces the inner elixir; martial cultivation produces the external elixir. However, the inner elixir always depends on the outer elixir, for action and stillness mutually engender each other. Proper cultivation naturally results in forming the ethereal fetus and returning to the primordial state. – Chang, 1932: 1

Interestingly, although Chang and the *Taiji Classics* share many verbatim and parallel passages, there are no traceable lineage links between his art and either Chen Village or Wuyang, the alleged site of the classics' find. In the "Author's Preface" to his 1919 *The Study of Taijiquan*, Sun Lutang is very explicit about taiji's potential for self-cultivation, and in a passage that reads like a Chinese Genesis says:

> At the dawn of the creation of heaven and earth, the original qi circulated freely. With the division and union of action and stillness, all creatures came into being, and this is the post-creation realm of form. The pre-creation original qi was wedded to the post-creation material world, and thus the post-creation substance contains the pre-creation original qi. Man, therefore, is a being who combines both the pre- and post-creation qi. However, once man acquired knowledge and desires, yin and yang were out of balance, and our post-creation qi gradually increased, resulting in the decline of yang and an overabundance of yin. Moreover, we are assailed by the six external qi—wind, cold, heat, dampness, dryness, and fire—and subject to the seven emotions. In this way, the body becomes daily weaker, and myriad illnesses appear. The ancients were concerned about this and experimented with herbs to eliminate illness, meditated to cultivate the mind, and fearing that movement and stillness would not be balanced, invented the martial arts to restore the subtle qi. – Sun, 1919: 1

Except for the concluding sentence, this passage could be the opening paragraph of any of a thousand tracts on inner elixir meditation, and clearly positions taijiquan as a method for realizing the Dao. Substituting the goal of supreme self-defense for immortality, however, Sun, in his *The True Essence of the Martial Arts* says:

> When one's art reaches the level of uniting emptiness with the dao, which is the true mind, it is transformed into the realm of the highest emptiness and highest void. When the mind is empty and without a single object, if suddenly something unexpected happens, even without hearing or seeing it, you can sense and avoid it. – Sun, 1924: 8

Nearly a century later, Sun Lutang's daughter, Sun Jianyun, echoes this same theme:

> One of the reasons why xingyi, bagua, and taiji have flourished during the 20th century is that they allow us to become one with the dao, that is, they are martial arts that are simultaneously Daoist arts.
> – Tong, 1999: 12

Radical new voices today, like Guo Tiefeng, however, are prepared to go beyond mere mystical union with the dao and boldly proclaim:

> Taijiquan is one of the paths to Daoist immortality and it gives practitioners an air of spiritual otherworldliness. . . . Taijiquan originated with Laozi and its goal is the attainment of immortality.
> – Guo, 1999: 28

This statement puts taijiquan in the service of a Daoism narrowly defined as the pursuit of immortality and is a throwback to Du Yuanhua, whose 1935 *Orthodox Taijiquan* insists,

> This art is a vehicle for cultivating the elixir and gaining longevity. After long practice, it can truly allow us to achieve the state of pure yang, that is, immortality. – Yan, 1997: 8

Although there are at least four different interpretations of the term "internal art" (*neijia*) in common usage today, taiji is considered "internal" because it works from the inside out, that is, training the qi rather than the muscles, bones, and ligaments and aims at developing intrinsic energy (*jin*) rather than brute strength (*li*). As a self-cultivation method, taijiquan has many things in common with other methods, as well as some unique features. The system almost always includes a form and usually push-hands. Like progressing from sheet music to memorization to improvisation, the form and push-hands are the scales, compositions, and duets of body mechanics, internal energy, and self-defense techniques. Ancillary exercises often include sitting meditation to focus on emptying the mind and opening the microcosmic orbit; standing meditation to raise the *yangqi*, lower the energetic center of gravity, and demonstrate how relaxation and abdominal breathing alter the perception of pain; acupressure massage to develop awareness of points and qi channels; and qigong to experience qi mobilization in repetitive single phrase exercises without the mental burden of memorization; and weapons to train qi extension beyond the body. More advanced work may include moving push-hands, fencing, free sparring, and grappling. Like sexual practices, all of these partnering exercises train coolness under fire and stillness in motion; scripts are left behind, and like dancers losing themselves in the music, one enters the realm of "soaring on the laws of the universe."

The path of natural movement is discovered by relaxing, listening inwardly, and slowing down, all of which takes us out of our conditioned mental and physical habits and allows us to drop into the Dao. The slow tempo, taiji's most distinctive external feature, slows the mind and breath, heightens awareness of gravity, momentum, and centrifugal force, and accelerates the strengthening of the legs. The body is emptied of tension and the mind of discursive thoughts and goals. In meditation, preconceptions stand in the way of enlightenment; in taijiquan, preconceptions cause the body to trip over the mind's intentions and prevent us from "forgetting ourselves and following the opponent." The fusion of body, mind, and breath in a moving meditation creates the perfect balance of excitation and relaxation required for the "flow" experience, and by centering the self in the radical present sets the stage for experiencing rare moments of spontaneity (*ziran*). Alignment creates the structural precondition for relaxation and optimizes the body mechanics for neutralizing or issuing energy, while emptying the body of tension allows the qi to concentrate and circulate. With both consciousness and qi rooted in center (*dantian*), the mind and extremities are relieved of leadership roles and practitioners can enjoy the "no-mind" experience of improvisational spontaneity—effortless, egoless, just so.

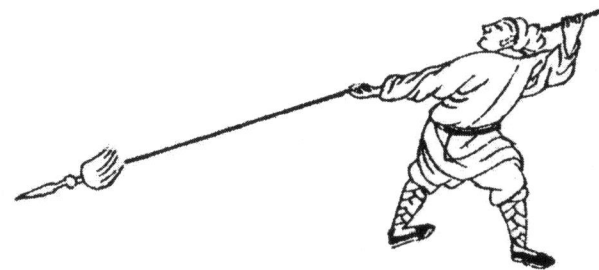

Qi Jiguang (1507–1587) entitled *Book of Effective Discipline*.

Whether couched in the terms of alchemy, cosmology, mythology, or medicine, all Chinese meditation texts are based on restoring body-mind harmony, or the heart-kidney axis, by focusing the mind in the lower abdomen. The injunction to "sink the qi to the dantian" appears in virtually every text of the Li Yiyu and Yang family redactions of the *Taiji Classics*, but nowhere in *Qi Jiguang's Boxing Classic*, Huang Baijia's *Internal School's Boxing Methods*, or the traditional Chen family material. The 18th and 19th centuries mark a turning point, then, in martial arts, when Chang Naizhou's writings and the *Taiji Classics* show the absorption of cultivation concepts into martial arts practice. Chen Xin's *Introduction to Chen Family Taijiquan* says, "Maintaining the focus in the center is what the Daoists refer to as gathering the *jing* and concentrating the qi so that the concentrated qi reverts to spirit" (Chen, 1934: 139). Chen and others like Zheng Manqing go further than dantian concentration and apply full microcosmic orbit meditation, based on a continuous circuit of qi circulation up the *du* (governing) and down the *ren* (controlling) channels, to taiji practice. It is only a small step then to bringing the entire channel system into the martial arts, with focus on specific acupuncture points and the use of various macrocosmic orbits to circulate the qi throughout the entire body. Other qigong techniques are enlisted by some taiji practitioners to demonstrate supernormal powers to attack acupuncture points (*dianxue*), withstand blows (*tieyi*), protect the genitals (*macangshen*), or issue energy through space (*lingkong faqi*). For taijiquan, and to some degree all the Chinese martial arts, to have adopted the language and methods of qigong and meditation is as natural as the Japanese martial arts borrowing from Zen. Although Western athletes may make use of prayer and psychology, it is the Western dance community that has evinced far greater interest in Indian yoga, Zen meditation, and Asian martial arts.

One of the perennial debates in Daoist meditation, and more broadly in Chinese philosophy, is whether to cultivate the mind (*xing, xin*) first, the body (*ming, shen*) first, or both simultaneously. This discussion is also sometimes framed as stillness (*jing*) versus action (*dong*), or the spiritual (*wen*) versus the martial (*wu*). Exponents of taijiquan have been uniquely well situated to champion the simultaneous cultivation position. Sitting meditators have often held that the *yangqi* sprouting in yin stillness is the pure prenatal yang, but have been criticized by qigong and sexual practitioners as fostering stagnation rather than stillness. Active practitioners, for their part, have sought to generate and mobilize large amounts of qi, but have been criticized for over stimulation and relying on the postnatal. By seeking "stillness in movement and movement in stillness" taijiquan has laid claim to the Golden Mean. This is brought out in a recent article by Feng Zhiqiang:

> Taijiquan is an internal martial art that simultaneously cultivates our intrinsic nature and life. Intrinsic nature and life may be called the heart and kidney.... This dual cultivation through taijiquan allows us to achieve an equilibrium of water and fire and harmony of yin and yang, which promotes the goal of health and longevity.   – Feng, 2000: 18

Dual cultivation may be considered orthodox in Daoist cultivation, but "paired practices" (*shuangxiu*) have been a persistent undercurrent for more than two thousand years. Usually associated with sexual practices, in the wider sense, it also encompasses any form of borrowing or exchanging qi with a partner. The "Yang Family Forty Chapters," attributed to Yang Banhou (1837–1892), contains a unique example of asexual paired practice within a martial arts context. Combining meditation's concept of the mating (*jiao*) of the male/yang consciousness principle with the female/yin physical principle in the body, together with sexual practice's concept of borrowing energy from a partner (*caizhan*) and applying this to martial arts sparring we hear:

> The male body belongs to yin, hence gathering (*cai*) the yin from one's own body or doing battle (*zhan*) with the female in one's own body is not as good as matching yin and yang between two males. This is a faster method of cultivating the body.

In solo meditation, the mind is anchored by the body and the body energized by the mind. In the martial meditation proposed by the Yang family material, the "battle of essences" is played out in the interaction of trigrams and phases represented by the "eight techniques" and "five steps." The text, whose title credits the work to Zhang Sanfeng, uses martial arts in the service of the "Great Learning's" call to "self-cultivation" (*xiushen*) to uncover Wang Yangming's "innate knowledge and ability" (*liangzhi liangneng*) and achieve the state of "sagehood or immortality" (*shengshen*). The technical details are expressed in the language of inner alchemy, and the tone can only be called religious—a martial mysticism promising the warrior the same fruits of self-cultivation as the sage.

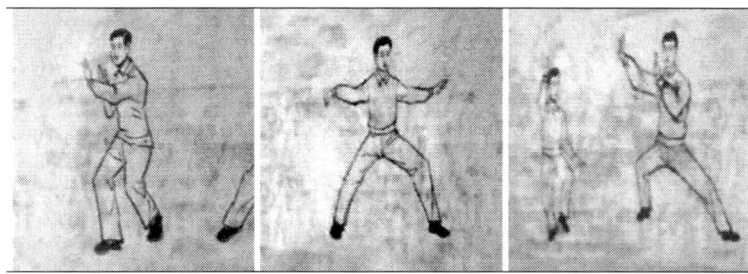

Depictions of Chen Taiji postures as seen on a wall in Chen Village.
Illustration courtesy of Stephan Berwick. www.truetaichi.com

Contra Zhang and Officialist History

The same Nationalist government that was prepared to consign traditional Chinese medicine to the dustbin of history and allow Western medicine to win the day tacitly cooperated in the construction of a mythos for taijiquan and created an infrastructure for its dissemination. By the early decades of the 20th century, taiji had its progenitor, its philosophy, its genealogy, a proliferation of styles, a stable of living masters, and an institutional base in the national and regional martial arts academies. If writers accepted Daoism as the state religion of taijiquan and Zhang Sanfeng as its chief god, they were free to expand the pantheon or embellish its lore and legends. During the early decades of the Republic (1911–1949) on the mainland, the strongest voices in opposition to this invented tradition came not from hard or other internal styles, but from leftist taiji enthusiasts who resented the art's abduction by conservative ideologues. Thus, with a mission to demystify taijiquan and return it to the people, Tang Hao visited Chen Village in the early 1930s, followed by fieldwork in the Wudang Mountains to locate descendants of Zhang Sanfeng and in Ningbo to find traces of the Internal School. He found nothing in the Wudang Mountains or Ningbo, but in Chen Village discovered form manuals that were clearly successors to Qi Jiguan's *Boxing Classic* and precursors to the Yang and subsequent forms. In the *Chen Family Biographies and Chen Family Genealogy*, he found entries stating that Chen Wangting, who served as a militia commander in Wen County in 1641 and retired after the fall of the Ming, was the creator of the family form, together with a poem attributed to Wangting saying that he choreographed martial arts forms in his retirement and always kept the *Huangting jing* by his side (Chen, 1933: 477; Tang/Gu, 1963: 7). Tang and collaborator Gu Liuxin acknowledge the Chen debt to Qi's *Boxing Classic*, as seen in the Chen form posture names and the "*Quangjing zongge*" (Poem on the Boxing Classic) but say that Chen's original contribution was the development of push-hands as a unique method of training tactile sensitivity and internal energy in sparring without protective gear. What Tang Hao found in Chen Village, then, was a copy of Qi's *Boxing Classic* and living family members who still practiced one of the several forms recorded in the family manuals; what he did not find were the "classics" or any written or oral tradition regarding Zhang Sanfeng or Wang Zongyue.

To close the gap between the Chen family forms and the "classics" theory, Tang asserted that Wang Zongyue, who is credited with writing some of the texts in the Wu/Li and Yang family corpuses, must have studied in Chen Village and summarized the principles of soft-style pugilism in these short compositions. Xu Zhen, also a modern-minded contemporary of Tang, could not accept that the Chen family developed taijiquan in isolation and so countered that Wang Zongyue must have been the transmitter who brought the art to Chen Village. Having discovered the cradle in Chen Village and giving taiji a humanistic genesis, Tang was somewhat credulous in accepting the authenticity of the "bookstall" manuscript he found in Beijing, and whose author, "Mr. Wang of Shanxi," he assumed to be Wang Zongyue, and the Chen family genealogy and biographies written or altered by Chen Xin. During the Mao era (1949–1976), idealistic accounts of human achievements were overturned as feudal dregs, a conspiracy to deprive the people of credit for producing knowledge with their own hands through trial and error. For Tang Hao, then, the prime mover is the masses. Qi Jiguang is a flesh and blood historical figure, and his form is a synthesis of the best features of sixteen popular styles he collected among the people. The Chen family is a flesh and blood grass roots family, and their family form is based on Qi's *Boxing Classic*. There is no need to kidnap a Daoist immortal and turn him into a martial artist and a patriot. Qi's credentials are impeccable: a patriotic general, a military reformer, a student, synthesizer, and standardizer of popular martial arts styles, and the most influential military mind since Sunzi. The changes—softening of the form and the addition of theory—in the transmission from Qi to Chen to Yang can all be explained by evolution.

Tang Hao's views held sway through the fifties, when the torch was passed to Gu Liuxin, who promoted Tang's thesis in a series of books, martial arts dictionaries, and even the *Chinese Encyclopedia*. Successors to Tang, Xu, and Gu still exist, but serious scholarship has been so marginalized by sensational historical fiction that, for example, a prefatory note by the editors of Wuhun to Mo Chaomai's *Study of the Late-Qing Manchu Princes* apologizes for the "dryness" of the article, that uses the *Draft History of the Qing Dynasty* to overturn the long held Yang family legend that Luchan taught taijiquan in the palace and garrison of a Manchu prince (Mo, 1997: 43). Wu Wenhan uses legitimate historical documents, such as *True Record of the Taiping Rebels' Attack on Huaiqing Prefecture*) and *Diary of the Defense of Huaiqing Prefecture* to demonstrate that Chen family accounts of the time and success of Chen led militia in repelling the rebels was exaggerated (Wu, 1995: 17). Yan Han calls for putting aside subjectivity, emotionalism, and sectarianism and a return to Marx's admonition: "Do not be concerned that your research conclusions fail to correspond to your subjective desires or popular theories but only that they reflect objective laws and historical fact" (Yan, 1999: 10). Pan Jianping compares the claims of the Neo-Zhang Sanfengists to the theory of "the divine right of kings" and restates Tang's gradualist approach in these words: "The formation of taijiquan is a synthesis of Ming dynasty martial arts, especially the thirty-two postures of Qi Jiguang's *Boxing Classic*, together with ancient qigong practices, channel theory, and proto-materialist yin-yang and five phases theory" (Pan, 1999: 51).

The pace of retiring errors in received wisdom is proceeding at a far slower rate than new fantasies are being churned out. In a strange convergence of Western orientalism and Chinese self-orientalization, many practitioners East and West would rather believe that they are participating in a practice with divine origins than a "synthesis" analyzed by intellectual historians; they would rather be part of something more romantic than mere human history, and so the voices of rationality grow smaller and smaller in a marketplace where fantasy is the ultimate product. Taiji religionist Li Zhaosheng's assertion that taijiquan cannot sustain itself without Daoist trappings and the promise of immortality takes the experience of the art out of the practitioner's sensorium and locates it in the realm of religion.

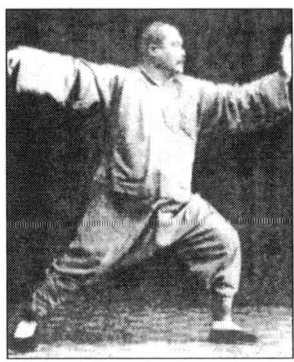

Yang Chengfu (1883–1936) in single whip posture.

The only expressed opposition to Mainland officialism during the 1950s through the 1970s came from cultural conservatives in Taiwan, Hong Kong, and overseas Chinese communities. The formula of most early 20th century taiji ideologues was patriotism, popularization, science, and mystification. The Communists eliminated only the mystification, using modern scholarship and science to explain taiji's history, theory, and practice. Myth deprived the people of their proud history, and lineage monopolized the knowledge that could benefit the whole nation. The psychosomatic state of relaxation in action induced by taiji practice is not described in terms of spiritual attainment but medicine and psychology. Conservative exponents of taiji believed that taiji's principles were consistent with Western science, but Western science was too crude to explain all taijiquan. For this, a knowledge of traditional medicine and meditation was necessary. In effect, this amounted to the essentialist position that you had to be Chinese to grasp the secrets of taijiquan. If science and history could explain all taijiquan, then anyone could master it, and it could no longer function as an ultimate refuge for Chinese identity. The thrust of arguments by cultural conservatives was that Chen Village was too marginal and the Chen family too undistinguished to create something as sublime as taijiquan—it could only have been created by an immortal. In the Chinese language postscript to Huang Wenshan's 1974 *Fundamentals of Tai Chi Chuan*, the author confesses to having been carried away in his youth by May Fourth Movement anti-feudal rhetoric and doubting Zhang Sanfeng, but after several decades of reflection has shaken off the May Fourth hangover and is coming home to Zhang (Huang, 1974: 515). If he was pushed one way by the May Fourth Movement, it is likely he was pushed the other by the Cultural Revolution. A reverse example is Wang Xinwu, whose 1930s *An Exposition of the Principles of Taijiquan* followed Song Shuming's fabricated lineage, but in the prefaces to his 1959 mainland and 1962 Hong Kong reprints allows that these tales were merely "myths" (Wang, 1959: n.p.; 1962: 2). Nevertheless, in communist and conservative, we see two different paths to national salvation: give the people faith in divine assistance or give them confidence in their own two hands.

Yang family spokesmen never denied their debt to Chen Village, but at the same time were at pains to construct a supernatural genesis for taijiquan. Chen Xin, for his part, strove to return the honor to his family by doctoring the family records and writing a book displaying encyclopedic mastery of medicine, cosmology, and meditation. Later generations of Chen family exponents obviously were comfortable with the official history of taijiquan and in so doing renounced any future claims to connection with Zhang Sanfeng. In exchange, they were allowed to glory in their ancestors. In the 1980s, Chen Xin's vision of the Chen family taking its rightful place in taiji history has been realized by a generation of Chen family members who have turned the village into a Mecca for training and competition and have made Chen Style taijquan the fastest growing style on the international circuit. Neighbors and rivals in Zhaobao, however, have taken the opposite tack and have thrown in with the Wudang camp. Thus, we can see that Cold War era taiji sectarianism, with divisions primarily along ideological and cultural lines, has given way today to the reemergence of lineage and free markets, with a return to family businesses and the rise of taiji tourism.

The Wudang–Zhaobao Axis

Until the recent Wudang revival, it was impossible for Daoism to reach out to taijiquan. Taiji was a lived practice, officially promoted for health and sport, although stripped of its feudal trappings of lineage, discipleship, and mythology. Daoism, however, which in the popular imagination had meant chiefly exorcists, recluses, talismans, idols, and elixirs, and in the Mao era smashed temples and defrocked priests, had no voice to reach out to taijiquan. Huang Zongxi's Zhang Sanfeng was "an alchemist from the Wudang Mountains" who "slew more than a hundred bandits," thus uniting the wizard and the warrior. The Shaolin monks may have practiced martial arts, but this was by no means typical for Buddhist monks. Our earliest records of shamanism depict exorcists brandishing weapons in a dance-like ritual to drive out demons, but the power here is magical and not technical. Likewise, Daoist immortal Lü Dongbin is pictured as a great swordsman, but this is an operatic caricature, having more to do with the romance of the sword than the fusion of qigong with martial arts. The unleashing of free market forces has now made it possible for the "Wudang" brand, formerly exploited by the Yang's of Hebei, to be brought back to its homeland in Hubei. As a center of Daoist activity, the Wudang Mountains, located in the northwest corner of Hubei Province, reached its peak in the early Ming but gradually declined, nearly disappearing by the late Qing. The Wudang Mountains are traditionally considered the site where Xuanwu (God of War), associated with the seven constellations of the northern sky and with the tortoise and snake, engaged in Daoist practices and attained immortality. He was elevated to the status of a celestial "emperor" (*di*) during the Yongle reign (1402–1424) of the Ming and thus became the logical choice to visit Zhang Sanfeng in a dream.

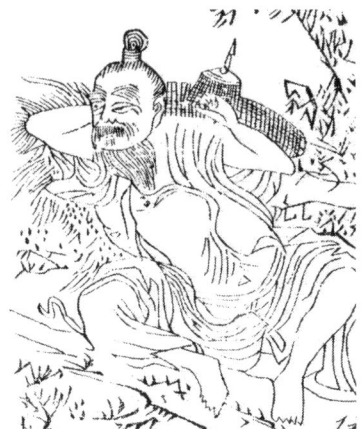

Illustration of Zhang Sanfeng taken from the *Collected Works of Zhang Sanfeng* (1844). Illustration courtesy of Douglas Wile.

Tang Hao's investigations in Wudang and Ningbo found no successors to Zhang Sanfeng or his Internal School. Recently, however, a number of practitioners have come forward claiming to be just that. It was not until after Mao's death that dissenters to the official view began to surface, and in 1980 the National Martial Arts Exhibition held in Wuhan featured a demonstration by Jin Zitao of a style allegedly preserved in the Wudang Mountains. Jin was subsequently invited by the Wuhan Physical Eduation Committee and the Hubei People's Publishing Company to teach in Wuhan and publish a book on the form whose name was shortened to *Wudang taiyi wuxingquan*. Jin moved to Danjiangkou, the nearest city to Wudang, and began to teach there. In 1982, the Wudang Martial Arts Research Association was founded in Danjiangkou, and by 1989 a coalition of Hubei martial arts groups, physical education institutes, research associations, and publishers petitioned the National Physical Education Committee for permission to research the "origins, varieties, and characteristics of Wudang martial arts." As a result, the topic was included as a panel in the academic conferences held in conjunction with planning for China's participation in the 1990 Olympics. They published their findings in a monograph entitled *Studies on Wudang Boxing* in 1992. Their conclusions may be summarized as follows:

1) Zhang Sanfeng was an historical figure.
2) he created a martial art.
3) the martial art he created is unique in its theory and technique.
4) the development of the Wudang School split into many paths, many levels, and many personalities; and
5) the theory that "Zhang Sanfeng did not exist" and that "The Wudang Mountains produced no martial art" is untrue.

Although the authors explain the paucity of credible records as, "Those who have realized the dao conceal their traces," nevertheless, they are prepared to assert that Zhang Sanfeng's birthplace was Yizhou and his dates 1247–1464, arriving at this by the same method that establishes the age of the world by adding the generations since Adam. That the state-run Beijing Physical Education Institute Press would put their imprimatur on a work that unflinchingly announces that Zhang Sanfeng lived 217 years shows how far we have come since the days of scientific socialism. The quality of the evidence marshaled for this study does not justify a claim that Zhang existed, let alone that he lived 217 years, but the study's sins go beyond mere wishful thinking to outright intellectual dishonesty. In Chapter Five, the very first expert witness called in defense of the Zhang Sanfeng theory is none other than Xu Zhen. The editors disingenuously quote from his 1930 *Brief Introduction to Chinese Martial Arts*: "The southern styles of martial arts originated with Zhang Sanfeng of the Wudang Mountains, and of these, taijiquan is the most important." Of all the sources cited in this chapter, Xu alone possesses credentials as a martial arts scholar; however, the authors of the *Studies on Wudang*

Boxing commit a serious sin of omission when they fail to mention that Xu completely reversed himself and publicly disavowed the Zhang Sanfeng theory in his more mature 1936 *A Study of the Truth of Taijiquan*:

> The martial arts abound in misrepresentations, but none surpass taijiquan in this regard. Originally, I failed to study the matter carefully and simply followed the view of one school as if it were fact. . . . The Chen family documents say nothing about Zhang Sanfeng creating taijiquan, and neither do the Wu family writings. In fact, Li Yiyu clearly states that the creator of taijiquan is unknown. . . . Zhang Sanfeng only appears in the Yang family writings and was clearly added by their followers.
> – Deng, 1980: 112

The tactic of quoting from Xu's earlier work was previewed in Wan Laiping and Yan Mei's 1989 *Wudang Taijiquan* (Wan, 1989: 1), published in Hubei under the sponsorship of the Hubei Physical Education Committee, and in fact, Wan's father, the famed Wan Laisheng's 1943 *Introduction to Original Taijiquan* was one of the pioneers in promoting the idea of a transmission independent of the Chens and Yangs. The three research associations who signed onto the publication of the *Studies on Wudang Boxing*, its 29 authors and editors, and the press who published it cannot have been unaware of Xu's retraction. Nevertheless, this is but one example of the egregious dishonesty that characterizes a book that is now the intellectual cornerstone of a commercial empire to capitalize on the Wudang mystique. These include the journal *Wudang* and the Danjiangkou Wudang Martial Arts Research Association, whose training facilities, guest accommodations, art gallery, and public relations center serve to "propagate Wudang culture at home and abroad." Independent origination of other martial arts with well-developed qigong internals is not impossible, as Chang Naizhou's form and writings amply demonstrate, but too many of the new pretenders are simply Yang wine in Yang bottles with antique Daoist labels. The undated early Republican Zhang Sanfeng's *Secret Transmissions on Taiji Elixir Cultivation*, showing a figure in ancient Daoist priest robes performing Yang Chengfu's form is a perfect example.

Jealous of Yang family success, the Chen family has mounted a more than eighty-year campaign to gain market share of taiji glory and profits. More recently, neighboring Zhaobao Town has made a bid to enter this market with capital based on the survival of Zhaobao taijiquan, a close cousin of the Chen Style, and the account of taiji history put forward by Du Yuanhua (1869–1938) in his 1935 *Orthodox Taijiquan*. Du was a student of Ren Changchun, who was a student of Chen Qingping (1795–1868). Du traces a transmission that extends all the way from Laozi, whom he credits with creating taijiquan, to contemporary Zhaobao masters. Accounts of Zhang Sanfeng variously place him in the Song, Yuan, or Ming dynasties, but interestingly Du allows only five generations between Laozi and Zhang. Of the immortal Zhang, he says:

> Zhang Sanfeng perfected this martial art to the level of the miraculous and his skill surpassed all others at that time. . . . His accomplishment in the martial arts is comparable to Confucius' in the realm of letters and sagehood.
> – Yan, 1996: 10

According to Du, Zhang's transmission was brought to Zhaobao by Jiang Fa, a shadowy and controversial figure in Chen and Yang folklore. Du paints Jiang as a native of Wenxian County, born in 1574 near Zhaobao, who went to study with Wang Linzhen in Shanxi and returned to foundd a lineage whose seventh generation master was Chen Qingping, the man whom Wu Yuxiang is said by Li Yiyu to have studied with for a month after his initial introduction to taijiquan by Yang Luchan. Placing Zhaobao in a direct line from Laozi, Zhang Sanfeng, and Jiang Fa effectively invalidates every other version of taiji history and every other lineage or style. Moreover, Zhaobao proponents have recently published a manuscript purported to have been copied in 1918 and containing writings on taijiquan from the first three generations of Jiang Fa's transmission. One of the texts is attributed to Jiang himself and is essentially identical with the *Treatise on Taijiquan* attributed to Zhang Sanfeng in the Yang family redaction of the classics. The rest are original, though whether they are of the vintage and authorship claimed is another matter (Yuan Baoshan, 1996: 3–5). If they are genuinely of the 16th and 17th centuries as claimed, they would be by far the oldest received documents on taijiquan and would supplant the existing "classics," which only exist in Li Yiyu's hand from the late 19th century. Zhaobao promoters point out that Zhaobao Town has been a prosperous commercial crossroads for over 2,500 years, and all of the texts have the name taiji in their titles, but they do not explain why neither the art nor the name were known to Qi Jiguang or Huang Zongxi, or how it dared to violate the imperial name taboo of the first Manchu emperor, Huang Taiji.

During the 1930s, national salvation was uppermost in the minds of Chinese intellectuals, and few failed to appreciate that spiritual resources would be as critical as material in determining China's fate. Qi Jiguang had already pronounced martial arts largely irrelevant to mass warfare in the 16th century, how much more so in an era of bombers, submarines, and nerve gas? A shared theme of all the martial arts publications from the 1930s through the 40s is that martial arts, in general, and taijiquan specifically, can promote the health of the nation and kindle a spirit of confidence and resistance. Some, seeing a deeper spiritual vacuum, presented it as a Daoist path to enlightenment. Du says, "The purpose of taijiquan is to cultivate the elixir and to demonstrate to the world that practicing this art can promote longevity, and after long training, allow us to attain pure yang, or immortality" (Yan, 1996: 11). This points out very vividly how far the inner alchemy vision of spirituality through self-deification differs from the Western worship of God or the Confucian worship of ancestors.

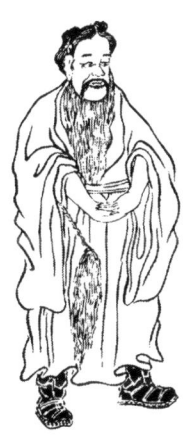

Zhang Sanfeng.

Zhang Sanfeng in Our Time

For sheer contentiousness, the Zhang Sanfeng case can only be compared to issues of racism, sexism, abortion, and homosexuality in American culture. At the dawn of the 21st century, the pendulum has once again swung towards the mythmakers. Western practitioners of taijiquan, with their monotheistic, atheistic, or "only begotten son" backgrounds are apt to view Zhang Sanfeng as simply an historical figure with some innocent Daoist embellishments. They are not likely to understand China's culture wars, polytheism, or embodied immortality. As a counterpoint to the dour Confucian scholar, the Chinese folk and artistic imaginations have populated novels, operas, and temples with sword slinging heroes like Sun Wukong, Guan Gong, and Lü Dongbin. Moreover, the custom of attributing the creation of martial arts to figures like Bodhidharma, Yue Fei, and Emperor Taizu of the Song makes it not surprising that Wang Zhengnan credited Zhang Sanfeng with creating the Internal School art.

The construction of the cult of Zhang Sanfeng during the Ming, the naming of Zhang as founder of the Internal School in the early Qing, the revival of the Zhang cult by the Sichuan Sect of Daoism in the mid-19th century, and the crediting of Zhang as creator of taijiquan in the early 20th century have all been noted by historians of Daoism and the martial arts. Now in the 21st century, we can report a renewed push, not simply to reassert Zhang's paternity in the taijiquan realm, but to refurbish his cult and to promote taijiquan as a religious path. What contemporary scholar Huang Zhaohan said in the 1970s and 80s of Qing dynasty Zhang Sanfeng cult promoters Wang Xiling (1664–1724) and Li Xiyue (c. 1796–1850) has proven to be surprisingly prophetic in the 1990s and beyond. In surveying the authenticity of works in the 1844 (reprinted 1906) *Complete Works of Zhang Sanfeng* compiled by Wang Xiling, Huang finds six forgeries, seven self-serving propaganda pieces for Li Xiyue's "Western Sect," and four pieces produced by planchette. He concludes that it would be a mistake to judge them by modern scholarly standards and offers the following perspective:

> Their research methods were uncritical, and they indiscriminately collected all materials whether historical, legendary, apocryphal, or mythological.... Only if later scholars are careful to use these materials critically will they arrive at the correct conclusions.... Regardless of expenditure of time and effort..... Because the object of their study was a Daoist and belongs to the category of Daoism, we cannot avoid the judgment that these are religious activities and that they were leading religious lives.
> – Huang, 1988: 110

This characterization applies perfectly to today's Neo-Zhang Sanfengists: their "research methods" are precisely the same, and their religious discourse every bit as ardent. Modern martial arts historians were once faced only with the task of extricating taijiquan from Zhang Sanfeng and scholars of the history of religion with showing the inauthenticity of the *Complete Works of Zhang Sanfeng*. The Neo-Zhang Sanfengists, however, require us to do both all over again. In his *Summary of Zhang Sanfeng's Inner Elixir Theory*, Yang Hongling plainly states: "As a kind of religious thought, Zhang Sanfeng's Daoist inner elixir theory is the product of social and historical conditions, together with Daoist theory and his own thinking and culture" (Yang, 1997: 28). The critical word here is "religious." Although containing no mention of martial arts, the reproduction of key *Complete Works of Zhang Sanfeng* meditation texts in today's martial arts journals, along with copious annotations, colloquial translations, and biographies of lineage successors fishes for converts to the cult of Zhang Sanfeng in a pool already familiar with his name.

It is obvious that the outpouring of religious sentiment toward Zhang Sanfeng that fills the pages of today's martial arts magazines is part of a broader "roots seeking" and "cultural reflection" movement in China. The basic message of the Zhang cultists is that socialism killed China's soul. One of the most passionate spokesmen for Zhang Sanfeng fundamentalism is Li Zhaosheng, who begins from the premise that Daoism is China's soul:

> Emperor Yingzong of the Song declared the fifteenth day of the second lunar month, Laozi's birthday, to be True Primordial Source Holiday. That is to say, it is only with the birth of Laozi that the Chinese people have a soul. This is the most ancient 'soul of China.'
> – Li, 1998: 6

The equation, then, is that Daoism is the soul of China, and taijiquan is the vehicle for its realization. Being a religion, though, health or ethics are not enough: we must have miracles. Therefore, Li Zhaosheng, who proclaims himself an 18th generation successor to the *Xiantian taijiquan* (Primordial taijiquan) style recounts an anecdote of his teacher Cai Xiang: Master Cai was collecting ginseng in the mountains when he spied a heroic figure in flowing robes performing a sword form among the trees. Spellbound, Cai continued to observe him from afar for several days. When he ventured to ask the personage his name, he was told that his surname was Zhang. Later, the figure appeared to him in a dream and revealed his identity: the immortal Zhang Sanfeng (Li, 1998: 7). A Zhang Sanfeng sighting in the 20th century, reported with absolute credulity on the eve of the 21st is the nicest capsule of post-modernism anyone could ask for. Although Li Zhaosheng himself does not claim to have seen Zhang Sanfeng, it has been his lifelong ambition as an artist and a Zhang devotee to create a worthy iconography for the immortal's veneration. Criticizing previous efforts as either too barbaric or too effete, he proposes to create a portrait combining traditional techniques, the principles of physiognomy, and even the best of Western influences to capture the otherworldly aura of the immortal. Portraiture as an act of piety, according to Li's description, then, has nothing in common with life drawing or photography, but involves seeing with the inner eye of faith.

The Confucian state had always viewed martial artists as troublemakers, but the Chinese Communists took up the self-strengthening theme of the 1890s and May Fourth Movement, giving state sponsorship to the martial arts as part of a national health and recreation program. In exchange for mass promotion, the martial arts were to give up secrecy and superstition. Nationally standardized and simplified forms replaced family transmissions, and training moved out of courtyards and backrooms into parks and gymnasiums. Though martial arts have joined the free market since the early 1980s, Li Zhaosheng resists any effort to secularize taijiquan, saying:

> Taijiquan, like other arts at that time, was transmitted by alchemists and recluses and later spread among the masses. . . . A martial art that seeks only to promote health is immature and cannot sustain itself. . . . "Internally upholding the way of inner alchemy" means that we can sprout feathers and ascend to heaven, attain life everlasting, cure the sick and infirm, and save all living things; "externally showing the point of the weapon" means that we possess the ultimate martial art technique and take killing evil people as our motto. . . . Those who say that everything is created by the laboring masses seem to be intelligent but on careful examination are not.   – Li, 1998: 6

Li's explicit opposition to the official policy of promoting martial arts for health, and his appeal to restoring them to the traditions of inner alchemy and knight-errantry, is essentially an anti-modernist position. In fact, his standard for historical validity is, "Only the descendants of the lineage are qualified to tell the story of its origins" (Li, 1996: 8). This flies in the face of modern scholarly notions of objectivity and the well-known tendency of styles to exaggerate their own lineages, while imposing an elitist and occultist definition on Daoism. However, at the same time as he champions Zhang Sanfeng as the creator of taijiquan, he denies the origination legends of xingyi and bagua, using opposite arguments. Xingyi, he says, was not created by Yue Fei, and bagua does not qualify as a true martial art because it cannot point to an immortal creator who preceded historical founder Dong Haichuan. In the end, he goes so far as to say that even taijiquan in its present form does not qualify as "a method for realizing the dao through the martial arts" because it "does not follow the acupuncture channels," as does Li's own style, the *Jouzhuan bapan youlongzhang* (Li, 1996: 9). Li insists that only the superficial aspects of the elixir teachings are made public through the martial arts, just as medicine is but a diluted version of the knowledge held by Daoist adepts and immortals and dispensed out of compassion for the masses. Li is thus willing to sell out taijiquan for the sake of promoting the new cult of Zhang Sanfeng. Fellow cultist Zheng Qing also holds that taijiquan is simply a debased version of a secret Daoist art:

> Taijiquan originally consisted of the external postures of the Daoist's "Taijimen jiugong taijishou," which included standing, sitting, and reclining postures. Because it features the internal principles of movement arising from stillness and advocates training through nonaction, when the qi channels within the body are activated, there is an internal power produced with movement. Practitioners will experience the sensation of a flow of qi that propels the body as it moves. This action is accompanied by a feeling of advancing with circular movements, and thus it is called "taijiquan." However, Zhang Sanfeng of the Ming felt that "Taijimen's" emphasis on non-action and the esoteric nature of the internal training, its secrecy among the five branches of Daoism, together with its requirement of open qi channels, spiritual enlightenment, and long dedication made it difficult for people to understand and accept. Therefore, he eliminated the difficult training and secrecy and presented some of the external postures of "Taijimen jiugong taijishou" to the world.   – Zheng, 1998: 40

It is difficult to know at this stage whether these efforts to pull taijiquan back into the shadows is a sincere religious impulse or simply cynical brandsmanship in a market that has reverted to family or Daoist lineage as a test of legitimacy rather than physical education diplomas or tournament trophies. Today, anticommunist progressives are still looking West, while anticommunist conservatives are still looking to Daoism. The government seems sensitive to progressive criticism but tolerant of reactionary, if it refrains from politics.

Li Zhaosheng's ingenuity as a marketing strategist is truly astonishing. He understands that some of the genies released by the communist government will be very difficult to put back in the lamp: the simplified characters and the Twenty-four Posture Taiji Short Form, for example. Recognizing that tens of millions of people already practice this form, Li has attempted to appropriate it for his own purposes, writing a manual (*pu*) in the archaic seven character rhymed couplet style, with all the old flowery language of inner alchemy, and declaring that its purpose is, "Using the *Yijing* to penetrate the great mystery and realize the dao; using the martial arts to illuminate the True and achieve enlightenment" (Li, 1997: 24). Li has thus not only created a counter-discourse but boldly appropriated the state's productions and recast them in an ancient mold, like dragging pottery in the dirt to create instant antiques. Evidence of fissures in the cult's consensus have already begun to appear, however, as Zhang Jie, who believes that Zhang Sanfeng is the reviver of a still older tradition rather than the creator of taijiquan, is taken to task by Li Shirong and Wu Tierong for weakening the Zhang genesis position and for accepting as authentic the transparently spurious Zhang Sanfeng's *Secret Transmissions on Taiji Elixir Cultivation*. They correctly point out that this counterfeit collection includes a supposedly ancient form that is identical with the Yang form in Chen Weiming's *Taijiquan shu*, and its *Treatise on the Necessity of Cultivating the Spirit and Concentrating the Qi in Practicing Taijiquan* was authored by Wu Tunan and published in his 1931 *Taijiquan* (Li and Wu, 1998: 26–27).

So far, we have examined attempts to link taijiquan with Daoism based on bald assertions and simple articles of faith. Another more sophisticated approach, however, deploys pseudo-scholarly methods, riddled with weak links and unwarranted leaps, to defend the paternity of Zhang Sanfeng.

Lu Dimin and Zhao Youbin use textual techniques, teasing out the seven character mnemonic verses embedded in the classics, attributing these to Zhang, and assigning the rest to Wang Zongyue's commentary or Wu Yuxiang's notes (Lu and Zhao, 1992: 7). Li Shirong supports this analysis but is careful to admit that Chen Wangting is indeed the creator of the Chen Style, which he accepts as valid, but derivative of the root "Thirteen Postures" transmitted by Zhang Sanfeng. He does not bother to refute the Li Yiyu "Postscript" assertion that the Wu brothers found the classics in a salt shop in Wuyang, Henan, but does insist that Yang received the complete version first, obliging Wu Yuxiang to copy some portions from Yang (Li, 2000: 10–13). Teasing classic from commentary is a standard scholarly procedure, but it cannot turn Zhang and Wang into bona fide historical figures or prevent Wu Yuxiang and Li Yiyu from writing the "classics" themselves, as some scholars have proposed.

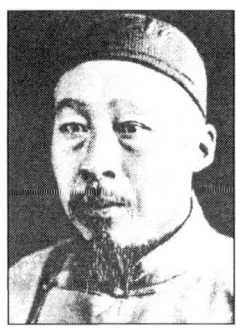

Chen Weiming (1881–1958).

In a 1999 article, Li Shirong, again attempting to appropriate the enemy's rhetoric, characterizes his own scholarly method, saying: "Its logic is consistent with dialectical materialism" (Le, 1999:6). Using this method he correctly challenges Tang Hao's assumption that the "Master Wang of Shanxi who lived during the Qianlong reign of the Qing" and authored the *Yinfu Spear Manual* is the same as Wang Zongyue. However, the basis for his skepticism is not the high probability that the *Yinfu Spear Manual* and accompanying biography found by Tang in the Beijing bookstalls is a forgery, but because to accept it would be to deny that Zhang Sanfeng and Wang Zongyue were both Ming figures. Again, asking the right question for the wrong reason, he calls Tang Hao's contention that Wang Zongyue received the four-line "Sparring Song" in Chen Village and elaborated it to six lines "pure nonsense." Certainly, too much of Tang's case rested on the shaky assumption of Wang Zongyue's historicity and Chen Wangting's creation of taijiquan, but Li Shirong's chief complaint is that Tang's dating would make Wang Zongyue two centuries too late to receive a direct transmission from Zhang Sanfeng. To weaken the Zhang Sanfeng authorship claims, Tang and Gu had cited the many parallels between the *Taiji Classics* and Zhou Dunyi's *Explanation of the Taiji Diagram* and the fact that this work was not published until 1757, too late to have influenced a Ming Daoist. Li, however, counters that Zhou received the interpretation of the taiji symbol from the Daoist immortal Chen Xiyi, and that it was independently handed down in Daoist circles until it reached Zhang Sanfeng, who was then inspired by it to create taijiquan. As further proof, he cites a diagram attributed to Wang Zongyue's student Jiang Fa and reproduced in handwritten manuscript form in a 1990 issue of *Wudang* magazine. He does not attempt to explain why this "Ming" manuscript is written in simplified characters. The release of old handwritten manuscripts attributed to the likes of Chen Changxing (Luchan's teacher), Wang Zongyue, and Jiang Fa is another aspect of the pseudo-scholarship phenomena. These are written in classical Chinese and contain large doses of Daoist jargon and channel theory, but the appearance of Western biomedical terms such as "blood pressure" (*xueya*) does not inspire confidence in their authenticity. If they were authentic, however, it would require us to throw out the existing corpus of "classics" and accept a whole new canon.

In the end, all of this can teach us nothing about the true origins of taijiquan, but a great deal about the contemporary intellectual milieu in China. Sima Nan, who has made it his personal mission to expose qigong cults, referred to the leader of one such cult as the "patriarch of a new religion," and Zhang Honglin refers to the qigong craze as "heretical cults." Taijiquan, at least, has had the decency to deify its invented ancestor and not a living exponent, but even socialism was not immune to the "cult of personality." Since it is difficult to use a capitalist discourse to undermine a "communist" regime that is privatizing everything in sight, and democracy is not perceived as a sure cure for poverty and corruption, it seems that only a religious movement can rally sufficient passion and numbers to challenge the regime. Taipings and Boxers are good examples from not-so-distant history, and the new Zhang Sanfeng cult shows that *Falun Dafa* (lit. "Great Law of the Wheel of Law"; also, *Falun Gong*) is not an isolated case. Paralleling the emergence of ethnic and provincial localism, defining "Chineseness" is no longer exclusively a monopoly of the state, but can be contested by special interests. Daoism wedded to taijiquan is once again resurrected as a carrier of Chineseness in an era of global economic integration. Instead of seeing this subculture as appealing to those who are left behind in the race to the modern, it may be that spiritual aspirations based on the work ethic of earned immortality through strenuous effort, and conferring a profound and secure sense of Chinese identity, may comport with the new entrepreneurial spirit in China in the same way that the Protestant ethic supported the rise of capitalism in the West. Certainly, for the subculture of Zhang Sanfeng cultists, the reconstruction era image of the proletarian "iron man" has given way to the myth of the Daoist immortal/warrior. Daoist chauvinism should never be underestimated, and we need only remind ourselves that some Daoist apologists have claimed that Buddhism sprang from seeds planted by Laozi when he rode westward on his ox.

Conclusion

The little old ladies in China's parks today, with their taiji swords, sly smiles, and twinkling eyes, probably care little about taiji's role in national self-strengthening, reviving the martial spirit, surviving Manchu, Western, and Japanese imperialism, post-modern religious fundamentalism, the ultimate fighting art, taiji tourism, cultural exports, identity politics, or the construction of masculinity. The martial arts politics of hard versus soft, of idealist versus materialist, and of scholarship versus religion will not trouble them. They probably never have fantasies about Zhang Sanfeng or dream of the God of War.

For non-Chinese practitioners, many of these concerns will likewise be irrelevant, but that does not mean that they do not have preconceptions of their own. Chinese ideologues have thought of taiji as a secret weapon in the epic struggle of civilizations; Western practitioners are more likely to think on the scale of the schoolyard or mean streets. Chinese martial arts missionaries and merchants in the West may see taiji as a vehicle for raising respect for Chinese culture, but Western practitioners are more likely to see their involvement in purely personal terms, consciously or unconsciously caught up in warrior dreams, the search for surrogate father figures, intentional community building, physical therapy, orientalism, or alternative spirituality.

Practitioners East and West have been polarized by the issue of whether taijiquan is essentially a fighting art or a moving meditation. Some are deadly serious about taiji as a fighting art, and some feel that taiji is to fighting what dance is to sex: ways to play with aggressive or erotic energy without going over the top. The Daoist-taiji connection in China was painstakingly constructed, and fiercely contested, but presented to the West as a fait accompli.

Leaving politics and scholarship aside, is taijiquan a good vehicle for exploring Chinese culture, and in particular Daoism? In China, the question has always been what did Daoism do for taiji, but in the West we can also ask what did taiji do for Daoism? How does it compare with language, history, literature, the arts, and travel as ways of exploring Chinese culture? To the extent that letting go, non-action, relaxing, egolessness, and no-mind must be actualized to perform the solo form or succeed in self-defense, dabbling in literature and philosophy cannot compare. Performance with the body is the essence of ritual and the reason why taijiquan can be such a powerful delivery system for the insights of Laozi, Zhuangzi, and the inner alchemists. As a theoretical model for explaining why taiji succeeds, Daoist philosophy is a perfect fit, but that does not mean that Daoism invented taiji—Pao Ding the butcher was not a Daoist.

Taijiquan and Daoism Glossary

Bian Renjie	卞人傑	Huang Zongxi	黃宗羲
caizhan	採戰	Jiang Fa	蔣發
Cantongqi	參同契參	jin	勁
Chang Naizhou	萇乃周	jing	靜
Chen Changxing	陳長興	li	力
Chen Fake	陳發科	liangzhi liangneng	良智良能
Chenshi taijiquan tushuo	陳氏太極拳圖說	lingkong faqi	凌空發氣
Chen Qingping	陳清苹	Li Shirong	李師融
Chenshi jiapu	陳氏家譜	Li Xiyue	李西月
Chenshi jiasheng	陳氏家乘	Li Yaxuan	李雅軒
Chen Wangting	陳王庭	Li Yiyu	李亦畬
Chen Weiming	陳微明	Li Zhaosheng	李兆生
Chen Xin	陳鑫	Lu Dimin	路迪民
"Da dao lun"	大道論	Lü Dongbin	呂洞賓
dianxue	點穴	Ma Yuannian	馬原年
Dong Yingjie	董英傑	Ma Yueliang	馬岳梁
Du Yuanhua	杜元化	ming	命
Feng Zhiqiang	馮志強	Neijia quanfa	內家拳法
Gan Fengchi	甘鳳池	Neijing	內經
Ge Hong	葛洪	Ningbo fuzhi	寧波府誌
Gu Liuxin	顧留馨	Pan Jianping	潘建平
Guoji lunlue	國技論略	Pao Ding	庖丁
Guo Tiefeng	郭鐵峰	Qi Jiguang	戚繼光
Hao Weizhen	郝微真	Qingshi gao	清史稿
He Hongming	何鴻明	Quanjing	拳經
Huang Baijia	黃百家	"Quanjing zongge"	拳經總歌
Huangting jing	黃庭經	Shaolin quanshu mijue	少林全數秘訣

Shaolin zongfa	少林宗法	Wudang taijiquan	武當太極拳
Shao Yong	紹雍	Wu Jianquan	吳鑑泉
Shen	神	Wushi taijiquan	吳氏太極拳
Shengshen	聖神	Wu Gongzao	吳公藻
Shen Nong	神農	Wu Tierong	吳鐵融
Shou Huai shilu	守懷實錄	Wu Tunan	吳圖南
shuangxiu	雙修	Wu Wenhan	吳文翰
Sun Lutang	孫祿堂	Wuyang	武陽
Sun Wukong	孫悟空	Wu Yuxiang	武禹襄
Taijimen jiugong taijishou	太極門九功太極手	xin	心
Taijiquan fa chanzong	太極拳法闡宗	xing	性
Taijiquan kaoxin lu	太極拳考信錄	Xu Yusheng	許禹生
Tiajiquan jiangyi	太極拳講義	Xuan Wu	玄武
Taijiquan shi tujie	太極拳勢圖解	"Xue taijiquan xu lianshen juqi lun"	學太極拳需煉神聚氣論
Taijiquan shiyi	太極拳釋義	Xu Zhen	許震
Taijiquan shiyong fa	太極拳使用法	Yang Banhou	楊班侯
Taijiquan shu	太極拳術	Yang Chengfu	楊澄甫
Taijiquan tiyong quanshu	太極拳體用全書	Yang Luchan	楊露禪
Taijiquan xue	太極拳學	Yang Shaohou	楊少侯
Taijiquan zhengzong	太極拳正宗	Yijing	易經
Taijiquan zhi yanjiu	太極拳之研究	Yue Fei	岳飛
Taijiquan zixiu xinfa	太極拳自修新法	Yuefei fan Huai shilu	粵匪犯壞實錄
Taijitu shuo	太極圖說	Zhang Sanfeng	張三豐
Taiji zhannian shisan qiang	太極沾黏十三槍	Zhang Sanfeng quanji	張三豐全集
Tang Hao	唐豪	Zhaobao	趙堡
Wan Laiping	萬賴平	Zhao Youbin	趙幼斌
Wang Xiling	王錫齡	Zheng Manqing	鄭曼青
Wang Xinwu	王新午	Zhengzi taijiquan shisan pian	鄭子太極拳十三篇
Wang Zhengnan	王征南	Zhuang Shen	莊申
Wang Zhengnan muzhi ming	王征南墓志銘	Zhuangzi	莊子
Wang Zongyue	王宗岳	Zhou Dunyi	周敦頤
wen	文		
wu	武		
Wudangquan zhi yanjiu	武當拳之研究		

Bibliography — English

Alter, J. (1992). *The wrestler's body: Identity and ideology in north India*. Berkeley: University of California Press.

Ames, R. (1993). The meaning of the body in classical Chinese thought. In T. Kasulis, et al., (Eds.), *Self as body in Asian theory and practice* (pp. 149–56). Albany, NY: State University of New York Press.

Ames, R. (1993). On the body as ritual practice. In T. Kasulis, et al. (Eds.), *Self as body in Asian theory and practice*. Albany, NY: State University of New York

Press.

Benthall, J. and Polhemus, T. (Eds.). (1975). *The body as a medium of expression*. London: Allen Lane.

Blacking, J. (Ed.). (1977). *The anthropology of the body*. New York: Academic Press.

Brownell, S. (1995). *Training the body for China: Sports in the moral order of the People's Republic*. Chicago and London: University of Chicago Press.

Csordas, T. (Ed.). (1994). *Embodiment and experience: The existential ground of culture and self*. Cambridge: Cambridge University Press.

Donohue, J. (1994). *Warrior dreams: Martial arts and the American imagination*. Westwood, CT: Bergin and Garvey.

Donohue, J. (1993). The ritual dimension of karate-do. *Journal of Ritual Studies* 7(1): 105–24.

Frank, A. (2000). "Kung fu fighters without history: Imagining tradition with Shanghai taijiquan players." Paper presented at Association for Asian Studies 2000 Annual Meeting as part of panel "Creating, Selling, and Remembering Martial Arts in Modern China."

Herman, D. (2000). "The commodification of chi: Remythologizing martial arts in the 20th century." Paper presented at Association for Asian Studies 2000 Annual Meeting as part of panel "Creating, selling, and remembering martial arts in modern China."

Hobshawn, E. and T. Ranger (Eds.) (1983). *The invention of tradition*. Cambridge: Cambridge University Press.

Kasulis, T., et al (Eds.). (1993). *Self as body in Asian theory and practice*. Albany: SUNY Press.

Kierman, F. and Fairbank, J. (Eds.) (1973). *Chinese ways in warfare*. Cambridge: Harvard University Press.

Kotkin, J. (1993). *Tribes: How race, religion, and identity determine success in the new global economy*. New York: Random House.

Law, J. (Ed.). (1995). *Religious reflections on the human body*. Bloomington: Indiana University Press.

Miura, Kunio (1989). The revival of qi: Qigong in contemporary China. In Kohn, L., and Yoshinobu, S. (Eds.), *Taoist Meditation and Longevity Techniques*, pp. 331–363. Ann Arbor: Center for Chinese Studies, The University of Michigan.

Morris, A. (2000). "National skills: Martial arts and the Nanjing state, 1928–1937." Paper presented at Association for Asian Studies 2000 Annual Meeting as part of panel, Creating, selling, and remember martial arts in modern China.

Oakes, T. (1998). *Tourism and modernity in China*. London and New York: Routledge.

Oakes, T. (August 2000). China's provincial identities: Reviving regionalism and reinventing 'Chineseness.' *The Journal of Asian Studies* 59(3): 667–692.

Ong, Aiwa (1999). *Flexible citizenship: The cultural logics of transnationality*. Durham, NC: Duke University Press.

Otis, T. (1994). The silenced body—The expressive Leib: On the dialectic of mind and life in Chinese cathartic healing. In T. Csordas, (Ed.), Embodiment and experience: The existential ground of culture and self. Cambridge: Cambridge University Press.

Rankin, M. (1986). *Elite activism and political transformation in China*. Stanford: Stanford University Press.

Rogoski, R. (2000). "Fists of Fury" or the Jingwu hui before Bruce Lee. Paper presented at Association for Asian Studies 2000 Annual Meeting as part of panel Creating, Selling, and Remembering Martial Arts in Modern China.

Seidel, A. (1970). A Taoist immortal of the Ming dynasty: Chang San-feng. In W. de Bary (Ed.), *Self and Society in Ming Thought*. New York: Columbia University Press.

Sharf, R. (1995). Whose Zen? Zen Nationalism Revisited. In J. Heisig and J. Maraldo, (Eds.), *Rude awakenings* (pp. 40–51). Honolulu: University of Hawaii Press.

Sivin, N. (1996). *Medicine, philosophy and religion in ancient China: Researches and reflections*. Alsershot, Great Britain: Variorum.

Stephenson, N. (1995). *The diamond age, or "A young lady's illustrated primer."* New York: Bantam.

Sutton, N. (1993). Gongfu, guoshu, and wushu: State appropriation of the martial arts in modern China. *Journal of Asian Martial Arts* 3(1): 102–14.

Tanaka, S. (1994). Imagining history: Inscribing belief in the nation. *Journal of Asian Studies,* 1: 24–44.

Victoria, B. (1997). *Zen at war*. New York: Weatherhill.

Wile, D. (2007). *Zheng Manqing's uncollected works on taijiquan, qigong, and health, with new biographical notes*. Milwaukee, WI: Sweet Ch'i Press.

Wile, D. (2000). *T'ai-chi's ancestors: The making of an internal martial art.* New City, NY: Sweet Ch'i Press.

Wile, D. (1996). *Lost t'ai-chi classics from the late Ch'ing dynasty*. Albany, NY: State University of New York Press.

Wile, D. (1985). *Cheng Man-ch'ing's advanced t'ai-chi form instructions, with selections on meditation, the I ching, medicine, and the arts*. Brooklyn, NY: Sweet Ch'i Press.

Wile, D. 1983. *Tai-chi touchstones: Yang family secret transmissions*. Brooklyn, NY: Sweet Ch'i Press.

Wile, D. (1982). *Master Cheng's thirteen chapters on t'ai-chi ch'uan*. Brooklyn, NY: Sweet Ch'i Press.

Xu Ben (1998). 'Modernity to Chineseness': The rise of nativist cultural theory in post-1989 China. *Positions: East Asia Cultures Critique,* 6(1): 203–37.

Xu Jian (1999). Body, discourse, and the cultural politics of contemporary Chinese qigong. *The Journal of Asian Studies,* 4: 961–91.

Yuasa Yasuo. (1987). *The Body: Toward an eastern mind-body theory*. Albany: State University of New York Press.

Zito, A. and T. Barlow, (Eds.). (1994). *Body, subject, and power in China.* Chicago: University of Chicago Press.

Bibliography — Chinese

Chang Naizhou (1936). *Changshi wuji shu* (Chang Naizhou's writings on martial arts). Xu Zhen (Ed.). Taiwan reprint, n.p., n.d. Xu Zhen preface, 1932; first published 1936.

Chen Bin (1989). Taijiquan yu daojiao guanxi bian. (Questions regarding the relationship between taijiquan and Daoism). *Zhonghua wushu* 5: 26–27.

Chen Changxing (1994). Taijiquan shida yaolun (Ten treatises on taijiquan). *Wuhun* 8: 44–45.

Chen Jifu (1935). *Chenshi taijiquan rumen zongjie* (General introduction to Chen family taijiquan). Taibei: Hualian Publishing House, 1980 reprint.

Chen Weiming (1925). *Taijiquan shu* (The art of taijiquan). Hong Kong: Xianggan Wushu Publishing House, n.d.

Chen Xin (1933). *Chenshi taijiquan tushuo* (Introduction to Chen family taijiquan). Hong Kong reprint: Chen Xiangji shuju, 1983; Author's preface, 1919; first published 1933.

Feng Fuming (1989). Guanyu 'taijiquan yuanliu' wenti de tongxin (An exchange of letters on the question of taijiquan's origins). *Wudang* 4: 22–24.

Fu Chengjiang (1991). Wudangquan yu Zhongguo gudai zhexue sixiang de guanxi (The relationship between Wudang boxing and ancient Chinese philosophy). *Wudang* 1: 35–38.

Fu Zhenlun (1983). Cong wushu de lishi fazhan kan wushu de shehui zuoyong (Looking at the social function of the martial arts from the point of view of their historical development). *Henan tiyu shiliao* 3: 1–4.

Gu Liuxin and Tang Hao (1963). *Taijiquan yanjiu* (Studies on taijiquan). Hong Kong: Bailing Publishing House.

Gu Liuxin and Tang Hao (1982). *Taijiquan shu* (The art of taijiquan). Shanghai: Jiaoyu Publishing House.

Guo Tiefeng (1999). Qigong dadao taijiquan (Qigong, the great dao, and taijiquan). *Jingwu* 3: 28–29.

Han Kang (1998). Taijiquan zaikao cong Wang Zhengnan shengping (Reexamining taijiquan from the point of view of the life of Wang Zhengnan). *Wudang* 4: 12.

Hao Chin (1988). Lun lishi shang tiyu yu zongjiao de guanxi (On the historical relationship between physical education and religion). *Tiyu wenshi* 4: 12–18.

Hao Chin (1990). Lun Zhongguo wushu dui daojiao wenhua de rongshe (On the absorption of Daoist culture into the martial arts). *Tiyu wenshi* 1: 7–11.

Hao Wen (1987). Zhouyi yu taijiquan shu (The *Yijing* and taijiquan). *Wulin* 3: 4–5.

He Hongming (1997). Yangshi taijiquan dingxing qian ceng de daomen gaoren zhidian (Yang Luchan received instruction from a Daoist before finalizing his form). *Wudang* 6: 34–35.

Huang Baijia. Neijia quanfa (Art of the internal school's boxing methods). *Zhaodai congshu*, Vol. 163.

Huang Zongxi. *Nanlei ji* (Collected works of Huang Zongxi). Shanghai: n.p., n.d.; photoreprint of 1680 edition.

Huang Zhaohan (1989). *Mingdai daoshi Zhang Sanfeng kao* (A study of the Ming dynasty Daoist Zhang Sanfeng). Taipei: Xuesheng Shuju.

Jiang Bailong, et al. (Eds.). (1992). *Wudangquan zhi yanjiu* (Studies on Wudang Boxing). Beijing: Beijing Tiyu Xueyuan Publishing House.

Jin Yiming (1936). Guoshu ying yi rujia wei zhengzong (Confucianism should be the true philosophy of the martial arts). *Guoshu zhoukan* 3: 156–57.

Kang Gewu (1983). Tansuo quanzhong yuanliu de fangfa (Methods in tracing the origins of martial arts styles). *Zhonghu wushu* 1: 43–44.

Kong De (1997). Zhang Sanfeng "Dadao lun" shuzhu (Zhang Sanfeng's "Treatise on the Great Dao" with annotations). *Wudang* 1: 39–41; 2: 38–40; 3: 42–44; 4: 37–39; 5: 38–39; 6: 38–39; 7: 40–41; 8: 39–40; 9: 35–36; 10: 38–40.

Li Jifang (1997). Chen Wangting 'yici' bian (Problems in Chen Wangting's 'Posthumous Poem'). *Tiyu wenshi* 3: 33–35.

Li Jinzhong (1989). Taojiao sixiang dui taijiquan de yingxiang (The influence of Daoism on taijiquan). *Zhonghua wushu* 1: 32–33.

Li Shirong (1998). Wang Zongyue, Wu Yuxiang liang quanpu de bijiao yu jianbie (Comparing and contrasting the martial arts manuals of Wang Zongyue and Wu Yuxiang). *Zhonghua wushu* 9: 10–13.

Li Shirong (2000). Zhang Sanfeng bu shi taiji bizu (Zhang Sanfeng is not the creator of taijiquan). *Jingwu* 6: 26–27.

Li Shirong (1999). 'Taijiquan lun' zhuzuo beijing ji niandai kaozheng (A study of the background and date of the author of the "Treatise on taijiquan"). *Wulin* 7: 4–10.

Li Zhaosheng (1998). Zhang Sanfeng zushi shengxiang xiezhen (Creating the holy image of master Zhang Sanfeng). *Wudang* 2: 6–8; 3: 4–5.

Li Zhaosheng (1996). Taijiquan shi xianxia jiandao fanhua yu su de xiuwei (Taijiquan is a spiritual practice of martial adepts that has filtered down to the common people). *Wudang* 8: 6–9.

Li Zheng (1999). Shilun taijiquan de 'shu' he 'dao' (A preliminary discussion of the technique and dao of taijiquan). *Wudang* 7: 19–20.

Li Zejian (1995). 'Taijiquan lun' de zuozhe shi shei? (Who is the author of the "Treatise on taijiquan?") *Wuhun* 2: 51.

Liang Qichao (1916). Zhongguo zhi wushidao (Japanese bushido). *Yinbingshi congshu, Vol. 7*. Shanghai: Commercial Press.

Liu Changlin (1987). Zhongguo gudai yinyang shuo (Ancient Chinese theories of yin and yang). *Wuhun* 4: 20–21.

Liu Junxiang (1988). Gudai zheli yu lunli dui Zhongguo wushu xingcheng he fazhan de yingxiang (The influence of ancient philosophy and ethics on the formation and development of Chinese martial arts). *Tiyu wenshi* 5: 51–56.

Lu Dimin (1996). 'Chenshi jiapu' pangzhu kao (A study of the annotations to the "Chen family geneology"). *Wudang* 9: 48–49.

Lu Dimin and Zhao Youbin (1992). *Yangshi taijiquan zhengzong* (Orthodox Yang style taijiquan). Beijing: Sanqin Publishing House.

Lu Zhaoming (1987). Wushu zhong de yinyang wuxing shuo (The yin-yang and five phases theories in the martial arts). *Tiyu wenshi* 4: 5–6.

Ma Guoxiang (1997). Caotan taijiquan de quanwai gong (A discussion of non-pugilistic elements in taijiquan). *Wuhun* 2: 12–13.

Ma Hong (1991). Taiji taijitu taijiquan (Taiji, the taiji symbol, and taijiquan). *Wulin* 2: 22–23.

Ma Hong (1998). Shilun daojia sixiang dui taijiquan de yingxiang (A preliminary discussion of the influence of Daoist thought on taijiquan). *Wudang* 3: 27–31.

Ma Yuannian (1998). Taijiquan he rujia sixiang (Taijiquan and Confucian thought). *Shaolin yu taiji* 11: 32–33.

Meng Naichang (1987). Taijiquan de zhexue jichu (The philosophical foundations of taijiquan). *Tiyu wenshi* 4: 47–52.

Meng Naichang (1990). Laozi yu taijiquan (Laozi and taijiquan). *Wudang* 1: 28–33.

Mo Chaomai (1999). Rujia wenhua yu wushu (Confucian culture and the martial arts). *Zhonghua wushu* 5: 38–40.

Mo Chaomai (1997). Baguazhang, taijiquan shi sheji zhi qingmo zhuwang kao (An examination of the involvement of the Manchu princes in the history of baguazhang and taijiquan). *Wuhun* 5: 43–44.

Niu Jia (1987). Taijiquan yu weiren zhi dao (Taijiquan and ethics). Zhonghua wushu 5: 43.

Qi Jiguang n.d. *Jixiao xinshu* (New and effective methods in military science). Ma Mingda (Ed.). Beijing: Renmin Tiyu Publishing House, 1986.

Qian Timing (1997). Taijiquan lilun tanyuan (An exploration of the theory of taijiquan). *Wudang* 5: 17–21.

Shan Zhongzi (1998). Guben 'taijiquan midian' (An ancient "Secret taijiquan classic"). *Wudang* 5: 21–22.

Sheng Qing. Zai fugu zhong qiu de jietuo (In search of an escape from the revivalist movement). *Wuhun* 3: 13.

Song Zhijian (1970). *Taijiquan xue* (The study of taijiquan). Taibei: Song Zhijian.

Su Jingcun (1989). Liang Qichao de shangwu sixiang yu minzu tiyu de xingjue (Liang Qichao's military thinking and the development of national physical education awareness). *Tiyu wenshi* 3: 22–25.

Su Xiaoqing (1988). Kang Youwei de tiyu sixiang ji qi chengyin (Kang Youwei's views on physical education and their background). *Tiyu wenshi* 1: 49–52.

Su Xiongfei (1975). Kongzi de tiyu kechenglun fangfalun ji qi pingjia (The role of physical education in Confucius' curriculum, its methodology, and an evaluation). *Tiyu xueshu yantaohui zhuankan*: 33–39.

Sun Lutang (n.d.). *Taijiquan xue* (The study of taijiquan). Hong Kong: Xianggang Wushu Publishing House, n.d.; preface dated 1919.

Tan Benlun (1991). Lun Wudang Songxi pai neijiaquan (On the Wudang Songxi lineage of the Internal School). *Wudang* 1: 15.

Tang Hao (1958). Jiu Zhongguo tiyu shi shang fuhui de Damo (Falsifications concerning the role of Bodhidharma in the history of Chinese physical education).

Zhongguo tiyu shi cankao ziliao, Vol. 4.

Tang Hao (1935). *Neijiaquan de yanjiu* (A study of the internal school). Hong Kong: Unicorn Press, 1969 reprint.

Tian Yongpeng (1988). Chuantong wushu yu gudai zongjiao yishi qiantan (A preliminary examination of traditional martial arts and ancient religious consciousness). *Tiyu wenshi* 3: 28–29.

Tong Xudong (1994). Sun Jianyun dashi fangtan lu (An interview with master Sun Jianyun). *Wuhun* 10: 36–37.

Tong Xudong (1990). Sun Jianyun xiansheng tan 'sanquan heyi' (Master Sun Jianyun discusses the unity of the three internal martial arts). *Jingwu* 12: 23.

Wang Huai (1992). Taojiao yangshengshu yu taijiquan (Daoist health practices and taijiquan). *Wudang* 4: 23–24, 26.

Wang Xinwu (n.d.) *Taijiquanfa chanzong* (The principles of taijiquan). Xian: Shaanxi Renmin Publishing House, 1959 (reprint); Hong Kong: Taiping shuju, 1962 reprint.

Wang Xian (1988). Yinyang xueshuo yu Zhongguo chuantong wushu (Yin-yang theory and traditional Chinese martial arts). *Tiyu wenshi* 2: 3, 21.

Wang Zixin (1988). Taijiquan zheyuan tan (An exploration of the philosophical sources of taijiquan). *Zhonghua wushu* 2: 11–13.

Wu Gongzao (1935). *Taijiquan jiangyi* (Commentaries on taijiquan). Shanghai: Shanghai Bookstore, 1991.

Wu Tunan (1991). *Wu Tunan taijiquan jingsui* (The essence of Wu Tunan taijiquan). Beijing: Renmin Tiyu Publishing House.

Wu Tunan (1984). *Taijiquan zhi yanjiu* (A study of taijiquan). Hong Kong: Commercial Press.

Wu Tunan (1928). *Taijiquan* (Taijiquan). Hong Kong: Jinhua Publishing House, n.d.

Wu Zhiqing (n.d.) *Taiji zhengzong* (Orthodox taijiquan). Shanghai: Shanghai Bookstore, 1986 (reprint); Hongkong: Jinhua Publishing House, n.d.

Wu Wenhan (1995). Yitiao yu Chengou wushu youguan de shiliao (An historical item on Chen Village martial arts). *Wuhun* 11: 17.

Xi Yuntai (1985). *Zhongguo wushu shi* (The history of Chinese martial arts): Beijing: Renmin Tiyu Publishing House.

Xu Zhen (1930). *Guoji lunlue* (Summary of the Chinese martial arts). Shanghai: Commercial Press.

Xu Zhen (1936). *Taijiquan kaoxin lu* (A study of the truth of taijiquan). Taipei: Zhenshanmei Publishing House, 1965 reprint.

Yan Han (1999). Taijiquan lishi shang zhi mi (A mystery in taijiquan's history). *Wulin* 8: 10–11.

Yang Chengfu (1931). *Taijiquan shiyong fa* (Self-defense applications of taijiquan). Taibei: Zhonghua Wushu Publishing House, 1974 reprint.

Yang Chengfu (1934). *Taijiquan tiyong quanshu* (Complete principles and applications of taijiquan). Taibei: Zhonghua Wushu Publishing House, 1975 reprint.

Yang Honglin (1996). Jianshu Zhang Sanfeng neidan lilun (A brief exposition of the theory of Zhang Sanfeng's inner elixir method). *Wudang* 4: 28–32.

Yang Shaoyu (1990). Shendao xuanxue yu wushu yundong (Mysticism, metaphysics, and the martial arts movement). *Wudang* 3: 21–30.

Yang Yong (1987). Xian you neijiaquan hou you Zhang Sanfeng (The internal school predates Zhang Sanfeng). *Tiyu wenshi* 4: 16.

Yu Jianhua (1986). Taijiquan lilun de zhexue jichu chutan (A preliminary discussion of the philosophical foundations of taijiquan theory). *Zhejiang tiyu kexue* 3: 10–13.

Yu Zhijun (1991). Wudang neijiaquan de quanli shi kexue haishi xuanxue (Is Wudang internal boxing theory science or metaphysics?). *Wudang* 6: 35–37.

Zeng Qingzong (1988). Taiji daojiao he shui: taijiquan zheli tansuo (Taiji, Daoism, and water: Tracing the philosophical principles of taijiquan). *Wulin* 4: 42–43.

Zeng Zhaoran (1960). *Taijiquan quanshu* (Complete taijiquan). Hong Kong: Youlian Publishing House.

Zhang Ruan (1988). Neijiaquan dashi Zhang Songxi shengping bianwu (Correcting errors in the biography of internal school master, Zhang Songxi). *Tiyu wenshi* 4: 28–30.

Zhang Weiyi (1988). Shixi rujia sixiang dui chuantong tiyu fazhan de ying-xiang (An analysis of the influence of Confucian thought on the development of physical education). *Tiyu wenshi* 1: 39–43.

Zhang Xuanhui (1984). Wuou youdu jue yichan neijia que you liuluquan (A unique legacy: the Internal School's Six Paths still exits). *Wulin* 5: 32.

Zheng Qing (1998). Taiji shuzhen (The truth about taijiquan). *Shaolin yu taiji* 4: 40–41.

Zheng Zhenkun (1988). Lun Huang Zongxi dui Zhonghua wushu de lishi gongxian (On Huang Zongxi's historical contribution to Chinese martial arts). *Tiyu wenshi* 6: 46–48.

Zhi Zi (1996). Fo Ru Dao huxiang yingxiang manyi (A discussion of the mutual influence of Buddhism, Confucianism, and Daoism). *Shaolin yu taiji* 4: 9.

Zhou Linyi (1975). Laozi sixiang yu tiyu benzhi (Laozi's thought and the nature of physical education). *Tiyu xueshu yantaohui zhuankan* 1: 40–48.

Zhou Weiliang (1991). Dui jianguo hou wushu shehui kexue lilun yanjiu de sikao. (An examination of social science theory in the martial arts since the founding of the People's Republic). *Wuhun* 4: 7–8.

Zunwozhai zhuren (n.d.). *Shaolin quanshu mijue* (Secrets of Shaolin boxing).

Taiji Ruler: Legacy of the Sleeping Immortal
by Kenneth S. Cohen, M.A., M.S.Th.

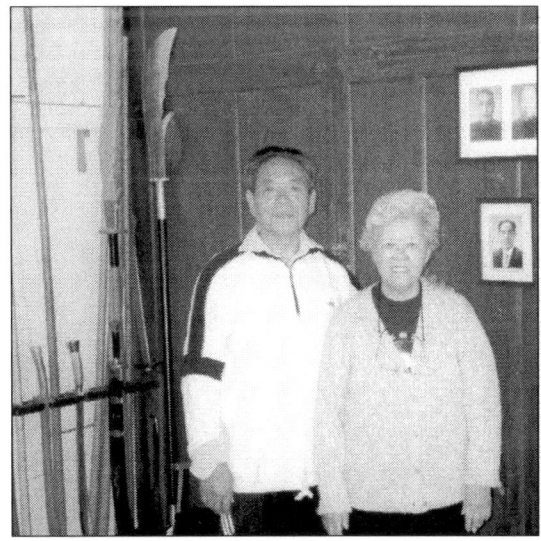

The author's primordial taiji ruler teachers,
Feng Zhiqiang and Madame Gao Fu.

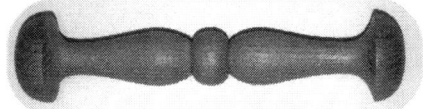

The classic taiji ruler.
All photographs courtesy of Kenneth S. Cohen.

Introduction

The taiji ruler (*chi*) is the name of a beautifully shaped foot-long wooden stick as well as the Daoist system of meditative postures and exercises (*qigong*) that may be performed while holding it. The ruler exercise is a powerful method of physical and spiritual cultivation (*xiu lian*) that increases the body's supply of qi, stimulates qi flow through the meridians and bodily tissues, and develops a tranquil state of awareness. It is suitable for men and women, young and old.

The taiji ruler is also called "taiji stick" (*taiji bang*), "The Needle Which Stills the Mind" (*ding xin zhen*), and "Heaven and Earth Precious Ruler" (*qian kun bao chi*). Since the mid-1950s, when the ruler was first taught publicly, it has also been known as "The Gentle Art of Taiji" (*taiji rou shu*) and "Prenatal Qigong Taiji Ruler" (*xiantian qigong taiji chi*). The word taiji means the blending of yin and yang and implies a state of harmony and balance. Although the taiji ruler and the popular taijiquan martial art both incorporate the philosophical principle of taiji, neither art is based on the other.

No one really knows the origin of the ruler exercise or the ruler itself. American qigong practitioner Richard M. Mooney believes that the shape of the ruler may be based on the shape of ancient Chinese sword handles, a hypothesis that cannot be proved or disproved (Mooney, no date).[1] Seidel notes that the legendary Daoist immortal Zhang Sanfeng is said to have always had a foot rule (*chi*) in his hands, "perhaps an early iconographic detail" (Seidel, 1970: 485). *The Complete Works of Zhang Sanfeng* (Zhang Sanfeng Quan Shu), a text transcribed mediumistically by planchette, explains that Zhang used the ruler "to cut open the primordial chaos" (Seidel, 1970: 517). Perhaps the ruler was a kind of Daoist scepter—like the Tibetan Buddhist dorje, a sign of spiritual authority. The Daoist priest is able to take the measurements of heaven and earth; he (or she) is aware of the true dimensions of the universe because his mind is free of the limitations of words. "The Dao that can be measured is not the immeasurable Dao."

The Transmission of the Ruler

The famed Daoist Chen Xiyi (ca. 906–989 CE) is considered the creator or first teacher of the ruler system. Chen Xiyi is the founder of several qigong systems that are still practiced today, including *Daoist Sleeping Practice* (*shui gong*, "ecstatic sleep" in Kohn, 1993: 271–276), *Daoyin for the Twenty-Four Seasonal Nodes* (Berk, 1979: 19–47; Zong and Li, 1990: 24–47), and a taijiquan-like qigong/martial art called *Six Harmonies Eight Methods* (Liu He Ba Fa, Foxx, 1995). In addition, Chen is credited with a system of *Yijing* interpretation, Daoist physiognomy, and one of the early representations of the taiji symbol. For comprehensive information about Chen Xiyi see Livia Kohn's *Chen Tuan: Discussions and Translations* (Kohn, 2001).

Daoist legends recorded at the beginning of the 19th century in the Le Shan District of Sichuan (near Mt. Emei) claim Chen Xiyi as one of the Six Patriarchs of the Hidden Immortals Sect of Daoism (Seidel, 1970: 511–513). In approximately the 4th century BCE, Laozi, the first patriarch, transmitted Daoist teachings to Yin Xi. Yin Xi must have achieved immortality because he was the teacher of the "Hemp Clad Daoist," Ma Yi, in the 4th century CE, eight hundred years later! During the 10th century, a young Daoist named Chen Tuan (later given the honorific "Chen Xiyi—the Unfathomable" by the first Song Emperor) studied alchemy with Ma Yi on Mount Hua, the Daoist sacred mountain in western China, becoming the fourth patriarch. Not long thereafter Chen taught Huo Long, the "Fire Dragon" Daoist, who became the teacher of Zhang Sanfeng. Chen Xiyi is also linked with Longmen Daoism and the teachings of Lu Dongpin, which he received from Liu Haichan (d. ca. 1050).

At least two lineages of taiji ruler have continued into the present, both tracing their origins to Chen Xiyi. In the first, Chen taught the ruler to his friend and chess partner Zhao Kuangyin, who later became the first emperor of the Song dynasty. The ruler was passed down as a precious family heirloom from one generation to the next. Eventually, it reached a descendant of the emperor named Zhao Zhongdao (1844–1962), the first person to teach it publicly (Xu, 1986: 45).

This story is supported by the majority of taiji ruler teachers with whom I have studied. However, Guan Yongnian, a disciple of Zhao, notes the lack of evidence linking the Song emperor with the ruler. Guan believes that a certain Wang Yongfu of Beijing was Zhao Zhongdao's first and perhaps only ruler teacher (Guan, 1984: ii). Zhao admits studying the ruler with Wang, which he notes in the preface to his first book, *The Gentle Art of Taiji Manual* (Taiji Rou Shu Shuo Ming Shu), published in 1928. Guan believes that, according to reliable evidence, Wang was the very first teacher of the ruler in China, and we have no way of knowing who, if anyone, preceded him. I will take the middle ground and assume that Zhao learned from both his family and from Wang. We may never know the full story.

In 1954 Zhao established The Supple Art of Taiji Health Society (*Taiji Rou Shu Jian Shen She*) in Beijing to teach the art publicly. Until 2000 all books or magazine articles about the ruler, whether in Chinese or western languages, represented only Zhao's lineage. The first book to mention the ruler was Zhao Zhongdao's 1928 work previously cited, followed by a limited-edition book titled *A Study of Taiji Ruler* published in 1961, and several other books (see Xu, 1986, 271–272 for a list of publications). Guan Yongnian's *Taiji Stick Qigong* published in 1984 was the first book published about the ruler in post-Communist China. My own writings, among the first in the West (Cohen, 1997, 1983a, 1983b) also explored the philosophy and techniques of Zhao's lineage, which I learned during the 1970s principally from Chan Bun-Piac[2] of Fujian, but also from Dan Farber (student of Qin Xu of Hong Kong) and Michael Mayer (student of Fong Ha, who teaches near San Francisco, California).

A second taiji ruler lineage was transmitted secretly from Daoist to Daoist and not taught publicly until the late 1990s (Feng and Wang, 2000: 200–205). Around 1820, a Daoist priest of unknown sect named Huo Chengguang, heir to Chen's system, traveled to Shanxi where he met a talented young martial artist named Peng Tingjun. After three years of diligent training, Peng became Huo's disciple. Peng taught the ruler to one of the greatest qigong masters of the 20th century, Hu Yaozhen (1879–1973). Hu was an esteemed practitioner of Chinese medicine, martial arts, and Daoism, and is generally considered "the father of modern qigong." He helped to standardize the term qigong as a substitute for the wide array of ancient words commonly used for Daoist qi cultivation (e.g. daoyin, yangsheng, neigong, tuna). Hu also coined the phrases "tranquil qigong" (*jinggong*) and "active qigong" (*donggong*) to distinguish qigong meditation from qigong exercise, and he was the first qigong practitioner to apply qigong in a clinical setting, laying the groundwork for the modern concept of medical qigong (*yigong*). He is the author of *Health Preserving Qigong, and Five Animal Frolics* (with co-author Jiao Guorui). Hu's qigong was introduced to western readers in Jiao Guorui's *Qigong Essentials for Health Promotion* (Jiao, 1988).

Hu's chief disciple and certainly his most famous was Chen Style taijiquan[3] Master Feng Zhiqiang (b. 1928). Feng studied with Hu for nine years. During the 1990s Feng combined Chen Style taijiquan (from Chen Fake), Liu He Xinyiquan[4] (from Hu Yaozhen), and qigong (from both Chen Fake and Hu Yaozhen) into a comprehensive qigong and martial arts system known as Chen Shi Xinyi Hunyuan Taiji (Chen Family Mind-Intent Primordial Taiji) or Hunyuan Taiji for short (Feng, 1998: 1999). The system includes various Chen Style taijiquan forms, applications, and weapons, and the following kinds of qigong: Hunyuan qigong, coiling silk (*chan si*) qigong, special Daoist taiji ruler, special Daoist taiji ball, taiji stick, and Six Character Formula (Meehan, 2000). Two of Feng's students have produced English language books based on Feng's qigong (Feng and Chen, 2001; Wang, ca. 2000). Hunyuan taiji has also been discussed in various journal articles (Meehan, 2000; Yang and Grubisich, 2000; Cohen, 2000). I had the opportunity to learn exercises from the Hunyuan taiji system with Madame Gao Fu (1916–2005), one of Feng's senior students, during the 1990s and with Grandmaster Feng during his visit to Seattle, Washington in July of 2001.

There are, however, certain riddles in the story of Feng's taiji ruler lineage. It seems that Hu Yaozhen learned the taiji ruler from both Peng Tingjun and Zhao Zhongdao, though I have not seen this fact mentioned in the published works of either Feng Zhiqiang or Feng's students. Hu Yaozhen wrote, "In the autumn of 1959 I studied taiji ruler with Master Zhao, and applied it in hospital clinics with great success" (Guan, 1984: 4). If Hu was already a long-time practitioner of Peng's ruler system, why did he not teach it to hospital patients? Hu Yaozhen's various books do not mention Peng's ruler, nor do his students, except for Feng Zhiqiang. Guan Yongnian, one of the finest authors on the ruler, learned qigong from both Zhao Zhongdao and Hu Yaozhen, but he attributes his ruler techniques entirely to Zhao (Guan, 1984: 1988). Did Feng, Hu's chief disciple, perhaps learn techniques from his Master that were hidden from both the public and from all of Hu's other students? Such a situation would not be without precedent. Even today, there are Chinese martial arts masters who believe they should teach the "secrets," their best techniques, only to their best student or to a very select group of disciples.

TAIJI RULER LINEAGES — PRINCIPAL FIGURES

Lineage A	Lineage B	Lineage C
Chen Xiyi	Chen Xiyi	Chen Xiyi
Zhao Kuangyin	X Generations	X Generations
X Generations	Wang Yongfu	Huo Chengguang
Zhao Zhongdao	Zhao Zhongdao	Peng Tingjun
		Hu Yaozhen
		Feng Zhiqiang

These various lineages are well represented in North America. I estimate that in 2007 there were at least 100 taiji ruler teachers who traced their systems to Zhao Zhongdao and another ten to twenty who learned from Feng Zhiqiang or his students. There are also a few American qigong teachers who have written about arts related to taiji ruler, but whose lineages are uncertain (Dunn, 1996; Stone, 1996).[5]

TALES OF
TAIJI RULER LUMINARIES

The Sleeping Immortal

Although many scholars believe that Chen Xiyi was born in 906 CE, the traditional date of his birth is 870, which means that when he died in 989, he was 118 years old. As a child, Chen enjoyed playing in a dried-up riverbed. One day, when he was four years old, a Daoist star goddess appeared—a mysterious lady dressed in green. She offered Chen her breast, nursed him and predicted that he would, from that day on, be free of desires and become exceptionally intelligent (See Zhang Lu, 1314: ch. 1; Kohn, 2001: 60, 91; Geil, 1926: 236–237). Chen is said to have had prodigious memory and was always seen with a book under his arm. He withdrew to a hermitage on Mount Wudang where for more than twenty years he abstained from grains[6] and refined his qi. *The Record of Chen Xiyi of Mount Hua* (Taihua Xiyi Zhi) contains the famous story of how Chen eventually arrived on Mount Hua:

> He once sat up during the night reciting the *Yijing* to the burning of incense, when five old men appeared. They had thick eyebrows and white hair, overall looking ancient and strange. They came along regularly to listen to his recitation. After several days of this, Tuan [Chen] decided to inquire who they were.
>
> The old men answered: "We are the dragons from Sun-Moon-Lake of this mountain. This area is the place that the God Xuanwu has selected for himself. Mount Hua, on the other hand, is where you should go to live as a recluse."
>
> On another day when the master practiced silent sitting, the five dragons suddenly appeared before him. They ordered him to close his eyes. They then, with him on their backs, rose up into the air and rode on the wind. Toward the end of the night, they reached Mount Hua where they deposited him on a flat rock.   – Kohn, 2001: 91

The five old men had vanished. Chen was standing by a beautiful pool of water called the "Five Dragon Pool." Chen settled in and restored a dilapidated Daoist monastery called Cloud Terrace Monastery (*Yuntai Guan*) where he spent the rest of his life. He visited the court three times, but always returned to his beloved mountain to wander, practice interior alchemy, gather herbs, and sleep. According to some accounts, Chen would sleep for months or even years at a time. When questioned about this, Chen said that dreams bring one to a mysterious reality in which the mind is free of desires and the world dissolves into breath. It is the realm of the immortals (Zhao Daoyi, ca. 1300; Kohn, 2001: 72–80). Chen described himself as "belonging to the wilderness of the mountains, like deer or boar" (Zhang Lu, 1314, trans. Kohn, 2001: 97).

Mount Hua is still closely associated with Chen. "To some extent the mountain as a whole is characterized as the domain of Chen Tuan, and one constantly runs into places associated with him" (Andersen, 1991: 350). Chen is believed to have designed the pavilion in the western courtyard of the Jade Spring Monastery (*Yuquan Yuan*) at the foot of Mount Hua. The nearby Xiyi cave has a Song Dynasty (960–1279 CE) statue of Chen in a reclining position, practicing his famous Sleeping Yoga. Chen was buried in a wooden coffin in Mount Hua's Xiyi Gorge. Geil reports that sometime before 1926, it was possible to see Chen's slightly reddish bones by climbing a chain to the coffin. But one day someone stole a heel bone. This infuriated the priests, who broke the chain to prevent future access (Geil, 1926: 259).

Zhao Zhongdao

Zhao Zhongdao was born November 18, 1844, in Fanyang, Dengbei. He died February 11, 1962, at age 118, coincidentally the same age at which Chen Xiyi ascended to the realm of the Immortals. Guan Yongnian believes that Zhao's famous longevity may have had as much to do with his personality as with his qigong. "He had an open minded and happy disposition and loved to make jokes. He got along easily with people. When he spoke, his voice was strong and deep like a great gong. He was charming, witty, and vivacious" (Guan, 1984: 1).

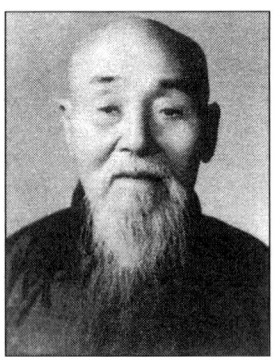

Zhao Zhongdao(1844–1962).

I am reminded of a video-taped interview I once saw of Wu Tunan, the famous taijiquan teacher and author. Wu was in his nineties and still actively teaching. The interviewer asked Wu if he attributed his longevity to taijiquan. Wu replied, "No. The reason for my long life is that I have a relaxed spirit. Taijiquan helps you to have a relaxed spirit."

The *Book of Tai Chi Ruler* (Xiantian Qigong Taiji Chi Quan Shu) has an excellent biographical sketch of Zhao Zhongdao, that I have partially translated below:

From his youth Zhao Zhongdao loved the martial arts and studied many different systems. His grandmother was heir to the Zhao family tradition of taiji ruler. One day, to awaken her grandson's interest in their family's secret treasure, she asked his martial arts instructor, "I hear that you can defeat people with your gongfu. Well then, why not try hitting me? And don't worry about killing me." Naturally the martial arts instructor was afraid of injuring the old lady and dared not raise a fist. However, just to humor her, he stepped close by and attempted to grab her. Grandmother Zhao raised her arm, and the instructor was thrown back ten paces. When he tried to grab her once more, again he was thrown. This was an example of the marvelous taiji ruler skills known as "adhering and following" and "using the supple to overcome the rigid." From this time on, young master Zhao trained under his grandmother's strict guidance. He thus began to study the prenatal qigong taiji ruler.

When the master was twenty-two, his grandmother reached the ripe old age of 108 and passed away without pain or illness. Before she died, she told her grandson, "Prenatal qigong taiji ruler is marvelous and unfathomable. I have benefited so much from it, more than I can express in words. You can only reap the benefits through sincere and long-term practice. Although it might not make you an immortal, it can certainly rid you of disease and increase your life span. Do not ignore it." The master followed his grandmother's advice and practiced unceasingly. When he was more than fifty years old, he was stronger than a youth and could easily lift a person off the ground with one hand.

While Zhao was living in Fanyang, an experienced Shaolin master became his disciple after being defeated by him. These were chaotic times in the northeast. The master protected his home using concealed "sleeve-arrows" (which were thrown by hand). However, since the art of concealed arrows was a method of inflicting harm rather than nurturing life, the master never transmitted it.

In 1933 when the master was eighty-nine, he moved to the capital. In 1940 at the age of ninety-six, the master was invited to dinner by the famous xingyiquan master Li Xingjie. Because Li lived more than three miles away, he hired a rickshaw, but the master wouldn't enter, saying instead, "You leave first. I'll follow behind." They arrived at the same time. The rickshaw boy's face was covered in sweat, but the master wasn't even panting. From that time on the master was nicknamed "Long Legs Zhao."

In 1954 the master established The Supple Art of Taiji Health Society and began to teach his treasured prenatal qigong taiji ruler publicly. At the same time, the master began using qigong healing methods to help many people who suffered from chronic illness and pain to become healthy and happy. Among these were patients with digestive ailments, diseases of the nervous system, insomnia, high blood pressure, and many with strange, unnamed conditions. Some patients were in critical condition and had already tried medicine and drugs without benefit. But upon experiencing the master's marvelous methods, not one failed to "return to spring-like vigor."

The Health Society was like a small hospital. Innumerable sick people were cured of their ills. It was also like a station for scientific research where scientists looked to Master Zhao for the secrets to human longevity and explored the reasons why so many patients were rid of disease.

At the age of 118, the master did not have "the appearance of a flickering lamp." Instead, he had a child's complexion and silvery hair. A reddish glow filled his face, and he could talk and chat easily. One glance and you knew this was an exceptional human being. On closer inspection, you discovered even more unusual characteristics: He had long ears, bright eyes, and a full set of healthy teeth (except for two that had once been chipped). His skin was clear and supple like a child's, his forehead unwrinkled, and he slept and ate like a young man.

In November of 1961, the master's friends and students gathered to celebrate his birthday. Forty-one days later he passed away.

– Xu, 1986, 48–51

Hu Yaozhen

Hu Yaozhen was born in Yuci in Shanxi Province in 1879. Not many details are known of his early life. He graduated from Shanxi Chuanzhi School of Chinese Medicine, studied Buddhist and Daoist meditation and qigong (including the five animal frolics of Hua Tuo, the Six Word Secret [*liu zi jue*], standing meditation [*zhanzhuang*], dantian cultivation, and taiji ruler), and learned the three famous internal styles (*nei jia quan*) of Chinese martial arts taijiquan, baguazhang, and Liu He Xingyiquan. Hu was especially known for his proficiency in Liu He Xingyiquan, an art he learned from Wang Fuyuan, disciple of Liu Qilan. In 1942, Hu became the President of the Shanxi Martial Arts Association.

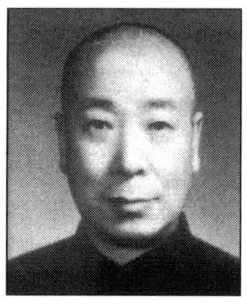

Hu Yaozhen (1879–1973).

Hu was a gentleman martial artist. He had what the Chinese call *wu de*, "martial virtue," that is high character and wisdom. He had an average build with delicate, almost effeminate hands, and a kind face that always bore a smile. His martial abilities were concealed, like "a steel bar wrapped in cotton," as the famous taijiquan expression goes. Hu was known as "A Single Finger Shakes Heaven and Earth" (*dan zhi zhen qian kun*) because of his alleged ability to defeat opponents by emitting qi from his index finger, without touching them.

Feng Zhiqiang's Hunyuan qigong recounts an exciting example of Hu's power. When Feng was twenty years old a friend introduced him to the famous master. Hu criticized Feng's previous martial arts training, telling him that he was relying on brute force rather than qi, a practice that was destroying his body. To demonstrate his point, he asked Feng to hit him with all his might. Feng took up the challenge. The moment he struck, he felt as though he hit a wall of qi. His force rebounded and he was thrown back nine feet, hitting a wall and breaking into a cold sweat. Yet, he was unharmed, and Master Hu was standing perfectly still as though nothing had happened. Now it was Master Hu's turn. Feng braced himself in a strong stance as Master Hu walked towards him with his index finger extended. Feng was suddenly overcome by a strange feeling.

> He did not know what it was but suddenly a strong force came out of the tip of Master Hu's finger. He felt a shock on his body as if being electrocuted. The whole body was bounced back and thrown backwards. He landed again on the same wall. "What kind of gongfu is this?" Master Hu smiled, "This is called internal qigong." It is called the 'Qi Gathered Into One Bullet and it comes out to one point." Suddenly Master Feng realized what he had heard before, "Single Finger Conquering the World." This is real! – Feng, 2001: 41

In 1953, Hu Yaozhen became the Vice President of the newly established Beijing Martial Arts Research Society, with his colleague Chen Fake as President. During the 1950s Hu combined qigong with acupuncture and moxibustion to successfully treat physician-referred patients. He presented his experiences at China's first major qigong conference in Beidaihe in 1959 and continued fully engaged in qigong, martial arts, medicine, and Daoist studies until his passing in 1973.

A Daoist Gymnasium

The taiji ruler is 10.5 inches long and made of willow, poplar, or any other sturdy, light, and porous wood. It is rounded at both ends so that it can fit comfortably in the palms, stimulating the important *laogong* acupuncture points. The porosity of the material allows the qi of the practitioner's hands to be conducted through the wood. Many practitioners sense that after regular daily practice, the Ruler becomes "charged" like a battery. There is an immediate influx of energy every time a practitioner holds the Ruler or begins the exercises.[7]

The foot long taiji ruler is the most important instrument traditionally used in the ruler system to enhance qi cultivation, but it is not the only one. The "gymnasium" of Chen Xiyi also includes a meter-long ruler, a wooden ball, a stone ball, a wooden board, a table, and a chair. The taiji ruler system includes the following practices:

1. *Supine Ruler:* While lying on the back with the upper arms on the ground, the practitioner holds the ruler above the navel and makes slow back and forth movements so that the ruler moves through the space between the chest and lower abdomen. This is considered an excellent practice to induce deep relaxation and for any student who is disabled, recovering from serious disease, or confined to a bed.

2. *Seated Ruler:* The practitioner sits in a chair with the feet flat on the ground. The hands make horizontal or vertical circles while holding the ruler or without the ruler. Many Daoists recommend chair meditation rather than the classical lotus posture done seated on the ground because uncrossed legs promote a more uninhibited flow of blood and qi and help Daoists realize their goal of "mind and body cultivated in balance" (*xing ming shuang xiu*).

3. *Standing Ruler:* The body stands perfectly still while holding the ruler at the level of any of the dantian energy centers. In the system of Feng Zhiqiang, the student may hold the ruler for five to ten minutes at the height of the "third eye" upper dantian, then navel middle dantian, and perineum (*hui yin*) lower dantian.

4. *Moving Ruler:* Various horizontal, vertical, and level circling movements are made either with or without the ruler. The moving ruler exercises are the foundation of the ruler system. They develop dantian qi and encourage healthy respiration.

5. *Taiji Wooden Ball:* An 8.5-inch diameter wooden ball is held between the hands at the height of the lower abdomen or rotated with either one or two hands or fingertips on a round wooden table. The tabletop is 23.5 inches in diameter, two inches thick, and slightly concave. This exercise is excellent for developing sensitivity in the fingers and hands and improving peripheral circulation.

6. *Taiji Stone Ball:* An 8.5-inch diameter stone ball is either held a short distance in front of each of the three dantians or slowly lifted from abdominal level to the height of the eyes. Most of my students practice this exercise with a sixteen-pound bowling ball, holding it for five

minutes at eyebrow, chest, and abdominal height. The benefits are similar to resistance training at the gym. Both the wooden and stone ball exercises are also practiced by students of Six Harmonies Eight Methods (*liuhebafa*), the martial art attributed to Chen Xiyi.

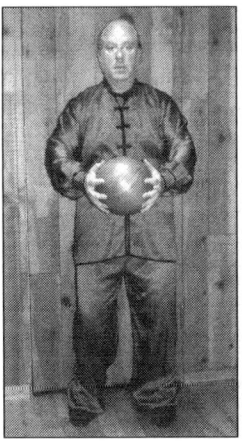
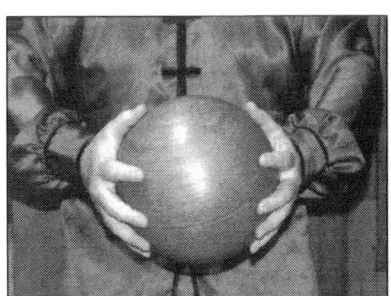

7. *Leaning on a Board:* This exercise uses a wooden board made of a pliable wood such as poplar, eight feet high, eight inches wide and less than an inch in thickness. It is buried approximately 2.5 feet into the ground. The practitioner stands with one foot slightly in front of the other and presses the board repeatedly with his fingers, each time causing it to flex slightly inwards. Leaning on a Board (*kao ban*) is excellent training for martial artists and massage therapists. The fingers fill with qi, and the practitioner learns to distinguish muscular force (*li*) from whole body internal force (*zheng ti jin*).

8. *Joined Hands:* Similar to the push hands (*tuishou*) exercises of taijiquan, two people face each other with their wrists lightly touching and through slow back and forth movements train their sensitivity and "listening" ability.

9. *Long Ruler:* The long ruler is about three feet long and shaped like the basic ruler. Two people face one another, each holding one end of the long ruler nestled in the palm with the other hand lightly supporting the ruler from underneath. Each person makes slow circling movements, one pushing the ruler slightly forward as the other yields in response. The long ruler trains and unifies the hands, eyes, mind, and intent.

A Lesson in Zhao Family Moving Taiji Ruler

To practice a basic taiji ruler exercise, stand with the left heel touching the instep of the right foot. This places the left foot several inches in front of the right.

The left foot is pointing very slightly to the left (about ten degrees off center), and the right foot is toe-out at a forty-five-degree angle. The feet are flat on the ground, the back straight, and the entire body is as relaxed as possible without being limp. Transfer your weight to the rear foot (the right), and step directly to the left with your left foot until the feet are shoulder-width apart. Be careful that as you move the left foot, you do not bring it forward or backward; the movement is entirely lateral. Thus, your left foot is still pointed forward a few inches in front of the right.

Now bend the knees until you cannot see your toes when you look down. The knees remain bent throughout the exercise. Incline your back slightly forward by bending at the waist, without slouching or bowing the spine. At this point your toes are no longer "hidden" by your knees. If you allow your hands to slide down the front of the thighs as you incline the back, you know that you have bent sufficiently when your fingertips are just above the kneecaps. Vary the posture as necessary to stay within your comfort zone. Do not incline the back if you have a spinal problem. The chest should feel soft and relaxed. Avoid lifting or puffing out the chest because this creates an unstable posture and forces qi to rise upwards, out of its primary reservoir, the abdominal dantian.

You are now in the basic taiji ruler posture. The posture naturally puts slight pressure on the lower abdomen, stimulating it to pump qi more strongly through the meridians. The posture may be modeled after the curled-up position of the embryo in the womb. The ruler exercise helps you contact the "prenatal qi," the clear, exuberant energy that you inherited from the universe, and which gives children their vitality. It also encourages "embryonic respiration" (*tai xi*), a state of ultra slow, quiet, and innocent breathing, like an infant who has not yet learned to interfere with nature's wisdom.[8]

Zhao Zhongdao Lineage Taiji Ruler

1a: The hands make small circling motions in front of the body, dipping three inches below the navel, then rising three inches above, in coordination with the weight rocking front and back. 1b: Close-up of the ruler hand position.

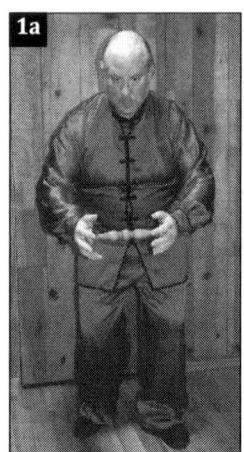
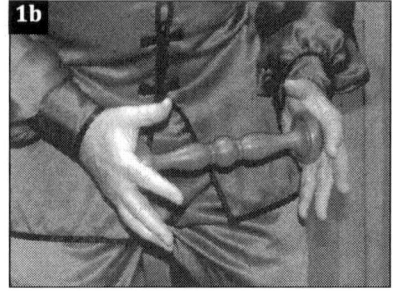

2a: The hands make level, horizontal circles at the height of the navel (as though wiping a table-top) in coordination with the weight rocking front and back. 2b: The hands continue making horizontal circles while holding an invisible ruler or ball between them, aware of the field of qi between the palms.

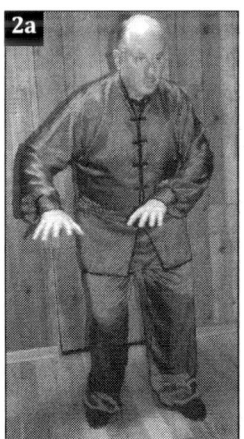 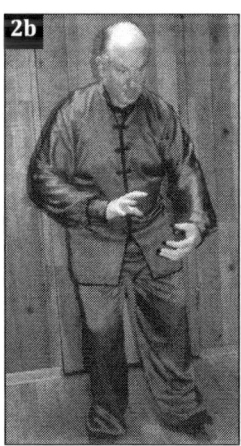

While maintaining the posture, place the hands about six inches in front of the navel, the palms facing each other approximately ten inches apart. If you have a ruler, hold it between the hands, parallel to the ground. The exercise may also be practiced effectively without it. Keep your shoulders and elbows relaxed and begin to rock your weight back and forth. Every time you rock forward the front foot presses flat on the ground, and the rear heel lifts slightly in the air. Every time you rock back, the rear foot is flat, and the front toe lifts slightly. The weight shifts only a little to and fro; soon you will feel like a rocking chair. As you rock, do not change the back's angle of inclination; maintain the taiji ruler posture throughout the exercise. Also do not let your body rise up and down. Keep the same amount of bend in the knees throughout the exercise. This helps qi to settle in the dantian. The alternate toe-heel lifting stimulates the important "bubbling spring" (*yong quan*) acupuncture points on the soles of the feet, the first point on the kidney meridian, through which qi from the earth enters the body.

As you continue rocking, lifting toe-heel, toe-heel, let the arms move in a counterclockwise vertical circle eight to ten inches in diameter. The navel is the center of your circle—that means you move your hands the same distance above and below the navel. If you are holding the ruler, you will naturally keep your hands the same distance apart while describing the circle. If you do not have a ruler, imagine that you are holding one or holding a ball of energy that you do not wish to drop. Gradually try to coordinate the circling of the hands with the rocking motion. Allow the momentum of forward and backward rocking to move your arms effortlessly. When you rock forward, your arms are gently propelled forward. As you rock back, your arms continue circling and are naturally drawn back. The eyes are open, with relaxed gaze. Keep the neck in line with the spine. Do not arch the neck to look straight ahead. Rather, because the back is inclined, you will naturally look toward the ground. Zhao Zhongdao says that you should breathe completely naturally and effortlessly. Do not try to coordinate your inhalations or exhalations with any particular part of the movement.

Rock back and forth thirty-six times, and then change sides, beginning with the other leg in front.

THE SPIRIT OF THE RULER

According to Zhao Zhongdao

Zhao Zhongdao advised that success in the ruler requires patience and perseverance. The exercise should be practiced for five to ten minutes every day at dawn and dusk. To deepen their practice, students should distinguish six qualities: "large, small, quick, slow, empty, full." The latter two terms refer to weight distribution and the active and passive quality of the hands and legs. A retreating movement or a part of the body that feels passive or weightless—such as a leg that rests lightly on the ground—is called "empty" (*xu*). An advancing or expansive gesture or a part of the body that feels active such as a leg that carries most of the body's weight is called "full" (*shi*). The upper body is relatively empty during qigong practice, while the lower body is full, heavy, and "rooted," recalling Laozi's "The sage empties the heart and fills the belly." Zhao Zhongdao said, "Use lightness to become heavy, small motion to generate big motion. Slowness is the key to speed. Strength is generated from suppleness" (Xu, 1986: 216). Zhao is suggesting that students pay attention to the quality of movement rather than the quantity (how big, how strong, how fast). A person who moves efficiently can tap all his or her potentials and reap what Zhao calls "the three benefits of the ruler: eliminating illness, strengthening the body, and longevity."

Zhao clearly considered taiji ruler to be a form of Daoist cultivation. He once said, "Taiji ruler is a standing form of seated meditation" (Xu, 1986: 201), that is, it incorporates all the principles and benefits of seated meditation plus the added benefits of qigong exercise. The ruler joins stillness and movement, suppleness with strength. "In the prenatal qigong taiji ruler, suppleness is found through inner stillness. Strength is cultivated through external movement. Inside, you are tranquil and still; outside you are moving." After diligent practice, "the mind becomes clear, the spirit settled... The mouth fills with saliva, the body's own elixir of longevity" (Xu, 1986: 67).

The practitioner cultivates the three treasures: sexual essence (*jing*), life force (*qi*), and spirit (*shen*). Zhao echoes classical Daoist theory when he writes that jing is more than bone marrow (with which it is associated in Chinese medicine), *qi* is more than breath, and spirit is more than consciousness; yet *jing, qi,* and *shen* are the essence of these three. We should cultivate the three treasures and not allow them to escape. The ears are the orifice or gate of *jing*. Jing leaves the gate when we pay too much attention to sound. The mouth is the gate of *qi*; to stabilize the *qi*, do not speak. The eyes are the gate of spirit; to collect the spirit and prevent its dispersal do not be entranced by appearances. "The human mind is a thing which moves. Do not let it move! Taiji ruler exercises train the mind. Yet the ruler does not require mental effort, only focused intent" (Xu, 1986: 67–68).

By focusing the mind on the abdominal area (*yi shou dantian*), the fire of spirit, which normally escapes upwards is made to descend. The water of sexual essence, which normally drains downwards, is stimulated to rise. Thus, fire and water join (Xu, 1986: 97). Opposing principles are integrated to create a state of inner harmony. Ultimately, one becomes aware of the original qi (*yuan qi*), the field of life force in which human beings live. Zhao writes, "Prenatal *qi* is the root of human life. People are unaware that they live amid *qi* just as fish are unaware that they live amidst water. The prenatal qi is just another name for original *qi*" (Xu, 1986: 97).

Feng Zhiqiang Lineage Primordial Taiji Ruler

Gathering qi to the dantian (1a–1d).
Pouring the qi, side to side (2a–2b).

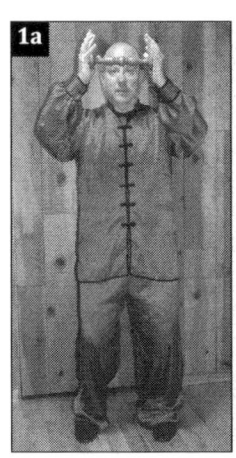
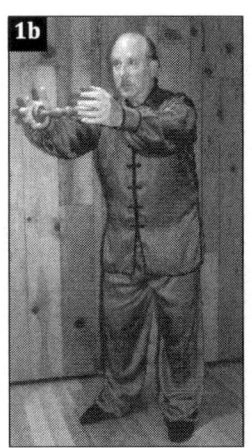
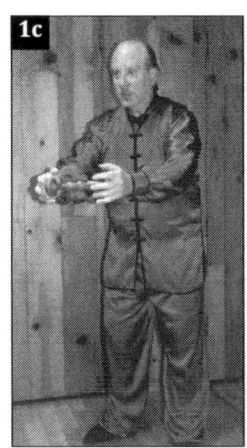
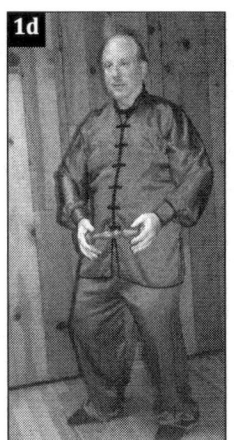
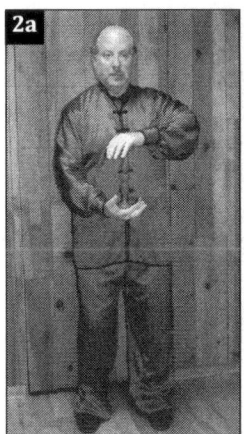
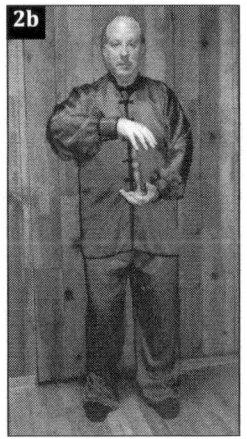

According to Feng Zhiqiang

Feng Zhiqiang's martial arts and qigong place a strong emphasis on dantian awareness and "dantian rotation" (*dantian nei zhuan*). The ruler exercises create a palpable sphere of energy in the abdomen that slowly turns and moves in harmony with one's actions. Sometimes the sphere rotates on an axis; sometimes the entire sphere orbits around the abdominal cavity, as though circling a central point between the navel and the "gate of life" acupuncture point (*ming men*, opposite the navel on the lower spine). From a health standpoint, the dantian sphere (*dantian qiu*) massages the internal organs and creates a feeling of energetic "fullness," corresponding to an actual increase in energy. I can personally testify that the skill of dantian rotation leads to a profound sense of well-being and an extraordinary increase in martial arts power. The ruler exercises also train the student to move qi through the lesser and greater heavenly circuits (*xiao zhou tian, da zhou tian*), the belt channel (*dai mai*) which circles the waist, and the meridians in the legs. Qi flow is also stimulated in the palms and fingers as it is poured from one hand to the other in side-to-side movements. As the energy channels (meridians) are cleared of obstructions, the current becomes stronger and clearer, like flowing water. Stagnant pockets of *qi*, like stagnant water, breed disease.

Feng Zhiqiang Lineage Primordial Taiji Ruler
Belt Channel Grinding the Millstone

While circling the ruler several times one
direction, then the other, the mind directs
qi around the waist (belt meridian).

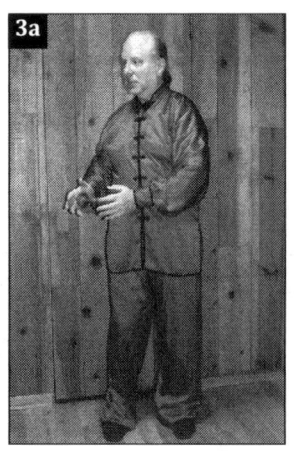
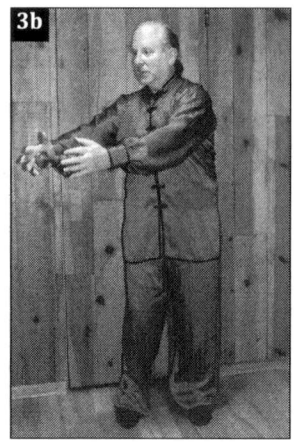
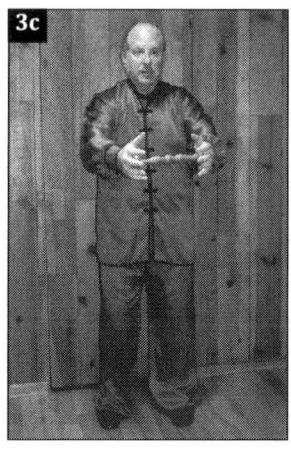

Feng Zhiqiang Lineage Primordial Taiji Ruler
Qi Rising and Descending the Leg

Move the ruler down the outside of one leg all the way to the foot, then up the inside of the same leg. Switch to the other side: down the outside of the leg to the foot, up the inside. Keep repeating, side to side, imagining that the qi field from the ruler is massaging the legs and clearing the energy channels (meridians).

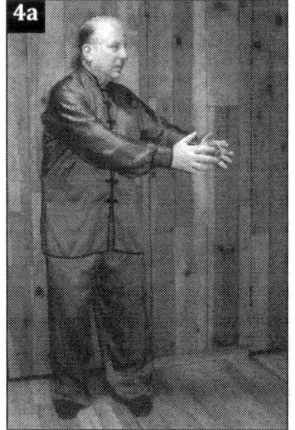
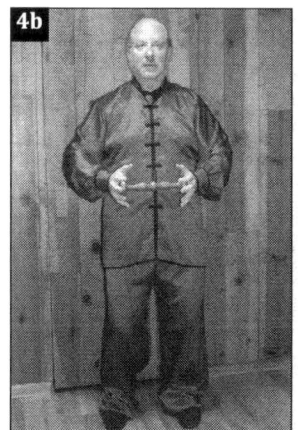
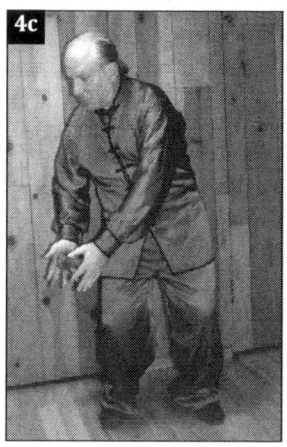

The ruler seems to emit a qi-field (*qi chang*) that affects the interior of the body. By holding the ruler several inches from the body and moving it in leisurely circles around the navel, the Ruler energetically massages the middle dantian and encourages the movement of jing, blood, and qi. In his July 2001 workshop in Seattle, Feng explained that jing and qi must be able to transform one into the other. Men store jing in the perineum. When jing moves to the "gate of life," it becomes jingqi, jing combined with qi. From there it moves horizontally across to the middle dantian behind the navel, where it becomes qi. For women, blood (*xue*) is the root of health. Blood is stored in the uterus. By practicing the ruler exercises in the abdominal region, blood is stimulated to rise to the gate of life, where it becomes xueqi, a combination of blood and qi. Then it proceeds to the middle dantian to become qi. Life is movement and transformation, and qigong encourages these processes.

Yet developing qi is a side effect of the ruler practice and does not represent the highest goal. Feng's writings and in-person instruction suggest three goals to the Hunyuan system, of which taiji ruler is a part:

1. **Awareness.** Feng constantly admonishes his students to focus on the yi, not the qi. Yi embraces the ideas of mindfulness, awareness, and focus (Cohen, 1999).
2. **Service.** During a dinner with Master Feng in July of 2001, I described a student of mine who had been diagnosed with widely metastasized terminal cancer. During the first class of an eight-week Hunyuan qigong course, she told me that she would probably not live to the end of the series. Eight weeks later she was in complete remission, and the remission lasted through the year in which I followed her case. When I finished the story, Master Feng stood up, placed his hand warmly on my shoulder and announced in a booming voice to the other dinner guests, "This is the highest goal of Hunyuan gong: to help others. Bravo!"
3. **The Dao.** Ultimately, the taiji ruler student become one with the Dao, also called the primordial qi of heaven and earth (*tian di hunyuan qi*). The practitioner learns to blend the qi of the body with the qi of the universe. In the *Daodejing* Laozi says, "The One gives birth to the two." Here duality returns to oneness.

▼●▼

CHINESE CHARACTER INDEX

An De Guan	安德觀
Baguazhang	八卦掌
Bao Jian Qigong	保健氣功
Bi qi	閉氣
Chan si	纏絲
Cheng Changxing	陳長興
Chen Fake	陳發科
Chen Shi Xinyi Hunyuan Taiji	陳式心意混元太極
Chen Tuan	陳摶
Chen Wangting	陳王廷
Chen Xiyi	陳希夷
Da zhou tian	大周天
Dai mai	帶脈
Dantian	丹田
Dantian nei zhuan	丹田內轉
Dantian qiu	丹田球
Dan zhi zhen qian kun	單指震乾坤
Daoyin	導引
Ding Xin Zhen	定心針
Dong gong	動功
Feng Zhiqiang	馮志強
Gao Fu	高郭

Guan Yongnian	關永年
Hu Yaozhen	胡耀真
Hui yin	會陰
Huo Chengguang	霍成廣
Huo Long	火龍
Jiao Guorui	焦國瑞
Ji Longfeng	姬隆風
Jing	精
Jing gong	精功
Kao ban	靠扳
Lao gong	勞宮
Le Shan	樂山
Li	力
Liu Haichan	劉海蟾
Liu He Ba Fa	六合八法
Liu He Xinyiquan	六合心意拳
Liu Qilan	劉奇蘭
Liu zi jue	六字訣
Li Xingjie	李興階
Lu Dongbin	呂洞賓
Ma Yi	痲衣
Ming men	命門
Nei jia quan	內家拳
Nei gong	內功
Peng Tingjun	彭庭俊
Qi	氣
Qian Kun Bao Chi	乾坤寶尺
Qi chang	氣場
Qigong	氣功
Qi qiu	氣球
Quan Jing	拳經
Shen	神
Shi	實
Shui gong	睡功
Si xi fei xi	似息非息
Sun Lutang	孫祿堂
Taiji bang	太極棒
Taiji chi	太極
Taiji Chi Yan Jiu	太極尺研究
Taijiquan	太極拳
Taiji Rou Shu	太極柔術
Taiji Rou Shu Jian Shen She	太極柔術健身社
Tai xi	胎息

Tian Di Huyuan Qi	天地混元氣
Tui shou	推手
Tuna	吐納
Wang Fuyuan	王福元
Wang Yongfu	王永福
Wu de	武德
Wu ming shi	無名師
Wu Qin Xi	五禽戲
Wu Quanyou	吳全佑
Wu Tunan	吳圖南
Wu Xing	五行
Xiantian qigong taiji chi	先天氣功太極尺
Xiao zhou tian	小周天
Xing ming shuang xiu	性命雙修
Xingyiquan	形意拳
Xiu lian	修
Xu	虛
Xue	血
Yang Luchan	楊露禪
Yang sheng	養生
Yi	意
Yi gong	醫功
Yin Xi	尹喜
Yin Xian Pai	隱仙派
Yi shou dantian	意守丹田
Yong quan	湧泉
Yuan qi	元氣
Yue Fei	岳飛
Yuquan Yuan	玉泉院
Zhang Sanfeng	張三丰
Zhang Sanfeng Quan Shu	張三丰全書
Zhanzhuang	站樁
Zhao Kuangyin	趙匡胤
Zhao Zhongdao	趙中道
Zheng ti jin	整體勁

Notes

[1] Daoists have always used the sword in dance-like fencing exercises and rituals for qigong and spiritual development. The fluid movements of the sword loosen the waist and nurture kidney-water. Ancient swords made of *tektite* (meteor) iron were wielded in ritual dances that helped the Daoist commune with the stars (Michel Strickmann, personal class notes, Berkeley, CA, 1979 and Schafer, 1977, 148–160), which, like the sword were thought to be expressions of the

element metal.

2. I began studying with "B.P." Chan (1922–2002)—Chan Bun-Piac in the Fujian dialect—in 1973. This exceptional teacher started learning Chinese martial arts, qigong, and Daoism at age ten. From an early age, he was a student of the famed Fujian White Crane Boxing and qigong master Chen Jingming. He also studied with Fung Lian-Dak (Northern Shaolin, starting in 1933), Liu Hing-Chow (baguazhang), Chow Chang-Hoon (xingyiquan), and Lui Chow-Munk (a student of Zhao Zhongdao in taiji ruler). In addition, Master Chan once mentioned to me that he was influenced by Daoist priests at the Monastery of Peaceful Virtue (An De Guan) in Fujian. Chan spent many years teaching in the Philippines and moved to New York City in the 1970s.

   A profoundly humble and dedicated teacher, Chan did not reveal his actual name to any of his early students. When asked his name, in Chinese or English, he would reply "Chan," equivalent to an American saying "Smith." He would not say what "B. P." stood for; nor would he write the Chinese characters for his name. Unlike many qigong instructors who wish to achieve status and recognition through their students, Master Chan was a "no name teacher" (*wu ming shi*). Once, when I questioned him about his name he said, "What do you want to learn—my name or the qigong? The Dao is nameless, people are originally nameless. Don't attach importance to names." When I asked Master Chan how I could explain my "lineage" to my students, he replied, "Teach when you truly know the art. Don't assume authority because of the name of your teacher." Only late in life did Master Chan reveal the pronunciation of B.P. and admit the names of his own teachers.

3. Chen family taijiquan is the first documented taijiquan style. It was created by General Chen Wangting early in the 17th century and transmitted within the Chen family until Chen Changxing (1771–1853) taught Yang Luchan (1799–1872). Yang established the Yang family style, the most popular style in the world today. Other styles of taijiquan are similarly named after the surnames of their founders: for example, Wu Style from Wu Quanyou (1834–1902) and Sun Style from Sun Lutang (1861–1932). Chen Style taijiquan consists of fluid, dynamic, coiling movements with changing rhythms. Whereas Yang Style moves like a stream, with an even and gentle pace, Chen Style is like an ocean, with crashing waves and slow retreating tides. Chen Style incorporates martial arts techniques from the Ming dynasty *Boxing Classic* (Quan Jing) as well as Daoist principles of health cultivation.

4. Liu He Xingyiquan, "Six Harmonies Mind Intent Boxing," is a variant name for Hebei style xingyiquan. Although legend attributes the art to General Yue Fei of the Northern Song Dynasty (960–1127), the first known practitioner was Ji Longfeng who learned it from a Daoist in the Zhongnan Mountains sometime between 1637 and 1661. Liu He Xinyiquan is a martial art with linear movements based on the five phases (*wu xing*). The wood exercise shoots like an arrow; the water technique coils like a stream, etc.

5 Terry Dunn, a well-known taijiquan and qigong instructor, does not include an acknowledgment section in his book (Dunn, 1996), nor does he list the taiji ruler teachers with whom he studied. The brief section on "Origins" attributes the ruler to Chen Xiyi but does not mention subsequent teachers such as Zhao or Feng (Dunn, 1996: 4–5). The various techniques described and photographed vary significantly from those of both Zhao Zhongdao and Feng Zhiqiang. All photographs in the book include the wooden ruler, correctly shaped. However, even in his "Advanced T'ai Chi Ruler Exercises" section (Dunn, 1996: 79–100) there is no mention of such traditional ruler practices as the taiji ball, long ruler, and joined hands.

Justin F. Stone created a series of exercises in 1974, based on "several little-known movements" that he learned from "an old Chinese man" (Stone, 1996: 12). The foot, arm, and body motions are too similar to taiji ruler to be mere coincidence. Yet they are too far from it to be based entirely on the ruler system. Stone never illustrates or discusses the wooden ruler or other instruments. He calls his art *T'ai Chi Chih*, which he translates as Taiji Knowledge or Taiji Knowing, and thus, he says, "Knowledge of the Supreme Ultimate" (Stone, 1996: 12). Is this a correct translation? Or did Stone confuse *ch'ih* (ruler) with *chih* (knowledge or wisdom), written so similarly in the Wade Giles system of romanization (in 1974, it was the standard method of representing Chinese in English)? Stone's T'ai Chi Chih has a large following in the United States. By 1996, he had accredited about 1,100 instructors (Stone, 1996: 13).

6 Avoiding grains was part of traditional Daoist dietetics. Grains weaken the qi and feed "the three worms" that inhabit the body's vital centers. As I explained in *The Way of Qigong* (Cohen, 1997: 299–302), grain avoidance probably meant "grain moderation." Professor Michel Strickmann once remarked to me (personal conversation, Berkeley, CA, 1979), "The Heavenly Master Daoist Sect required five pecks of rice as an initiation fee. What do you think they did with all that rice? Dump it in a landfill?" Daoists realized that excessive carbohydrates lower vitality, producing what today's scientists call insulin resistance, a state in which the cells are energy starved.

7 Here I differ from the view presented by Guan Yongnian in his *Taiji Stick Qigong* (Taiji Bang Qigong). Guan believes that the wooden ruler is no more than a helpful adjunct and that any wooden stick can be used (Guan, 1984: 13). However, I agree wholeheartedly with Guan that the benefits of ruler practice can only be achieved by following the principles of good qigong (correct posture, movement, intent, etc.).

8 Embryonic respiration is sometimes described as "like breathing, but not breathing" (*sixi feixi*) or "stopping the breath" (*bi qi*) because relative to the habitual breathing patterns of most people, the breath seems to have stopped. It is entirely effortless and so soft that a down feather held in front of the nostrils does not move. The respiratory rate slows down from the average of seventeen breaths per minute to about three, creating a state of profound peace and

restfulness. (For further information on the philosophy, science, and practice of embryonic respiration see Cohen, 1997: 111–129.)

Bibliography

Andersen, P. (1991). A visit to Huashan. *Cahiers d'Extrême-Asie* 5, 349–354.

Berk, W. (Ed.). (1979). *Chinese healing arts: Internal kung-fu*. Culver City, CA: Peace Press. Drawn largely from John Dudgeon, M.D. (1895). *The beverages of the Chinese; Kung-fu or tauist medical gymnastics*. Tientsin, China: The Tiantsin Press.

Chen, Hongjen (Ed.). (1964). *Xian tian qigong taiji chi* (Prenatal qigong taiji ruler). Taibei: Hualian Publishers.

Cohen, K. (1983a, January). The tai chi ruler, part I: The history. *Inside Kung Fu Magazine*, 79–81.

Cohen, K. (1983b). The t'ai chi ruler, part II: The technique. *Inside Kung Fu Yearbook*, 51–53.

Cohen, K. (1997). *The way of qigong: The art and science of Chinese energy healing*. NY: Ballantine Books.

Cohen, K. (1999, Fall). The role of intention in cross-cultural healing traditions. *Bridges 10*(3), 8–11.

Cohen, K. (2000, Winter). Hunyuan: Tracing life to its root. *The Dragon's Mouth: Journal of the British Taoist Association*, 2–4.

Dunn, T. (1996). *T'ai chi ruler: Chinese yoga for health and longevity*. St. Paul, MN: Dragon Door Publications.

Feng, Zhiqiang (1998). *Chen shi xinyi Hunyuan taiji jiao cheng* (A course in Chen family mind-intent primordial taijiquan). Beijing: Qingdao Chu Ban She.

Feng, Zhiqiang (no date). *Chen shi xinyi hunyuan taijiquan jiao cai* (Teaching materials for Chen family mind-intent primordial taijiquan). No place.

Feng, Zhiqiang (1999). *Hunyuan taiji*. Beijing: Nei Bu Fa Xing.

Feng, Zhiqiang with Chen Zhonghua (Trans.). (2001). *Hunyuan qigong*. Edmonton, Alberta: Hunyuantaiji Academy.

Feng, Zhiqiang with Wang Fengming (Ed.). (no date). *Special Taoist taiji stick and ruler qigong*. No place.

Foxx, Khan (1995). Hua yo t'ai chi ch'uan: The kung fu of six combinations and eight methods. Unpublished Manuscript.

Geil, W. (1926). *The sacred five of China*. New York: Houghton Mifflin Company.

Guan, Yongnian (1984). *Taiji bang qigong* (Taiji stick qigong). Beijing: Ren Min Ti Yu Chu Ban She.

Guan, Yongnian (1988). Taiji bang qigong (Taiji stick qigong). In Li Yongdeng (Ed.), *Zhi bing yang sheng qigong tu jie* (Curing disease and nourishing life qigong illustrated) (pp. 69–75). Hong Kong: Guangdeng Ren Min Chu Ban She.

Hu, Yaozhen with Jiao, Guorui (no date). *Wu qin xi* (Five animal frolics). Hong Kong: Xin Wen Shu Dian.

Hu, Yaozhen (no date). *Bao jian qigong* (Qigong for health). Hong Kong: Nan Tong Tu Shu Gong Si.

Jiao, Guogrui (1988). *Qigong essentials for health promotion*. Beijing: China Reconstructs Press.

Kohn, L. (Ed) (1993). *The Taoist experience: An anthology*. Albany, NY: State University of New York.

Kohn, L. (2001). *Chen Tuan: Discussions and translations*. Magdalena, NM: Three Pines Press.

Meehan, J. (2000). The Hun Yuan t'ai chi system. *T'ai Chi 24*(6), 17–23.

Mooney, R. (no date). Taiji ruler system. www.cyberkwoon.com/alma/martial/texts taiji_ruler.html

Schafer, E. (1977). *Pacing the void: T'ang approaches to the stars*. Berkeley, CA: University of California Press.

Seidel, A. (1970). A Taoist immortal of the Ming Dynasty: Chang San-feng. In *Wm. Theodore de Bary and the Conference on Ming Thought, Self and Society in Ming Thought* (pp. 483–531). NY: Columbia University Press.

Stone, J. (1996). *T'ai chi chih!: Joy thru movement*. Fort Yates, ND: Good Karma Publishing.

Xu, Leiyu (Ed.). (1986). *Xian tian qigong taiji chi quan shu: The book of tai chi ruler with complete details*. Hong Kong: The Institute of Inborn Physical Endowment of Chi Kung Tai Chi Ruler.

Yang, Yang, and Grubisich, S. (2000). Feng Zhiqiang on integrating mind and body. *T'ai Chi 24*(3), 10–21.

Zhang, Lu (Ed.). (1314). *Taihua Xiyi zhi* (Record of Chen Xiyi of Mount Hua). Dao Zang 306, fasc. 160. (See Kohn, 2001, 91–107).

Zhao, Daoyi (ca. 1300). Lishi zhenxian tidao tongjian houji (Supplement to the Comprehensive mirror on successive generations of spirit immortals and those who embody the Dao) *Dao Zang* 298, fasc. 150. (See Kohn, 2001, 60–90).

Zhao, Zhongdao (1928). *Taiji rou shu shuo ming shu* (The gentle art of taiji manual). Guandong Yin Shu Guan.

Zong, Wu, and Li, Mao (1990). *Exercises illustrated: Ancient way to keep fit*. Hong Kong: Hai Feng Publishing.

Chenjiagou: The History of the Taiji Village
by David Gaffney, B.A.

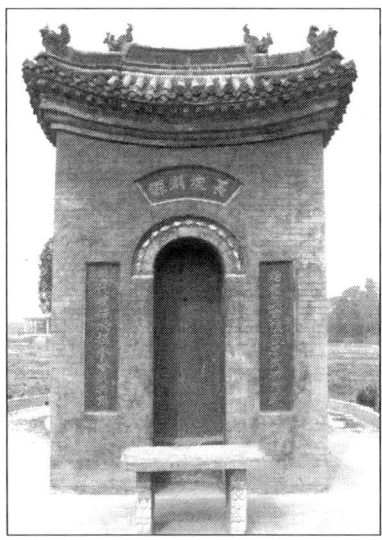

Memorial to Chen Bu – Patriarch of the Chen family
and founder of Chenjiagou.
All photographs courtesy of David Gaffney

Introduction

Chenjiagou (Chen Family Ditch), alongside the Shaolin Temple and Wudang Mountain, is one of the most significant martial arts locations in China and is often referred to simply as the "Taiji Village." It is located in Henan Province, central China, and is surrounded by four large cities: Xinxiang to the east, Zhengzhou to the south, Luoyang to the west, and Jiaozuo to the north. An examination of Chenjiagou's history shows how difficult it has been for the village to preserve its legacy. A combination of political, social, and environmental factors has conspired to challenge taijiquan's very survival in its birthplace.

Traditional Community

To chart the experience of generations of taijiquan practitioners in Chenjiagou in any kind of meaningful way, one must consider how they perceived the world. To Western eyes, Chenjiagou, like many remote rural communities throughout the world, seems to give off a sense of timeless permanence. Each generation of the Chen clan preserved and built upon the family art passed down to them. In *Understanding Folk Religion*, the author captures this sense: "Emphasis on membership in a greater family provides people with a strong sense of identity. Including ancestors provides a sense of stability and continuity" (Heibert, 1999: 179). Ancestor worship served to strengthen ties of kinship to the extent that within traditional Chinese social organization, the concept of the patrilineal family is taken to be the essential cohesive unit in society. Blood kinship is unquestionably the social tie of greatest significance (Hucker, 1975: 57).

Chen Bu's Journey to Chenjiagou

While taijiquan was widely acknowledged to be created in the late 17th century, the Chenjiagou villagers trace their ancestry back to Chen Bu, the historical patriarch of the Chen clan. Chen Bu founded the village during the turbulent early years of the Ming Dynasty (1368–1644). It was a time of war, devastation, and chaos as the previous Yuan Dynasty (1271–1368) was coming to an end. Law and order were non-existent, and the population lived in poverty and fear. The warrior Zhu Yuanzhang emerged victorious and took control of China, establishing the Ming Dynasty.

During a raid in Huaiqing Prefecture (today's Qinyang city, which in those days governed eight counties, including Wen County where Chenjiagou is located), Zhu Yuanzhang's men were met with fierce resistance by Yuan General Tien Moer and sustained huge casualties. However, a single prefecture could not hold off sustained attacks from Zhu's vast army. It was finally defeated by lack of supplies and reinforcements, and the few remaining Yuan soldiers dispersed (Chen, 2004: 1).

The consequences for the region were catastrophic. "After Zhu Yuanzhang ascended the throne, he turned his anger on the common people of Huaiqing Prefecture, accusing them of helping the resistance against the imperial soldiers. He sent his solders to 'clean' Huaiqing three times by slaying all the innocent people. It is said that after the Ming soldiers finished pillaging a place, they often placed money, food, cloths, etc. at the crossroad in the center of a village. If these items were picked up, a new search would ensue. Although people went into hiding with their families, eight to nine out of ten did not manage to escape the massacre. After the three 'cleansings' of the prefecture and its eight counties, an area of several thousand square kilometers were littered with blood and bodies. Almost no crops could be seen and not a single rooster could be heard in the thousand villages" (Chen, 2004: 1).

Records of the period tell of the implementation of a policy of mass migration and wasteland reclamation. A migration office was established in Shanxi Province, and local inhabitants were compelled to relocate to sparsely populated areas devastated by the war (one of which was Huaiqing Prefecture). One of those forced to move was Chen Bu. According to Chen Xiaowang, Chen Bu "originated from Dongtuhe Village, Hezhou (today's Jincheng County), Shanxi. In the first year of Hongwu [1367], Chen Bu with his whole family fled from famine to Hongdong. In the fifth year of Hongwu (1372), he was among the ones who were forced by government officials to move to Henan's Huaiqing Prefecture" (Chen, X., 2004: 1).

Since the traditional starting point for all migrations was beneath a scholar tree (*huaishu*, sophora sinensis), the saying persists today that the Chen family ancestors came from "Shanxi Hongdong Big Scholar Tree" (Gaffney and

Sim, 2002: 10).

Chen Bu settled on a wide fertile flood plain in southeastern Huaiqing Prefecture, with the Yellow River (*Huanghe*) to the south and the Taihang Mountains to the north. A village was gradually established that was named Chen Bu's Village (*Chen Bu Zhuang*). The village bears his name to this day, though it is now part of Wen County instead of Qinyang.

The village, however, proved less than ideal as it was on low lying ground and prone to flooding. Chen Bu moved about five kilometers to the east, to Green Wind Ridge (*Qing Feng Ling*). The new place was named Chang Yang Village after a temple there. Chen Bu soon led an attack to destroy a nearby bandit stronghold that had been terrorizing the area. Chen Bu's reputation grew, and he established a martial arts school to train the villagers.

Despite his many heroic exploits, the way the village eventually acquired its name is somewhat prosaic. "Areas on both sides of the Yellow River were frequently flooded. Many failed attempts were made to deepen the river. Parallel drainage ditches, therefore, were created to help deal with floodwaters. These came to be associated with families. Chen Bu's family name gave Chang Yang Village its modern name of Chenjiagou, meaning 'Chen Family Ditch'" (Gaffney and Sim, 2002).

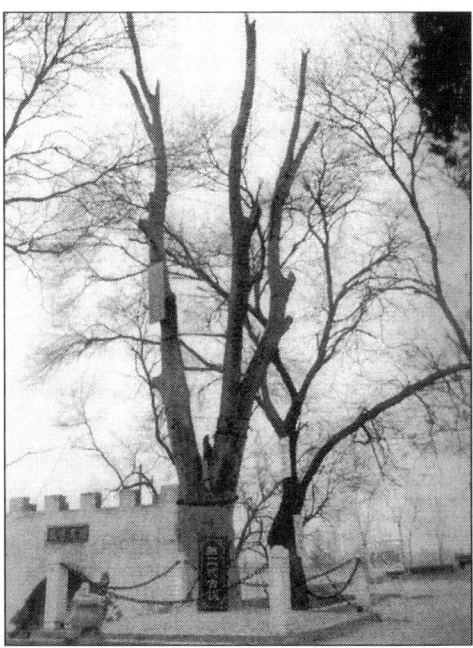
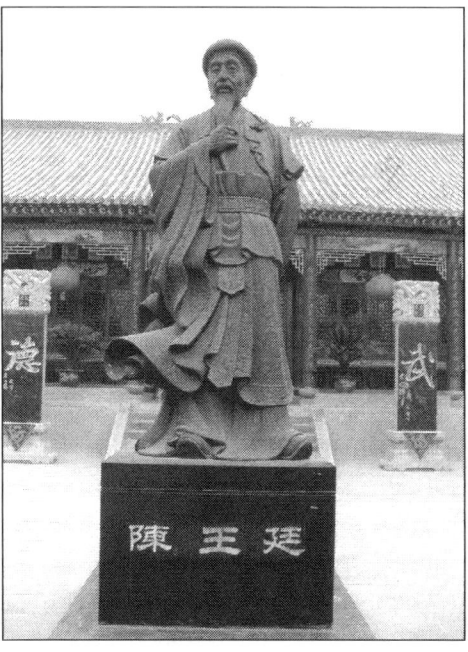

The "Scholar Tree" in Shanxi province from which
Chen Bu began his migration to Henan Province.
Right, statue of taijiquan creator Chen Wangting.

The Birth of Taijiquan

While the art of taijiquan had yet to make an appearance, the Chen clan's martial tradition continued. It seems likely that the martial art practiced was external in nature. "The close proximity of the village to the Shaolin Temple gives credence to the theory that it may have been some form of Shaolin boxing. The Chen family was famous for several generations for their cannon fist boxing (*paochuiquan*) and was known as the Paochui Chen family (*paohcui Chen jia*) (Gaffney and Sim, 2002: 10–11).

Detailed historical records of people, events, and martial arts started from the time of Chen Wangting (1600–1680). According to Annals of Huaiqing Prefecture, Wen County Annals, and Anping County Annals, in 1641, before the fall of the Ming dynasty, Chen Wangting was a military officer and was commander of the Wen County garrison force. The *Genealogy of Chen Families* states that at the end of the Ming dynasty, Chen Wangting was already famous for his martial skills, "having once defeated more than 1000 bandits and was a born warrior, as can be proven by the sword he used in combat" (Gaffney and Sim, 2002: 12).

Some three centuries earlier, Emperor Hongwu (imperial name of Ming dynasty founder Zhu Yuanzhang) had established a powerful military machine with a million-man standing army. This was divided into basic garrison units (*wei*) of roughly five thousand men that were further subdivided into smaller companies (*so*). For major campaigns, soldiers were assembled from *wei* and so from the four corners of the country under the instruction of commanders from the capital. By Chen Wangting's time, however, the *wei-so* system had become a bureaucratic nightmare.

"The *wei-so* standing army declined in strength and fighting ability. It was supplemented by local militiamen, then by conscripts from the general population, and finally in the last Ming century by recruited mercenaries in awesome numbers. In the last Ming decades, the military rolls swelled to a reported total of four million men. But they were poorly equipped, ill-trained, and irregularly fed and clothed; only a small fraction of the total can have been effective soldiers" (Hucker, 1975: 327).

Chen Wangting was fiercely loyal to the Ming dynasty and its fall ended any ambitions of advancement he held. Consequently, he retired to Chenjiagou where he lived out the rest of his days. It is not hard to imagine the frustration that this warrior, pensioned off at the peak of his powers, must have felt. It was during this period that he began to compile a unique form of martial art combining various disciplines and assimilating the essence of many martial skills existing at the time.

In developing his new art, Chen Wangting appears to have been heavily influenced by the famous general and outstanding military strategist Qi Jiguang (1528–1587). Qi was most famous for defending China against rampaging pirates from Japan. He also defeated Mongolian invaders from the north. His tactics involved feigning weakness and retreating before the enemy. After leading them far inland and lulling them into a false sense of superiority, Qi's forces overwhelmed the invaders in a sudden and decisive counterattack (Millinger and Fang, 1976: 220–224). Chen Wangting adopted this as taijiquan's central tenet of "not meeting strength with strength" and "leading an opponent into emptiness."

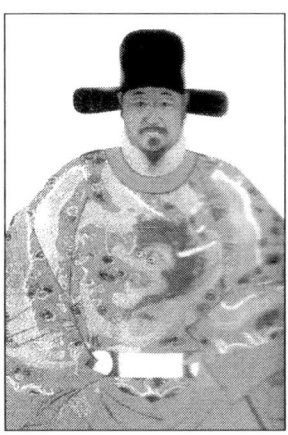

General Qi Jiguang – the general
whose book on military strategy provided
inspiration for the new art of taijiquan.

Between 1559 and 1561, General Qi compiled his classic text on strategy and martial arts, *New Book of Effective Techniques* (Ji Qiao Xinshu). This comprehensive manual is comprised of fourteen chapters with four dedicated to the practice of gongfu/wushu. The most widely quoted chapter is the "Boxing Canon" (*Quan Jing*), which depicts an effective and powerful repertoire assimilating the arts of sixteen different martial systems of the time (Gaffney and Sim, 2002: 15). Like Chen Wangting later, Qi placed great emphasis on martial effectiveness, deriding the use of "flowery fists and embroidered legs" (movements that are spectacular to look at, but of no practical use).

"Chen Wangting and Qi Jiguang were not of the same dynasty, but Chen admired Qi's patriotism and the way he had absorbed the best of the various martial schools. He was especially influenced by Qi's arrangement of the different martial systems. Society was in turmoil during the period of Chen Wangting's middle age, and the country was being invaded by foreigners. Unable to do his duty for the country and unable to fulfill his ambitions, Chen Wangting retired to the village with his constant companion, the *Huangting Jing* (The Yellow Chamber's Internal and External Canon) with the intention of organizing the different martial arts systems of his time. In this way Chen Wangting, following Qi Jiguang, is renowned for the research and collation of folk martial arts. This was the base from where he later created taijiquan" (Chen, 2004: 3).

Chen, however, did more than simply incorporate the essential theories of Qi Jiguang. His new system was highly innovative adding the novel concepts of hiding firmness in softness and using different movements to overcome the opponent's unpredictable and changing moves, thereby raising external fighting skills to a higher level. Power is generated from within, with the use of "internal energy to become outward strength." This theory is embodied in Chen's *Song of the Boxing Canon*: "Actions are varied and executed in a way that is completely unpredictable to the opponent, and I rely on twining movements and numerous hand-touching actions. 'Hand-touching' denotes the close contact of the arms to develop sensitivity to react quickly—nobody knows me, while I alone know everybody'" (Chen, 2004: 3).

In a poem written not long before his death, Chen Wangting reflected: "Sighing for past years when I was strong and sharp. Sweeping away dangerous obstacles without fear! All the favors bestowed on me by the emperor are in vain. Now old and fragile, I am left only with the book of Huang Ting for company. In moments of listlessness, I study martial arts. In times of activity, I cultivate the land. In leisure I teach disciples and descendants so that they may be worthy members of society" (Gaffney and Sim, 2002: 12–13).

Chen Changxing — Breaking with Tradition

Up until the time of Chen Changxing (1771–1853), the fourteenth generation of the Chen clan, taijiquan was a closely guarded family secret. Chen Changxing carried out escort duties to neighboring bandit lands, particularly in Shandong Province. His words revealed a no-nonsense approach to combat that balanced the physical and psychological aspects necessary to be successful. For example, in his *Important Words on Martial Applications*, Chen Changxing wrote: "To get the upper hand in fighting, look around and examine the shape of the ground. Hands must be fast, feet light. Examine the opponent's movements like a cat. Heart (mind) must be in order and clear. . . . If the hands arrive and the body also arrives [at the same moment], then defeating the enemy is like smashing a weed" (Chen X., 1990: 226).

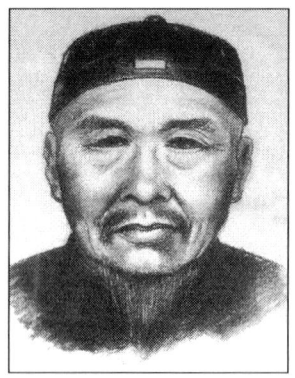

Chen Changxing
– the first person to teach taijiquan
to someone outside the Chen clan.

Chen Changxing seems to have been a practical individual not afraid to break with tradition. The original art passed down from Chen Wangting's time had five boxing routines that Chen Changxing synthesized into what is known today as the old frame first routine (*laojia yilu*) and second routine (*laojia erlu*), also known as the cannon fist form (*paochui*). These make up the foundation forms from which subsequent generations of Chen Village practitioners have developed their capabilities (Chen X., 2003). The change from the original forms represents the biggest change of all in the evolution of Chen taijiquan.

Chen Changxing's second momentous break with tradition was to teach taijiquan to Yang Luchan (1799-1871)—the first time the art had been transmitted to someone outside the Chen clan. While today this may not sound so startling, at the time, the significance of the clan cannot be over-emphasized. In fact, the secrecy of the rural family clans is an important reason why many family martial systems were able to develop their own unique characteristics and flavor. A vital condition for the development of the many local fighting systems was the patriarchal family system. The primary importance traditionally placed on the family, it's setting itself strictly apart from other clans, and its autonomous way of life preserved the distinctive family combat systems over generations (but also often led to the gradual stagnation and eventual disappearance of many family systems). Outsiders were strictly excluded from learning clan secrets. By breaking this taboo, Chen paved the way for the development of the widely practiced Yang Style taijiquan and thereon to other taiji styles.

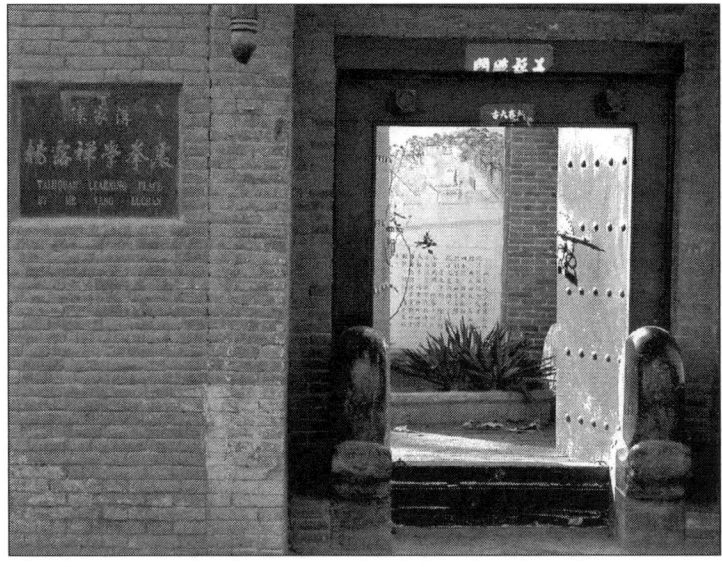

Doorway leading to the courtyard where Chen Changxing taught Yang Luchan, creator of Yang Style taijiquan.

Today, when most people practice martial arts for sport, health, and recreation, it is easy to lose sight of the life and death seriousness of martial skill in the past. A *Shaolin Yu Taiji* magazine article refers to Wu Wenhan's book *The Complete Book of the Essence and Applications of Wu [Yuxiang] Style Taijiquan* that contains a fascinating insight into Chen taijiquan's combat history. It relates two official government documents that record the defense of Huaiqing County (where Chenjiagou is located) against the Taiping Rebellion army in 1853. One is entitled "Veritable Record of Taiping Army Attacking Huaiqing County," written by Tian

Guilin, who was responsible for "defending the western town" in Huaiqing. The other is the "Daily Records of Huaiqing Defense," compiled by local schoolteacher Ye Zhiji (Jian, G., 2002).

Neither Tian nor Ye were taijiquan practitioners. Both were government officials, and hence their accounts can be considered somewhat objective descriptions of the events. According to the documents, once the Taiping army crossed the Yellow River and attacked Huaiqing County, the local militia was defeated and dispersed, and government troops escaped. Of all the villages, only Chenjiagou resisted. In his "Veritable Record Under the 29th Day of the 5th Month," Tian notes:

> The head of the thieves (i.e. Taiping rebels) called Big Headed Ram (Datou Yang) invaded Chenjiagou. This thief was extremely bold and strong; he was able to carry two big canons under his arms and swiftly attack the town. The battles that destroyed whole towns were conducted under the command of this thief. Fortunately, Chen Zhongshen and Chen Jishen, two brothers from Chenjiagou, were very skilled in using spears and long poles. They used long poles to pull Big Headed Ram down from the horse, and then they cut his head off. The thieves got very angry, and the whole group went on to Zhaobao Jie burning everything, then to Henei and villages around Baofeng, and no soldiers came to their rescue [of these areas, fortunately Chen Zhongshen and others managed to escape]. – Jian, G., 2002

The documents stated that only the inhabitants of Chenjiagou took an active part in the resistance against the Taiping rebels. This would imply that, unlike the other villages in the area, Chenjiagou had a stronger martial tradition and used it to defend itself (Jian G., 2002).

The Modern Era

During the early years of the 20th century, taijiquan practice in Chenjiagou reached its zenith, with almost everyone in the village training in the art. At the same time, the establishment of a taijiquan school and a more formalized teaching syllabus led to the development of many famous practitioners. To express their respect for the family art, the villagers reconstructed many of the dwellings of famous practitioners of the past and built many taijiquan related structures (Wang, J., 2006: 4).

However, the good times were not to last and the fall of the Qing dynasty in 1912 brought a resurgence of regional warlordism to many parts of China, including Henan Province (Hucker, 1975: 328). On top of this, much of China suffered a period of devastating natural disasters. During the early 1920's, much of Henan Province, along with the neighboring provinces of Shandong, Shanxi, Shaanxi, and Hebei, suffered a catastrophic period of famine caused by the severe droughts of 1919. In *The Search for Modern China*, Jonathan Spence described a shattered scene: "In farm villages . . . the combination of withered crops and inadequate government relief was disastrous: at least 500,000 people died, and out of an estimated 48.8 million in these five provinces, over 19.8 million were declared destitute" (Spence, 1999: 298–299). Villagers were reduced to eating straw and leaves and epidemics such as typhus cut a swathe through many too frail to fight back.

The disastrous combination of events meant that the numbers of people practicing taijiquan in the village was getting less and less as people left the village to escape the hardships. In 1928, Chen Fake (1887–1957), a 17th-generation Chen clan master, went to Beijing to teach at the request of his nephew, Chen Zhaopei. In those days, travel was difficult, and Beijing must have seemed like the other side of the world to villagers most of whom had spent their entire lives in the village. One can imagine the somber mood the night before he was to leave when Chen Fake went to the family temple to bid farewell to his fellow villagers and demonstrate his taijiquan one last time. Chen Liqing, a noted small frame (*xiaojia*) practitioner was a young child at the time and witnessed the event. She recalled, "Chen Fake demonstrated laojia yilu. During the emitting power (*fajing*) movements, you could hear the power from the wind created that made the candle-flames flicker. At that time, the temple was made of mud and, when he stamped his foot, five of the roof tiles were dislodged and came down. One person tried to test his strength and was bounced off the wall. When he finished, he saluted those present in the room" (Chen, L., 2005).

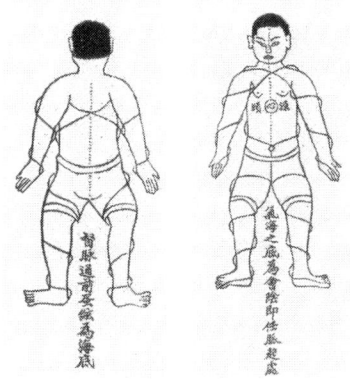

Chen taijiquan's silk reeling energy depicted in Chen Xin's
Illustrated Explanation of Chen Taijiquan.

Chen Zhaopei, who had left the village shortly before Chen Fake to teach taijiquan throughout China, was deeply troubled that there was no one left in the village to transmit taijiquan to the next generation. He had learned taijiquan from several renowned masters, including his uncles Chen Fadou and Chen Fake, and village elders Chen Yanxi and Chen Xin. In 1958, after retiring, the 65-year-old Zhaopei assumed the daunting responsibility himself, returning home to Chenjiagou to revive the practice of taijiquan.

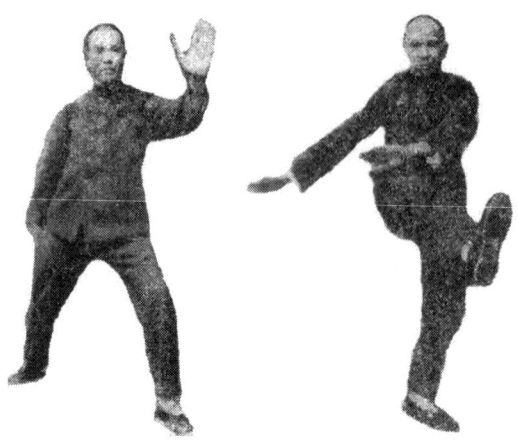

Chen Zhaopei – the teacher who revived taijiquan practice in Chenjiagou.

Chen Zhaopei's son, Chen Kesen recalled his father's decision to pick up the mantle of preserving taijiquan in its birthplace: "He willingly returned to the spartan village life of Chenjiagou. After he returned to the village, he set up a taijiquan school in his own home, bearing all of the costs himself. At the same time, he also set up a training class in the county town, Wenxian, teaching members of the government, the workers and staff of the Mining School, as well as coaching the teachers and students. There was a vigorous renaissance of taijiquan in old Wenxian. Who knew that this good scene would not last for long" (Chen, 1993)?

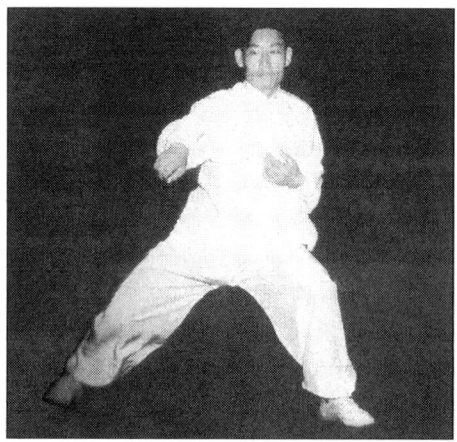

An early picture of Chen Xiaowang –
19th generation standard bearer.

Chen Zhaopei set about improving and tightening the standards of Chen tajiquan in the village, bringing under his tutelage many new devotees. The resurrection of the dwindling Chen family taijiquan is generally attributed to this period. His most celebrated disciples today are Chen Xiaowang, Wang Xi'an, Zhu Tiancai, and Chen Zhenglei, described collectively as the "Four Buddha's Warriors" by a journalist in the early 1980's. All were sent out to take part in various competitions and demonstrations, slowly increasing Chen taijiquan's profile (Zhu, 2000). The combination of his affectionate and easy-going nature and serious attitude to training attracted many students. Reminiscing about this period, Chen Xiaowang remembered: "at that time, learning from my uncle Chen Zhaopei was very grueling" (Chen, X., 2005: 76).

The Impact of the Cultural Revolution

In 1966, Mao Zedong and his close supporters instigated the Cultural Revolution, an immense and distorted movement that for ten years inflicted fear and anarchy on China. By arousing peasant-powered mass violence, Mao let loose a whirlwind of social turmoil. Individuals deemed to be a "four bad-categories element" (*silei fenzi*) were labeled as "bad class" and suffered severe discrimination. The four groups were defined as: landlord, rich peasant, counterrevolutionary, and rotten element. Throughout the countryside, anyone unlucky enough to be branded within these categories was shown little mercy in the highly emotional environment during the "Maoist struggle sessions." In *The Class System in Rural China: A Case Study,* Jonathan Unger documented the creation of caste-like pariah groups and their maltreatment during the post-revolutionary period. His study focused upon a small rural community in Guangdong Province (coincidentally also called Chen Village) with many similarities to Chenjiagou: "As a symbol of polluted status, during the 1960s and 1970s the dozen or so elderly 'four bad elements'... had to sweep dung from the village square before mass meetings were held there. To symbolize further that most of them were irredeemably among the damned, they were not permitted to attend any political sessions or participate in Mao study groups" (Unger, 1984: 121–141).

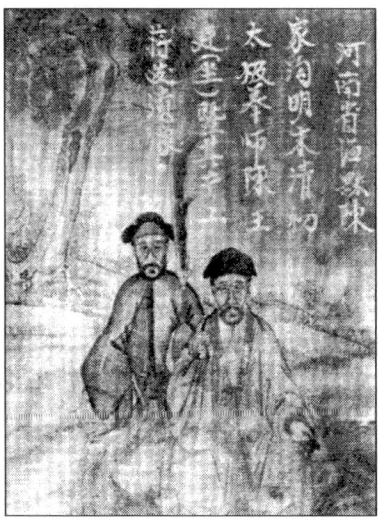

Copy of a painting of Chen Wangting
lost during the Cultural Revolution.

At its heart, the Cultural Revolution demanded a comprehensive assault on the "four old" elements within Chinese society: "old customs, old habits, old culture, and old thinking" (Spence, 1999: 575). During this period, the Red Guard burned many historic taijiquan documents. One story recounts how Wang Xi'an was deeply upset to see the destruction of such irreplaceable manuscripts. Coming into possession of one such document, Wang wrapped it in plastic and plastered it into the ceiling of his home. Discovery of his actions could have had dire consequences both to himself and his family.

During the Cultural Revolution and the period of civil unrest just preceding it, most taijiquan related structures in the village were destroyed (Wang, J., 2006: 6). The location of Chen Changxing's grave was lost with the removal of its headstone and a number of priceless artifacts were lost, including Chen Wangting's sword and a portrait of Chen Wangting with Jiang Fa. Disastrously for taijiquan's progress, many taiji experts suffered greatly throughout this time.

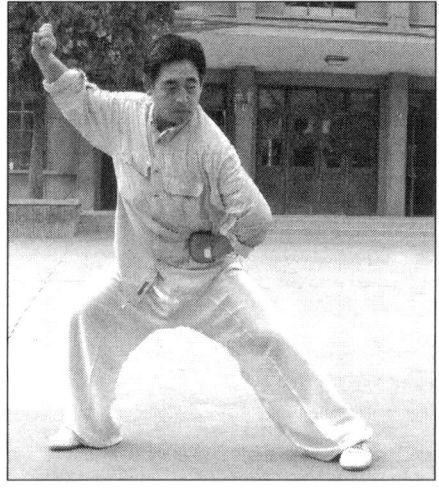

Avove: Chen Xiaoxing – Principal of Chenjiagou Taijiquan School.
Following two photos: Training in the Chenjiagou Taijiquan School courtyard.

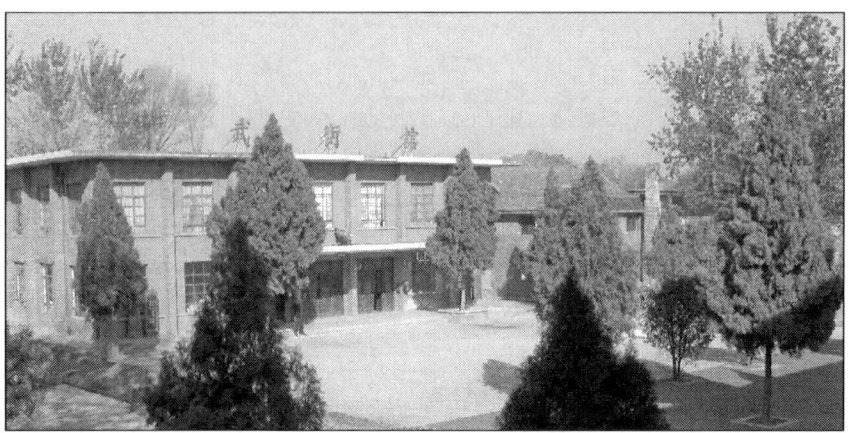

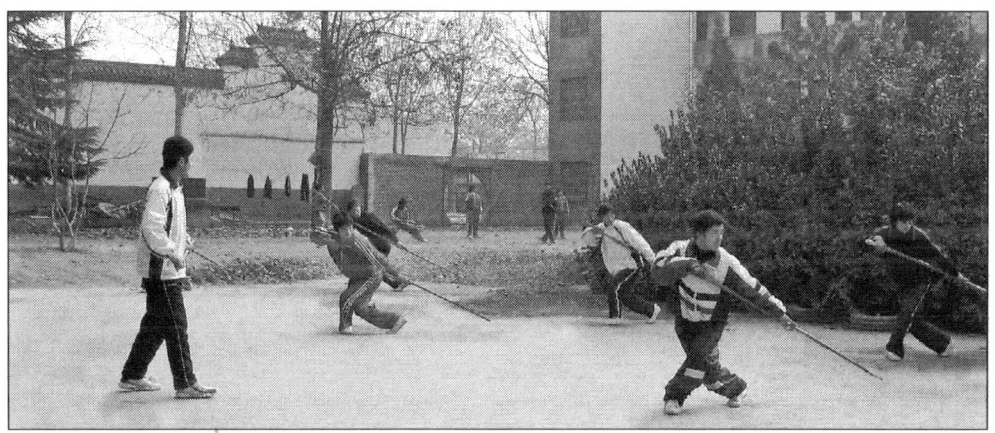

The combination of incessant Maoist indoctrination with hard labor was the norm in villages all over China throughout the Cultural Revolution. Chen Xiaoxing, the principal of the Chenjiagou Taijiquan School, recalled how he was required to work twelve hours a day in a brick factory (Chen, X., 2003). Chen Kesen recalled how his father, Chen Zhaopei, was persecuted and subjected to humiliating public "struggle sessions" during the Cultural Revolution, but courageously taught secretly at night. The courage of his prized disciples led him to compose the following verse: "At eighty years I teach taiji, without concern for whether the road ahead is bad or good. The wind howls, the rain beats down, and the difficulties are many. I delight in seeing the next generation of successors filling my home village" (Chen K., 1993).

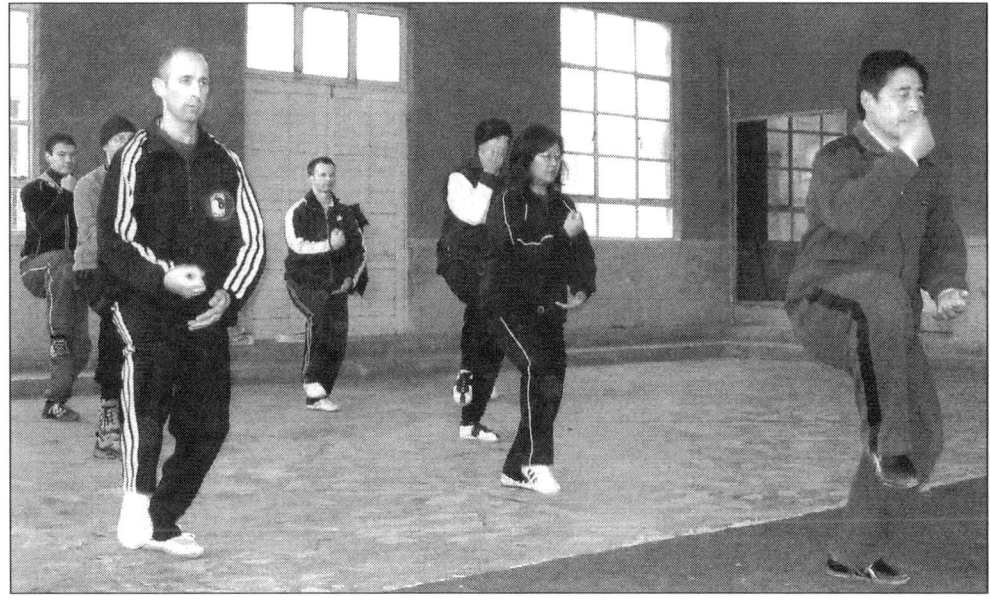

Training the posture Buddha's
warrior attendant pounds mortar.
Chen Xiaoxing at front.

In a radio interview conducted in the United Kingdom for BBC Radio's "Eastern Horizon," Chen Zhenglei (one of the four Buddha's Warriors) explained: "The biggest setback for taijiquan and all martial arts was during the Cultural Revolution when people were not able to practice freely and martial arts became outlawed. Taijiquan and other martial arts diminished in China. When China opened its gates again to the rest of the world, its rich culture was promoted and martial arts became standardized and simplified in the process. This had its pros and cons—it allows more people to learn, but this ultimately dilutes and changes the virtues of the traditional form" (Feng, 2004: 33–34).

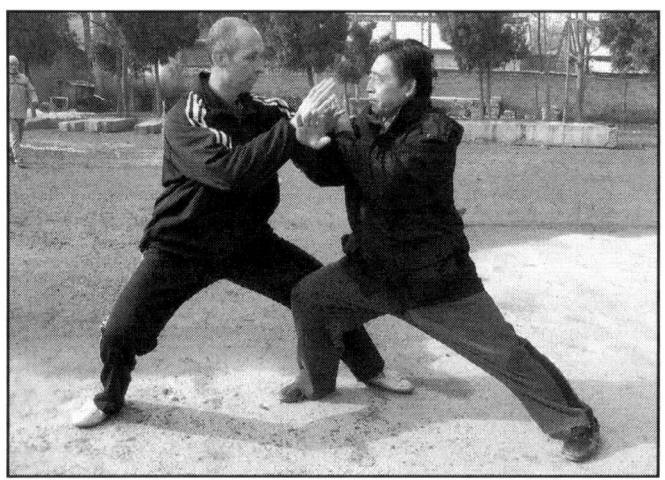

The author pushing hands with Chen Xiaoxing.

However, from the mid-1970's, the political climate began to soften, and the outlook became brighter for taijiquan in Chenjiagou. In 1974, the eighteenth-generation standard-bearer, Chen Zhaokui, son of Chen Fake, returned to the village to teach the new frame (*xinjia*). In 1978, a host of new writings was given wide circulation through the state-controlled press. "Focusing on the horrors and tragedies experienced by many in the Cultural Revolution, this 'literature of the wounded,' as it was called, stimulated debate and reflection about China's past and its prospects. Signs seemed to point to a cultural thaw, among which one could include the convening of a conference (in far-off Kunming in Yunnan admittedly) to study the long-taboo subject of comparative religion, with papers delivered on Buddhism and Daoism, Islam and Christianity" (Spence, 1999: 621).

Opening Up of China

Chen Style taijiquan has enjoyed a surge of popularity around the world in the last few decades. As the current generation of masters from Chenjiagou finally got the opportunity to travel and demonstrate their skills, more and more people have been exposed to the traditional village art. Before, to many, taijiquan was synonymous with the more widely seen Yang Style with its characteristic slow movements and even tempo, or the various government approved versions of taiji e.g. Simplified 24-Step, etc.

Since the change of national policy and the opening up of China's economy, the district government has begun the process of building up Chenjiagou again. As the birthplace of taijiquan, the village carries with it profound cultural and historical significance of interest not just in China, but to the world over. Plans are afoot to develop Chenjiagou as a tourist attraction. In recent years, the district government has invited architects from Beijing to survey and plan projects. At present, nothing definite has been decided and the only officially designated tourist attractions in the village are the Taiji Temple and the house where Yang Luchan learned taijiquan (Chen, B., 2005).

Twentieth-generation practitioner Chen Bing optimistically looks forward to the day when Chenjiagou and taijiquan will go out into the international arena on a scale to match the nearby Shaolin Temple. However, he notes the caveat of the need for higher-level government support: "If the central government takes an interest, then the steps toward development will be much lighter. Individual influence is small and if you just rely on the villagers, teachers, and instructors, the development will be much slower and smaller. You need the infrastructure behind it and at the moment the climate is favorable" (Chen, B., 2005).

References

Chen, B. (2005, Sep 12). Personal interview conducted in Chenjiagou by members of Chenjiagou Taijiquan GB (Great Britain).

Chen, K. (1993 Apr 22). My father, Chen Zhaopei, *Henan Sports Journal*. Downloaded from website: www.chenstyle.com.

Chen, L. (2005). Interview downloaded from website: www.chenjiagou.net.

Chen, X. (2003 Dec 5). Personal interview conducted in Chenjiagou by members of Chenjiagou Taijiquan GB (Great Britain).

Chen, X. (2005). China's living treasure. *Chinatown – the Magazine*, No. 18: 75–77.

Chen, X. (2004). *Chen family taijiquan of China*. Zhengzhou, Henan, China: Henan People's Publishing.

Chen, X. (1990). *Chen Style Taijiquan transmitted through generations*. Beijing, China: People's Sports Publishing.

Chen, Z. (n.d.). Eastern Horizon, BBC Radio program interview.

Feng, N. (2004). Chen Zhenglei. *Chinatown – the Magazine*, No. 8: 33–34.

Gaffney, D. and Sim, D. (2002). *Chen Style Taijiquan: The source of taiji boxing*. Berkeley, CA: North Atlantic Books.

Hiebert, P., Shaw, R., and Tienou, T. (1999). *Understanding folk religion*. Grand Rapids, MI: Baker Books.

Hucker, C. (1975). *China's imperial past: An introduction to Chinese history and culture*. Stanford, CA: Stanford University Press.

Jian, G. (2002). The small frame of Chen style taijiquan. *Shaolin Yu Taiji*, 9. Downloaded from website: www.taiji-bg.com.

Millinger, J. and Fang C. (1976). *Ch'i Chi-kuang, in Dictionary of Ming biography, 1368–1644*. Goodrich, L. and Fang, C. (Eds.). New York City, NY: Columbia University Press.

Spence, J. (1999). *The search for modern China*. New York City, NY: Norton.

Unger, J. (1984). *The class system in rural China: A case study in class and social stratification in post-revolution China*. Watson, J. (Ed.). Cambridge, UK: Cambridge University Press.

Wang, J., et al. (2006). *Chenjiagou research*. Zhengzhou, Henan, China: Henan Agricultural University Research Centre.

Zhu, T. (2000, Aug. 17). Personal interview conducted in Singapore by members of Chenjiagou Taijiquan GB (Great Britain).

Zheng Manqing: The Memorial Hall and Legacy of the Master of Five Excellences in Taiwan
by Russ Mason, M.A.

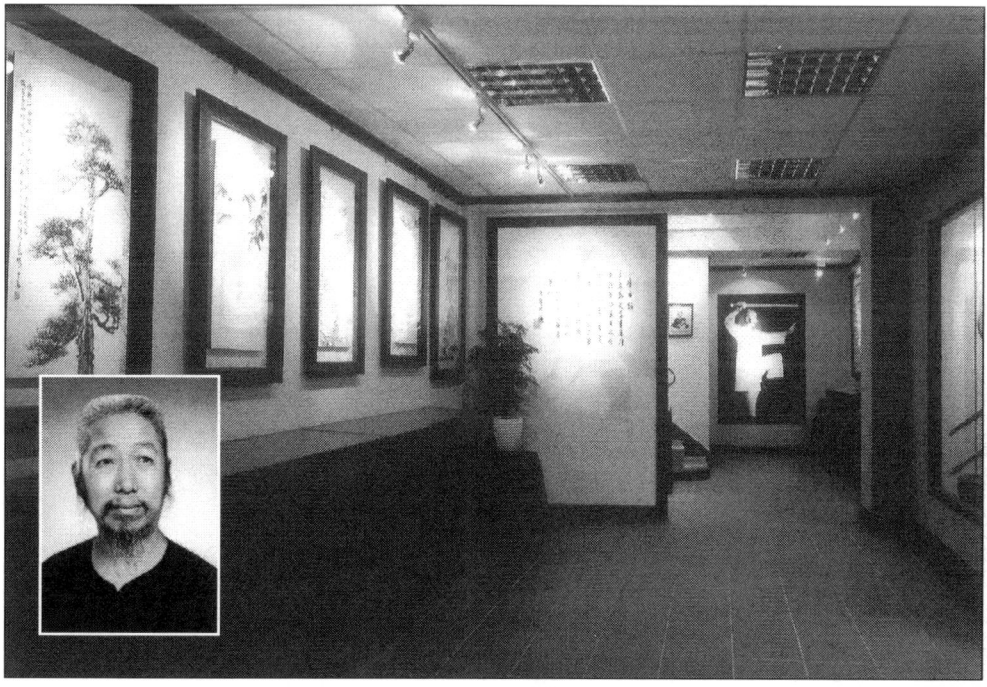

Inset photo of Professor Zheng courtesy of Robert W. Smith. The large exhibit room in the downstairs area of the Zheng Manqing Memorial Hall. It displays several paintings and photographs of Professor Zheng. Photo courtesy of Yuan Weiming.

Introduction

Professor Zheng Manqing (Cheng Man-ch'ing) has been called a "taiji genius" and a "multifaceted savant" (Smith, 1999: 201). A living bridge between ancient China and contemporary Western society, Zheng embodied the ideal of the cultivated Chinese gentleman of the literati class. In old China, a scholar needed a thorough knowledge of the literary classics, calligraphy, and poetry in order to pass the imperial civil service examinations, which were still in place during Zheng's childhood at the end of the Qing dynasty (1644–1911). These requirements of public office shaped the Chinese concept of education. Beyond these accomplishments a cultured man was expected to be familiar with painting, the game of Go (*Weiqi*), and other classical arts (Barnstone and Chou, 1996: xii). Zheng excelled in all these arts. Moreover, following the Confucian ideal, Zheng blended the martial arts with the fine arts, for Confucius taught that without martial training (e.g., archery and charioteering) one could not master the mental discipline necessary for the civil arts (e.g., propriety, music, mathematics, and writing) (Zheng, 1985: 14).

Professor Zheng is known as the Master of Five Excellences, referring to his outstanding abilities in traditional Chinese medicine, martial arts, and fine arts (painting, poetry, and calligraphy). One American researcher has written that, in order to properly evaluate Zheng's accomplishments in the Chinese milieu, a westerner must begin by imagining a person who has made extraordinary contributions in classical scholarship, literary theory, and criticism. In addition, such a person is: "an Olympic boxer, president of a national medical association, distinguished poet and professor of literature, and [one whose] paintings hang in the Louvre" (Wile, 2007: 2). How did Professor Zheng establish a reputation of such stature that it is deserving of a memorial?

The following sections will present a concise biographical sketch of Zheng's early personal life, his academic and professional successes, and his training and accomplishments in the field of martial arts. The focus will be on his work in Taiwan, the growth of his Taibei school, and the posthumous establishment of the memorial hall currently housed in his former residence.

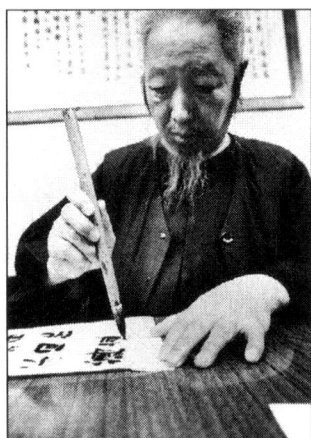

Professor Zheng completes a poem. Photo courtesy of Ken van Sickle.

Early Life

Born in Yongjia County (now the Lucheng District of Wenzhou) in Zhejiang Province, Zheng Yue[1] grew up the youngest child in a family of humble means. His father died while he was still young, and life was hard. Yet, even as a child, Zheng's interest in calligraphy, painting, poetry, and medicinal herbs was encouraged and nurtured by his mother and maternal aunt. Yue was a precocious child with a keen and inquiring intellect who had memorized the Confucian classics by age nine. Then, after suffering a fracture of the skull in an accident, he spent two days and nights in a coma. A teacher of martial arts treated the boy with mountain herbs, and he regained consciousness but had completely lost his memory and was in a near vegetative state. His mother apprenticed Zheng soon after to local painter, Wang Xiangchan.[2] The simple, repetitive work of grinding ink proved therapeutic, and within five years the young artist had not only recovered his mental acuity but had also mastered the skill of painting well enough to begin supporting himself and his family by selling his own works.

Academic and Professional Success

In 1916 the famed poet Lu Chengbei provided an introduction for the budding artist that led to further study in painting, poetry, and calligraphy in Hangzhou (Wile, 2007: 16). Three years later, at the tender age of seventeen, Zheng traveled to Beijing, where he met and was befriended by several elder painters and poets, winning their respect through his intelligence and skill. All around him young thinkers caught up in the May Fourth reform movement and the early days of the new republic were questioning the ancient ways, but Zheng's *guanxi* (social connections) with members of the older generation, developed through participation in these traditional artistic circles, led to an invitation to teach poetry at Yuwen University in Beijing (cir. 1919). Shortly afterward, Zheng received a recommendation to teach at National Jinan University in Shanghai from none other than Cai Yuanpei (1868–1940), one of the highest-ranking and most influential educators of the early Republican era (Davis, 1996: 40, 53). Cai was chancellor of Beijing University at that time. It is reasonable to assume that Cai's personal support opened doors and helped to propel the younger man's rapid rise in academia.

After his move south from the capital, Zheng became director of the painting department at the Shanghai School of Fine Arts and was also instrumental in establishing the College of Culture and Art there. But his responsibilities in Shanghai did not prevent him from mounting a solo art exhibition at Waterside (*Shuixie*) Pavilion in Beijing's Central Park, and in 1925, together with such colleagues as the famous artist Zhang Daqian, founding the Xiaohan Painting Society (Wile, 2007: 16). He also traveled to Japan to do research on the fine arts for the Chinese Ministry of Education (Davis, 1996: 40).

Zheng's students relate an anecdote[3] that clearly illustrates the young professor's artistic ability at this time in his career, as well as his photographic memory.

Once, while attending a dinner party at the home of the mayor of Shanghai, Zheng became fascinated by a hanging scroll created by a famous master of rattan painting. Stepping aside from the gathering of distinguished guests, he gazed long at the scroll, lost in admiration. When it was suggested that he might borrow the painting in order to study it in the privacy of his home, the young artist declined, saying that such extended study was unnecessary, as he had already committed the scene to memory. The next day Zheng presented a replica of the painting to his host. Mayor Wu was amazed to see that the replica painted by Zheng matched the original in every detail and was, in itself, a masterful work of art. After this, word of Zheng's artistic genius spread throughout Shanghai.

Some sources suggest Zheng's move to the south may have been partially motivated by health concerns, as he was already suffering from tuberculosis, which was aggravated by the northern Beijing climate as well as by the ubiquitous chalk dust of the classroom environment.[4] During his time in Shanghai, Zheng began to devote himself to a more serious study of Chinese medicine. Building on the foundational knowledge of herbal remedies gained from his mother, Zheng sought and gained tuition from Dr. Song You'an, a famous practitioner from Anhui Province who was persuaded to come out of retirement to provide a personal apprenticeship. Much later, Zheng practiced herbal medicine full time, eventually serving as president of the National Chinese Medical Association (Davis, 1996: 41). In addition to being named to the National Assembly for the Construction of the Constitution in 1946, Zheng was one year later elected to the National Assembly to represent the community of doctors of traditional Chinese medicine, a position he held until the end of his life (Cheng, 1971: 238).

Zheng Manqing was widely recognized as a man of great and varied accomplishments, so much so that Lin Sen (1868–1943), the Chairman of the Nationalist government at the time of the Sino-Japanese War, presented Zheng with a calligraphic inscription conferring upon him the title "Master of Five Arts."[5]

At the age of forty Zheng married Ding Yidu (known in the US as Madame Juliana T. Cheng), the daughter of General Ding Muhan, founder of the Chinese Air Force Bureau. Madame Zheng had been a student of medicine at Beijing University, and her specialty of medical practice became obstetrics. The couple would have five children.

Martial Accomplishments

Perhaps because of his childhood health concerns, Zheng early on studied exercises such as *baduanjin* and *yijin* (Davis, 1996: 40). He had also practiced taijiquan intermittently beginning in 1923 to bolster his weak physique, but each time his physical condition would improve, he would leave off practice to devote himself to other endeavors.[6] After Zheng's tuberculosis progressed to the point of coughing up blood, he committed himself to persevere in a daily exercise regimen. Zheng received an introduction to the famous master Yang Chengfu and credited the practice of Yang Style taijiquan with his complete recovery from the life-threatening illness (Cheng, 1971: 238, Cheng, 1985: 64; and Yang, 1934/2005: 2).

In his own book, Yang Zhenji (Yang Chengfu's second son; b. 1921) emphasized the fact that Zheng was his father's disciple, and that Zheng was the scholar who transcribed Yang Chengfu's 1934 book, *The Essence and Applications of Taijiquan* (*Taijiquan tiyong quanshu*) (Yang, 1993: 250). In addition to being chosen to record Yang's teaching, Zheng was further honored by being asked to write a preface for the master's book.[7]

One of Yang Chengfu's senior-most students was Li Yaxuan. Li's student, Yan Changkong, writes that after the Maoist victory, subsequent editions of Yang's book censored Zheng's name and preface for political reasons. This was due to his connections with Chiang Kai-shek. However, after thirty years of blackout, Zheng's name and biography are once again appearing in mainland publications (Wile, 2007: 15, 32; Davis, 1996: 48). Yan also recorded Li's statement that Yang gave

Zheng private instruction in inner cultivation (*neigong*), which helped him comprehend the subtler elements of the art. Yan, citing Li Yaxuan's high standards, went on to note that Li's praise for Zheng's insights and skills was "truly a rare thing" (Wile, 2007: 33, 35).

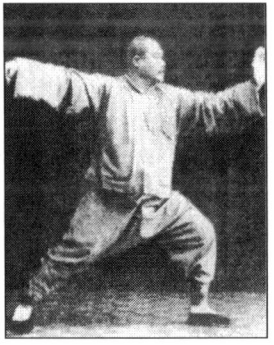 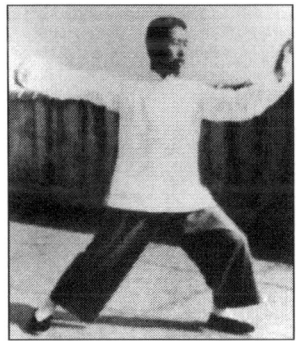 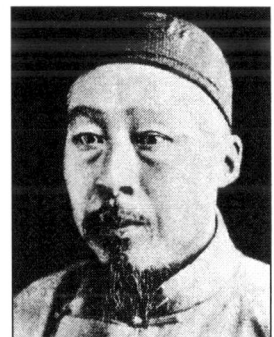

Left to right: Yang Chengfu (ca. 1933) and his student Zheng Manqing (ca. 1948) show the posture of single whip. Chen Weiming, a senior student of Yang Chengfu and a classmate, friend, and supporter of Zheng Manqing.

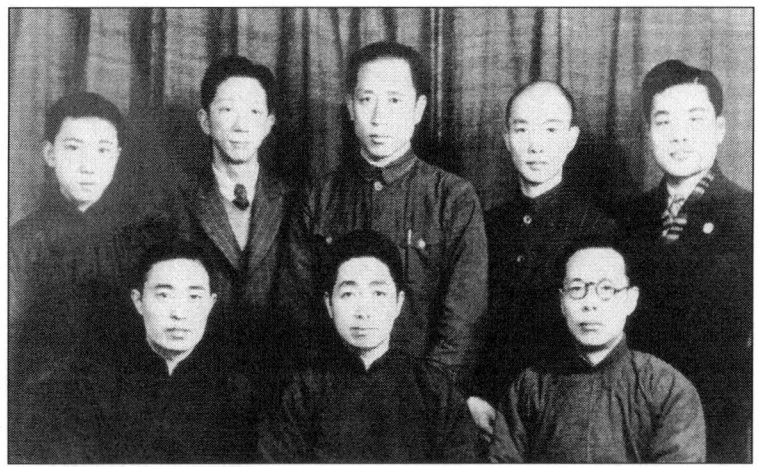

Professor Zheng Manqing (center front) in China in 1943 with a group of students: directly behind Zheng is Zhang Zigang; in the rear row, far right with scarf, is Guo Qingfang, Western boxing lightweight champion of China in the late 1930s. Photo courtesy of Guo Qingfang.

Another of Yang's most famous students was Chen Weiming (1881–1958). Chen was not only a senior student of Yang Chengfu, but also a scholar and writer who had himself represented Yang's teachings in print.[8] After the Sino-Japanese war, Zheng took the early manuscript of his own text, *Master Zheng's Thirteen Treatises on Taijiquan*, to Chen to see whether it would meet with his senior classmate's approval (Cheng, 1965/1999: 9). Zheng felt that both his book and his approach to taijiquan were merely a continuation of Yang's own teaching and earlier text, *Essence and Applications of Taijiquan*. Chen approved of Zheng's work and urged its publication, even offering to write a preface (Cheng, 1985: 108; Cheng, 1965/1999: 9). Chen wrote in his preface to the book that, during the years of Zheng's study, when Madame Yang (née Hou) fell ill, Zheng used his knowledge of herbal medicine to treat her, saving her life. Chen writes: "Master Yang was so thankful that he taught [Zheng] all the secret oral transmissions. No one else had ever heard them" (Wile, 1985: 1). Chen supported Zheng's conviction that an overarching principle of Yang Style taijiquan is commitment to the twin principle: sink-relax (*chen song*), something that would come to be a distinguishing characteristic of Zheng's approach to taijiquan.[9]

Fu Zhongwen (1903–1994, nephew, disciple, and teaching assistant of Yang Chengfu) stated that Zheng established his reputation in the 1930s in Yang's circle because of his deep interest in *tuishou* (pushing hands) and his enthusiastic training with the most skilled seniors (Yu and Sharp, 1993: 45–46). After developing his skill by working with Yang and his senior students, Zheng went on to meet a number of public and private challenges, some involving British and American military personnel and others with well-regarded Chinese boxers. The fact that Zheng served as head of the Hunan Martial Arts Academy (as well as serving on the faculty of two other military academies) and the fact that he won the respect of the seasoned military officers he worked with attest to the functionality of his skills.[10] On the mainland, Zheng was called upon in 1933 to teach taijiquan to Nationalist troops at the Central Military Academy (formerly known as Huangpu). Later, during the Sino-Japanese War, he taught in Sichuan for the Central Military Training Group (Davis, 1996: 41). In 1938, as director of the provincial government's Hunan Martial Arts Academy, Zheng was responsible for training hundreds of officers in only two months' time. Under these circumstances he was forced to simplify th Yang Style long form by eliminating repetitions, eventually settling on thirty-seven as the standard number of postures for his version of the solo exercise.[11]

Arrival in Taiwan

After the surrender of Japan in 1945, full-scale civil war reerupted in China between the Nationalist forces of Generalissimo Chiang Kai-shek (the Guomindang) and the Maoists. After the communist victory on the mainland in 1949, Zheng immigrated to Taiwan with the Guomindang. Eventually, he settled in a house on Zhongxing Road in Yunghe, a suburb of Chiang Kai-shek's capital city, Taibei. He would dub the place Xi Chang Lou, which could be interpreted "Tower of Long Evening" or "Long Night Lodge" (Wile, 2007: 52). There he concentrated on practicing medicine, later opening a taijiquan school on the top floor of Zhongshan Hall at the request of Taibei mayor You Mijian (Wile, 2007: 18). In Taiwan, Zheng taught his thirty-seven-posture simplified form (*jianyi taijiquan*) publicly to civilians.

After establishing himself as a physician in Taiwan, Zheng accepted his first student on the island in the art of taijiquan. Benjamin Lo, a young university student, came for medical treatment and was advised to practice taijiquan so his body could develop the strength needed to absorb the prescribed herbal medications (Davis and Mann, 1996: 50).[12] Beginning in 1949, Lo went to Professor Zheng's home each day to learn taijiquan in the traditional way, perfecting the form posture by posture. He would later come to the United States, where he has taught Zheng's method since 1974. Soon after Lo began to study, Liu Xiheng bowed as a disciple to Zheng, followed by Xu Yizhong and others. As the master's fame spread throughout the island, many more students were added, most coming with previous training in the martial arts and, in the traditional way, by personal introduction. Zheng established the Shizhong Study Society (Shizhong Xueshe)[13] in 1949 for the promotion of taijiquan (Davis, 1996: 43; Wile, 2007: 7; see also the Shizhong webpage).

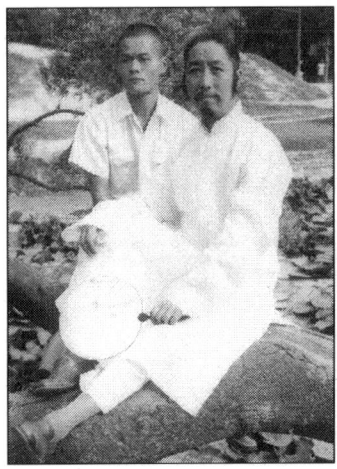 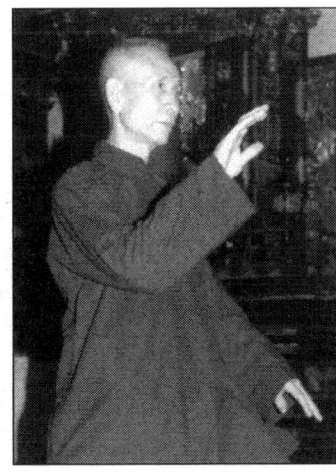

Left: Zheng Manqing with his first student in Taiwan, Benjamin Lo, in the botanical garden, Taibei, 1951. Photo courtesy of Benjamin Lo.
Right: Liu Xiheng shows brush knee twist step. Photo courtesy of Liu Xiheng.

In addition to heading his own school, the Shizhong Study Society, Zheng was a member of the Chinese Taijiquan Club (*Zhong Guo Taijiquan Ju Le Bu*), formally established on March 27, 1960. National assembly member Chen Panling (who was also head of the ROC Chinese Boxing Association) served as chief commissioner. In addition to Zheng and Chen, other well-known members included Wang Yannian, Xiong Yanghe, Guo Lianyin, and Han Qingtang. Later, in 1963, an expanded version of the club, known as the Taijiquan Academic Research Committee, was established under the auspices of the Sino-American Cultural and Economic Association, with Zheng serving as a consultant (Fairchild and Lin, 2007: 2–3).

During the period between 1959 and 1962, American martial arts historian Robert W. Smith was assigned a CIA post in Taiwan as intelligence advisor to the admiral of the US Pacific Fleet. His research into the practice and history of Chinese martial arts led him to Zheng's door and, eventually, to a lifelong commitment to Zheng's taijiquan method.[14] As Zheng's first Western student, Smith did much to publicize "the Professor" (as he was respectfully addressed by his students) in the West. In 1964 Zheng traveled abroad, first to Paris and then to the United States, where he exhibited his paintings at the Cernuschi Museum of Chinese Art and the Republic of China pavilion of the New York World's Fair, respectively.[15] After establishing a residence in New York City, Zheng received the title director of fine arts, the Republic of China Cultural Renaissance Movement, American Branch from the Chiang Kai-shek government (Davis, 1996: 46). There he established an American branch of his Shizhong School to promote taijiquan, as well as other forms of traditional Chinese arts and culture. Leaving Liu Xiheng in charge of his school in Taiwan in his absence (Davis, 1996: 54), Zheng would balance his time between his homes in New York and Taibei over the next ten years. During this period, he exhibited paintings at the FAR Gallery in 1968 and at the Hudson River Museum in 1973 and authored some of his most profound works, including commentaries on the *Daodejing*, the *Yijing*, and the Confucian classics of the *Analects*, the *Great Learning*, and the *Doctrine of the Mean* (Cheng, 1971/1981: 239; Davis, 1996: 46). At this time in his life, Zheng led flourishing taijiquan schools in both America and the Republic of China. His work did much to popularize taijiquan in the West and Taiwan, and to establish the international reputation of his thirty-seven-posture simplified Yang Style short form. Professor Zheng was particularly noted in the international martial arts community for his remarkable skill in push-hands (*tuishou*).

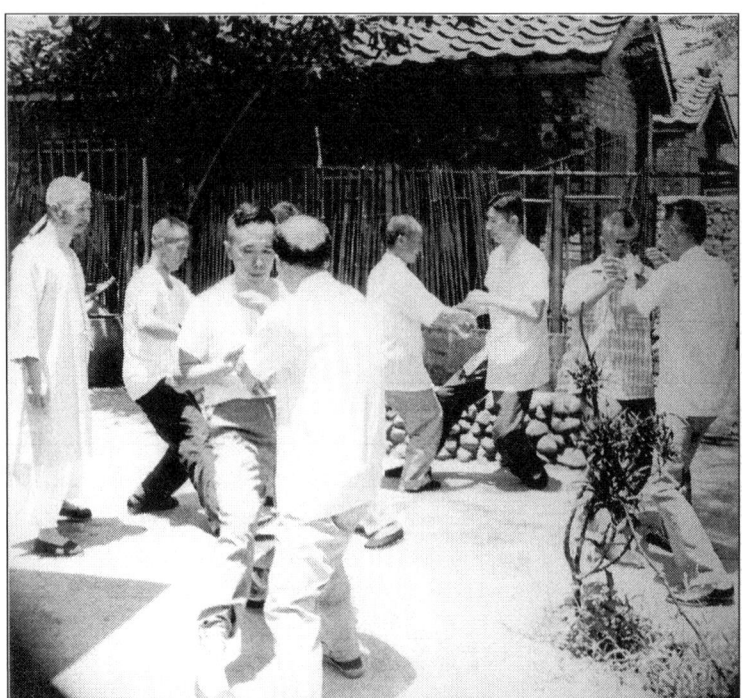 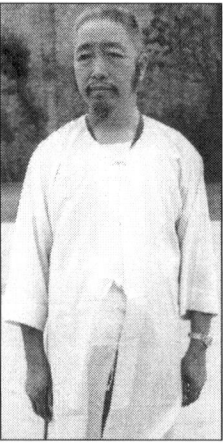

Left: Professor Zheng watches students push-hands at his residence in Yonghe.
Right: Zheng Manqing (1902–1975).

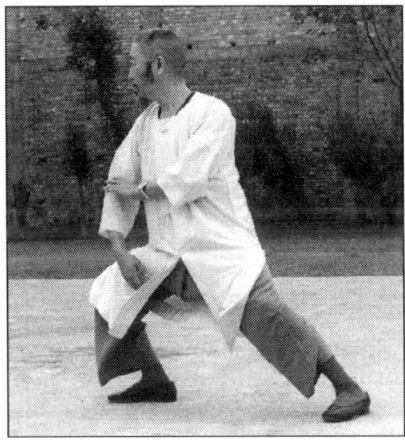 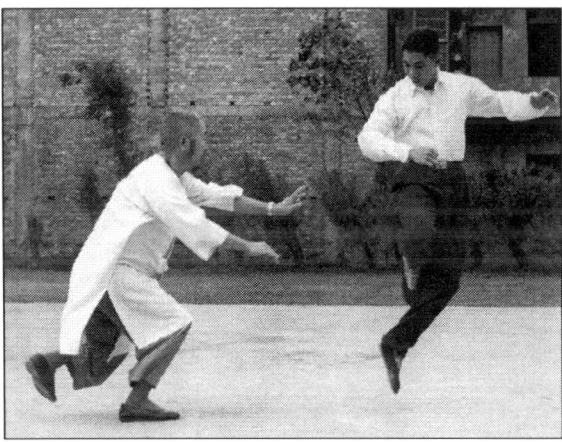

Left: In the posture shoulder stroke. Repelling an attacker.
Note the cross-substantial push: rooted right foot and active left hand.

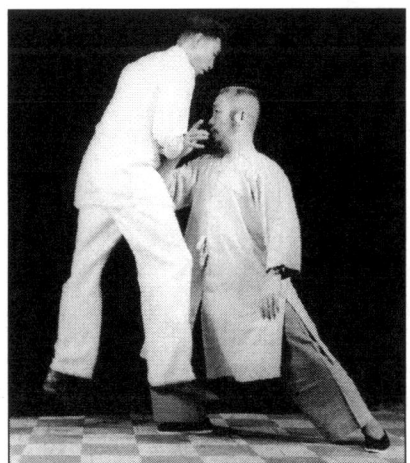 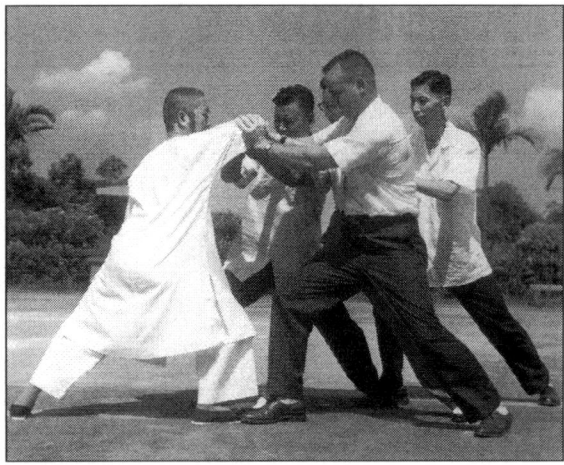

Left: Zheng Manqing uproots William C. C. Chen.
Note the relaxed hands and the effective *tifang* (lit: lift/let-go).
Withstands the push of four men (Taiwan, c. 1960). Photos courtesy of Robert W. Smith.

Zheng's Death and Legacy in Taiwan

Zheng died on March 26, 1975, from the effects of a cerebral hemorrhage suffered at his home in Taibei (Wile, 2007: 19). The Master of the Five Excellences funeral was attended by hundreds, including distinguished representatives from his many fields of endeavor, students, and government officials. Memorials were also held in Singapore and New York City (Davis 1996: 48).

Upon Professor Zheng's passing, Liu Xihong succeeded him as president of the Taibei Shizhong Study Society in 1975 and served in this capacity, heading up taijiquan instruction at the school, until his retirement in 1986. His classmate, Xu Yizhong, served as president after that. In addition, in 1993 Xu was elected first committee chairman of a new organization, the Master Zheng Taijiquan Study Association. Chairman Xu served the first two consecutive terms at this post. Ke

Qihua served as third committee chairman from 1999 until his passing in 2001, with Ju Hongbin of Gaoxiong finishing out his term.[16] Following this, Xu Yizhong returned to the post and continues to serve in this capacity at the present time. Current advisors to the association include two names familiar to the American taijiquan community: Benjamin P. Lo and William C. C. Chen. With the assistance of his able advisors and instructors, the association chairman, Xu Yizhong, is tireless in his efforts to promote Professor Zheng's simplified taijiquan in Taiwan and around the world.

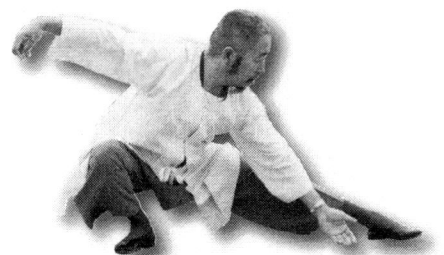

Zheng shows the posture squatting single whip.

Among the special events organized by the association was the hundredth anniversary celebration of Professor Zheng Manqing's birth. This week-long event was celebrated in August of 2000 and featured panel discussions, martial arts demonstrations, a tournament, and an exhibition of Zheng's paintings and calligraphy on loan from the National Palace Museum.[17]

Today simplified taijiquan has come full circle, as one of Zheng's senior students in Taiwan, Chairman Xu Yizhong, traveled in October of 2006 to Nankai University in Tianjin on the Chinese mainland to teach the form at the request of that university's martial arts (*wushu*) community. Nankai University's curriculum currently offers an ongoing course to research Professor Zheng's simplified taijiquan, and other such programs are in the discussion stage. In addition, the Beijing University of Physical Education and related organizations have expressed interest in publishing Zheng's instructional books on taijiquan.[18]

Establishment of the Zheng Manqing Memorial Hall

In the years following Professor Zheng's passing, Madame Juliana T. Zheng and her family continued to divide their time between the United States and Taiwan, using the old home place on Zhongxing Road in Yonghe as a base during their visits to Taibei. After Madame Zheng's passing in January 2005, it was decided that a portion of the family residence would be refurbished and converted to a memorial hall for the preservation of Professor Zheng's artifacts and legacy. After much work on the part of the family, students, Chairman Xu Yizhong, and the association, the opening ceremony of the Zheng Manqing Memorial Hall was celebrated on June 25, 2006. Due to space limitations and the number of guests, the ceremony was held in the gymnasium of the Taibei Wuchang Junior High School (the current location of taijiquan classes offered by the Shizhong Study Society).

In attendance were five hundred people, including noted artists, poets, philosophers, and the head of the Taiwan National Taijiquan Association, Zhan Deshen.

Xu Chongming (the first chair advisor of the Zhengzi Taijiquan Study Association) made a report of Master Zheng's history in Taiwan, and Chou Bozi (the vice chairman of the committee) presented a golden key to the new memorial hall facility.[19] In November of 2006, this author visited the memorial hall. The photographic tour of the Zheng Manqing Memorial Hall outlined here is presented with the permission of Chairman Xu and the assistance of the association staff and others. Visitors to the memorial are welcome and may receive further information by visiting www.37taichi.org.tw. In addition, plans are under consideration to offer overseas memberships in the association.

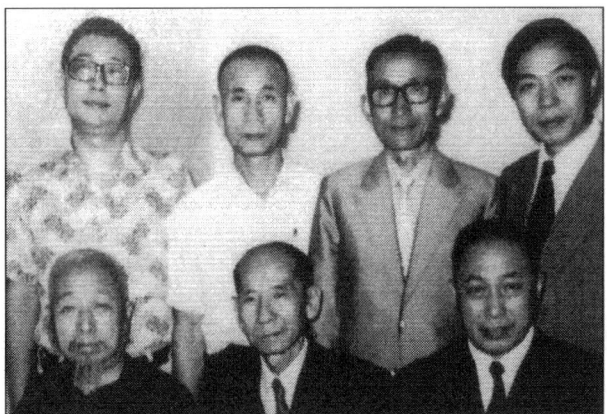
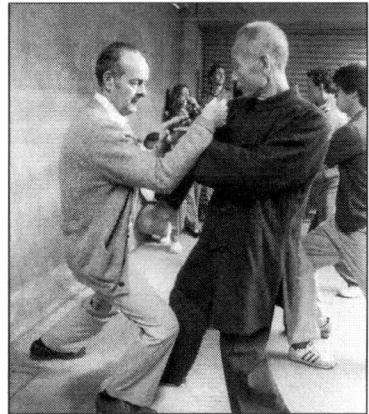

Above, left: Zheng with friends and senior students. First row, left to right: Zheng, Mr. Hong (friend and legal advisor from Hong Kong), and Wang Yannian. Back row, left to right: Mr. Yang (a lawyer friend), Liu Xiheng (first president of the association), the late Tao Bingxiang (d. 2006), and Xu Yizhong (current president of the association). Right: Liu Xiheng and Robert W. Smith push hands in Taibei (1983). Photo courtesy of Robert W. Smith.

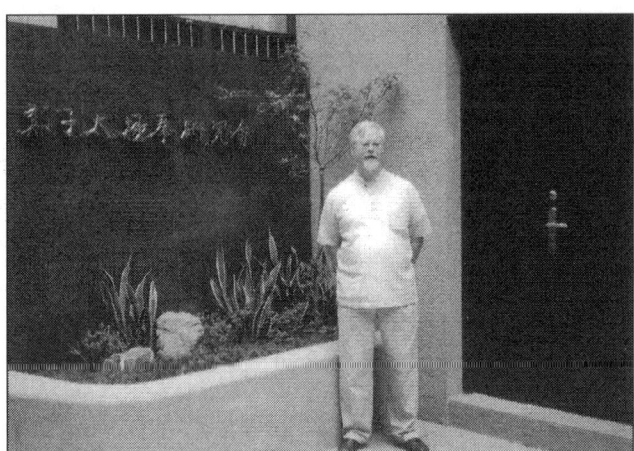
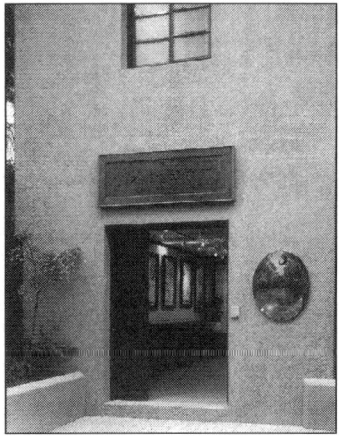

Danny Emerick stands outside the door to the memorial hall at the Professor's old residence. The entranceway with sign above reading Zheng Manqing Memorial Hall. Photos by R. Mason.

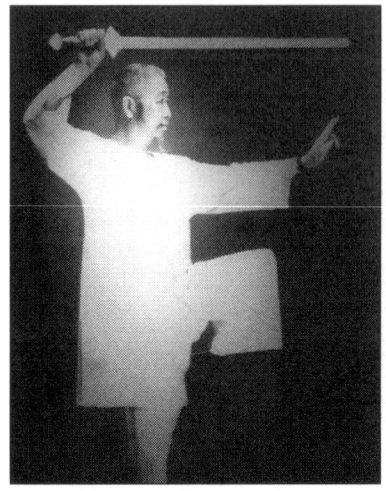
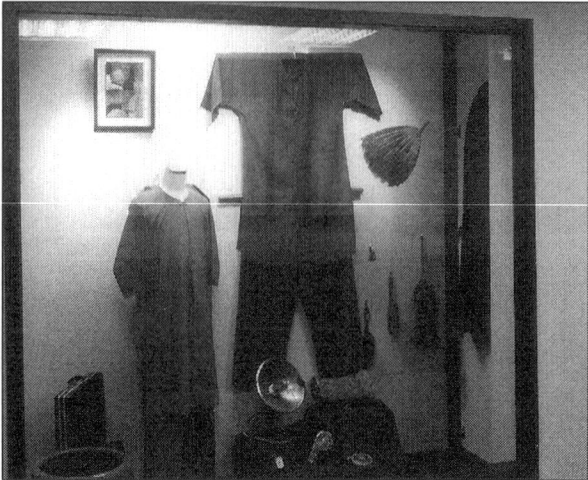

Above left: Zheng with sword in the posture of major literary star (*da kui xing*). Photo by R. Mason. Right: A display case containing Zheng's personal artifacts. Next to this is also a brief lineage chart, and a chronology of his life. Photo courtesy of Yuan Weiming.

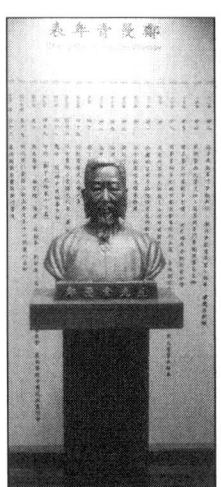
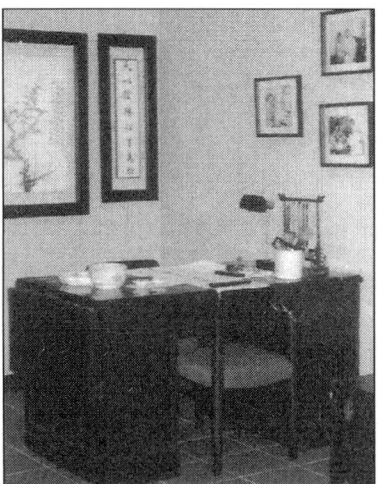
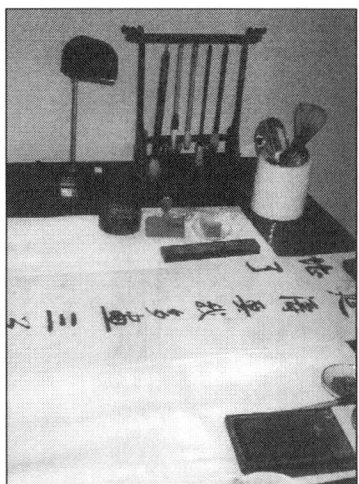

Above left: This life-size bronze bust of Professor Zheng stands in a small alcove with a chronology of his major life events. Center and right: Zheng's desk and details of the desktop showing inkstone, brushes, calligraphy, and personal name seal (chop). Photos by R. Mason.

Zheng Manqing's *Zuo You Ming*

As one enters the front door of the memorial hall, straight ahead and toward the left wall is a large panel displaying a 1949 photograph of Zheng in the single-whip posture. Overlaid on the photo is his *zuo you ming* calligraphy. The terms *zuo you* literally translate "seat right hand," and ming can be interpreted "inscription," "tablet," or "motto." Therefore, the phrase "*zuo you ming*" could refer to something that is carved and kept close at hand for constant reference, as in "words to live by." Written in the terse, classical style, the verses of Zheng's poem resonate with literary allusion and could be interpreted in various ways. The gist of the motto goes something like this:

Allow the hands to be led lightly and humbly.
Allow the feet to be heavy, stepping with dignity.
Hang straight; hang straight! Be poised and upright.
Speak sparingly, directly, and with great care.
Be forgiving and generous; out of a centered heart, give back.
Be loyal, tolerant, and patient in your dealings.
Let your attitude toward others be temperate.
Repent, and correct your errors with silent contemplation.

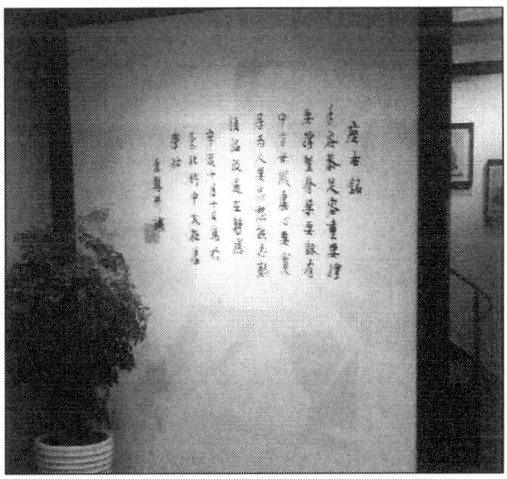

Zheng's *zuo you ming* calligraphy superimposed over a photo of him in the posture single whip. Photos by R. Mason. Below, left to right: Red scrolls constituting a matching couplet. Blossoming bough flanked by a matching couplet. Above these is a wooden plaque with Zheng's Tower of Long Evening calligraphy. All photos by R. Mason.

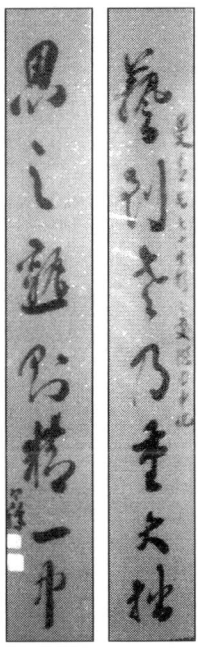

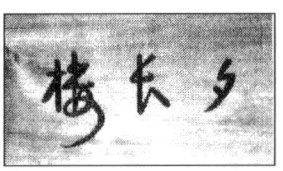

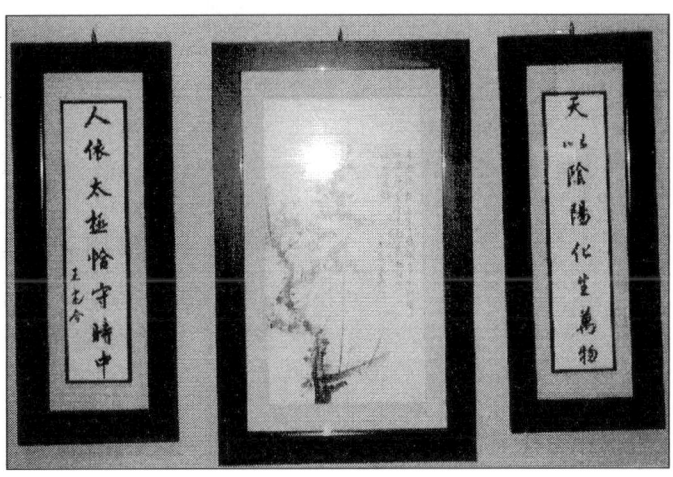

Matching Couplet Red Scrolls

Upstairs, on either side of the entryway between the conference room and Professor Zheng's office, hang two red vertical scrolls of verse. The pair constitutes a poem of a special structure called *duilian*. In such paired scrolls, the Chinese phrasing and grammar must match exactly; therefore, the creation of this type of verse is very demanding. The two sections of the couplet depicted here read something like this:

> When you ponder deeply, you will reach high
> competency in the area of your special skill.
> When your artistic skill has reached maturity,
> you will plumb the depths of great simplicity.

Matching Couplet with Blossoming Bough

Behind Professor Zheng's desk hangs a painting of a blossoming bough. Above the painting is a wooden plaque with the inscription "Tower of Long Evening" (*Xi Chang Lou*), Zheng's nickname for his study. On either side of the painting is another couplet. The couplet reads:

> Heaven creates all living things from yin and yang.
> All humanity depends upon taiji to safeguard Shizhong.

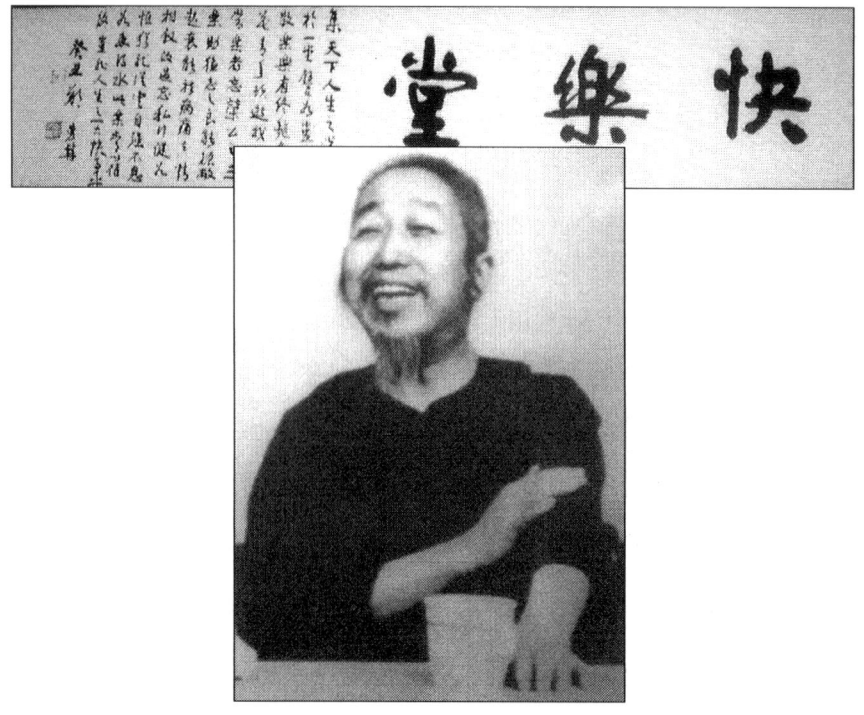

"Hall of Happiness" calligraphy. Professor Zheng expounds with a smile. Photo by R. Mason.

The Hall of Happiness

On this broad, horizontal work of calligraphy, Professor Zheng's beautiful brushwork showcases his poem "The Hall of Happiness" ("*Tang Le Kuai*"). The text of the poem appears below as translated by Tam Gibbs:

> May the joy that is everlasting gather in this hall. Not the joy of a sumptuous feast, which slips away even as we leave the table; nor that which music brings—it is only of a limited duration. Beauty and a pretty face are like flowers; they bloom for a while, then die. Even our youth slips swiftly away and is gone. No; enduring happiness is not in these, nor in the three joys of Tung Kung. We may as well forget them, for the joy I mean is worlds away from these. It is the joy of continuous growth, of helping to develop in ourselves and others the talents and abilities with which we were born—the gifts of heaven to mortal men. It is to revive the exhausted and to rejuvenate that which is in decline so that we are enabled to dispel sickness and suffering. Let true affection and happy concourse abide in this hall. Let us here correct our past mistakes and lose preoccupation with self. With the constancy of the planets in their courses or of the dragon in his cloud-wrapped path, let us enter the land of health and ever after walk within its bounds. Let us fortify ourselves against weakness and learn to be self-reliant, without ever a moment's lapse. Then our resolution will become the very air we breathe, the world we live in; then we will be as happy as a fish in crystal waters. This is the joy which lasts, that we can carry with us to the end of our days. And tell me, if you can; what greater happiness can life bestow?

Ying Erpo's Stylized Calligraphy of Zheng Kung

Hanging in the larger ground-floor room to the left of the display case is a specialized piece of artwork created by Ying Erpo. It consists of a stylized character for the family name Zheng in the form of a painting of Professor Zheng preparing to perform the posture turn body and sweep lotus with leg. The figure is like a riddle, with various parts of the body made up of stylized strokes from the character. The inscription to the right of the image reads:

> Taijiquan's founder Zhang Sanfeng's
> true successor Master Zheng Manqing's
> 'name-character' is here stylized into this
> figure in memory of the inauguration of
> the Master Zheng Manqing Memorial Hall
> on this 25th day of June (Zheng's birthday)
> in the year 2006.

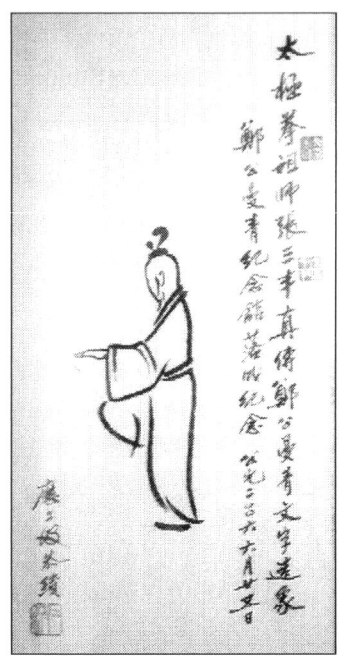 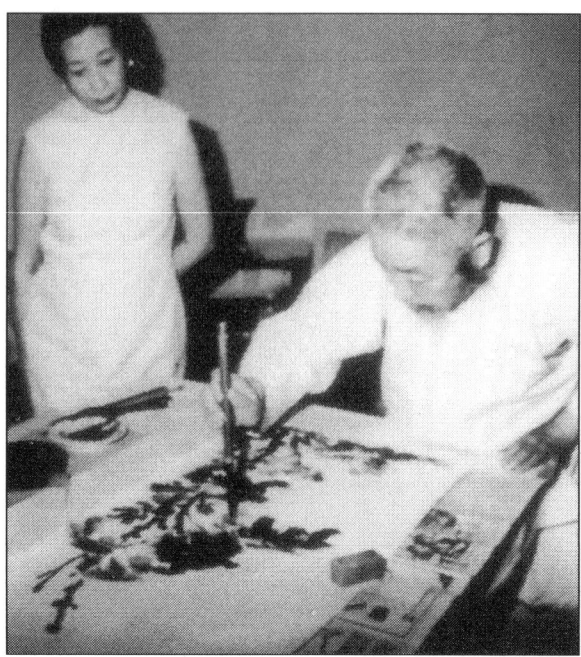

Above left: Ying Erpo's stylized painting of the character *zheng* (鄭).
Photo by R. Mason. The inscription to the bottom left reads:
"Respectfully drawn by Ying Erpo." [1]

Above right: Professor Zheng does brushwork as Madame Zheng looks on.
Courtesy of the Zheng Manqing Memorial Hall.

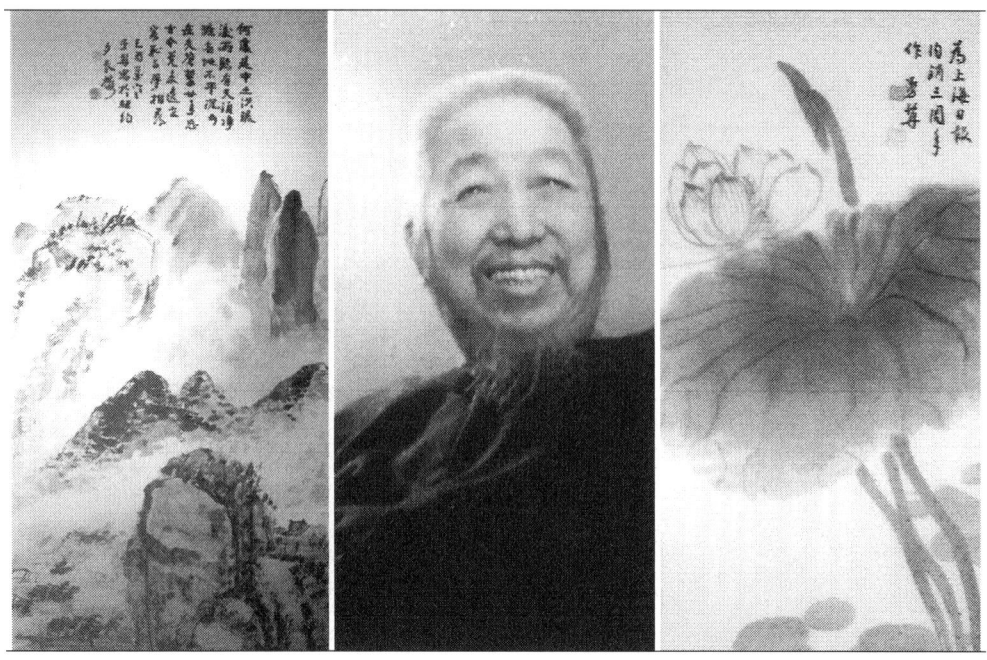

Examples of Professor Zheng's paintings:
a mountain landscape (left) and a single lotus (right). Center: Zheng relaxing.

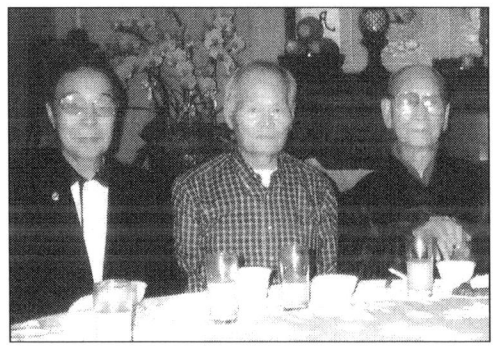 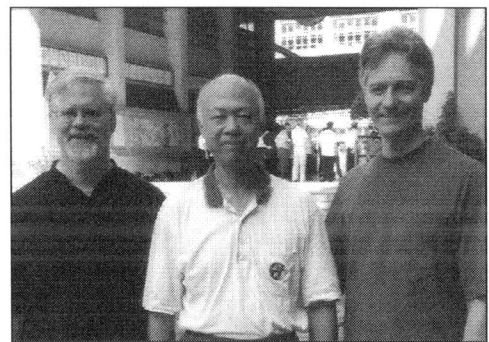

Left: Three of Professor Zheng's most senior students, left to right: current president Xu Yizhong, association advisor Benjamin Lo, and first president Liu Xiheng. Photo courtesy of Danny Emerick. Right: Shizhong instructor Yuan Weiming with Danny Emerick and the author. Taijiquan classes at Wu Chang Junior High School facility are in progress in the background.

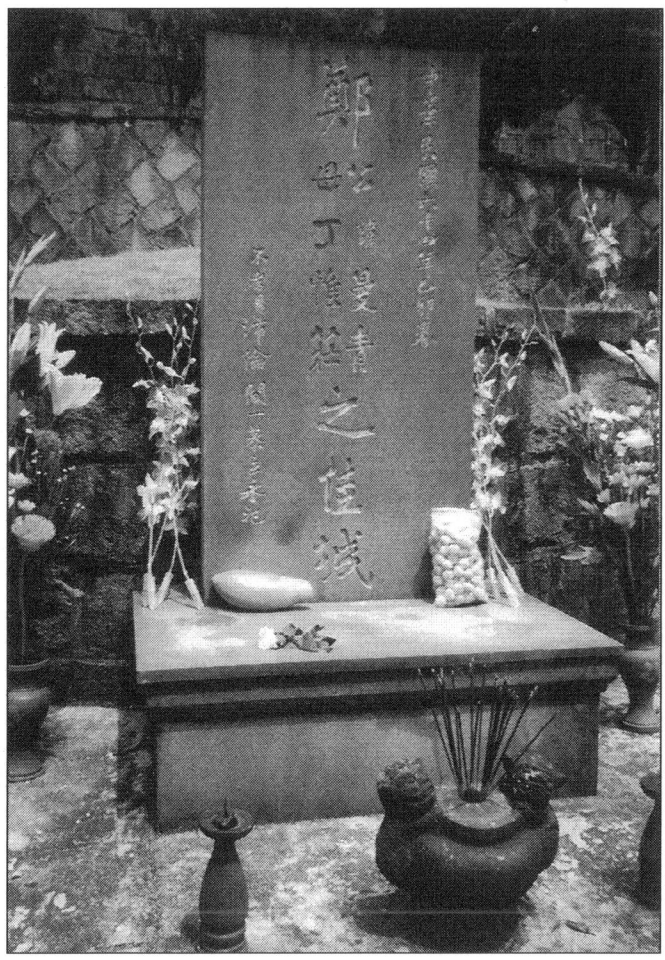

Professor Zheng Manqing's tombstone, Taibei, Taiwan. Photo courtesy of Mark Westcott.

Glossary

Chen Zhicheng (William C. C.)	陳至誠	Shi Zhong Xueshe	时中學社
Chen Panling	陳泮嶺	Tang Le Kuai	堂樂快
Chen Weiming	陳微明	Tao Bingxiang	陶炳祥
duilian	對聯	tuishou	推手
Fu Zhongwen	傅鈡文	Xiong Yanghe	熊養和
guanxi	關係	Xu Yizhung	徐憶中
Li Yaxuan	李雅軒	Yang Chengfu	楊澄甫
Liang Tongcai	梁棟材	Yang Jianho	楊健侯
Lin Sen	林森	Yang Shaohou	楊少侯
Liu Xiheng	劉錫亨	Yonghe City	永和市
Luo Bangzhen (Benjamin Lo)	羅邦楨	Zheng Manqing	鄭曼青
neigong	內功	Zheng Yue	鄭岳
Zheng Manqing Jinian Guan		鄭曼青 紀念 館	

Acknowledgements

Thanks are in order to all those who contributed to this project in ways large and small. Xu Yizhong gave his enthusiastic support and gracious permission to use photographs and materials. Benjamin Lo, Robert W. Smith, Liu Xiheng, Yuan Weiming, and Danny Emerick provided photos and other assistance, as did Monica Chen, Julia Fairchild, Ken Van Sickle, Mark Westcott, and others. A special debt of gratitude is owed Nick Tan and Jeff Herrod (as well as other researchers noted in the bibliography) for help with the translation of source materials. Readers' corrections are welcome. The author would like to acknowledge the late Tam Gibbs and to thank Ed Young and Maggie Newman for their help and encouragement. For more information on the Master Zheng Taijiquan Study Association, please contact via their website: www.37taichi@yahoo.com.tw.

Notes

[1] Although Yue was his given name, later in life Zheng would adopt the sobriquet Manqing. Other nicknames and titles would be conferred upon him by others, and he would adopt a variety of pen names. See Yan Changkong's "Recollections of Zheng" (Wile, 2007: 32), Min Xiaoji's comments in his brief biography of "Man-Jan" (Cheng, 1985: 13–15), and Barbara Davis (1996: 39) for more biographical details.

[2] Professor Zheng's American assistant and translator, Tam Gibbs, provides details in the brief biography of Zheng appended to his translation of Zheng's commentary on *Laozi* (Cheng, 1971: 237). Barbara Davis cites the *Great Dictionary of Names and Aliases of Contemporary and Modern China* as a source of details on Wang Xiangchan, whose given name was Ruyuan and who was known for his flower and plant paintings, the specialization that would become Zheng's

forte (Davis, 1996: 39, 53).

3   This story was related to the author by Benjamin Lo in a conversation on April 29, 2007. A version of the story also appears in an article by Xu Yizhong, translated into English by Douglas Wile (2007: 29).

4   See Liang Tongcai's remarks recorded by Robert W. Smith (1974: 29) and Professor Zheng's own writings on his recovery from lung disease (Cheng, 1985: 64).

5   See Yan Changkong's remarks (Wile, 2007: 32).

6   Zheng discusses his early, sporadic practice and his ultimate commitment and perseverance in his book (Cheng, 1962: 25), as well as in his preface to Yang Chengfu's *Essence and Applications of Taijiquan* (Yang, 1934/2005, 1–2).

7   The fact that Zheng worked with Yang Chengfu, transcribing the master's words for his final literary opus, has been acknowledged by Yang's sons, as well as other independent sources. Gu Liuxin, the president of the Shanghai Martial Arts Association, states the fact of Zheng's contribution in his introduction to Yang Zhenduo's book on Yang Style taijiquan (Yang, 1988: 8). Prefaces written by Yang Shouzhong and Zheng Manqing, as well as a discussion of Zheng's contributions to the wording and presentation of Yang Chengfu's teaching, may be read in Louis Swaim's 2005 English translation of Yang's masterwork (Yang, 1934/2005). See also (Mason, 2006) for a review of Swaim's translation. The Taiwan edition of Yang Zhengguo's book, *Yang Style Tai Chi Clearly Explained*, contains a preface by Zheng's student Xu Yizhong.

8   See Chen's 1929 work, translated into English in 1985 by Benjamin Lo and Robert W. Smith, in which Chen presents the teaching of his master, Yang Chengfu(Chen, 1929/1985: 11–12).

9   Like Chen Weiming, Zheng insisted that in real taijiquan one must not use even the slightest force; one must have utter faith in the principle of relaxing body and mind totally (Cheng and Smith, 1967: 101). Following Yang Chengfu, Chen Weiming also wrote that those who insist on using force never obtain the essence of taijiquan: "They can't believe that at the limit of suppleness lies a different quality of strength" (Chen, 1929/1985: 18). Yang Chengfu told Zheng continuously that he must relax completely, not using the slightest force to defend himself. Only by "investing in loss" in this way can one manifest Laozi's maxim that "The soft and pliable will defeat the hard and strong" (Cheng, 1985: 22, 87–88). Yang Chengfu's emphasis on softness reiterates the teaching of his own father, Yang Jianhou: "The first step in learning taijiquan martial applications is learning how to be light and agile. That means without muscular force" (Yang, 2001: 3), which in turn echoes the words of the *Taiji Classics*: "The softest will become the strongest" (Lo/Inn/Amacker/Foe, 1979: 19, 32, 37, 46, etc.).

10 In an interview (Mason, 2001) Robert W. Smith noted that, in his personal experience with taijiquan exponents, there was no one equal to Zheng. Smith hastened to add, however, that in saying this he was not maintaining that Zheng was the best in China. By Zheng's own admission, others even in the Yang

Chengfu circle such as Li Yaxuan and Zhang Qinlin were superior to him in tuishou (Mason, 2001, Vol. 10, No. 1: 42). For accounts of Zheng's challenge matches, see Zheng's writings, as well as articles and books by others, particularly Liang Tongcai, Robert W. Smith, and Douglas Wile. Liang Tongcai claimed to have studied with fifteen different teachers of taijiquan, including direct students of Yang Chienhou, Yang Banhou, and Yang Shaohou, yet, like Smith, Liang maintained that Zheng was the greatest master of taijiquan he had ever personally encountered. Other evidence supports the legitimacy of Zheng's skills (see Hayward, 1993: 94; Wile, 2007: 24–25; Smith, 1974/1990: 37–42, Smith, 1999: 196–197, 304; Smith, 1995, Vol. 4, No. 3, etc.).

[11] Zheng discusses his reasons for abbreviating the Yang family form in his essay entitled "Taijiquan and Physical Education" in the section "In Martial Arts Seek Quality Not Quantity" (Wile, 2007: 103–104, see also p. 80) and also in his 1965 work (Cheng, 1965/1999: 9). Zheng's use of the number thirty-seven is noteworthy and not without precedent. Chen Weiming, in his 1929 text, selected photos of a number of important postures for practice, citing as precedent that "Long ago [Xu Xianbing] taught an exercise of thirty-seven-postures, discrete and unconnected" (Chen, 1929/1985: 12). Yang Banhou refers to the thirty-seven postures of Yang Style taijiquan in his song "Nine Key Secrets of Taijiquan" (Yang, 2001: 7). [Xu Longhou] offers one theory of taiji's origin in which there was a hermit named [Xu Xuanbing] who lived in Anhuei Province during the Tang dynasty and created a style of taijiquan named Thirty-Seven, after the movements of his form (see Smith, 1974/1990: 115; and Jou, 1981/1991: 8–9). Although Zheng does not explain the significance of the number, one may assume it is noteworthy, as varied listings of postures appear in the books authored by Zheng, yet the total number always works out to thirty-seven (see the translator's introduction, Cheng, 1965/1999: x).

[12] See Davis and Mann's (1996) informative interview with Benjamin Lo, Professor Zheng's first student in Taiwan and standard-bearer in the United States.

[13] The name *Shizhong* (*Shih Chung*, as it was first Romanized in Taibei, or *Shr Jung* as it was later transliterated by the American branch in New York City) refers to the ideas of correct timing and balance and resonates with literary allusions to the *Doctrine of the Mean* and other classics of traditional Chinese literature and philosophy, with which Zheng was well versed.

[14] See Robert W. Smith's classic text (1974/1990), and the follow-up memoir (1999), for details on that pioneering martial historian's adventures in Taiwan. See also Mason (2001) for an extensive interview with Smith.

[15] For details see translator Tam Gibbs's "Brief Biography of Professor M.C. Cheng" in the Professor's commentary on Laozi (Cheng, 1971/1981: 239).

[16] According to an internet announcement circulated by Bill Law of the Melbourne Cheng Zi Taichi Chuan Study Association (2/15/02), Ju Hongbin, who teaches extensively in southern Taiwan as well as at the Taibei Shizhong, dedicated a separate memorial hall to the memory of Zheng in Gaoxiong on September 23,

2001. The flat is located at 2/F, 255 Ming Hua Rd., in the Gu Shan District of Gaoxiong.

[17] In 1982 the National Palace Museum, in cooperation with Madame Zheng, put on a special retrospective exhibit of more than two dozen of Professor Zheng's paintings and calligraphic works. This was an outstanding honor, as the museum rarely featured the work of modern artists. A catalogue of prints was published along with a preface previously written by Madame Chiang Kai-shek, who had been a painting student of Professor Zheng (Davis, 1996: 48).

[18] For more information see "Interview with Grand Master Hsu Yee Chung," edited by Massimiliano Biondi and published on the Study Society webpage at: www.37taichi.org.tw

[19] More details of the opening ceremony may be found in the *Zheng Manqing Memorial Hall Donors' Record* booklet, published by the association in 2007.

Bibliography

Barnstone T., and Chou, P. (1996). *The art of writing: Teachings of the Chinese masters*. Boston: Shambhala.

Biondi, M. (2006). Interview with grand master Hsu Yee Chung. Published on the Shizhong Study Society webpage at www.37taichi.org.tw

Chen, W. (1929/1985). *T'ai chi ch'uan ta wen: Questions and answers on t'ai chi ch'uan* (B. Lo, and R. Smith, Trans.). Berkeley, CA: North Atlantic Books.

Cheng, M. (1962). *T'ai chi ch'uan: A simplified method of calisthenics for health and self-defense*. Taibei: Shizhong Taijiquan Center.

Cheng, M. (1965/1999). *Master Cheng's new method of tai chi ch'uan self-cultivation* (M. Hennessy, Trans.). Berkeley, CA: Frog, Ltd.

Cheng, M., and Smith, R. (1967/2004). *T'ai chi*. Rutland, VT: Charles E. Tuttle. Cheng, M. (1971/1981). *Lao-tzu: My words are very easy to understand* (T. Gibbs, Trans.). Berkeley, CA: North Atlantic Books.

Cheng, M. (1985). *Cheng Tzu's thirteen treatises on t'ai chi ch'uan* (B. Lo and M. Inn, Trans.). Richmond, CA: North Atlantic Books.

Cheng, M. (1996). T'ai chi ch'uan: A simplified method of calisthenics for health and self-defense. [Video]. Ashville, NC: Cho San. 1

Chengtzu Tai-Chi Chuan Research Association, (2007). Cheng Man-ch'ing Ji Nien Guan donors' record. Taibei, Taiwan.

Davis, B. (1996). In search of a unified Dao: Zheng Manqing's life and contributions to taijiquan. *Journal of Asian Martial Arts*, 5(2), 36–59.

Davis, D., and Mann, L. (1996). Conservator of the Taiji classics: An interview with Benjamin Pang Jeng Lo. *Journal of Asian Martial Arts*, 5(4), 46–67.

Fairchild, J., and Lin, G. (2007). The beginnings, growth, and development of taijiquan in Taiwan: An interview with Chairman Wang Yennien. Taibei, Taiwan: Yennien Shanghao, published on the Yennien Daoguan website.

Hayward, R. (1993). *T'ai-chi ch'uan: Lessons with master T. T. Liang*. St. Paul, MN: Shukuang Press.

Jou, T. (1981/1991). *The Tao of tai-chi chuan: Way to rejuvenation*. Warwick, NY: Tai Chi Foundation.

Lo, B., Inn, M., Amacker, R., and Foe, S. (1979). *The essence of t'ai chi ch'uan: The literary tradition*. Richmond, CA: North Atlantic Books.

Mason, R. (2001). Fifty years in the fighting arts: An interview with Robert W. Smith. *Journal of Asian Martial Arts, 10*(1), 36–73.

Mason, R. (2006). Review of the book Yang Chengfu: The essence and applications of taijiquan. *Journal of Asian Martial Arts, 15*(3), 92–93.

Smith, R. (1974/1990). *Chinese boxing: Masters and methods*. Berkeley, CA: North Atlantic Books.

Smith, R. (1975). A master passes: A tribute to Cheng Man-ch'ing. *Shr Jung newsletter, 1*(1), 2–7.

Smith, R. (1995). Remembering Zheng Manqing: Some sketches from his life. *Journal of Asian Martial Arts, 4*(3), 46–59.

Smith, R. (1999). *Martial musings: A portrayal of martial arts in the 20th century*. Erie, PA: Via Media.

Wile, D. (1985). *Cheng Man-Ch'ing's advanced t'ai-chi form instructions*. Brooklyn, NY: Sweet Ch'i Press.

Wile, D. (2007). *Zheng Manqing's uncollected writings on taijiquan, qigong, and health, with new biographical notes*. Milwaukee, WI: Sweet Ch'i Press.

Yang, C. (1934/2005). *Yang Chengfu: The essence and applications of taijiquan* (L. Swaim, Trans.). Berkeley, CA: North Atlantic Books.

Yang, J. (2001). *Tai chi secrets of the Yang style*. Boston, MA: YMAA Publication Center. Yang, Z. (1988). *Yang style taijiquan*. Hong Kong: Hai Feng Publishing Co. and Beijing, China: Morning Glory Press.

Yang, Z. (1993). *Yang Cheng Fu shi tai ji quan*. Guangxi Province, China: Guangxi Minzu.

Yu, W., and Sharp, G. (1993). Fu Zhongwen: A Yang family legend. *Inside kung-fu*, April 1993, 44–46.

A Comprehensive Introduction to Sun Family Taiji Boxing Theory and Applications
by Jake Burroughs, B.A.

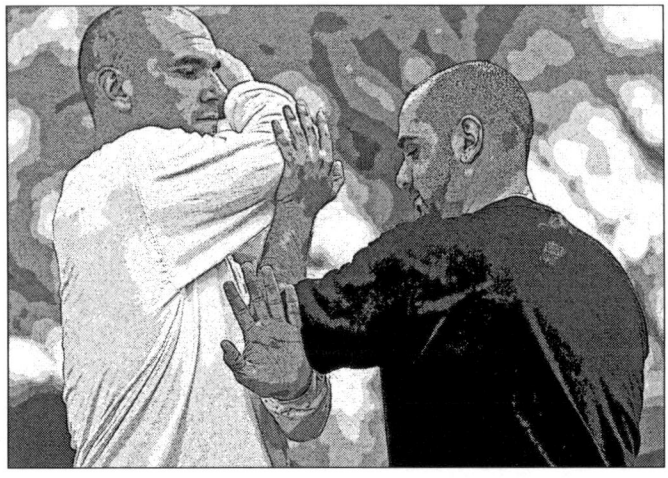

All photographs by Dana Benjamin. www.dkbimages.com

Introduction

Sun family taiji boxing is the most recently developed system of traditional taiji practiced today. Created by the legendary boxer Sun Lutang (1861–1933) during the golden years of Chinese pugilism, this martial art represents the culmination of over fifty years of martial experience compressed into one art form. According to his daughter, Sun Jianyun (1913–2003), of all his accomplishments Master Sun considered his taiji to be his "crowning achievement" within his lifetime—considering all of his accolades this is quite a statement to make. The following pages present the influential historical setting in which Sun Lutang developed his unique style and detail the fundamental principles upon which it was based.

Historical Setting

Sun Lutang was born in 1861 near Baoding in Hebei Province. His birth name was Sun Fuquan, and later in his life he took the name Han Zhai. Lutang was a name given to him by his bagua teacher Cheng Tinghua (1848–1900) in Sun's early 20's. Sun Lutang was a sick, weak child. Being born into a family of poverty it was common to see Sun on the streets begging for money. Eventually Sun discovered the arts of bajiquan and Shaolinquan, quickly progressing in these arts due to rigid practice sessions and hard work. As time progressed Sun dedicated himself to the arts of xingyiquan and baguazhang with the most combat-oriented teachers available. Guo Yunshen (1822–1898) and Li Kuiyuan taught him xingyi, while Cheng

Tinghua tutored Sun in bagua. It did not take Sun long to master these arts, and eventually his reputation as a fighter spread throughout Asia. Even though Sun Lutang was small in size, he accepted any and all challenges, earning victories over *shuai chiao* (Chinese wrestling) players, as well as judo players from Japan.

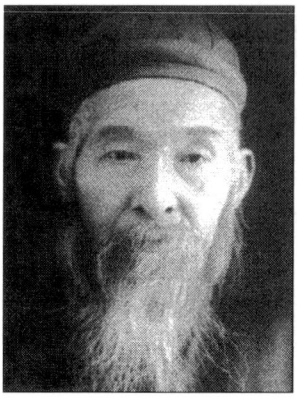

Sun Lutang (1861–1933).

It is beyond the scope of this chapter to delve into all the details of Sun's extensive martial history. Suffice it to say that throughout the years Sun Lutang trained hundreds of fighters in xingyi and bagua, and also worked as a bodyguard where he acquired invaluable real world, hand-to-hand combat experience. Via these encounters, Sun refined his boxing and grappling skills, being meticulous in his notetaking and study of combat theory and application. He honed his own techniques accordingly with scrupulous detail to ensure he did not alter the principles of the traditional arts yet made sure that the techniques he taught (as well as practiced) were efficient, accurate, and applicable. For a more detailed account of Sun Lutang's life history please refer to Tim Cartmell's translation of Sun's *A Study of Taijiquan* (2003, North Atlantic Books).

While visiting Beijing in the summer of 1914, the famous taiji teacher Hao Weizhen (1842–1920) fell ill. Sun invited Hao to stay with him so that he could help the teacher recover his health. Many people believe that Sun healed Hao, but Sun actually just took care of him—bringing the doctor to the house to treat him, running to fill herbal prescriptions, helping to feed Hao, etc.

When Hao recuperated, he taught Sun the Wu Yuxiang (1812–1880) taijiquan system as a token of gratitude. Already an accomplished master in his own right, Sun must have seen great benefit in learning this system—he immersed himself in practice day and night. After several years of intensive study, Sun decided to create his own system of taiji. He removed techniques he felt were useless and repetitive, and included many characteristics of bagua and xingyi that he had mastered over decades of practice. Sun Jianyun explained, "Sun Taiji has baguazhang's stepping method, xingyiquan's leg and waist methods, and taijiquan's body softness" (Cartmel, personal communication).

> "Sun's taijiquan emphasizes the importance of skill, sensitivity, and technique over the developmentof exceptional strength or speed."
> – Tim Cartmell, personal communication

Foundational Training

Sun Taiji follows the same sequence of movements in its form as the other taiji systems, and shares the major principles, such as Taiji's thirteen postures. Yet Sun Taiji is distinctive in that the practice of the form duplicates exactly how the techniques are applied in combat. Other styles of taiji tend to divide their study into form practice, then separate drills to develop applied martial theory and applications, whereas Sun Taiji combines all these aspects into one comprehensive martial system. Hence there is only one traditional form that is under eight minutes long when practiced in full. Though push hands (*tui shou*) is practiced within the Sun Taiji system, more emphasis is put on the actual application of force and technique with uncooperative partners, such as sparring and/or grappling drills. One must remember that push hands was originally much more combative in nature than what is commonly seen in today's martial society. Various levels would be taught from basic attempts to disrupt an opponent's balance, to all out wrestling incorporating joint immobilizations and strikes. Today some of these aspects are absent from taiji groups in an attempt to make push hands 'safer.' Unfortunately, many of these teachers are missing the core ideas being taught in push hands type training.

All too often students become overwhelmed and confused with extensive curriculums. This is where Sun's genius comes into play: he developed the form to replicate fighting as much as one can for solo form practice. One example can be found within the footwork.

Sun Taiji employs the follow-up step from xingyi (the same footwork can be found in fencing, western boxing, and folk wrestling), which immediately trains whole body power. The upright stance (fighting posture), coupled with the rhythm of one foot advancing followed by the rear foot, and back again is unique to the Sun Taiji system, as other systems of thought emphasize low postures to build strength and flexibility. The use of whole-body power is integral to any combat-oriented system, for if a practitioner weighs 180 pounds it is far more advantageous to use the full 180 pounds of mass, coupled with the velocity of the technique, than just to use the strength of an isolated appendage. This unification of body and technique is the epitome of force equals mass, times acceleration (F=MA), and is a vital trademark of Sun Taiji.

As stated earlier, Sun incorporated the circular footwork of bagua into his system of taiji. This afforded the practitioner circular mobility in technique, coupled with the linear footwork borrowed from xingyi. Bagua's stepping theory stresses constant changing, always trying to get to the opponent's back or side (the safest place to be in a fight where one's opponent cannot strike them), staying tight to the body and disrupting the opponent's center of balance. Once the opponent's center has been compromised, a throw, strike, joint manipulation, or kick can be applied. The bagua influence is most evident in the taiji technique of Repulse Monkey, which is akin to the single palm change.

Though these aspects of xingyi and bagua were incorporated into Sun Taiji, Sun Lutang maintained the taiji framework and principles as taught to him by Hao Weizhen. Redirection of force, sticking, and manipulating weak angles are all characteristics of taijiquan. Beyond the solo form and sparring/grappling practice, the curriculum also covered taiji's thirteen postures. These are not solo movements per se, but rather principles found throughout the form used to apply force in combat regardless of whether one is striking, or grappling (kicks and knees are included in striking, as joint manipulation is included into grappling in this instance). Broken down into the eight energies of force, the first four being the most prevalent, and then the five stepping methods, I offer a brief explanation for each as follows:

FOUR DIRECTIONS (*si zheng*)

1. Ward off (*peng*): this represents any kind of rising energy generated by the body. Supported from below or to lift upward much like the hull of a boat supports the weight of the cargo when in water.
2. Rollback (*lu*): redirecting energy in a wedge-like manner, bringing force around the body, and maintaining central equilibrium (*zhong ding*) by turning around the center of the body.
3. Press (*ji*): applied straight into the opponent's body with a squeezing type of force that is sudden, not maintained. One analogy Tim Cartmell uses is like throwing a pebble onto the head of a drum.
4. Push or Press Downward (*an*): force applied in a downward trajectory generated by the whole body, not just the arms.

FOUR CORNERS (*si au*)

1. Pluck (*cai*): Much like when one tries to pick an apple from the tree: if one simply pulls on it, the stem does not break free. But once the slack is taken out of the pliable branch, all one needs to do is give it a quick jerk and the stem snaps off.
2. Split (*lie*): Where the upper body goes one direction, and the lower body is led in the opposite direction. One visualization is the mechanics of a dead bolt lock where the one set of gears moves in one direction, while the other set is moved in the opposite direction.
3. Elbow (*zhou*): This concept is conveyed by using the elbow in any way possible from a strike, to coupling it with a throw or takedown. No one specific technique is localized; this is a general theory of applying the elbow.
4. Lean (*kao*): can be applied with any part of the body other than the arms or legs. Essentially to lean on, or into an opponent with one's own body. Think of it as a body stroke.

FIVE STEPPING METHODS (*wu ba fa*)
1. Forward Advance (*qian jin*): simply means to step forward.
2. Backward Retreat (*hou tui*): means just what the name implies, to step backwards.
3. Look Left (*zuo gu*): simply means to move to the left.
4. Gaze Right (*you pan*): to shift to the right.
5. Central Equilibrium (*zhong ding*): where one has one's weight/balance (equilibrium) centered evenly, where one is most stable.

Another unique facet of Sun Taiji is the *kai-he* movement found at the closing of each section within the form. Throughout the form there is a series of movements where the practitioner aligns the body, and "opens and closes" (*kai-he*) the shoulder girdle. One example of Sun's genius was that he knew people practicing a long form could not maintain proper structural integrity throughout, so he added these checkpoints to assist in proper structure to act as a reminder. Structure is key to martial usage, not to mention general overall health maintenance throughout daily life. In the martial sense if one does not have structure, then one cannot absorb, nor issue force efficiently. Keep in mind it is no different than building a house; no matter how well-built the frame is, without a solid foundation the frame will crumble to the earth.

Stillness in Motion

One of the first things a practitioner learns in the study of Sun Taiji is the *wuji* (carefree) posture. When practicing the form, the student starts in *wuji*, and ends in *wuji*. Wuji is not a static pose, but rather a set of alignments used to ensure proper physical structure is attained and maintained. Some points of reference in regard to wuji:

CAREFREE POSTURE (*wuji zhuang*)
- Head is suspended from the crown as if being extended by a balloon attached to a string connected to the crown. This draws in the chin, preventing the chin from protruding, as well as properly extending the cervical vertebrae. Some of the classics refer to this alignment as "tucking the ears."
- Shoulders are rounded and relaxed, ensuring the chest does not stick out, nor does it slouch. The shoulder blades should feel as if they are going to slough off the back.
- Sternum is kept up as if a hook is underneath it, gently pulling up.
- Pelvic girdle has a quality of floating in a fishbowl. This means that the pelvis should not be tucked, nor should the butt be sticking out. There should be no left or right flexion, either. Relaxed and ready to move in any direction.
- Knees are slightly bent and tracking the toes, which means wherever the

toes point, the knees should be pointing in the exact same direction. Otherwise, a sheering force is put on the knee and can do quite a bit of damage to the soft tissue supporting the knee.
- Feet are flat on the ground, weight evenly distributed with a slight shift towards the balls of the feet.
- Arms are relaxed at the sides with the hands open and slightly curved as if palming a basketball.

The open/closing action done at the close of each section within the form is essentially a wuji checkpoint that allows the practitioner to check the posture without interrupting the flow of practice. The only physical difference is with open/closing the arms are maintained in front of the body as if holding a ball at chest height, instead of the arms at the sides as in the posture of *wuji*.

According to Sun Jianyun, her father had the students stand in the three powers posture (*santi shi*) more so than *wuji*. Santi is from the xingyi boxing school and is basically a more combative version of *wuji*. In the *santi* posture, the student stands in more of a combat posture with a lead arm and leg, maintaining the same pointers found above with *wuji*, but with more of a martial intent and focus. The goal with santi training is to relax in a combative posture, engaging only the skeletal muscles to stand in the proper posture. The characteristics practiced in *santi* are found throughout the Sun Taiji form: again, posture and structure being key to the proper usage of combat-oriented martial arts—not to mention all the positive health benefits gained from proper posture throughout daily living!

Other than *wuji* and *santi*, there are not many basics in Sun Taiji. Again, everything the student needs is found within the framework of the form and the practice of applications that are extrapolated from the movements of the form. Sun Lutang had a wonderful reputation throughout China so most of the very experienced, knowledgeable martial artists that trained under Sun were already quite well-versed in the basics of martial combat from their previous training.

Taiji as Combative Art

The structure and flow of the form also attests to Sun's intelligent design. The techniques that one would most often use in combat were repeated throughout the entire form, for example too lazy to tie coat, hands strum the pipa, single whip, repulse monkey, and brush knee twist step. Brush knee twist step, and single whip alone were the initial movements in every section of the form! The easier techniques were also usually practiced towards the beginning of the form, with the more challenging maneuvers reserved for the final couple of sections.

This is a prime example why many traditionalists take exception to modern wushu variations on forms, because techniques are in a certain order, placed carefully within the form that act as keys integral to unlocking the usage of the movement. For instance, certain footwork patterns in the solo form are indicators as to how one should apply a kick in combat. If the player does not step to this specific angle, the kick is rendered useless.

All systems of taiji are combative in nature, training to issue maximum force while using minimal effort, and as much as 80% of the techniques practiced are grappling (or counter-grappling) in nature. Sun Lutang fought many high-level grappling experts in his time (Sun's birthplace, Baoding, was famous for its wrestlers), so by the time he developed Sun Taiji he was well versed in grappling and counter-grappling techniques and the theory on which they are based. As it is today, it was 120 years ago when two combatants engaging in hand-to-hand combat used strikes to close the distance and encounter their opponent. Once contact was made (usually in what is now called the "clinch range") the most proficient fighters used their grappling skills to throw, sweep, or takedown their opponent. This strategy afforded several benefits for the fighter as any kind of throw is extremely destructive in nature. By utilizing proper technique and leverage, a smaller, weaker fighter can have an advantage over a larger, stronger opponent. This may not be the case if he chooses to stand and trade blows with his opponent, since the larger, stronger fighter will more likely prevail. That is simple physics. Also keep in mind that at the time, the majority of average civilians in China were laborers who relied on their hands to earn money. A broken hand or foot caused by a fight (or practice for that matter) rendered a person not only injured, but also took him out of work for a period.

Throws and the variations such as sweeps, takedowns, and joint manipulation techniques were preferred because they could be practiced without having to "pull" one's technique (as in the case with strikes), and in actual combat a throw on the hard ground can decisively end a confrontation. It should come as no surprise to the taiji student, or any martial artist for that matter, that the majority of techniques in Sun Taiji are grappling-based. This is human nature.

One needs to look no further than to watch two untrained people fight. Inevitably one will initiate contact with strikes, while the other will try to protect himself by bringing his arms up to cover his head and face, while simultaneously trying to grab and hold his opponent in an effort to control the strikes that are overwhelming him. Once this is accomplished, the opponents are in the "clinch" range. Strikes are limited within the clinch so grappling takes precedence as one closes with the opponent, enabling one to join mutual centers of gravity. Once one has joined these centers of gravity, it becomes much easier to manipulate the opponent's "dead angle" (the angle representing the weakest directions in which a person can be put off-balance). In combat we are constantly trying to control our opponent's dead angle, while concurrently attempting to hide our own.

Sun Lutang realized that the nature of true combat fell within these parameters and was mindful of including close quarter combat theory and application into his system of taiji. This was already second nature to him as his xingyi training included many *kao die* (literally "knock downs") type takedowns which are quick and percussive. Also, he learned bagua from Cheng Tinghua, whose foundation was in shuai chiao (Chinese wrestling/grappling), and who was considered one of the best wrestlers of his era. This is not to say striking and kicking are not practiced in the art, as they certainly are very well represented; however, I simply wish to shed some light on the role of grappling in traditional Chinese martial arts.

TECHNICAL SECTION
Rollback / Elbow Strike

1a)   White sets up his attack with a quick back-fist type strike (it is the intention to get the opponent to react, hence the big movement of the back-fist), which of course black blocks.

1b-c) White uses his left hand to parry black's block, while simultaneously stepping through with his left foot. White has his hand "hooked" onto black's elbow crease so that when black pushes back against white's pressure, it assists white in executing the upward elbow (*zhou*). Usually this elbow lands because of the speed and aggressiveness of the technique, but for argument's sake black deflects the incoming elbow.

1d)   Again using the pressure from black's defense, white applies rollback by bringing black's arm across his body. It may be necessary to shift or lean slightly back while parrying the opponent's arm. That is fine as long as one's structure is not compromised.

1e)   White finishes with a simple projection, but really any number of techniques can be applied here.

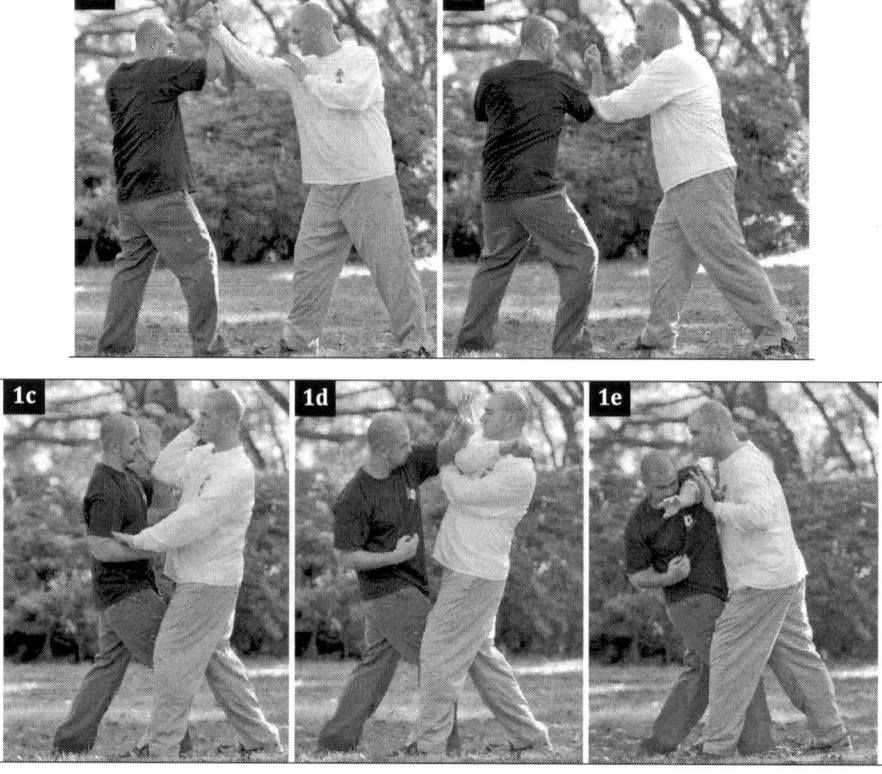

Reverse Angle of Elbow Strike – Rollback

2a-d) Close up and reverse angle to previous technique.

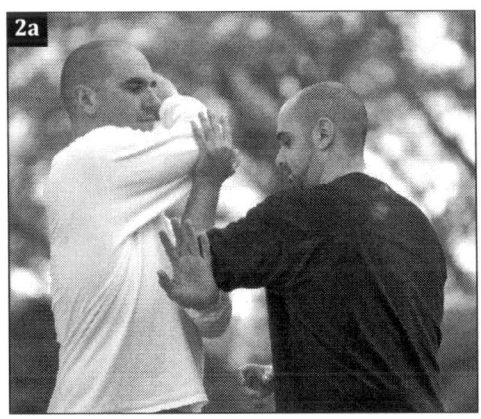

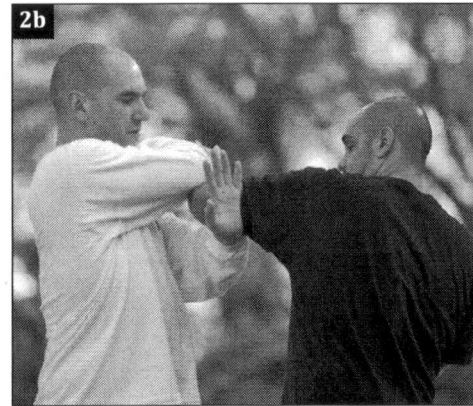

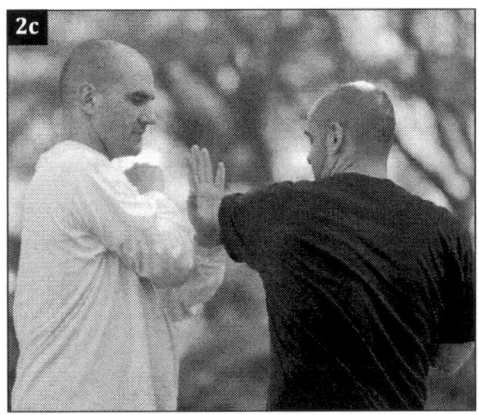

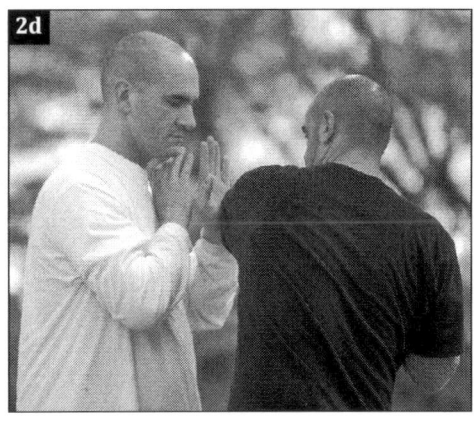

Joint Manipulation

3a) Here is a joint manipulation application utilizing the splitting principle (*lie*). Tim (black) and Jake (white) are jockeying for position in grappling range. Neither has a better position yet notice how black's right arm is on the inside gate of white's left arm.

3b) Black obtains wrist control with his left hand and sets up the arm drag with his right hand. Notice black reaching high (superior) on white's tricep for the arm drag.

3c) Black switches his grip by sliding along white's arm. As black brings white's arm across his body (to black's right), black's right hand slips down to obtain wrist control, while his left hand slides up just superior to the elbow joint. This is obviously done quickly and decisively, but arm drags are deceiving to their victims in that by the time one notices their position has been compromised—it is too late.

3d) Black maneuvers under white's arm, extending it, applying pressure at the fulcrum, which is white's elbow, using white's arm as a lever. Notice how black has also twisted white's arm to black's right. This rotation tightens the joint lock by taking all the slack out of the arm.

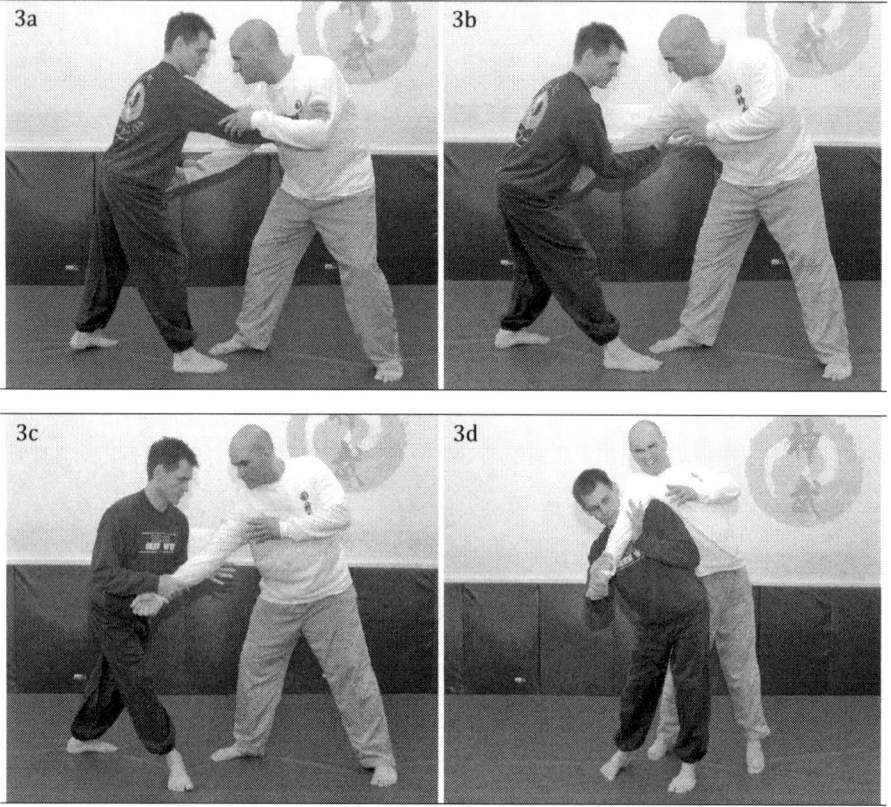

Single Whip

4a-b) White attacks black from behind and puts him in an over-arm bear hug. Black lowers his center of gravity.

4c) Black lifts on the elbows by using his legs, not the strength of his arms.

4d-e) Black steps behind white with his left leg. It is key to keep close contact with the opponent here. This is where black joins centers. Without doing so, black would not be able to disrupt a bigger, stronger opponent's structure. To finish the takedown, black simply turns to his left and white falls from the pressure of black's turn, coupled with the fact that white's mobility is compromised because black has stepped behind him.

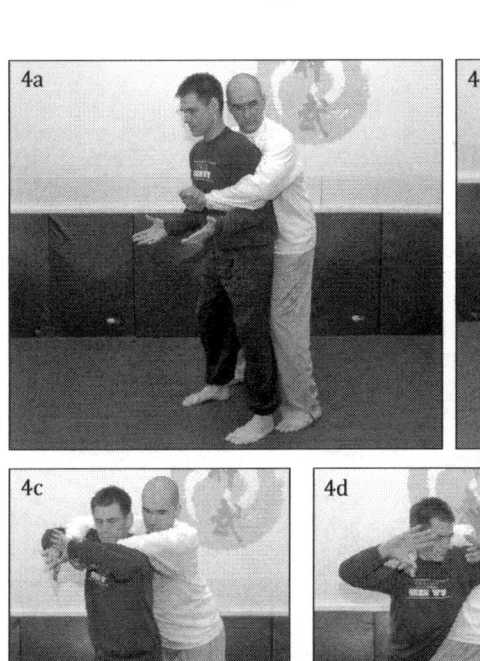
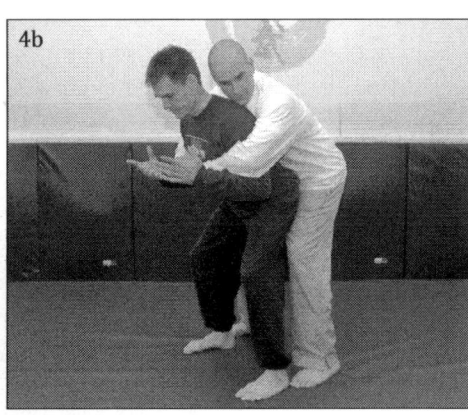
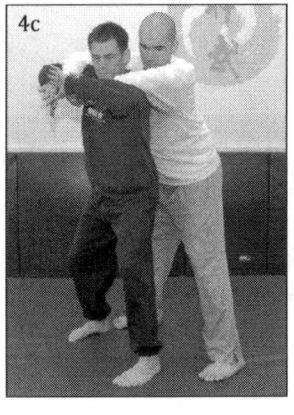
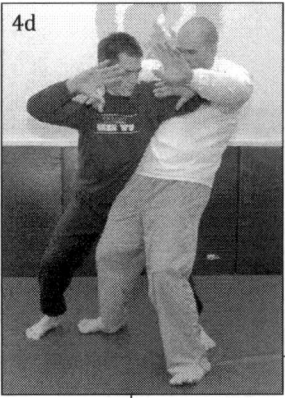

Fist Under Elbow

5a) Black offers a right lead jab, which white slips (*zuo gu*, or "look left").

5b) White strikes low with a straight punch to black's ribs ("fist under elbow").

5c) Black drops his right elbow to block, or possibly as a reaction to white's strike.

5d) White steps behind black, taking his left hand and draping it (thumb down) onto black's eyebrow ridge. Again, notice the proximity of the bodies, joining centers once again.

5e) White simply turns his body to the left using a classic "eyebrow mop" type technique as a follow-up. White has superior leverage the closer to the top of black's head he gets, again blocking black from stepping out by using white's left leg. It is very important to use a spiral type of action with the "eyebrow mop" takedown, not just turning in a circle.

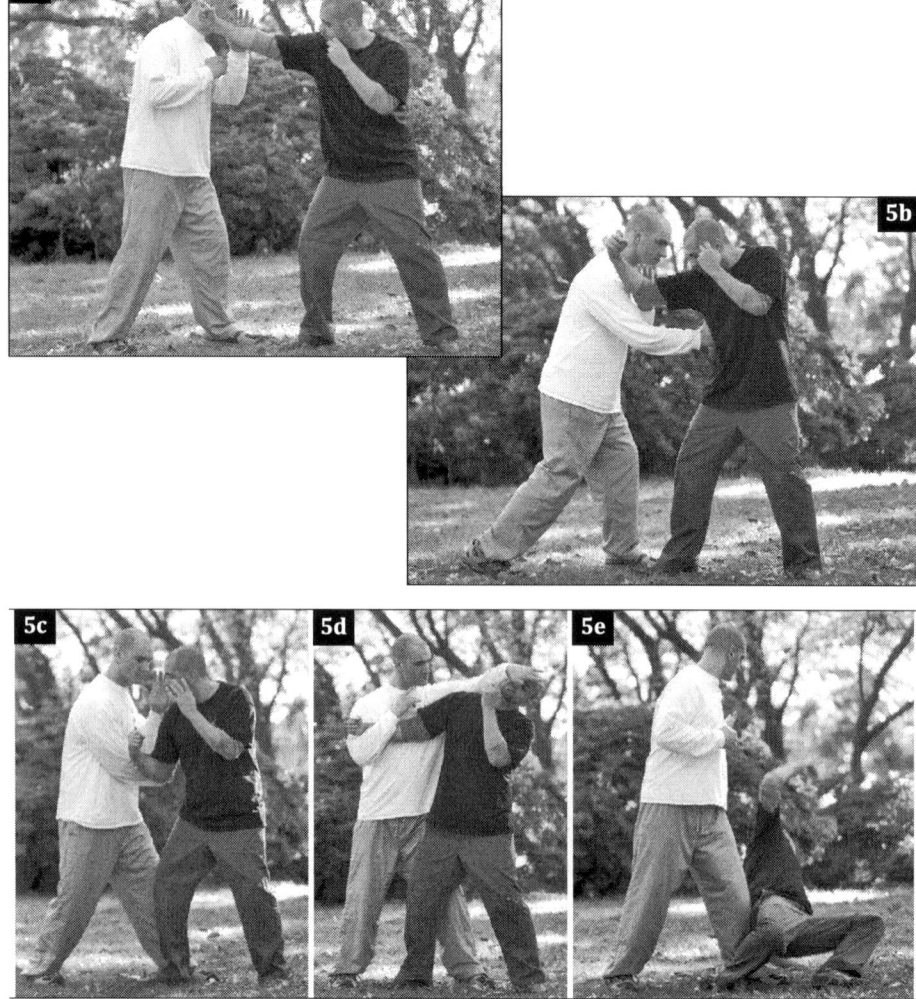

Open and Closed Fighting Postures

6a) The ending postures for each section of the routine, as divided by Tim Cartmell; open-close (*kai-he*) is used to realign and reposition the student ensuring the chest is up, head suspended, shoulder blades relaxed, elbows in and down, hands up, all the attributes of *wuji* stance but with the hands held in a fighting position.

6b) *Kai-he* is the standard fighting position: hands up protecting the head, elbows down and in protecting the body, eyes forward, weight distributed 50/50 on the legs, weight towards the balls of the feet, knees bent and relaxed, and intent forward.

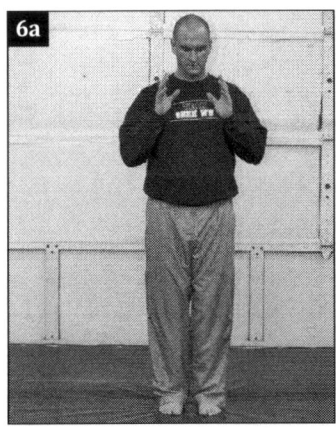
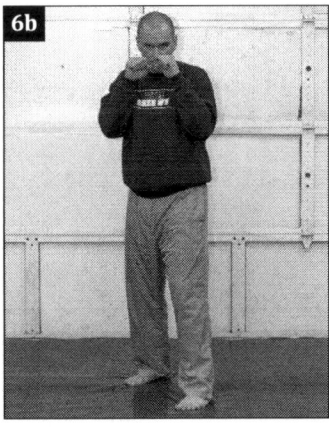

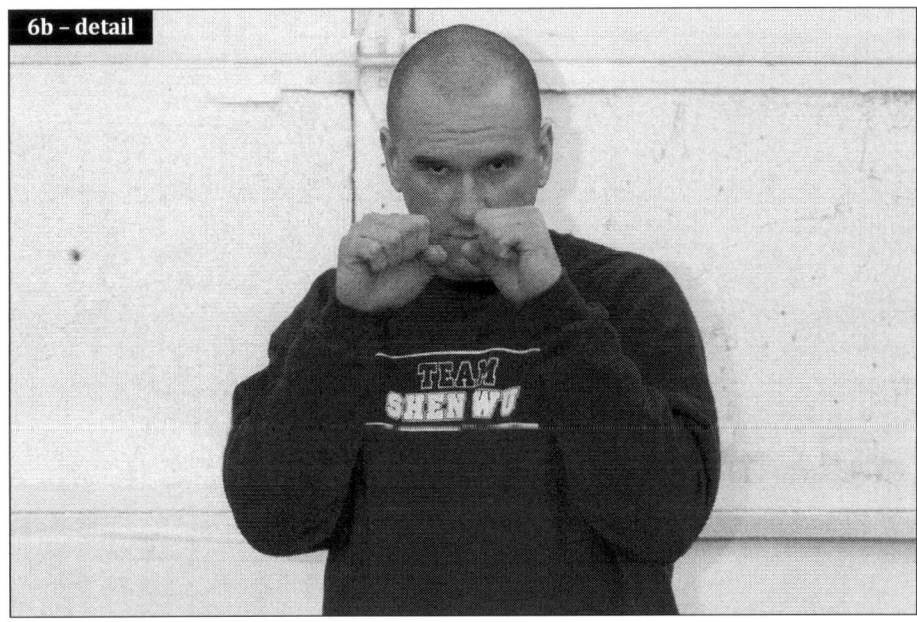

Part Wild Horse's Mane

7a)   Here black initiates a lead arm hook, which white steps off-line to avoid (you pan, or "gaze right") while simultaneously striking with a cross-palm strike.

7b)   White quickly steps in and behind black with his left leg, while keeping his left arm taut, thus disrupting black's structure. Notice there is no gap between the two bodies.

7c)   Exploiting black's dead angle, white simply shifts his weight forward to complete the takedown. It is not necessary for white to turn the body or push with the arm. Positioning the body correctly (with no gaps) joins centers with the opponent. White's leg prevents black from stepping out, and the pressure into black's dead angle is what creates the takedown.

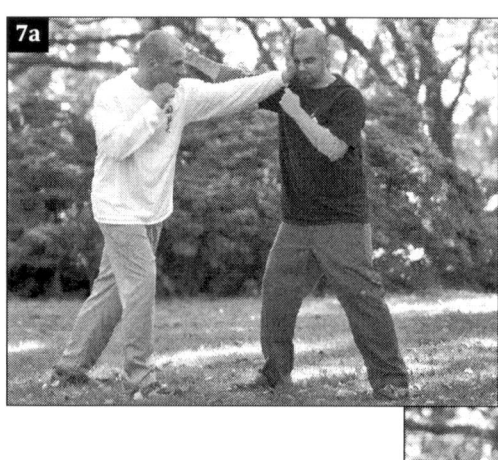

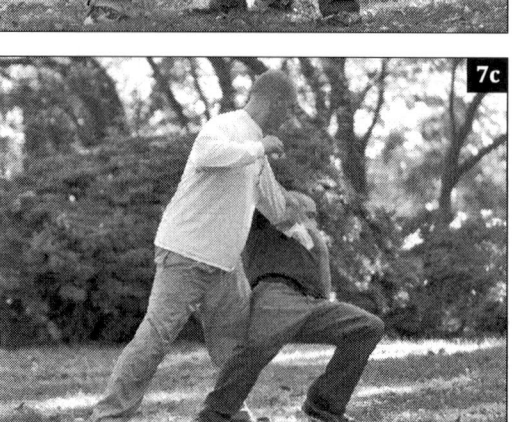

Repulse Monkey

8a-b) Black and white square-off in a right lead closed stance. White initiates with a lead arm hook which black covers, and counters with a lead arm palm strike in an effort to get white to react with a block.

8c) Black quickly swings his right arm over, down, and through to obtain his right underhook. Simultaneously black's left arm clamps down over top of white's arm, and black has left arm control at the elbow, squeezing white's arm in-between his body and his left arm. Notice here how black has also toed in his right foot setting up the throw.

8d) Black turns to his left, pulling on white's right elbow, lifting with his underhook, and slipping his hip in under white's center of gravity for the hip throw.

8e) Black finishes with a devastating throw, which flows nicely into a superior position with white's arm extended, and a knee on white's ribs. Black can strike, work to submit with an arm bar, or continue the fight on the ground. Repulse monkey is repeated twice in the Sun Taiji set emphasizing the importance, and applicability of this technique. The influence of Sun's bagua is found here as repulse monkey is essentially the same movement/ technique as the single palm change in Sun bagua.

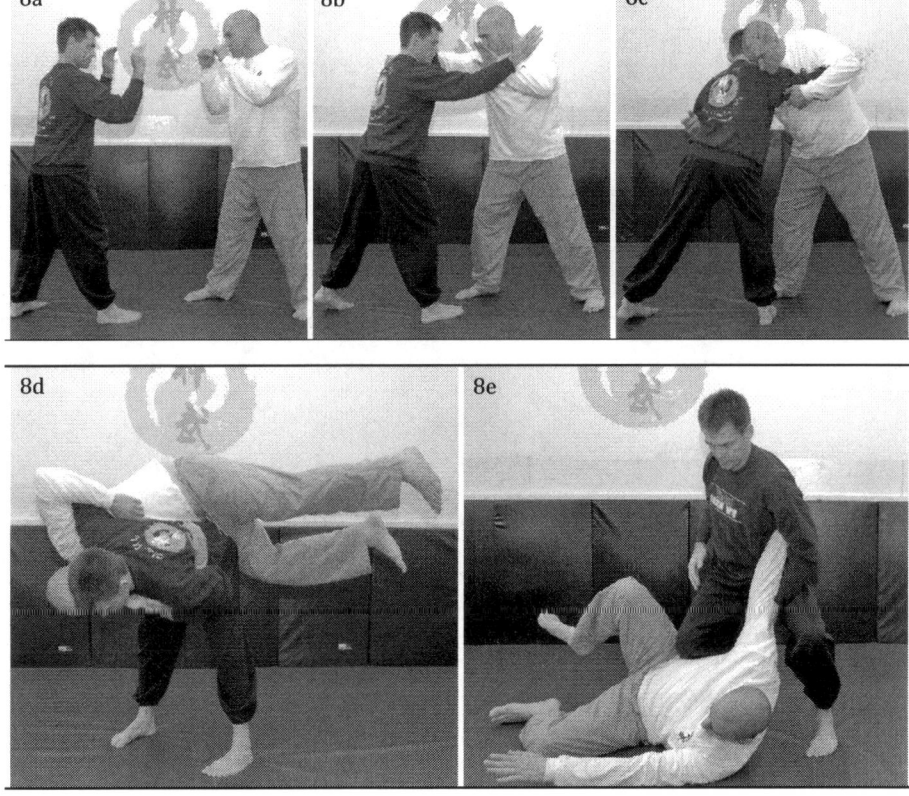

Lotus Kick

9a-b) Black and white square off in an open posture, where white throws a lead arm committed jab, which black quickly slips and parries.

9c) Black throws a left hand towards white's face to get him to react with his left hand. Since black is grabbing white's right hand it is natural instinct for white to pull back on his arm when it is grabbed.

9d) Black shoots his right hand across white's body and uses his right hip as a leverage point. By pivoting and twisting in this manner, white's structure is compromised.

9e-f) Black finishes by stepping his right leg behind white and using a combination.

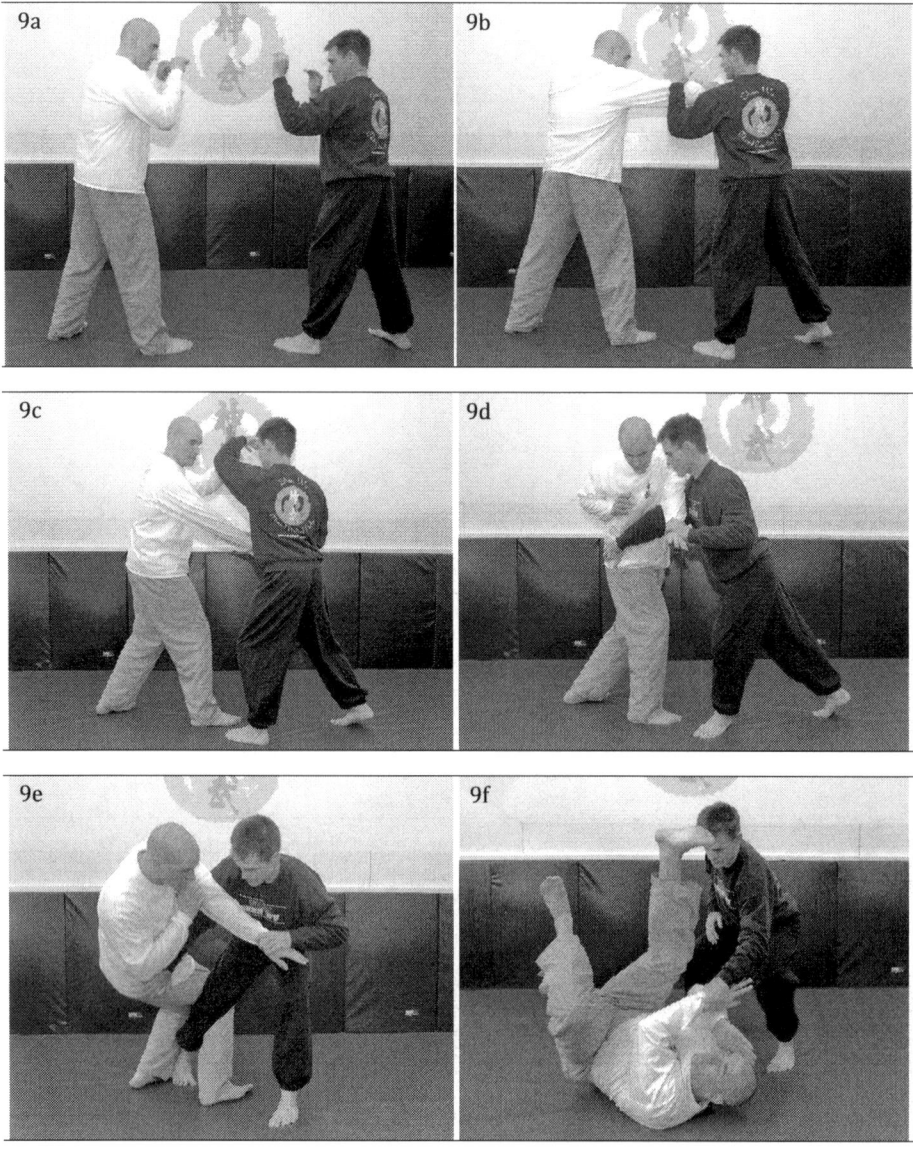

Step to the Seven Stars

10a) Step to the seven stars is an entry technique to get inside your opponent's guard. Here white simply does a basic palm strike to black's head causing him to react with a basic block.

10b) White steps forward and weaves his left hand under black's block, opening his guard.

10c) This creates an opening where white can again execute any application, but here employs an elbow technique (remember taiji is a close-quarter fighting system, so elbows, knees, and grappling are heavily emphasized).

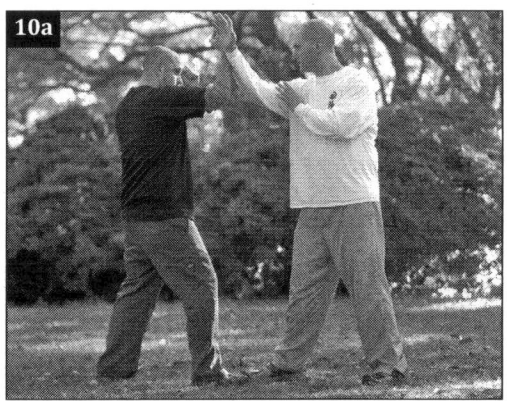

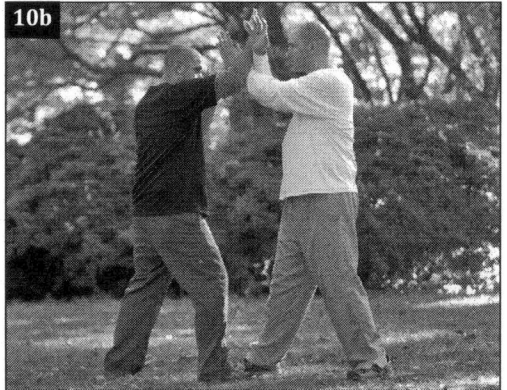

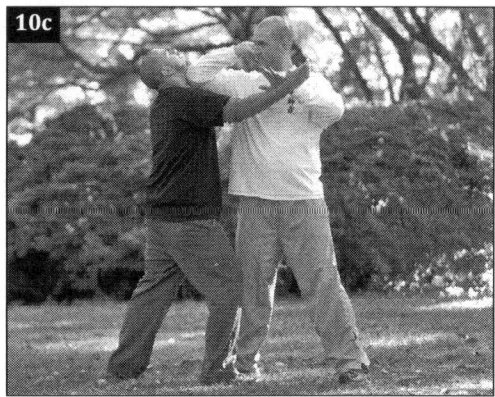

Turn the Body – Ambush the Tiger

11a) Black attacks with a lead arm palm strike, which white quickly blocks.

11b) Black checks white's block, and throw's another palm strike towards white's face causing him to block with his left arm now.

11c) Black pulls white's left arm across his body, maintaining wrist control on white's right wrist. Notice how black has toed in his right foot in preparation for the throw and has white's weight towards his heels to circumvent any counter measures.

11d) Crossing white's arm, keeping them extended, and loading him onto his back like a sack of potatoes, black now shoots in his hip getting under white's center of gravity and joins centers.

11e) To finish the throw, black loads the weight of white onto him, straightens his leg and turns his right shoulder in the direction toward his left foot. Be careful; your partner has no way of slapping out from this very large, hard throw!

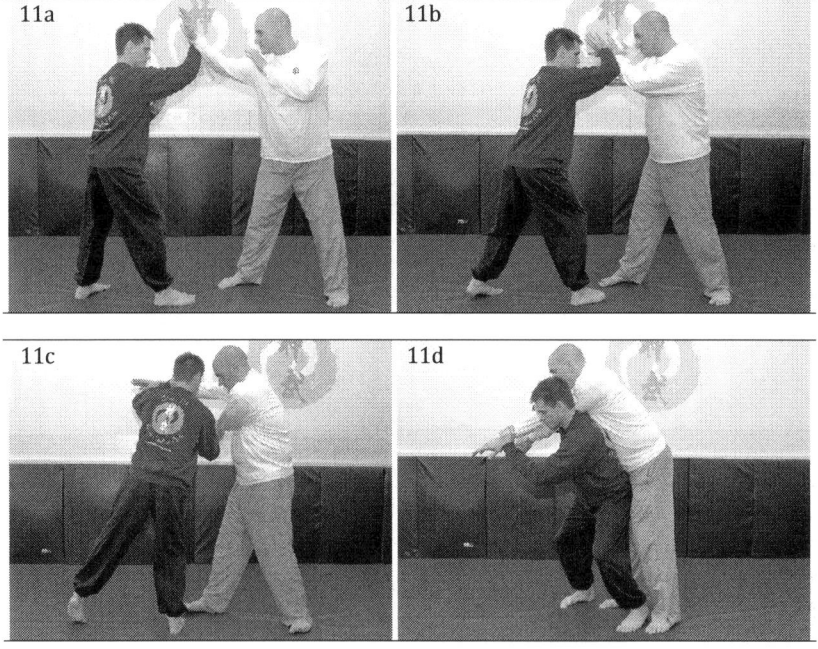

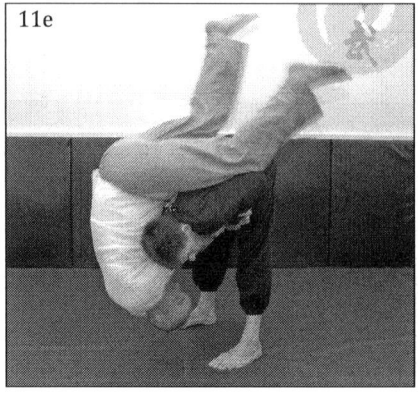

Be careful with this throw as your partner has no way of slapping out from this very large, hard throw!

Not Just for Fighters

The recent popularity of practicing taiji as a meditative, yoga-like exercise was non-existent in Sun Lutang's lifetime. That is not to say Sun Taiji cannot be practiced by those looking to reap the rewards of non-combative aspects of the art. The upright posture and high stance are ideal for those with back, knee, or hip problems. The complete form takes less than ten minutes to perform so it does not necessarily require a lot of energy, yet the faster pace in which Sun Taiji is practiced offers a light cardiovascular workout as well. The movements are simple, easy to remember, and are low impact for those with health issues or the elderly. The emphasis on correct posture, and the repeated twisting and bending of the waist is wonderful exercise for the body's core. Remember, any physical exercise will harvest positive results, and any exercise is better than none. Sun Taiji can be practiced with as little, or as much, intensity as the practitioner desires.

Sun Taiji is a complete martial system and can be adapted to almost anyone. It is a beautiful form, as well as an effective martial art. Maintaining many familiar aspects of the internal arts (*neijia*) while simultaneously creating a new approach to the study of taiji, Sun Lutang was truly ahead of his time with the creation of Sun Taijiquan. Though rare in the West, Sun Taiji is gaining in popularity as more teachers are offering lessons, seminars, and classes throughout the United States, and Europe. It is my hope that Sun Taiji is made available to more people throughout the world, as it is a wonderful martial art with bountiful health benefits.

Glossary

Baoding	保定	Santi Shi	三體式
Cheng Tinghua	程廷華	Sun Family Taijiquan	孫家太極拳
Guo Yunshen	郭雲深	Sun Fuquan	孫福全
Hao Weizhen	郝為真	Sun Jianyun	孫劍雲
he	合	Sun Lutang	孫祿堂
kai	開	Wu Yuxiang	武禹襄
Li Kuiyuan	李魁元	Wuji	無極

Acknowledgments

The author would like to thank Tim Cartmell for his diligent teachings, never ending patience, and forthright approach to the study and teaching of the Chinese martial arts. Also, thanks to Tim and Anthony Natale for assistance in the application photographs. Plus, deep gratitude to Dana Benjamin for her amazing work with photographs in all the authors works, and her support and input behind the scenes.

Xiong Style Taiji in Taiwan: Historical Development and a Photographic Exposé Featuring Master Lin Jianhong

by Michael A. DeMarco, M.A.

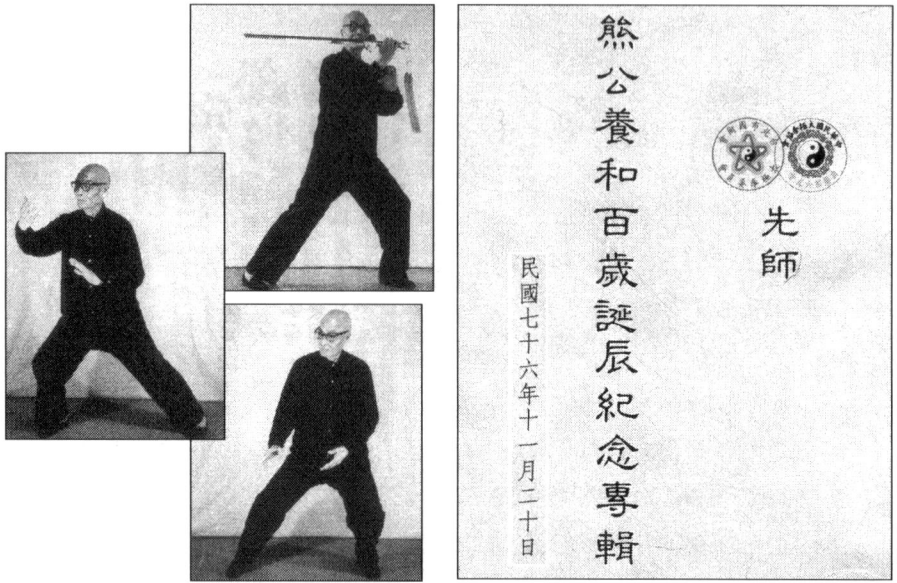

Photographs of Xiong Yanghe alongside the cover of a special commemorative edition published for his 100th birthday anniversary ("Commemorative," 1987). Photographs from the author's collection. Photographs courtesy of Robert Lin-I Yu, except where noted.

Introduction

In the thickly branched tree representing taijiquan's growth over the centuries, some branches are stronger than others, and some hold higher positions than others. This chapter introduces a relatively rare branch in the Yang Family tradition that is associated with Xiong Yanghe (1888–1981). Before delving into aspects of what is now called the Xiong Style, we must first ask ourselves what we can learn from studying the lives of main lineage representatives. How can their theories and practices of taiji influence our overall understanding of the art? Hopefully such research can offer a better historical perspective while enriching both our understanding and practice of the art.

The following text presents aspects of lineage that play a role in formulating a definition of taijiquan. Following a general overview of the early Yang Family lineage, we will look closely at the two main branches that stem directly from the Yang Style founder, Yang Luchan (1799–1872), his sons and grandsons, who were so influential in the initial growth of taiji in China. Since the focus of this chapter is on Xiong Style, it is necessary to look at Xiong's teachers and these main predecessors who formed the main trunk of the taiji evolutionary tree.

China's socio-political setting during the lives of Yang Luchan and Xiong Yanghe was rife with foreign invasions and civil strife. This difficult period—marred by the decaying decades of the last dynasty (Qing, 1644–1911) and the following decades up to the founding of the People's Republic of China in 1949—presents an overwhelming wealth of information that played into the thoughts and actions of each taiji master mentioned above. Each master has his own story to tell. This chapter is a brief synopsis of Xiong Yanghe's story, supplemented with information and photographic illustrations provided by Mr. Lin Jianhong, a leading Xiong Style instructor teaching today in Taipei, Taiwan.

The Question of Taiji Lineage

Many newcomers are thrilled to begin learning taiji. If they have a decent teacher and a growing interest in the art, they eventually delve deeper into its history, theory, and practice. However, they soon find themselves entangled in a mesh of lineage lines. Who taught whom? What are the differences between the original Chen Family Style and evolving branches? What did the main instructors actually teach versus the curricula taught by their students in following generations? In the end, what do we really learn from the academic grasp of lineages, names, dates, and a stock of stories which may be true or false?

When we approach taijiquan's history, we are usually given our initial glimpse through our first teacher. This provides an introduction to taiji. Depending on the teacher, the art may be totally focused on its health nurturing aspects suitable for aged retirees in their quest to keep fit. Some teachers focus on it as a fighting art, suitable for bodyguards, military, and police. Others can teach both aspects of the art in varied proportions.

There are other layers to consider in our desire to understand taiji. All teachers have unique qualities in their form and function: movements, stances, fighting techniques, and applied skills. It is easy to see great differences among beginning students in their awkward execution of taiji forms, but even teachers of the same lineage and generation exhibit their own individual flavors, although it may be in the most subtle ways. Of course, it is important to discern the dissimilarity in movements as either a variant application performed according to taiji principles, or an incorrect movement based on faulty understanding of application and performed contrary to the taiji principles.

Often the more we learn about taiji the more confusing it gets! There is an old tale that originated in India that may offer some help in our view of taiji lineages and practice. It is the story of six blind men who were asked to describe the nature of an elephant, with each person feeling the elephant's various body parts, such as its tusk, tail, trunk, leg, ear, or side. Of course, all their conclusions vary because of their different perspectives. The "elephant" they envisioned appeared like a spear, wall, snake, tree, fan or rope. They may endlessly argue over their viewpoints or use them to better understand what an elephant really is in its completeness.

If we really seek to know taiji thoroughly, we need to go beyond relative half-truths to get a broader perspective. A study of the leading standard-bearers of each main lineage is certainly helpful for the broad view. On a more detailed level, we can look closely at the main teachers within one specific lineage. The learning process takes many years, and we eventually see how our concept of taiji continually evolves.

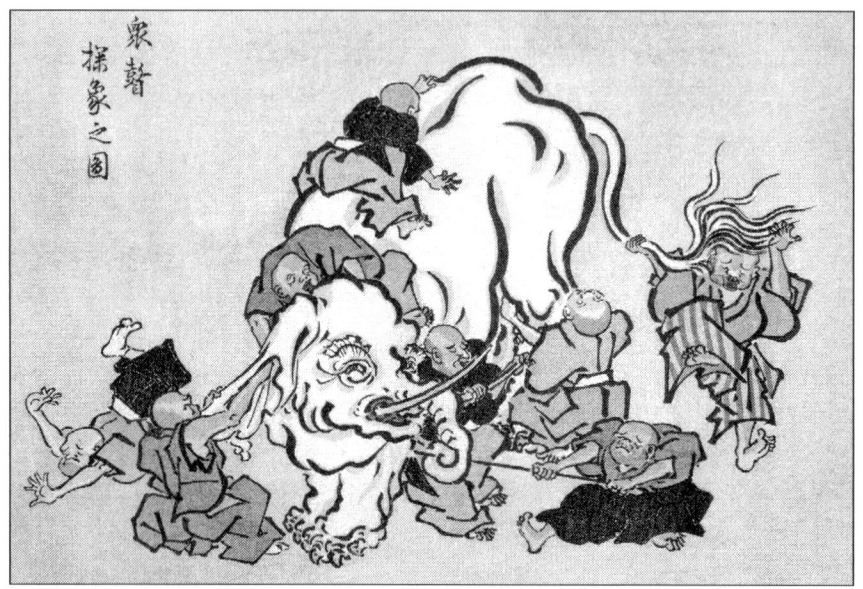

Blind Monks Examining an Elephant by Itcho Hanabusa
Japanese Ukiyo-e print illustration from Buddhist parable
showing blind monks examining an elephant. Dated 1888.
Library of Congress. Call # Illus. in H67 [Asian RR]

Early Yang Style Lineage Representatives

Yang Luchan was born in 1799 in Yongnian County, Hebei Province. Although he was a man of humble origins and illiterate, he loved martial arts. He probably studied Shaolin boxing when very young but later was drawn to the Chen Village in Henan Province with the desire to study Chen Family Taijiquan. Although there are a number of stories regarding Luchan's study in Chen Village, the most probable themes are: 1) he worked as a servant and studied Chen Taiji under Chen Changxing (1771–1853) for most likely ten years or so, becoming extraordinarily proficient in the art, 2) he returned to his home village and taught the art to many there, and 3) moved to Beijing where he gained a reputation as "Invincible Yang" and taught the Manchu royal family and bodyguards. Of course, his unique flavor of taiji became known as the Yang Style.

Whether factual or fictional, stories regarding Yang Luchan leave no doubt that he possessed fighting skills of the highest order. What he taught and to whom is another matter. It certainly would be logical for him to follow ancient precedent and teach the higher aspects of the art only to those closest to him.

When Yang Luchan died in 1872, two of his sons carried on the family's taiji tradition. Both were naturally gifted, mentally and physically, to receive full transmission of their father's knowledge, and both practiced with dedication under a demanding training regimen. The brothers came to exhibit very different personalities. Yang Banhou (1837–1890), the elder son, had a character often described as hard and fierce, which manifested in his love of sparring. The younger son, Yang Jianhou (1839–1917), was friendly and gentle, a personality which attracted a large number of students.

Although Yang Shaohou (1862–1930) was the first son of Yang Jianhou, Shaohou studied primarily with his uncle, Yang Banhou. Shaohou followed his uncle in temperament and fighting style. Both were harsh teachers and only a relatively small number of students became dedicated disciples. It seems they used the combative elements of Yang Luchan's methods as the main guideline for their own practice, which included high speed execution of techniques, jumps, and varied kicks, as well as the psychological use of expressions and vocal sound. As Douglas Wile writes: "Writings tracing their origins to Yang [Banhou] are our closest link to Yang [Luchan] and to the richness of the art before it moved into the mainstream of Chinese culture in the twentieth century" (Wile, 1996: 93).

Yang Jianhou's second son was Yang Chengfu (1883–1936). He and his brother Shaohou taught taijiquan at the Beijing Physical Culture Research Institute from 1914 until 1928. They were pioneers in bringing instruction to the general public. Chengfu moved to Shanghai in 1928 and taught many. Over the years, Chengfu's particular style became the most widespread. He eliminated some of the more vigorous techniques from the long routine and taught others to practice at a slow, even tempo. Although he certainly retained the teachings of his father, uncle, and grandfather, Chengfu's public style became popular for its health nurturing benefits.

Lineage Chart Early Yang Family

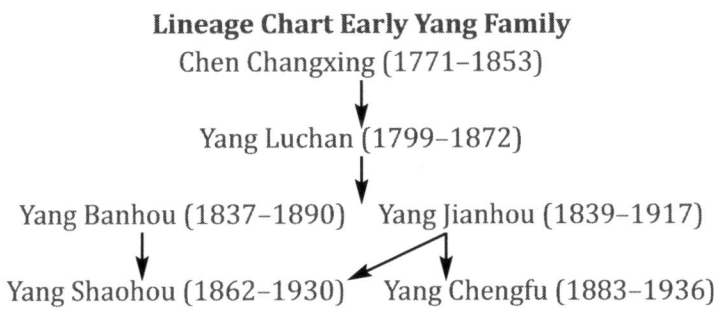

The five Yang family members discussed in the preceding paragraphs lived during a time of drastic change in China. Their lives cover 137 years, from the birth of Yang Luchan in 1799 to the death of Yang Chengfu in 1936. A brief overview of Chinese history during this period will be helpful for understanding the development of taijiquan, as well as other Chinese martial arts that have become popular in the modern era. The realities of those decades influenced the ways the early taiji masters viewed their art, how they taught, and to whom they would transmit their knowledge and skills.

The Effect of Time and Place for Early Yang Style Taiji

What inspired Yang Luchan to study martial arts? Was Chen Family boxing very different from other family styles developed in other villages? Actually, to have a group of villagers with a common surname practicing boxing within their courtyards was not a rare phenomenon in the latter half of the Qing Dynasty (1644–1911). Philip Kuhn (1970) details the growth of local militia, rebels, bandit groups, and secret societies in his excellent work, *Rebellion and Its Enemies in Late Imperial China: Militarization and Social Structure, 1796–1864*. Chen Village is only one example of a village that built up their walls and fighting tradition for protection from attack and theft from outsiders, such as local bandits.

There are "... two basic types of militia institutions in Chinese society—those born of state prescription and those born of the needs of natural social units..." (Kuhn, 1970: 35). The rise of local defense groups became more and more important as the Qing government and its military and police structures fragmented under internal and external pressures. Their rise was in direct response to the unstable socio-political climate.

In the 18th century there was a growing domestic discontent throughout China as the population increased to a point where food production could not keep pace. "Population growth inevitably surpassed increased food production, and the standard of living began to decline. Spreading corruption and indolence in government made conditions worse" (Hucker, 1975: 302). Besides an antiforeign sentiment for the Manchu rulers who conquered China and ruled from 1644 to 1911, the general population felt the government had lost the Mandate of Heaven and were unfit to rule. Popular uprisings became endemic, erupting into major social upheavals such as the rebellion by the White Lotus Society (1793–1804). Even more devastating was the Taiping Rebellion (1851–1864) in which nearly thirty million lost their lives bringing destruction to fifteen provinces (Wakeman, 1977: 156). By the mid-19th century, in some provinces "two-thirds of the population was reported dead or missing" (Wakeman, 1977: 155).

For centuries, China had thought itself to be the most civilized state in the world. However, rebellions, famine, and floods took a great toll on the government and society during the 19th century. China's image of itself gradually changed. It was no longer a country of strength and wealth, and foreign countries took advantage of this frailty. With the intrusion of European traders and missionaries, China soon felt its weakness regarding modern ways of warfare and international business. Over the decades, the Portuguese, Dutch, British, French, Americans, Russians, and Japanese applied more pressure on China as they tried to profit through unequal trade agreements, acquisition of port cities, opium trafficking, and a siphoning off the dwindling reserves of silver. Foreign powers took advantage of a China that had already been weakened from within.

In parallel with a long list of internal rebellions is a list of wars with foreign countries, such as the Opium War (1839–1842), the Anglo-Chinese War (1856–1860), and the Sino-French War (1884–1885). The foreign encroachments were destructive, but their real significance lies in the resulting treaties, which were unequal in that they gave great advantage to the foreign powers at a high cost to the Chinese. The Sino-Japanese War (1884–1895) provided a "profound psychological shock," since it "did more than any other crisis to force the Chinese to evaluate their own strengths and weaknesses" (Wakeman, 1977: 192). Above all, each treaty humiliated the Chinese, and many started to seek solutions to resolve the problems caused by the decades of internal strife and foreign influence.

During the latter half of the 19th century, many political and intellectual leaders were engaged in discussing ways to restore the Qing Imperial system or a new political system through "self-strengthening." It seems most of the attempts either failed or made matters worse. For example, one idea was to use the resentment against imperialist expansion to encourage the Boxer Uprising (1900–1901) against foreign embassies. This was doomed to failure. "Thousands of young men began to practice the stylized exercises of Shaolin and [bagua] boxing—exercises that were supposed to release their [qi] (pneuma) and invest them with strength so awesome that it repelled foreign bullets" (Wakeman, 1977: 217). Even a Chinese military general "simply scoffed at their claims of invulnerability to firearms," and "put fiifty Boxers of the Golden Belt Society to the test by lining them up against a wall and shooting them" (Wakeman, 1977: 218). The Boxers' leader was caught and decapitated. Their defeat brought new demands upon the Chinese and resulted in even greater loss of power.

As the Beijing government was losing control of the provinces, there was a corresponding growth of power in local areas, often associated with the provinces themselves. Frederic Wakeman notes that "the provincial governors of the early 1900s, took on more and more of the military and fiscal functions that had once belonged to the central government" (Wakeman, 1977: 232). In nearly half of China's provinces "military men became governors immediately after the [Wuhan Revolution (1911)], or within the following two or three months. Moreover, the troops in the various provinces... were largely recruited from within the provinces in which they served; their loyalties were strongly provincial and personal, so that provincial military leaders had, in effect, personal armies at their disposal...." (Sheridan, 1977: 147).

As private armies developed—some small and some large—warfare increased. "Between 1916 and 1928, the struggle among independent militarists—warlords—tore China into fragments, and the formal political machinery of the republic that had succeeded the monarchy—the parliament, ministries, and so forth—became largely irrelevant to the realities of Chinese political life. At the head of their personal armies, the warlords dominated districts, provinces, and regions, and warred with neighboring generals for additional territory and revenues" (Sheridan, 1977: 20).

War was endemic during this Warlord Period (1916–1928). One writer has "counted more than 400 large and small civil wars in the province of Szechwan alone" (Sheridan, 1977: 88). With such chaos in the land, how would it be possible to reintegrate China under a modern, unified national government? Each warlord faction operated according to his own interests and political ends. One interesting aspect of note is how soldiers were trained. Decorum varied greatly according to group. Some warlords demanded that troops be highly trained while acting with utmost compassion toward the general population. Their honorable code of discipline stressed good treatment toward all and maintaining personal restraint from vices associated with soldiers of poor character. General Feng Yuxiang (1882–1948), for example, "demanded extraordinary physical fitness, and subjected his officers and men to constant and rigorous training to achieve it. . . . He prohibited drinking, gambling, visiting prostitutes, even swearing" (Sheridan, 1977: 74). At the other end of the spectrum were other warlords and their troops who drank alcohol, raped, and robbed at will.

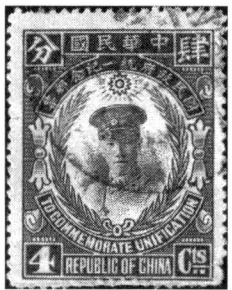

Postage stamp issued by the Republic of China
"To Commemorate Unification," bearing the portrait of
Generalissimo Chiang Kai-shek. Courtesy of iStockphoto.com.

Amid the dynamic political and military flux of the warlord period, loyalties often shifted between warlords, as well as their officers and troops (Sheridan, 1977: 58). A few factions grew strong while many became weak and disintegrated or were absorbed. Eventually there were two main political parties contending for supremacy: the Nationalists (Guomintang) under the leadership of General Chiang Kai-shek (1887–1975), and the Chinese Communist Party, under Mao Zedong (1893–1976). Initially they worked together to end the warlord period and drive out the Japanese, but their differences in political ideology brought on an inevitable civil war (1927–1949).

Chiang Kai-shek, raised during the warlord period, had learned "to revolve all his politics about the concept of force . . . He had grown up in a time of treachery and violence . . . . There were few standards of human decency his warlord contemporaries did not violate. They obeyed no law but power . . ." (Schurmann and Schell, 1967: 236). Mao also faced this hard reality, and his often-quoted statement is: "Political power grows out of the barrel of a gun." Chiang and Mao fought it out until the Communists emerged victorious in 1949.

A "protracted revolutionary transformation" lasted for more than a century, "but in many ways the critical period was the 37 years, 1912–1949, from the fall of the monarchy and founding of a republic to the establishment of the People's Republic of China by the Communists. During this republican period, disintegration and disorder were at their maximum" (Sheridan, 1977: 4). All of the early Yang Style Taijiquan masters lived during this revolutionary transformation, and there are some common factors in their lives that influenced their teaching.

The greatest single factor in taijiquan's development was its association with defense. There were centuries of banditry, small- and large-scale rebellions, and secret society activities throughout China. Particularly, rural areas lacked protection by the national army or police, so martial arts training was utilized for regional and local defense. The Chen Village is only one example of how a family style martial art developed within a walled village, although it is a famous example. It is the site of the original Chen Family Style Taijiquan, which was famed for its superior boxing system. Chen family representatives, such as Chen Changxing (1771–1853) and Chen Gengyun (1799–1872), were employed as elite bodyguards and for cargo transport security personnel; Chen Yenxi (1848–1929) trained the son of the first Republican president Yuan Shikai and was also the family bodyguard for scholar-official Du Youmei in Boai, Henan. Du's son, Du Yuzi (1886–1990) became a disciple of Chen Yenxi.

Fear is a great motivator. People had to protect their food stocks as well as their lives. Many trained hard and often. They also feared a shift in loyalties, so they were cautious about whom they taught. Usually the ties were personal (teaching family or village members) and, under circumstances involving a larger area, ties would be provincial, where common dialect and social customs reinforced some bonding.

The decades of great social change brought changes in relationships. Chen Style moved outside its home village, and others, such as Yang Luchan, came to learn Chen Taiji. Luchan and his son Banhou taught Manchu imperial guards and garrison troops. Some teaching was done privately and some publicly. "When asked why the [Guangping] students of the Yang family showed both hard and soft techniques in their style, whereas the [Beijing] students showed only soft techniques, [Banhou] replied that the [Beijing] students were mainly wealthy aristocrats, and that, after all, there was a difference between Chinese and Manchus, implying a policy of passive resistance to the alien dynasty by imparting only half of taijiquan transmission" (Wile, 1983: ix).

When Yang Chengfu was born (1883), his grandfather Luchan had already been dead eleven years, and his uncle Banhou died when Chengfu was nine. As a result, Chengfu's training was somewhat different than that of his brother Yang Shaohou. Shaohou and Banhou were noted for their rough boxing. Internationally, Shaohou's style is not as well-known as Yang Chengfu's. The difficulties surrounding his life led him to commit suicide in 1930 (Yun, 2006: 55).

The lives of the Chen Style and early Yang Style Taiji masters reflect their times. The leading figures were highly involved with defense on a local, provincial, and sometimes national level. The need for true, highly effective martial skills was ingrained in the consciousness of all facing life and death struggles in their daily lives. Famed martial art teachers, like Yang Luchan, were placed in a quandary between the desire to keep their highest knowledge from "outsiders" and the wish to help close family members and friends. They also had to make a living during difficult times.

There was another motivation for teaching that is often overlooked. It involves the many decades of humiliating treatment at the hands of foreign countries which forced China to give concessions away while losing their own land, wealth, and dignity. The Chinese became known as the "sick man of Asia." That phrase features in the Bruce Lee film Fist of Fury (1971), and the Jet Li film *Fearless* (2006). The idea of teaching martial arts for health fit in well with the "self-strengthening" movement in the early 20th century. The country needed to become strong, as did its people.

Xiong Yanghe and His Unique Contributions to Taijiquan
Early on, Yang Luchan and his sons were exhibiting different modes of instruction. They had an array of students: family members, military officials, Manchu guards, other martial art instructors, the affluent and the peasant. Each held the Yang Family tradition and could tailor their instruction according to the student-teacher relationship.

Personalities also played a role in teaching methods as well as in the selection of students. There were polar yin-yang characteristics shown between Yang Banhou (yang) and Yang Jianhou (yin), and in the following generation between Yang Shaohou (yang) and Yang Chengfu (yin)! Shaohou's style was physically and mentally demanding, plus he would not pull punches with his students. Yang Chengfu's style became the most popular because of his more pleasing character and teaching methods. The slower tempo and modifications he made were suitable for a greater number of people, such as the elderly. His teaching had a great impact on national "self-strengthening" by bringing health to thousands.

What is Xiong Yanghe's place in this development? Within the Yang Taiji linage, he took his teachings to Taiwan following the exodus of the Chinese Nationalists to Taiwan in 1949 and became a major influence in the spread of taiji throughout the island. When he passed away in 1981, he and his senior disciples had taught over ten thousand students. His style continues to spread via his disciples, and his unique system is now referred to as Xiong Style Taiji. Xiong's story proves interesting for his unique place in taiji as well as his personal life.

Xiong was born on September 29, 1888, in Jiangsu Province, in Funing County. His father, Xiong Weizhen, passed the provincial examination (*juren* military degree) during the late Qing Dynasty. Yanghe studied martial arts first with his father, then his father hired instructors for his young son: at age 12, a Shaolin master named Liu He and his disciple Liu Zhongfang came to teach; at age 15, Master Yin Wanbang for Jiangnan Eight Harmonies Boxing system. These had a martial influence from Gan Fengchi. When Xiong was 20, "Miraculous Hand" Tang Dianqing (1850–1926) was hired to teach. These teachers provided young Xiong with an excellent foundation in Shaolin boxing and may have given Xiong his first exposure to taijiquan.

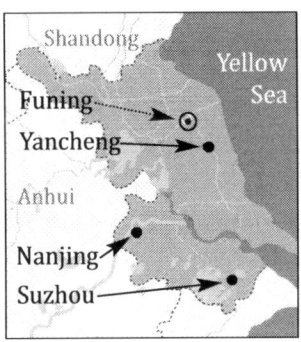

Xiong had hands-on fighting experience as he helped his father maintain township security. He found himself all too often fighting with gangsters. When he was 19 years old, he was the local boxing champion in the "no holds barred" competitions held on raised platforms (*leitai*), as seen in the movie *Fearless*. Because of his powerful kicks, Xiong earned the nickname of "Funing Legs." Such experiences gave him boxing insights, but he was destined to enrich his martial arts by contacts made through his work.

When Xiong was 23 years old, he began a career in the military, which dealt with security and military operations. At 29, he was Adjunct Director of the Anhui Province government office, and at 35 he went on to a management position in the Funing County garrisons. During this period, Xiong met Old Frame Yang Style Taijiquan master Hu Puan (1878–1947), who became his most influential teacher. Hu's nickname was "Hu Hu," meaning "Tiger Hu."

Hu was born in Anhui Province, Jing County. He served as the Department Chief of Jiangsu Province Civil Administration. As a sinologist well-known for his books and poetry, Hu taught at Shanghai University. While in Shanghai, he had an opportunity to meet and study with a number of high caliber taiji masters. He practiced daily starting at 6:00am for over 18 years, until he became disabled by a stroke and resulting paralysis.[1]

Who was Hu's primary taiji teacher? Sources differ, stating he studied with:

1) Chen Weiming (1881–1958) [2]
2) Yang Jianhou (1839–1917) [3]
3) Yang Chengfu (1883–1936) [4]
4) Yang Shaohou (1862–1930) [5]
5) Le Huanzhi (1899–1960) [6]

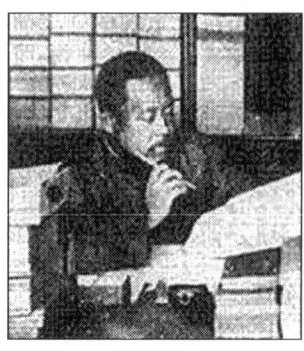

At his desk, Hu Puan (1878–1947) was famed as a China scholar and taijiquan master. — www.taiji.net.cn

Most statements regarding Hu Puan's teachers simply say that he studied with this particular person or that one. Furthermore, there are questions about the length of time that Hu studied with his teachers. What could he have learned from them? One reference says "Yang Chengfu and disciple Mr. Hu Puan . . . compared notes together, making a thorough study of taijiquan, gaining thorough and penetrating insights into taiji gongfu."[7] To state that Hu was Yang Chengfu's "disciple" is a strong statement. Unfortunately, I have not found solid evidence to substantiate this pronouncement.

Hu Puan probably met all these teachers and may have studied with each to different degrees. But it is interesting to note that he spoke so highly of Le Huanzhi (1899–1960), who was from Gushi County in Henan. Le was a medical doctor and a senior disciple of Dong Yingjie (1898–1961). In his published memoir, Hu wrote that Le's taijiquan is extremely fine. Hu wrote that—from his own push hands experience with Yang Chengfu, Sun Lutang, Wu Jianquan, and Le Huanzhi—Le proved superior, and his touch was highly effective yet had an undetectable source, "like passing clouds and flowing water," "as not having matter."[8]

Because the sources are obscure, it is difficult to know from whom Hu Puan received his taijiquan instruction. Also, the lineage for Xiong has not been evenly defined. There are a few sources that state that Xiong was a disciple of Yang Shaohou.[9] This seems to be an assumption based primarily on what Xiong taught. However, both Xiong and Hu Puan probably had some contact with Yang Shaohou. What we do know for sure is that, in his autobiography (1962), Xiong himself only mentions Hu Puan in regard to the transmission of the Yang Style Old Frame. This does not negate the possibility that Xiong met other Yang Style Taiji masters or learned their methods via Hu Puan.

Xiong may have "studied thoroughly with Hu Puan," but he no doubt did have good relations with other taijiquan masters.[10] One source states that Xiong had the chance to meet Yang Jianhou while staying in Beijing for official business. It gave him the opportunity to seek advice about taijiquan, especially regarding the two-person routine call *sanshou* ("dispersing hands"). At this time, Xiong studied wholeheartedly and was able to grasp the deeper mysteries of the art.[11] Yet another source mentions that Yang Jianhou taught in Funing County, and Xiong sought his advice for the sanshou practice.[12] Liang Dongcai (aka, T. T. Liang) states that Yang Jianhou taught Xiong sanshou. Liang also maintains that nobody could have possibly learned it from Yang Chengfu, because his father Yang Jianhou died before he could teach it to him (Hayward, 2000: 61).

Since Xiong had to take part in policy discussions falling within the range of his official military duties, he had a great opportunity to meet many people who were highly skilled in a variety of martial traditions. They could compare their studies and benefit by observing the full scope of Chinese martial arts. Over the decades, Xiong received a solid grounding in Northern and Southern Shaolin and taijiquan from his personal teachers and from contact with others through his military career. Here are some highlights from his career:[13]

Age	Position
39	Regimental Commander, Revolutionary Army
40	Jiangsu Province Funing County Public Security Bureau Chief, and concurrent position as Production Brigade Chief
49	Jiangsu Province Funing County Magistrate
52	Security Major General Brigade Commander
53	Security Assistant Commandant
54	Security Major General Commander
58	Major General Group Commander
60	Deputy Commanding Officer, Military Headquarters

In 1949, the Nationalist Party under Chiang Kai-shek retreated to Taiwan, and the Communist Party established the People's Republic of China (PRC) on the mainland. Xiong resigned and moved to Taiwan when "nearly 600,000 Nationalist troops and their dependents withdrew from the mainland to Taiwan."[14] It is commonly said that part of this migratory wave included four famed "Big Dogs" of taijiquan: Zheng Manqing (1901–1975), Guo Lianying, Shi Diaomei and Xiong Yanghe.

After settling in Yilan city in 1953, Xiong tirelessly taught taiji. Eventually, Xiong Style practitioners came to number over 10,000. Xiong's most significant contribution to taiji's legacy is the through preservation and transmission of Yang Taijiquan as a fighting art and exercise system, most notably being the two-person practice of sanshou. In addition, his books leave a detailed record of the system.

Even in his twilight years, Xiong was up daily at 4:30 am to start his day, which included his regular taiji classes. In addition to chanting Buddhist scriptures, practicing brush calligraphy, and reading military history, he wrote books, which leave a detailed record of the taiji system for following generations. He was a Buddhist who treated his disciples with a fatherly affection. He died on October 29, 1981 in Yilan Yuan Shan Rongmin Hospital at the age of 94.

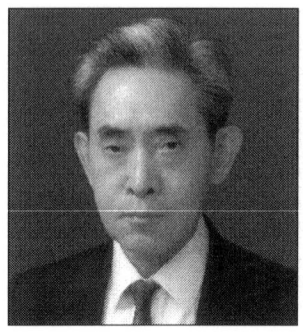 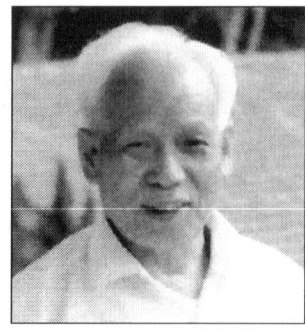

Left: Master Guo Tingxian (1923–2002) was one of Xiong Yanghe's top disciples, and the teacher of Lin Jianhong. Photograph courtesy of Lin Jianhong. Right: Master Yang Qingyu (1915–2002) was one of Xiong Yanghe's longtime students and close confidant. Born in Henan, he served in the military and moved to Taiwan. Photograph by M. DeMarco.

Xiong Yanghe's Curriculum as Presented by Lin Jianhong

On the Neijia Formosa website, David Chesser writes this regarding Xiong's curriculum: "This amount of training makes it the most complete version of taiji practiced on the island. I simply haven't found anything that compares to it."[15] In order to present some of Xiong Yanghe's system in this anthology, photographs were provided by Robert Yu, who contacted Master Lin Jianhong during a visit to Taiwan in October of 2006.

Master Lin Jianhong studied under Guo Tingxian, a top Xiong Yanghe disciple. Through Guo, Lin also learned Hua Tuo's Five Animal Frolics. Lin teaches in the Taipei area, including Liberty Square (formerly called the Chiang Kai-shek Memorial Square). Mr. Robert Yu visited Master Lin's class three times, saying that Lin and his students were refreshing to meet, "open, friendly and competent" people (R. Yu, personal communication, November 3, 2006). Yu provided over 100 photographs and reference materials for this article. Now in his mid-50s, Master Lin enjoys teaching, usually with the help of his assistant Ms. Ye Jinxiu, as shown on the following pages.

XIONG STYLE CURRICULUM

- Yang Family Old Frame Xiong Style Taijiquan　　楊家老架熊氏太極拳
- Taiji Basic (standing) Post　　太極基本樁
- Taiji Qigong　　太極氣功
- Push hands (tuishou)　　推手
- Dispersing Hands (sanshou)　　散手
- Taiji sword　　太極劍
- knife　　刀
- stick　　棍
- staff　　桿
- paired swords (two-person)　　對劍

- paired knives (two-person) 對刀
- paired sticks (two-person) 對桿
- paired staves (two-person) 對棍
- Six Directions Flower Spear (Liulu Huaqiang) 六路花槍
- Spring and Autumn broadsword 春秋大刀
- double swords 雙劍
- Mizong Boxing 秘宗拳【迷蹤拳】
- Four Gates Hong Boxing 四門洪拳
- Young Hong Boxing 小洪拳
- Sunlight Palm (Ziyang Zhang Deng) 曦陽掌等
- and more

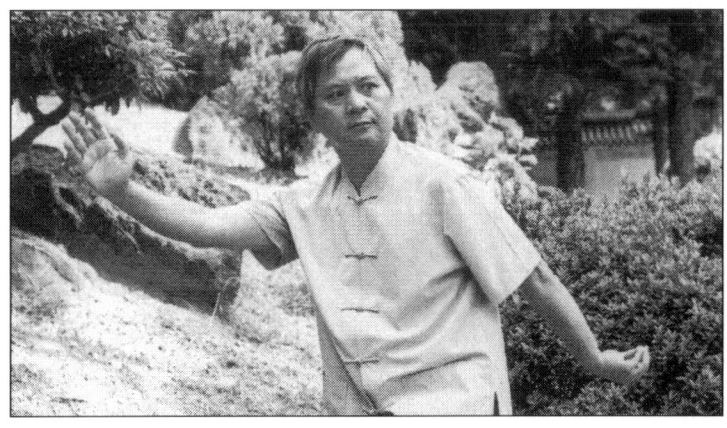

Lin Jianhong

LONG FORM SOLO ROUTINE

Selected postures from the traditional long routine consisting of 111 postures。
1) Beginning posture 2) Ward-off left

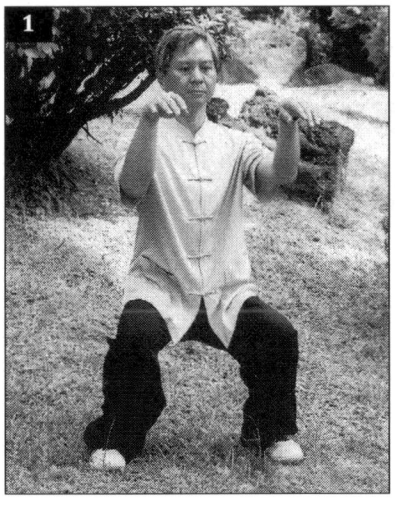
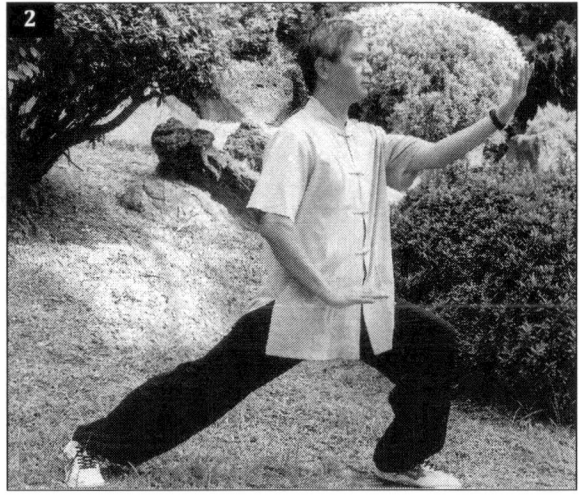

3) Ward Off right 4) Rollback

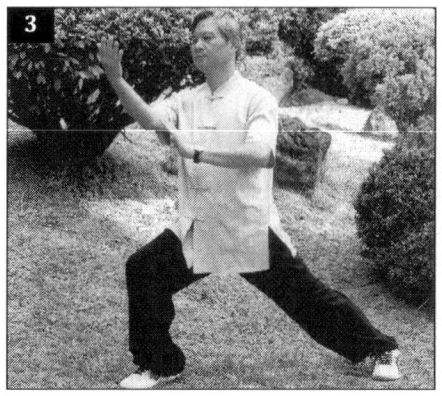 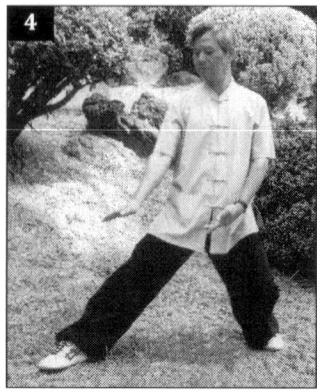

5) Press 6) Double Elbow

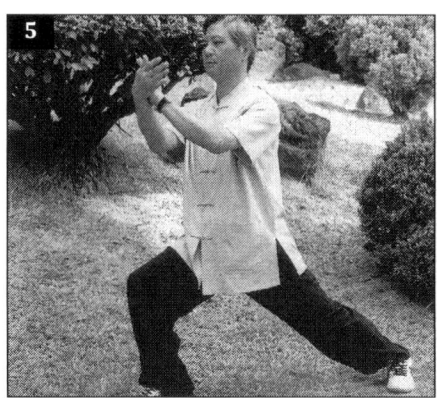 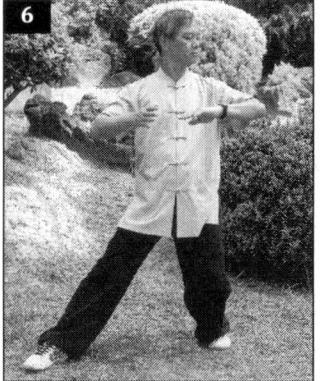

7) Single Whip 8) Raise Hands

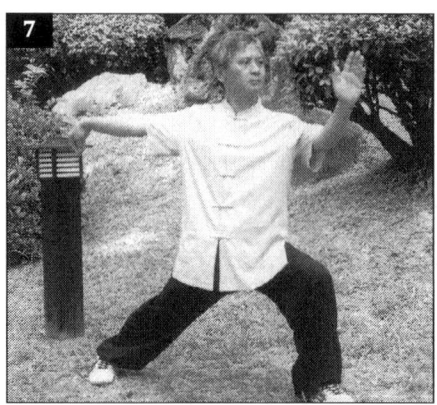 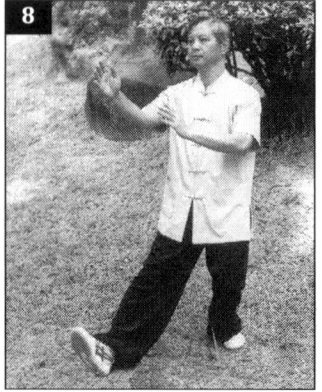

9) Rooster Stands on One Leg 10) Snake Creeps Down

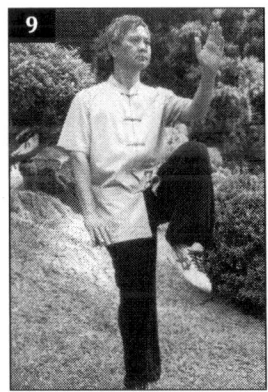 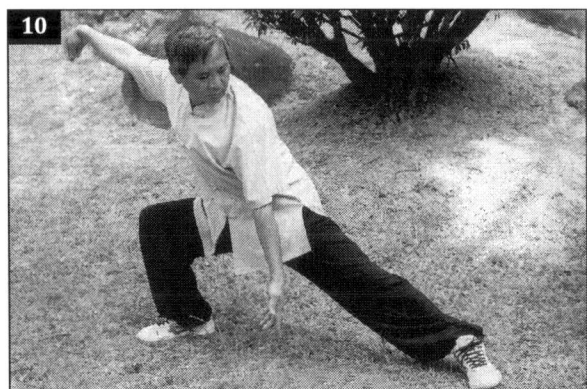

11) Ride Tiger

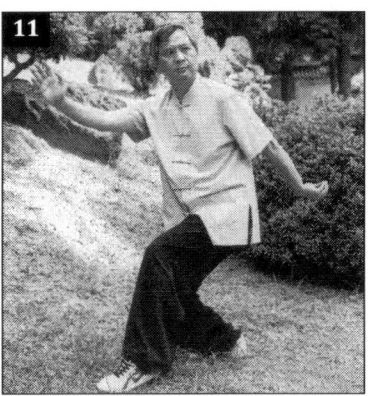

12) Bend Bow Shoot Tiger

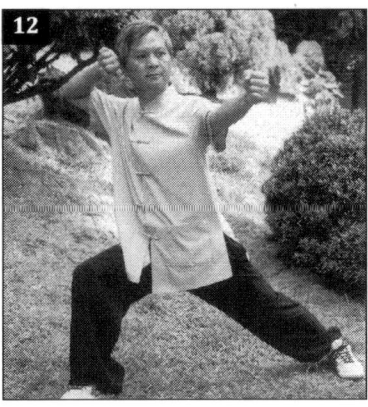

Five Animal Frolics

A superb way to cultivate taijiquan principles is to devote a few minutes a day to these exercises. Master Lin was fortunate to learn this system from Guo Tingxian. Mr. Lin's student, Ms. Ye Jinxiu, leads the group.

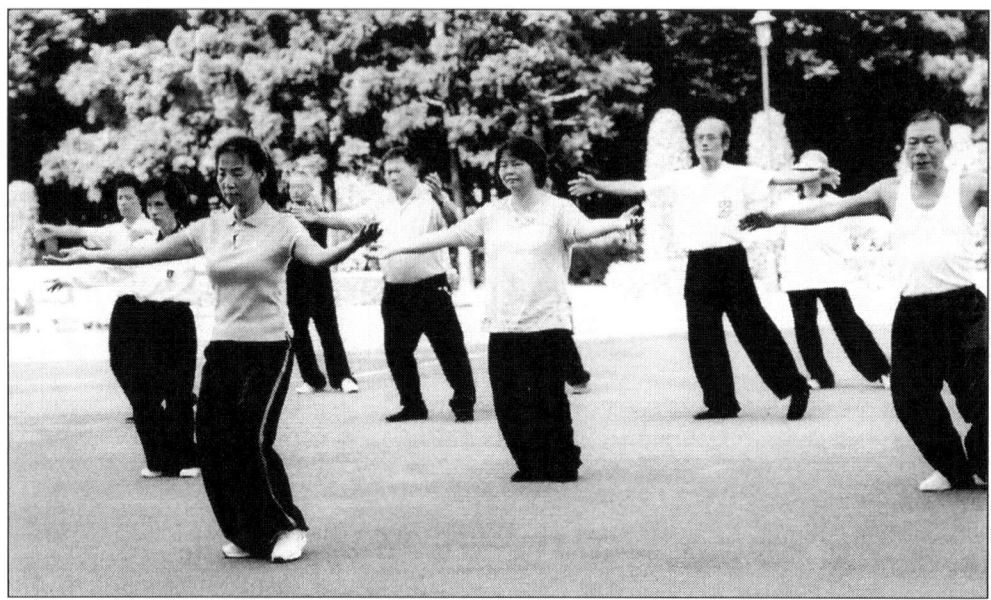

Long Form Solo Routine Group Practice

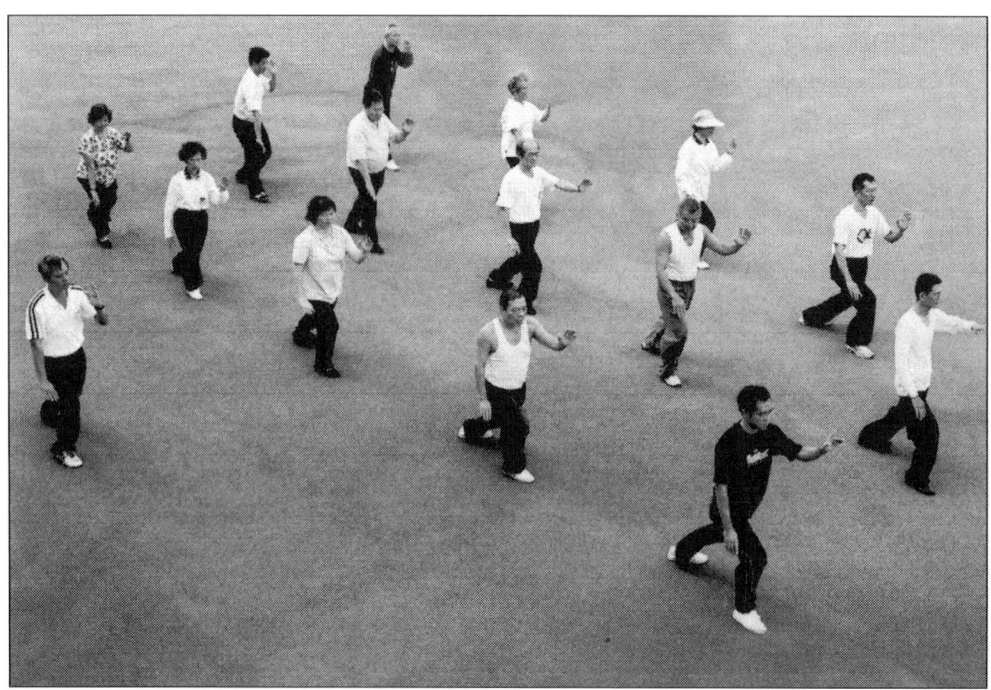

Long Form Solo Routine Group Practice

Mr. Lin closely observes each student during practice sessions and later suggests ways to improve their practice.

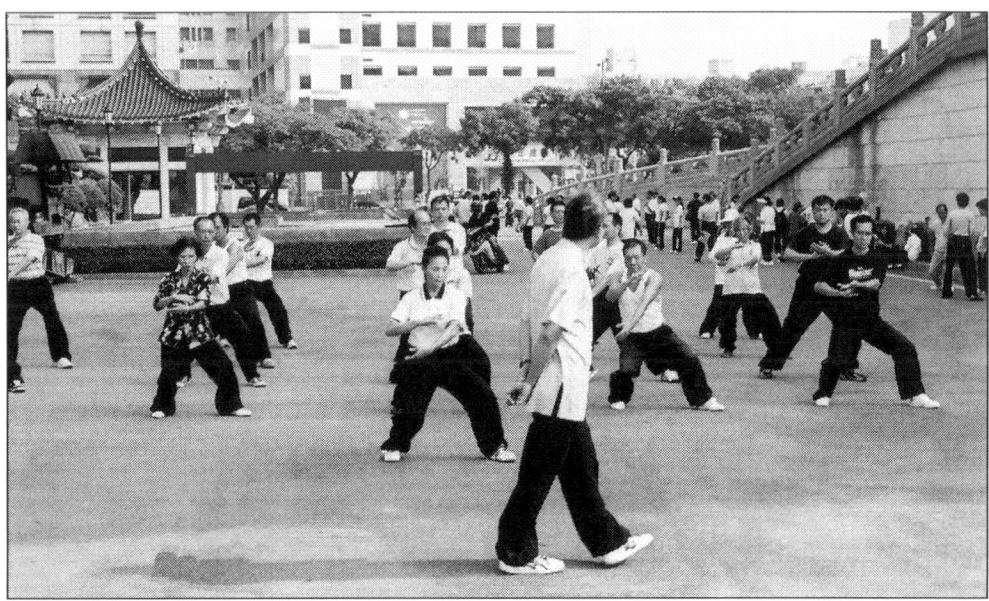

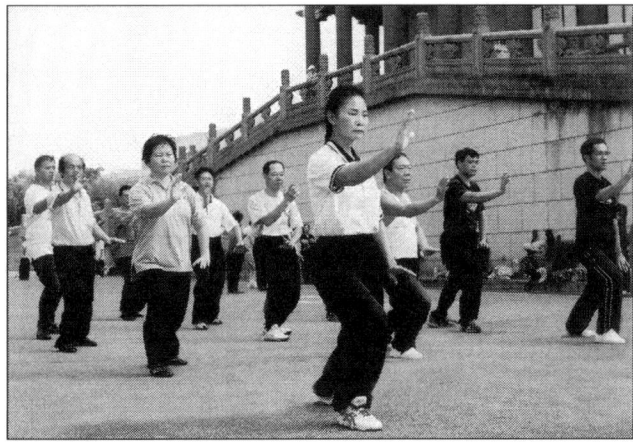 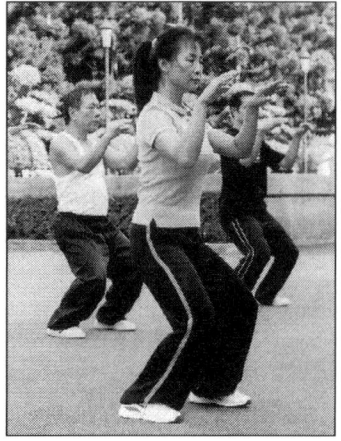

Master Lin teaches a variety of students at different locations and class times. Most want to learn taiji for health purposes and the good comradery. Others, usually younger students, delve into the fighting traditions. Regardless, if you study Xiong Style, you will get a mixture of both due to the completeness of this traditional system.

Staff

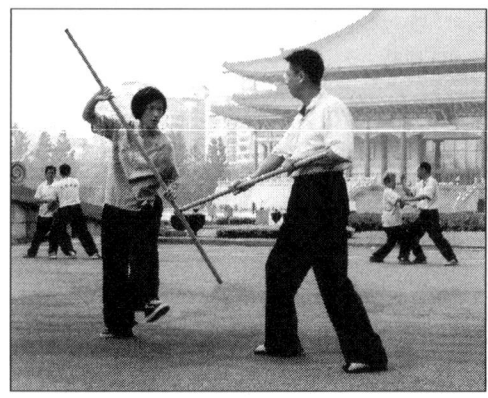
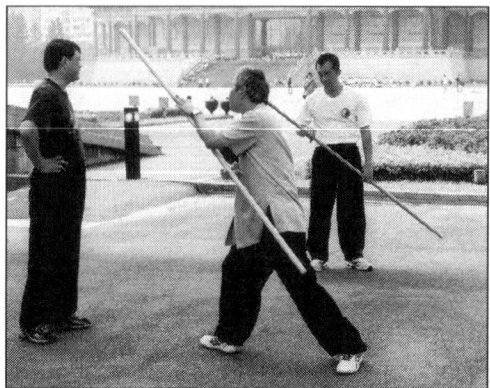
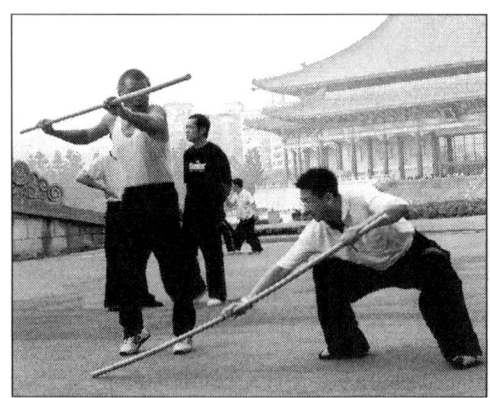
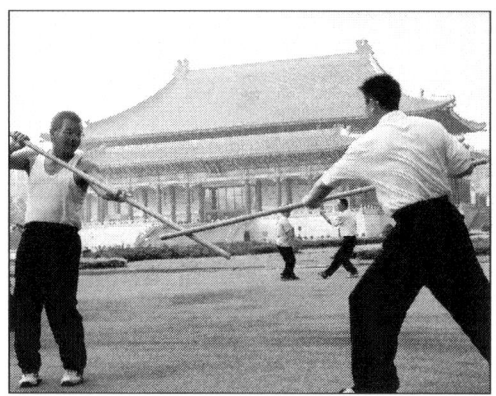

Broadsword

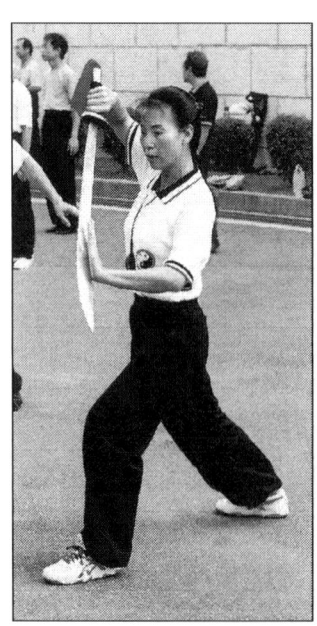
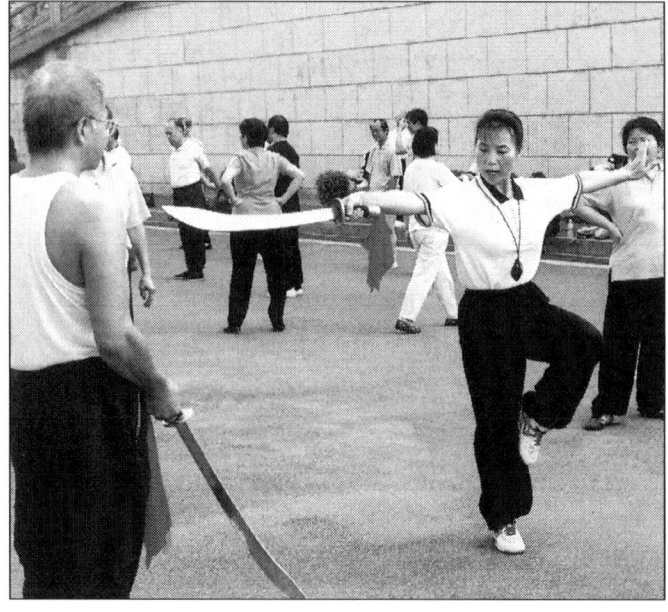

Sanshou

"Dispersing Hands" is a two-person routine designed to give advanced students a realistic feel for taiji as a combative art. It can be practiced at various speeds and includes functions from the solo form as well as others derived from Chen Family Style. It seems Grandmaster Xiong learned this from Hu Puan, but there is probably a link to Yang Jianhou as well. Contact is never broken during sanshou practice.

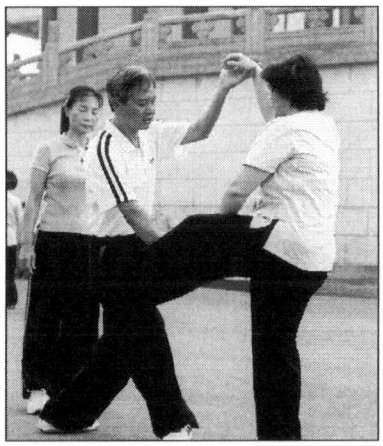

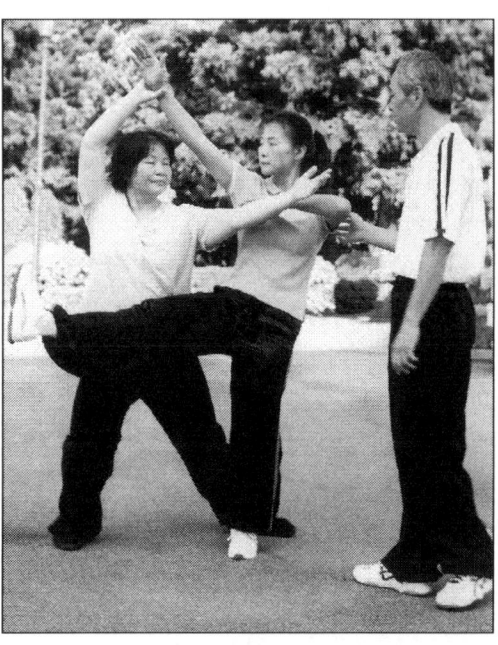

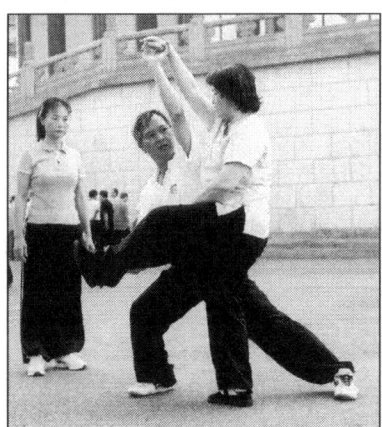

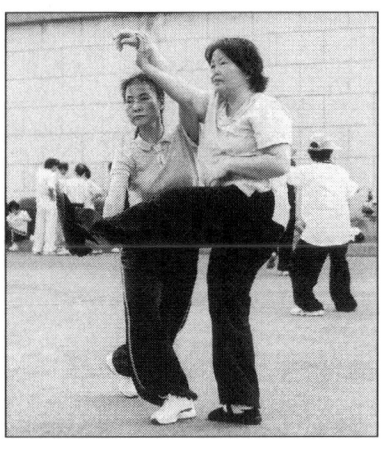

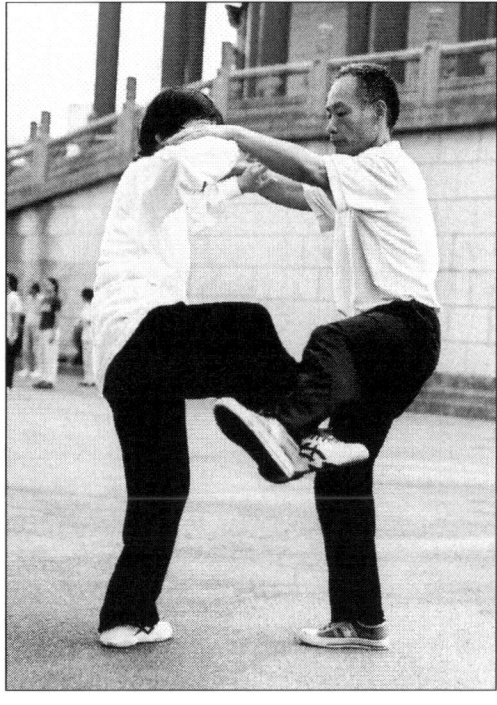

Concluding Remarks on Xiong Style Taijiquan

Like the story of the blind men examining an elephant, this chapter can only represent the author's personal findings limited by a relative lack of reference materials, the difficulty in translating Chinese texts accurately, and time available for research. I take responsibility for any shortcomings and welcome any helpful feedback. Hopefully, despite such limitations, the material presented here can broaden the perspective on taijiquan, considering the historical setting where the art was developed by the leading Yang Family lineage representatives.

We have found that there were two major factors influencing early Yang Style development. The first is the nearly incomprehensible violence from the downfall of the Qing dynasty to the founding of the Peoples' Republic of China, especially during the Republican Period (1911-1949) that soaked the Chinese soil with blood when disorder was at a maximum. It was a time when many sought out superior fighting methods and practiced as if their lives depended upon it. It is no surprise that taijiquan was a desirable system to learn and that it migrated from a small village to be practiced by bodyguards in major cities where military and security personnel were found.

The other major factor influencing taiji's history stems from the exhaustion felt by the country and its population after centuries of rebellions and foreign interventions. Years of struggle, defeat, and humiliation inspired a growing sense of nationalism and an era of "self-strengthening" for the country. One way to cure the "sick man of Asia" was to spread taiji for health: it was found to be highly effective as a form of exercise, no special gear or facility was required, and it was inexpensive when practiced in groups. Millions are healthier because of it.

If we keep in mind the two influences mentioned above while looking at the early Yang Style lineage, a special interrelationship unfolds between taiji and Chinese social history. Between the birth of Yang Luchan and the death of Xiong Yanghe, factions of China's population fought for survival for 150 years before finally emerging as a nation at peace. No doubt Yang Luchan's taiji was a fighting art, but what did it look like? How did he practice? What was the depth of his knowledge?

Most taiji styles today have evolved away from their martial roots. This evolution paralleled the decline of violence in China and the growing social and political stability. At its highest levels, taiji as a fighting art has always been transmitted to a relatively small number of people. Teaching en masse for public health has reached millions. As a result, a vast majority of taiji practitioners know form, but little of function. The reasons one has for learning taiji affects how the form is practiced and looks. We cannot see how Yang Luchan practiced, but the system preserved by Xiong Yanghe seems to be a good indicator and is valued for preserving a great tradition in Taiwan that was nearly lost during the Communist Cultural Revolution (1966-1976), a social movement that included a crusade to rid China of "old ways of thinking," such as those exhibited in the traditional martial arts.

Xiong Style offers combative elements that were necessary during the extreme chaos found in China during the early Yang Family transmissions of the art. Yang Luchan studied Chen Style and aspects of this are reflected in Xiong Style too: stances are often low and wide, applications are effective, training methods in push-hands and sanshou are practical, and the inclusion of weaponry is encompassing. Even though Xiong's system retains the old Yang flavor, he lived forty years longer than Yang Chengfu, and into the post-1949 era. He was motivated to teach for two reasons. He taught close students taiji as a fighting art and as an exercise for health and longevity. Thousands of other students were taught basically for "self-strengthening."

This brief overview of Xiong Style helps define and give meaning to the words "taijiquan." Taiji is not just an exercise and not only a fighting art. It is both, and its dual nature is inherent in the teachings of true masters. One who has mastered Xiong's system, or the early Yang Family systems, can impart the theory and knowledge applicable in both areas as a combative art and exercise system. The mix is largely determined by the teacher-student relationship and the motives involved. Yang Family Xiong Style Taijiquan gives us an unique opportunity to look back in time when the template of Yang Style was forged. As the system thrives in Taiwan under Xiong's disciples and their own disciples—teachers such as Lin Jianhong and Lin Chaolai—we see that the old system has been preserved, while even spreading outside Taiwan to benefit others. It's a taste of "old wine in a new bottle."

Acknowledgments

The impetus for this article came from Mr. Robert Lin-I Yu, a noted baguazhang and xingyi instructor (disciple of Hong Yixiang, Zhou Jincai, and others in Taiwan). From his home in Madison, Wisconsin, Yu called to say he would be returning to Taiwan in October (2006) to conduct martial arts research and visit relatives. "Would you like me to do anything for you while there?" My only response was that, if he wished, he could contact Mr. Lin Shengxuan (one of my Xiong Style Taiji classmates) and any other Xiong Style instructor he could find. He followed up and returned to the U.S. with a huge stack of photographs, notes, copies of handwritten documents, books, and unpublished manuscripts from Xiong Style instructors. A special thanks to these two fine gentlemen for the friendship and support, and to Master Lin Jianghong, Ms. Ye Jinxiu, and fellow students for kindly participating.

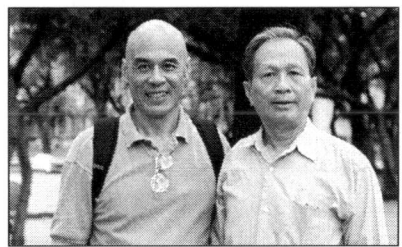

Robert Yu and Lin Shengxuanin 228 Memorial Park.

Short List of Xiong Students

Cao Zenghua	曹增華	Lin Xianghua	林祥華
Chen Deyang	陳德洋	Lu Yuxuan	陸雨軒
Chen Huang	陳皇	Lü Zhenzhong	呂振忠
Chen Xiaoyin	陳曉寅	Meng Shanfu	孟善夫
Chen Xinggui	陳興桂	Qiu Shuzhou	裘署舟
Chen Zhenhe	陳珍和	Rao Shunchen	饒舜臣
Guo Tingxian	郭廷獻	Yang Qingyu	楊清玉
Huang Guozhi	黃國治	Ye Shiyi	葉式意
Huang Qinglin	黃清麟	Yu Xianquan	俞賢詮
Jan Tiangong	天拱	Wan Xiaoyan	萬小燕
Li Guoguang	李國光	Wang Jingzhi	王靜之
Li Rixin	李日新	Wang Juemin	王覺民
Lin Chaolai	林朝來	Wei Guang	魏廣
Lin Lianfu	林連富	Zhang Nan	張楠
Lin Lianzhi	林連祬	Zhang Zhongping	張仲平
Lin Qingzhi	林清智	Zou Xueyuan	鄒學元

Other Xiong Students

Liang Dongcai	梁棟材	(Liang Tsung Tsai)
Liu Chenhuan		(Abraham Liu)
Tao Bingxiang	陶恦祥	(Tao Ping-Siang)
Zhong Dazhen	鍾大振	(Tchoung Ta-tchen)

People Mentioned in the Article

Chen Changxing	陳長興	Hu Puan	胡扑安
Chen Yanxi	陳延熙	Le Huanzhi	乐奂之
Chen Weiming	陳微明	Lin Jianhong	林建宏
Dong Yingjie	董英杰	Lin Shengxuan	林聖軒
Du Yuze	杜毓澤	Liu He	劉和
Gan Fengchi	甘鳳池	Liu Zhongfang	劉仲仿
Guo Lianying	郭連英	Shi Diaomei	施調梅

Places

Anhui Province	安徽省	Guangping County	廣平縣
Chen Village	陳家溝	Gushi County	固始縣
Funing County	阜寧縣	Hebei Province	河北省

References for Website Sources

1. http://yuehuanzhi.blog.sohu.com
2. www.taiji.net.cn/liu/wlys/200712/6426.shtml; http://yuehuanzhi.blog.sohu.com
3. http://blog.udn.com/article/trackback.jsp?uid=wang6196192001&aid=107787
4. http://tw.myblog.yahoo.com/q3taichi/article?mid=23&sc=1
5. http://library.taiwanschoolnet.org
6. http://yuehuanzhi.blog.sohu.com; www.xici.net/u6819319/d19792891.htm
7. http://tw.myblog.yahoo.com/q3taichi/profile
8. www.xici.net/u6819319/d19792891.htm
9. www.dotaichi.com
10. http://blog.sina.com.tw/lkk_blog/article.php?pbgid=36074&entryid=320007
11. http://www.lin-gi.com.tw/discuss/Viewtopic.asp? Subject ID=7135&Sign=150
12. http://tw.myblog.yahoo.com/jin_cang/article?mid=1003&prev=2170&next=554&=f&fid=3
13. http://blog.udn.com/wang6196192001/1067085
14. http://taiwanreview.nat.gov.tw/fp.asp?xItem=589&CtNode=128
15. http://chessman71.wordpress.com/2006/05/15/yang-shao-hous-taiji/)

References – Chinese

Anonymous (1987). *Mr. Xiong's 100th birthday commemorative special edition.* (n.p.).

Anonymous (1984). *National arts master Xiong Yanghe commemorative collection.* (n.p.).

Lin, Caolai (2007). Yang family old frame Xiong style taijiquan. DVD. Yilan, Taiwan: Chin-yu Martial Art Study Association.

Yang, Qingyu (1976). Xiong style taijiquan long form, push-hands, and sword form. Private film collection.

Yang, Qingyu (1988). Autobiography. Self-published.

Yang, Qingyu (n.d.). *A brief biography of Xiong Yanghe.* Self-published.

Xiong, Y.H. (1962). *Autobiography.* Self-published.

Xiong, Y.H. (1963). *The taijiquan explained.* Taipei: Taiwan China Book Printing House.

Xiong, Y.H. (1971). *Taiji swordsmanship illustrated.* Yilan, Taiwan: Lu Feng Printing and Publishing House.

Xiong, Y.H. (1975). *The taijiquan explained.* 3rd edition. Taipei: Huge Distribution Planning Company.

References – English

Hucker, C. (1975). *China's imperial past: An introduction to Chinese history and culture*. Stanford, CA: Stanford University Press.

DeMarco, M. (1992). The origin and evolution of taijiquan. *Journal of Asian Martial Arts, 1*(1): 8–25.

Gallagher, P. (2007). *Drawing silk: Masters' secrets for successful tai chi practice*. Charleston, SC: BookSurge.

Hayward, R. (2000). *T'ai-chi ch'uan: Lessons with master T.T. Liang*. St. Paul, MN: Shu-Kuang Press.

Kuhn, P. (1970). Rebellion and Its Enemies in Late Imperial China: Militarization and Social Structure, 1796~1864. Cambridge, MA: Harvard University Press.

Kurland, H. (May 1998). "Hsiung Yang-Ho's san shou form." *T'ai chi Ch'uan and Wellness Newsletter*. Downloaded July 16, 2009.

Kurland, H. (2003). "History of a rare t'ai-chi form: San shou." http://www.selfgrowth.com/articles/Kurland3.html. Downloaded July 16, 2009.

Lu, S. (Yun, Z., Trans.) (2006). *Combat techniques of taiji, xingyi, and bagua*. Berkeley, CA: Blue Snake Books.

Olson, S. (1999). *T'ai chi thirteen sword: A sword master's manual*. Burbank, CA: Multi-Media Books.

Olson, S. (1999). *T'ai chi sensing-hands: A complete guide to t'ai chi t'ui-shou training from original Yang Family records*. Burbank, CA: Multi-Media Books.

Olson, S. (1992). *The teachings of master T.T. Liang: Imagination becomes reality, the complete guide to the 150-posture solo form*. St. Paul, MN: Dragon Door Publications.

Russell, J. (2004). *The tai chi two-person dance: Tai chi with a partner*. Berkeley, CA: North Atlantic Books.

Sheridan, J. (1977). *China in Disintegration: The Republican Era in Chinese history 1912–1949*. New York: The Free Press.

Schurmann, F. and Schell, O. (1967). *Republican China: Nationalism, war, and the rise of Communism 1911–1949*. New York: Vintage Book.

Wakeman, F. (1977). *The fall of imperial China*. New York: The Free Press.

Wile, D. (1996). *T'ai-chi touchstones: Yang family secret transmissions*. Brooklyn, NY: Sweet Chi Press.

Xiong Yanghe Photographs

As part of its goal to maintain cultural records, Taiwan's National Digital Archives Program (see www.ndap.org.tw) has digital photographs of Xiong Yanghe in the collection which can be viewed in thumbnail and large format (view at http:/ digitalarchives.tw).

• 54 •
Throwing Techniques in the Internal Martial Arts:
An Elucidation of the Guiding Principle of 'Sticking & Following'
by Tim Cartmell, B.A.

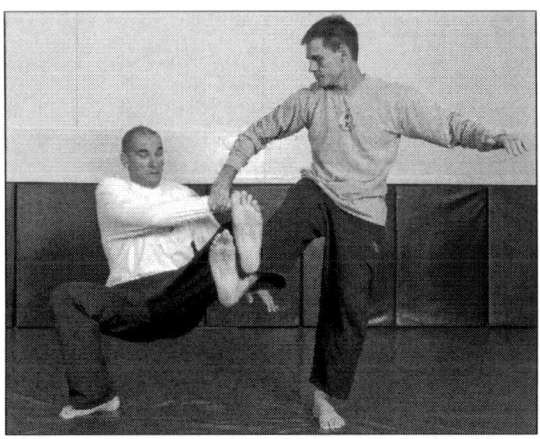

Jake Burroughts, left, and the author practicing techniques using the principles of sticking and following. All photographs by Dana Benjamin.

Abstract

This article explains the key concepts of "sticking and following" as they apply to the throwing methods of the Chinese internal martial arts. The concepts are defined, explained and illustrated with practical examples of sample techniques from each of the three orthodox internal styles: xingyiquan, taijiquan and baguazhang. The theory and application of sticking and following determine the strategy and mechanics of all internal arts techniques, as well as set the techniques of these styles apart from similar techniques in unrelated styles. An understanding of sticking and following provides direct insight into the essence of the Chinese internal martial arts.

Introduction

One could argue that throws are throws, no matter the style. All throws and takedowns are executed in fundamentally the same way. Excepting minor details in method, this assertion is true: there are only so many ways to put an opponent on the ground. All types of throws are based on leverage, manipulation of mass, removal of support, and the use of momentum and gravity. There are, however, some concrete differences in the ways throws are set up and executed in different styles. Among styles, the variation in throwing techniques is found in four broad areas: entries, grips, body method, and strategy of application. The Chinese internal styles have unique variations of common throws, based on a unique strategy of application.

Entries will primarily be determined by the ability or desirability of using striking techniques, the types of throws preferred, and the relative positioning of the fighters. The threat of strikes, type of clothing, uniform or lack thereof, and types of throws to be applied will be the primary determinate of the grips. The presence of weapons will also greatly influence the above variables, but we will limit this discussion to unarmed fighting. The thrower's body method (here we are most concerned with the methods of generating force, including mobility in footwork, level change, types of power and particular use of rhythm) will also greatly influence the types of throws used. Finally, the chosen strategy of application will have the greatest influence on throwing methods, including the types of entries and grips used, as well as the methods of generating force.

This article is concerned with the throws used in the three most popular styles of Chinese internal martial arts (CIMA), xingyiquan, baguazhang and taijiquan. The throws used in the CIMA are similar to comparable throws found in other styles and are heavily influenced by *shuaijiao* (Chinese wrestling). What makes the throwing methods of the CIMA styles unique is their emphasis on the principle of "sticking and following." Sticking and following can be viewed as the underlying strategy of the entire throwing method of all three internal styles, and is therefore the strongest influence on the entries, grips and body method used.

Sticking and Following

The name "sticking and following" (*zhannian / liansui*) is used to describe a united strategic concept of technical application in the CIMA. Although most often associated with the various arts of taijiquan, the principle applies to the other internal styles as well. A central tenet of the internal styles is the avoidance of the use of force directly against a stronger force. The corollary to this tenet is the concept of "borrowing force," that is, using an attacker's force to one's advantage. The means of borrowing an opponent's force is realized within the skills of sticking and following. The stick and follow skill set is so important the CIMA have evolved a number of specific training exercises designed exclusively to foster the skill (variations of the popular "push hands" practice being the most recognizable). The concept of sticking and following evolved from the most basic paradox of personal combat, how to develop a method that allows a smaller and weaker man to defeat a heavier and stronger opponent.

Let's go into the definition of the terms "stick" and "follow" as they apply to the CIMA. "Sticking" implies a consistency of contact, and by extension, contact from which the opponent cannot escape. Imagine fly paper stuck to your hand that passively thwarts all effort to shake it off. Or for a more universal image, imagine walking in a pool. No matter the direction you move, the water yields to your advance without losing contact while following your advance without the slightest gap in pressure. It is impossible to escape the ubiquitous and constant contact pressure of the water, yet the nature of the water is "passive." Similarly, the Internal fighter's contact with his opponent is "passive" in the sense of non-opposition of the opponent's force. To "stick" is not the same as to resist. The constant adherence to the opponent is made active when the concept of "following" is included as well. Although the internal fighter seeks to maintain constant contact without opposition of force, he must also actively follow the opponent to maintain contact while seeking the most advantageous position.

Another way of understanding sticking and following is through the idea of "filling in the gaps." Wherever there is space, the Internal fighter enters to fill the gap. A very important part of filling in the gaps is the amount of surface area covered. In general, the more surface area one is able to contact, the more control and potential for power one will have. For example, you would have exponentially more control over an opponent if you wrapped your arms around him and pulled him tightly against you in a body lock (bear hug) as opposed to holding his wrist with your fingertips at arm's length. In most cases, the more surface area of your body in contact with the opponent (from a superior position) the more control you will have, the less effort you will need to effect your technique, and the less likely your opponent will be able to escape or counter.

Finally, it is very important to realize sticking and following can and should be done with any and all parts of your body. Not only the arms and legs, but all parts of the torso and even the head can be used to maintain contact, control the opponent and issue force where appropriate. Many times, potentially successful throws are thwarted by a lack of committed contact or gaps in pressure. Space you are not controlling is space your opponent can use to escape.

Entries

Obviously, it is impossible to throw an opponent without making contact, and contrary to striking techniques, contact must be of a continuous duration at least until the throw is completed. How best to make contact and set up the throw is the subject of entries. Entering into and setting up a technique will be determined by several variables, including the combination of throws with striking techniques, the particular set of techniques to be applied, and opportunities based on the combatants reactions and relative positions. Leaving aside sport fights with specific rules, entering into a throw in an actual fight will have as a primary consideration the safety of the fighter as he enters. For the purposes of this article, we'll assume the CIMA fighter is facing a ready and capable opponent, face on, in a hands up fight.

In general, all-in fights will begin with blows before the fighters close to grappling range. Although many confrontations start with attempts at grabbing or begin from extreme close range before strikes are thrown, being struck is always a concern at any range. The strategic preference for the CIMA styles is close range. It is important to note that being at close range doesn't preclude striking but will always include wrestling. The internal fighter not only wants to get close; he wants to get close and obtain a superior position as efficiently as possible ("superior positions" are those which provide a great margin of safety from blows and allow one to apply most or all of one's body power with superior leverage). At its most basic level, this involves avoiding being stuck or ending up in an inferior position.

From the point of view of a fighter, fights will start in one of two ways; either you will take the offensive and attack first, or your opponent will attack first, and you will react defensively. There is a popular stereotypical idea that internal styles are "soft" and internal stylists prefer to wait passively while an opponent attacks first in order to take advantage of his force. This is not true. While it is absolutely necessary to learn how to deal with incoming aggressive force while reacting defensively, this is not preferred. The preferred strategy of entry is to attack first, causing the opponent to react and then using his reaction to one's own advantage. The fighter who acts and continues to act maintains an advantage over the fighter who is forced to continually react. One simply cannot win a fight while on defense.

With our strategy of preemptive attack in mind, let's look at the specifics of entries. Because of the threat of blows, the internal fighter in general will not simply charge directly in to obtain grips. Rushing in towards a ready opponent leaves one too vulnerable to being struck. Even the popular and effective strike high, level change and shoot for the legs strategy popular in MMA is not seen in CIMA entries. Again, the threat of being struck (or cut if the opponent is armed) disallows this type of entry from the CIMA repertoire. When facing an opponent whose hands are up and ready to fight, the CIMA fighter needs to make contact, control or clear the opponent's hands, and obtain contact in a superior position. In order to make first contact and force the opponent to react, the CIMA fighter prefers to attack with strikes or a combination of feints and strikes to elicit a response from the opponent, and will enter into a superior position as the situation allows. Another important point of strategy is that the CIMA fighter will seek to maintain continuous pressure and contact after initial contact is made, conforming to the master strategy of sticking and following.

Grips

The term "grips" is used here is the broad sense of contact with an opponent and is not limited to grasping with the hands. The configuration of contact and the amount of control it affords will directly determine the particular throwing technique that is appropriate to the situation. Fights are dynamic, and points of contact will change as the fight goes on. The strategy of the CIMA fighter is to continually seek greater and greater control. Application of Sticking and Following is crucial to success in obtaining, maintaining and improving control. As mentioned above, the more surface area of one's body that is in contact with an opponent, in a superior position, the greater the degree of control over the opponent, and the less overall effort needed to apply a technique. The CIMA fighter will train to use all parts of his body to connect with and apply force to an opponent. One point of interest is that, in contrast to most Western styles of wrestling, CIMA techniques rarely include locking the hands together. Although locking one's hands together in a closed grip may provide a stronger static hold, the principle of Sticking and

Following is better served with the hands free to move independently of one another.

From the instant of initial contact, the CIMA fighter seeks to maintain contact and pressure, while ever seeking to improve position and control. This calls for a type of "dynamic gripping" that allows the fighter to maintain contact pressure while not being stuck to a single place. The general flow of pressure is inward toward the opponent's center of gravity, and sometimes tangentially to turn or pull the opponent's center of gravity. The goal is control. Most CIMA throwing techniques will be completed from body-to-body contact, attempting to throw an opponent with wrist or elbow control alone is seen comparatively less (it should be noted that joint locking techniques (*qinna*) applied to the extremities will often result in a fall, but this is a secondary effect of their primary purpose of breaking or dislocating a joint).

Body Method

All types of martial arts have evolved specific methods of developing power. Without power, there is no "martial art." The way a martial artist develops and applies power is generally referred to as "body method" (*shen fa*). Body method will include the movements of the torso and limbs, displacement through space (including footwork and level change) and the rhythm of the body as a whole. The types of power developed are primarily determined by the strategy of application of technique. When creating methods of developing power, it is only logical to work backward from the goal to its means of completion. Since the goal of any martial discipline worthy of the moniker "art" is to impart a method that allows the weaker to defeat the stronger, the body method of the CIMA is, by necessity, based on the principle of sticking and following.

Most throws are very similar in terms of mechanics. For a specific throw to be executed efficiently, fulcrums must be placed in the correct place and power must be applied in the right direction. These fundamental conditions cannot be altered if the throw is to "work" in an efficient manner. How a fighter moves into position and how he develops power will differ however, and these differences in body method will show the most pronounced variance between the CIMA and other styles of martial art.

Let's take a more in-depth look at the body method of Chinese internal martial arts. Although there is some variation in the methods of movement and force development, some principles of body movement remain constant among the various CIMA styles (these principles are not exclusive to CIMA however and can be found in a number of other martial styles). First and foremost, all styles of CIMA place a heavy emphasis on developing "whole body power" (*zheng ti jing*). Whole body power refers to generating force with the strongest muscles of the body, radiating this force outward through the torso and extremities while each successive part of the body contributes to and magnifies the force until it is issued outward into the target. Inherent in the concept is the idea of using the weight of one's entire body mass as much as possible. The strongest muscles of the body, and the muscles primarily concerned with the initial and most powerful generation of force all have one end attached to the pelvis. Whole body power originates from there. To generate and magnify force from the center outward, force must move in a wave-like fashion. Since all points of a wave have force, any part of the body may be used to apply force to the opponent. This facet of the body method is very important to the CIMA fighter's ability to stick and follow his opponent with any part of his body. This is a clear example of the principle of sticking and following dictating the type of body method necessary to apply CIMA techniques successfully.

Strategy

As discussed above, in order to qualify as a martial "art" the guiding principle of development must be the creation of strategies and techniques that provide a method for the smaller and weaker fighter to overcome the larger and stronger. The first principle that emerges from this demand is the futility of opposing a stronger force directly with a weaker force. It is often said in regard to CIMA technique that one should never use "force against force." This is incorrect. Force will always be applied against some resistant force, even in the absence of conscious resistance on the part of an opponent, it will still be necessary to overcome the inherent resistance of the opponent's weight, no matter how mechanically efficient the technique. It should be properly stated that force should never be used directly against a greater force. If your own force is sufficient to overcome the resistant force of an opponent, your force can be efficiently applied, even if the opponent resists. Sticking to an opponent by its very nature requires that some level of force must be constantly applied, like water flowing downstream, not necessarily attempting to overcome the opponent's force yet not retreating from any level of resistance. The ultimate goal is the application of one's total wholebody power toward a "dead angle" (*si jiao*), an angle from which the opponent cannot offer resistance.

This brings us to the next point; while sticking and following an opponent, what do we do when his resistant force becomes greater than our applied force? This study is found in the principle of "transformation" (*zhou hua*). The overall goal is to borrow the opponent's force and transform it into our own force. This principle in application can be seen in various forms, from the "push when pulled/ pull when pushed" concept popular in many throwing arts to more subtle methods of unbalancing and controlling the opponent that are barely noticeable until it is too late for him to counter. In taijiquan, this concept is referred to as "no letting go and no resistance" (*bu diu bu ding*). Simply stated, when the opponent's resistant force threatens to overcome your sticking force and cause you to become resistant to the point of rigidity, you yield to the force without disjoining at that specific point of contact. Conversely all other points of contact (or potential contact) continue to pressure in toward the opponent's center, ever seeking greater control. This is the combination of sticking and following in practical application.

One other result of the sticking and following strategy is the goal of closing the distance and entering into clinch range as soon as practically possible. The longer the CIMA fighter stays in a neutral position, toe-to-toe for example, the greater the possibility he will be struck or taken down. In real fights in general, prolonged exchanges are not a good idea, and one should seek to end the fight or escape danger as quickly as possible. Whether the CIMA fighter uses the preferred strategy and initiates with an attack, or the opponent attacks and he is forced to defend, the CIMA fighter will seek to maintain contact and pressure on the opponent as he seeks a superior angle, more contact and greater control. So important is the strategy of closing in on an opponent that many of the drills found in the CIMA will start from the contact position, much less time is spent initiating attacks from long range. Here again, the various push hands drills so often emphasized in the internal styles are prime examples of the heavy emphasis on close range, close contact fighting.

BAGUAZHANG TECHNIQUES
Shoulder Throw
1a The fighters are on guard, the baguazhang fighter in grey.
1b Grey moves forward and attacks with a crashing palm strike. White defends with his right arm. The strike allows Grey to establish a connection with his opponent.

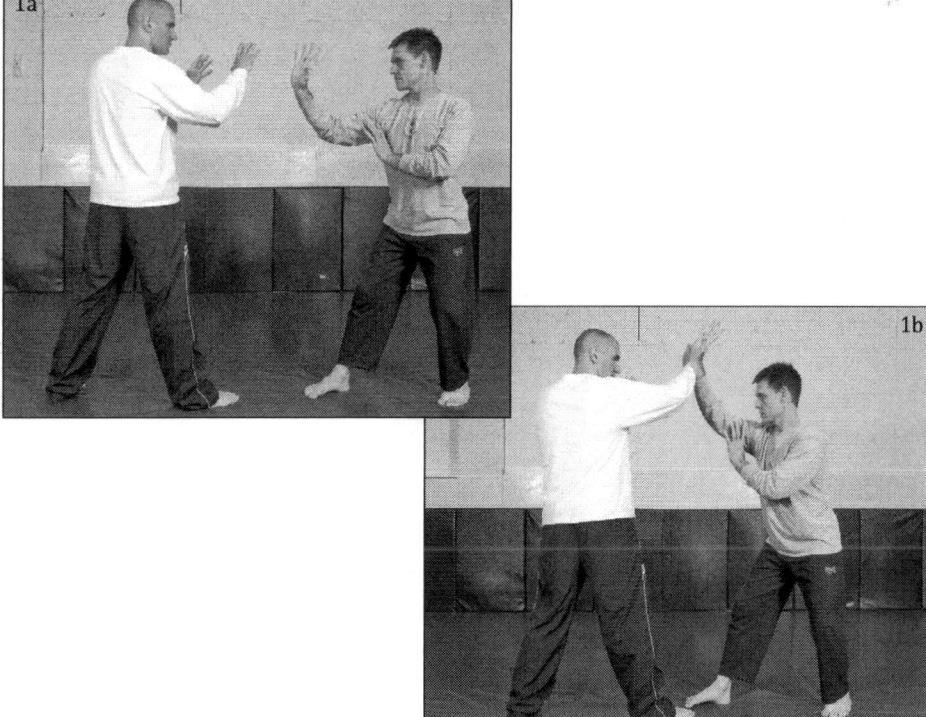

1c Maintaining contact and constant forward sticking pressure, Grey clears White's arm with his left arm and moves in with a right elbow strike.
1d As White deflects the elbow strike downward, Grey continues to follow White's movement and moves in with a shoulder strike to White's chest.
1e Maintaining pressure, Grey spins counterclockwise on his right foot and swings his left leg back as he pulls White's right arm tightly over his right shoulder. Grey lowers his hips below White's hips and contacts his entire back.
1f Grey shifts his weight forward and straightens his legs as he bows to throw White over his shoulder.
1g As White lands, Grey continues to stick and follow the movement maintaining control over his downed opponent.

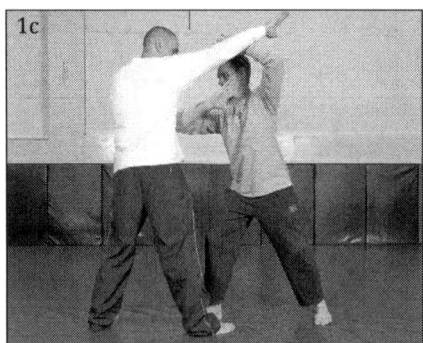
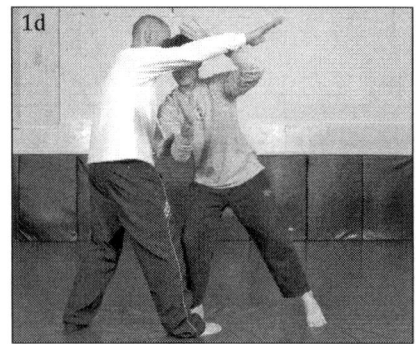
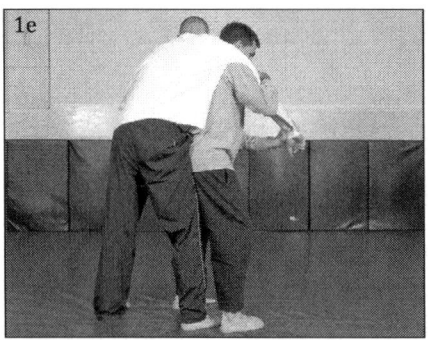
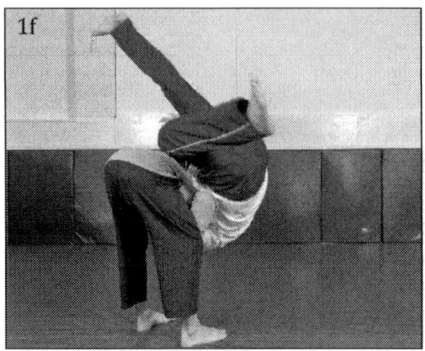
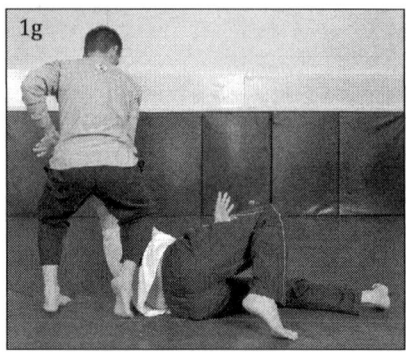

Follow-Up Technique: "T" Shape Shoulder Separation

2a White counters the throw by moving his hips back and pushing against Grey's lower back.

2b Maintaining his grips, Grey follows White's motion and turns with White's defensive force. Grey turns clockwise, sticks tightly to White's shoulder with his head and threads his right arm up from below White's arm. The force bends White's arm 90°.

2c Grey steps up with his left foot and grabs the top of his left wrist with his right hand, locking White's shoulder into his torso.

2d Maintaining his connection to White's center through the lock, Grey simply lowers his level, causing White to fall straight onto his back.

2e Grey continues sticking to White as he follows him to the ground. Grey drops his right knee onto White's side to control his torso as he twists White's upper arm counterclockwise to dislocate the shoulder.

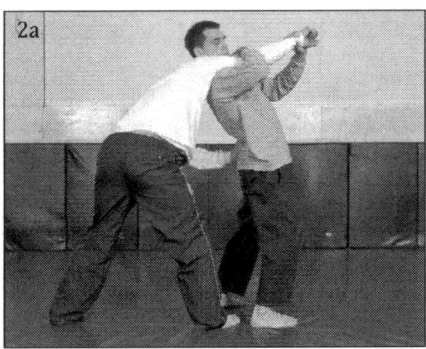 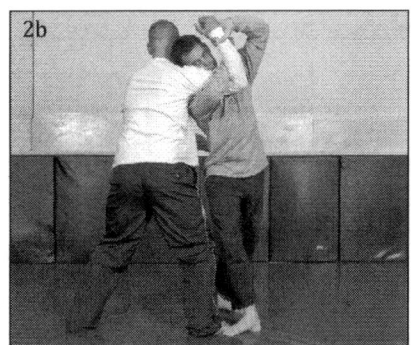

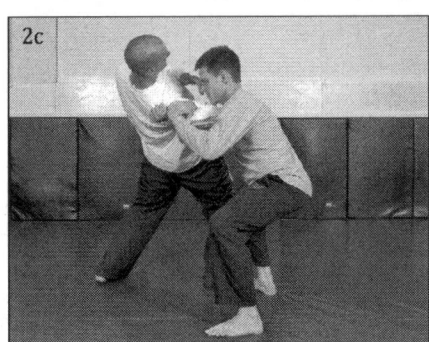 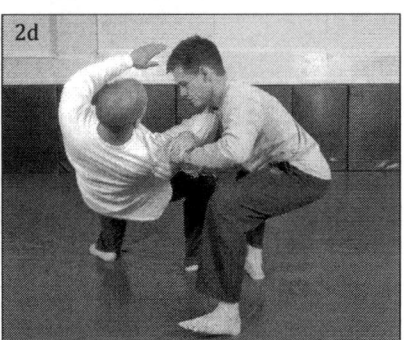

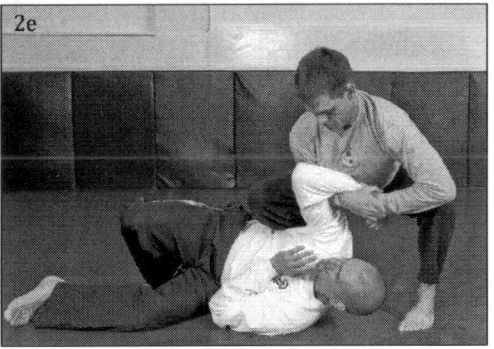

Baguazhang "Ban" Eyebrow Mopping

3a The fighters come to the on-guard position.

3b White attacks with a right straight punch. Grey responds by slipping to his left and covering his head with his right arm as the punch goes by.

3c Turning to his right, Grey maintains his initial contact and wraps his right arm over the top of White's right arm. At the same time, Grey strikes White in the right side of the head with a left backhand palm strike. Grey maintains contact after the strike and adheres to the side of White's head.

3d Grey pushes White's head in a counterclockwise circle as he lowers his weight, causing White to arch over backward.

3e Grey continues the downward spiraling pressure and brings White to the ground.

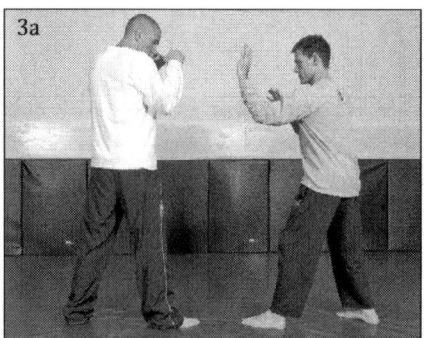
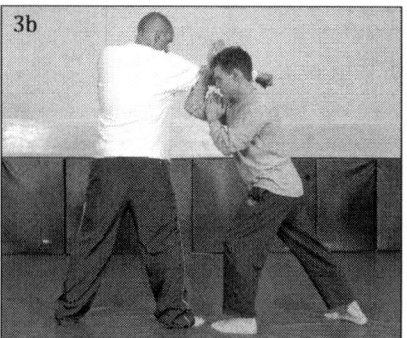
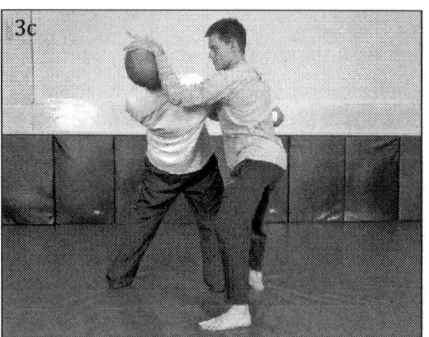
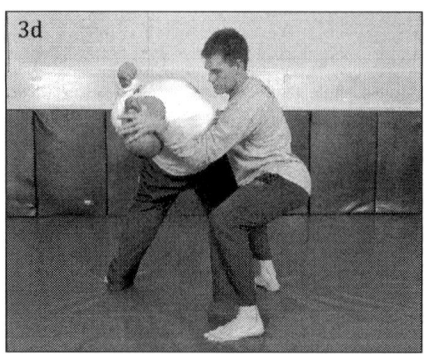
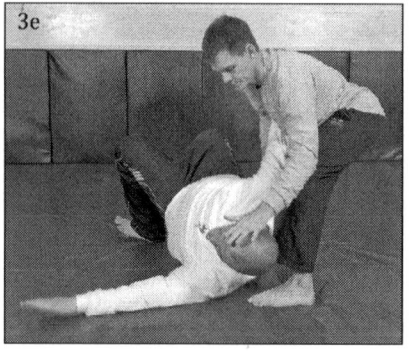

Follow-Up Technique: "Kua" Hip Throw

4a White counters the eyebrow mop by turning his head and pulling his right arm back.

4b White continues to escape by pulling his right arm free and stepping back with his right leg. Grey follows White's motion and sticks to his right arm with his left palm. Grey simultaneously steps up with his right foot and under hooks White's left arm with his right. Note that Grey has maintained constant forward, sticking pressure with is whole body.

4c Continuing his forward pressure, Grey steps forward with his right foot and turns his hips counterclockwise below White's hips. Grey simultaneously pulls White's right arm down to break his posture.

4d Grey shifts his weight forward, straightens his legs and bows to throw White over his right hip.

4e White lands at Grey's feet.

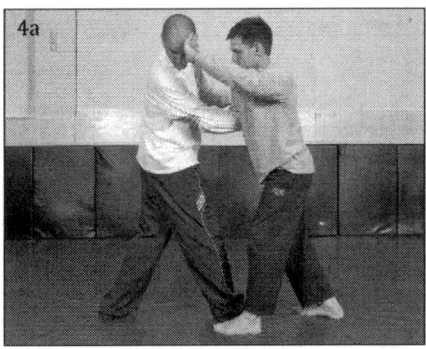
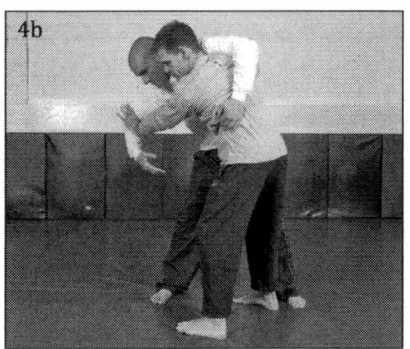
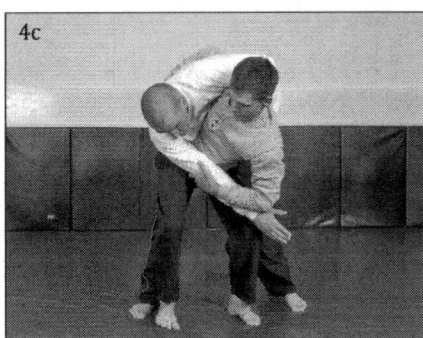
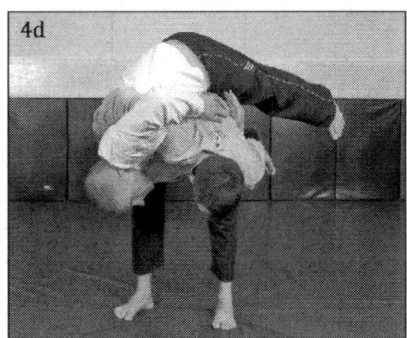
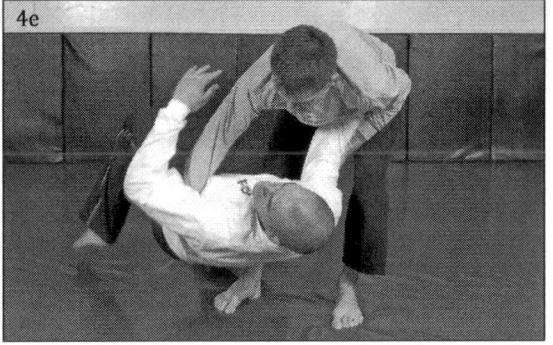

Xingyiquan Techniques

"Open the Window to View the Moon" Takedown

5a The fighters square off.

5b White begins to launch a right hook at Grey's head. Grey immediately responds by driving forward as he covers his head with his right arm in the "Tiger Hugs its Head" position.

5c Intercepting White's force early, Grey drives his elbow into White's chest.

5d Maintaining his sticking pressure, Grey moves in and wraps his right arm across the front of White's chest, trapping White's right arm to prevent a possible counterattack. It is important to note Grey uses his position and momentum to begin to displace White's hips toward White's right.

5e Continuing to stick to White with his whole body, Grey turns clockwise and begins to lower his level as he grabs outside White's right knee to prevent

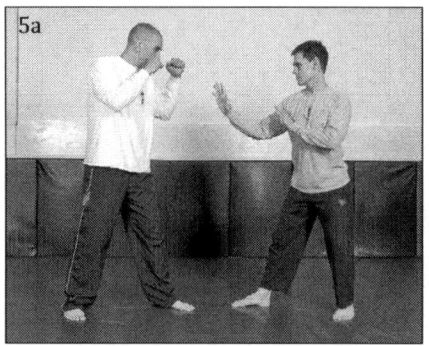
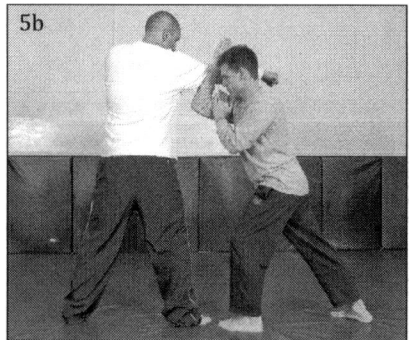
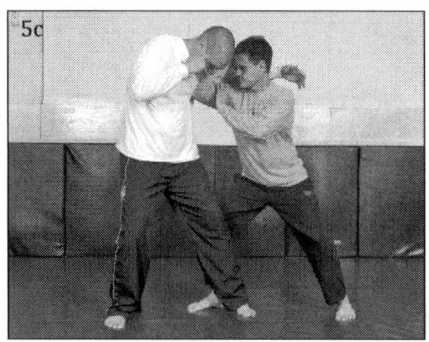
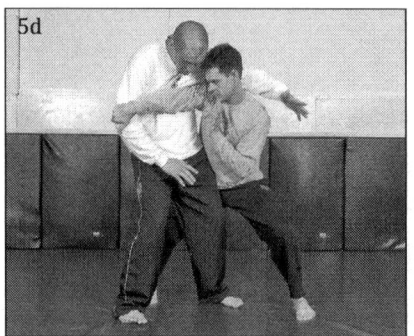
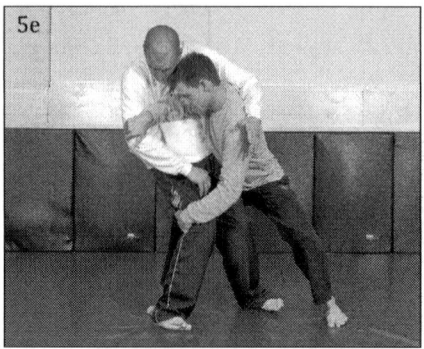
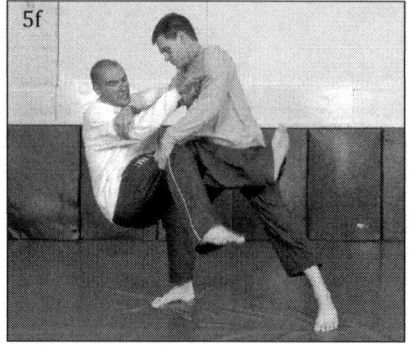

White's escape.

5f Grey completes the takedown by driving through White and throwing him to his rear. The throw is affected with the sticking pressure of Grey's entire body as he displaces White completely off his base.

Follow-Up Technique: "Wing Blows the Lotus Leaves" Foot Sweep

6a White escapes the "Open the Window to View the Moon" takedown by shuffling away as Grey enters.

6b Grey maintains control by following White's motion while sliding his right hand down White's right forearm to catch his wrist.

6c Grey now pulls White's wrist to his left rear as he simultaneously sweeps White's left foot forward.

6d White falls on his back.

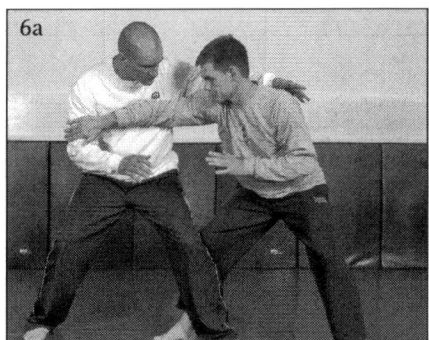
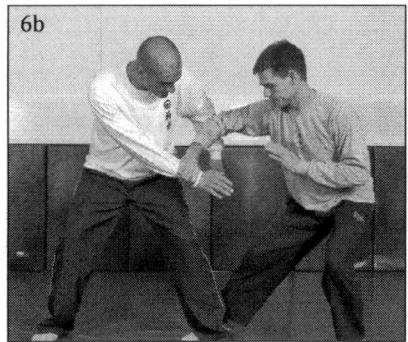
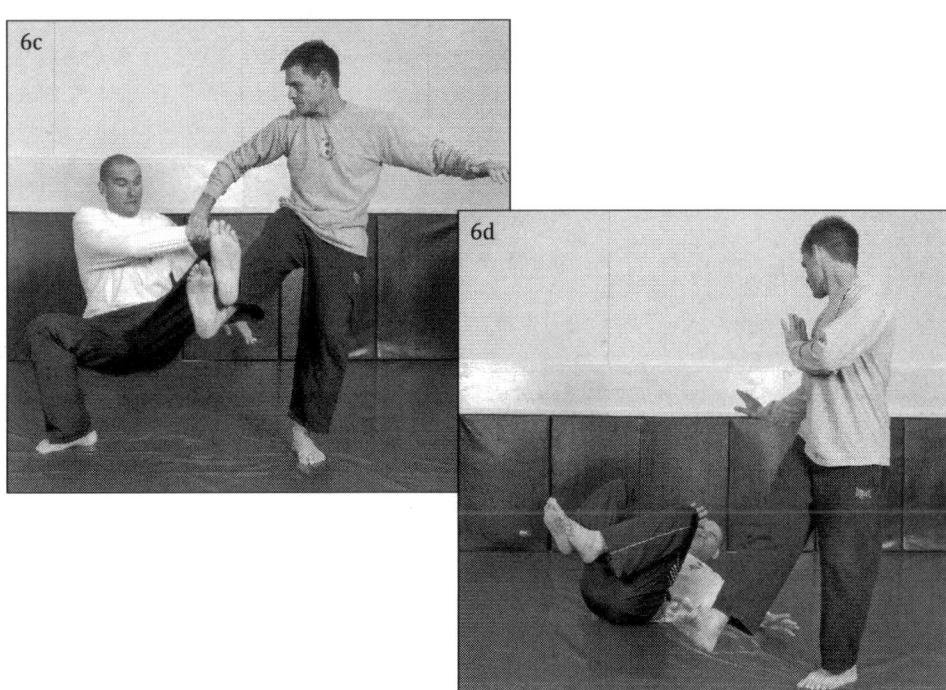

Monkey Technique

7a The fighters square off.

7b White throws a left straight punch. Grey slips the punch to the outside and simultaneously checks White's arm as he palms White in the face. Notice Grey has moved his body in as close as possible and sticks to White with his arms and chest.

7c Maintaining contact with his left hand, Grey slides his hand around to the back of White's neck and pulls down on his head as he simultaneously knees White in the ribs. Note that Grey also has his chest adhering to White's left side.

7d Continuing the downward pull on Grey's head, Grey lowers his left foot, turns his body counterclockwise and leans his body weight into White. Grey immediately presses his right hip into White's left hip and slides his right leg between White's legs. As he steps in, Grey wraps his right arm around the back of White's left leg.

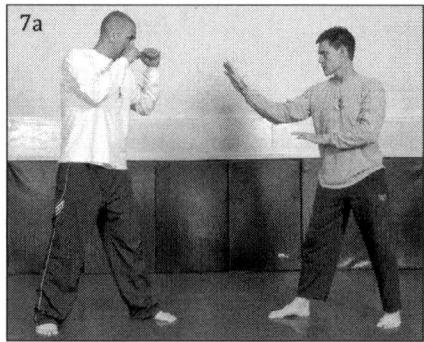

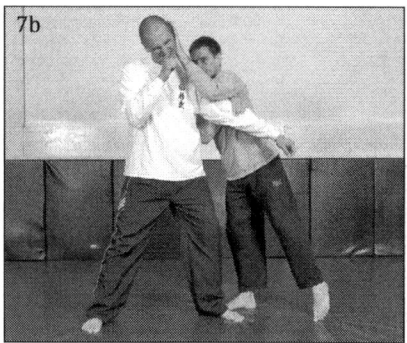

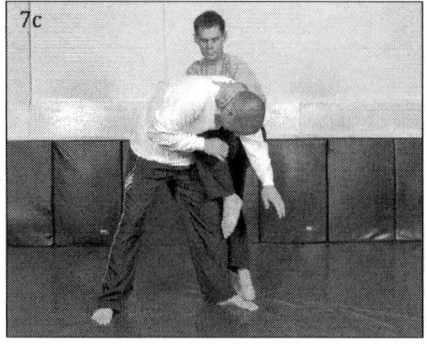

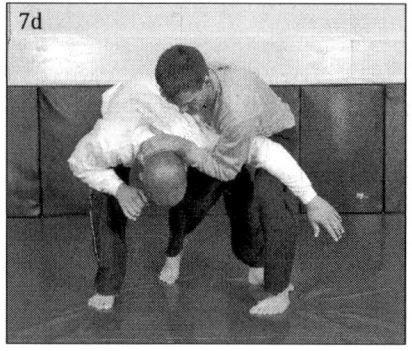

7e Grey continues turning counterclockwise as he pulls down on White's head while lifting his leg. White is flipped over forward. This technique is an illustration of the sticking and following method applied when strikes and throws are used in combination. There is never a loss of contact as the Internal fighter flows between percussive, grappling, and throwing techniques.

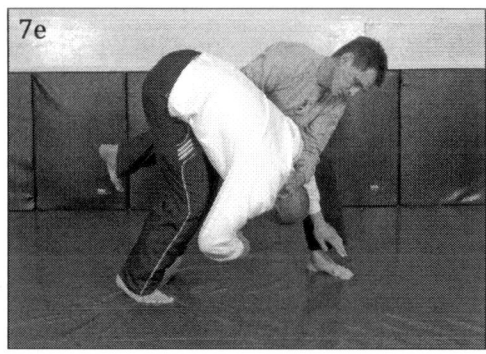

TAIJIQUAN TECHNIQUES

Zhaobao Taijiquan "Lazy About Tying Clothes" Takedown

8a The fighters are in the on guard position.
8b Grey initiates the encounter and moves forward with a right palm strike. White defends with his right arm.

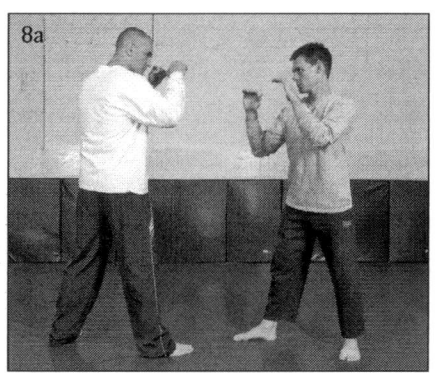

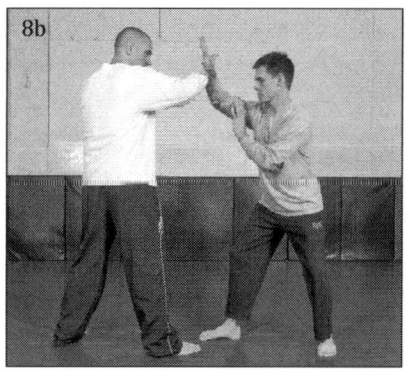

8c Maintaining contact, Grey grabs White's right wrist and "plucks" his arm downward, passing the arm underneath his left armpit. Grey then wraps up White's right arm as he steps forward with his left foot. Notice Grey has made contact with his shoulders and chest.

8d Grey now turns counterclockwise and pulls White off-balance with his body weight. Grey simultaneously slides his right palm up the front of White's chest as he rotates his hips clockwise, pressing the back of his right hip into the back of White's right hip while Grey's right leg moves behind White's right leg.

8e Grey displaces White's hips with his own as he turns counterclockwise and lowers his weight.

8f Grey continues the motion and pushes White's unstable body to the ground with his right hand.

8g Grey follows White down and maintains control.

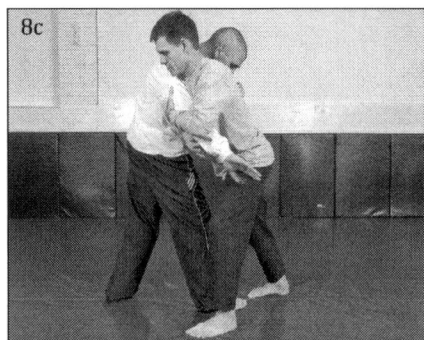
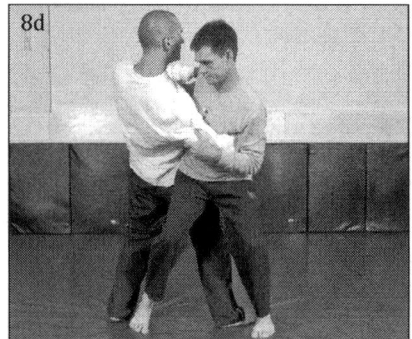
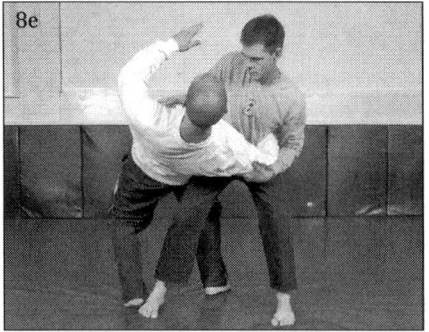
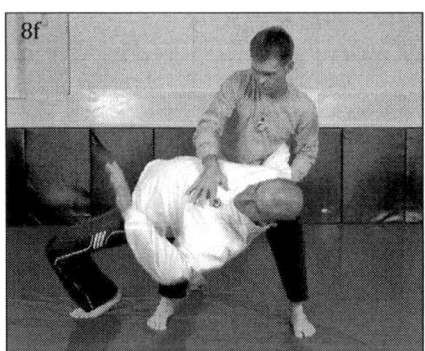
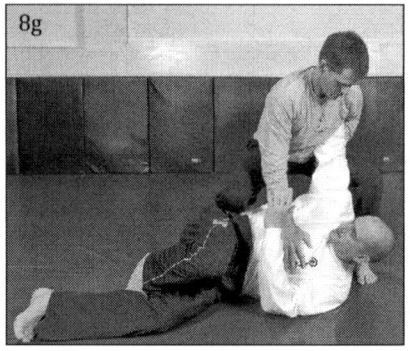

Follow-Up Technique

9a Grey steps behind White for the "Lazy About Tying Clothes" takedown.

9b White escapes the throw by stepping back with his right foot. Grey follows White's motion and sticks to him with his upper body.

9c Turning counterclockwise, Grey shuffles his left foot forward and pulls White's right arm to his left and down with his body weight as he begins to step back between White's legs with his right leg.

9d Maintaining his upper body connection, Grey sags his weight downward and begins to sit back over his right leg. Notice Grey has wrapped White's left lower leg behind his knee.

9e Grey sits back into White's left leg. The pressure against the inside of White's knee causes him to fall backward.

9f The throw is completed as White lands on his back.

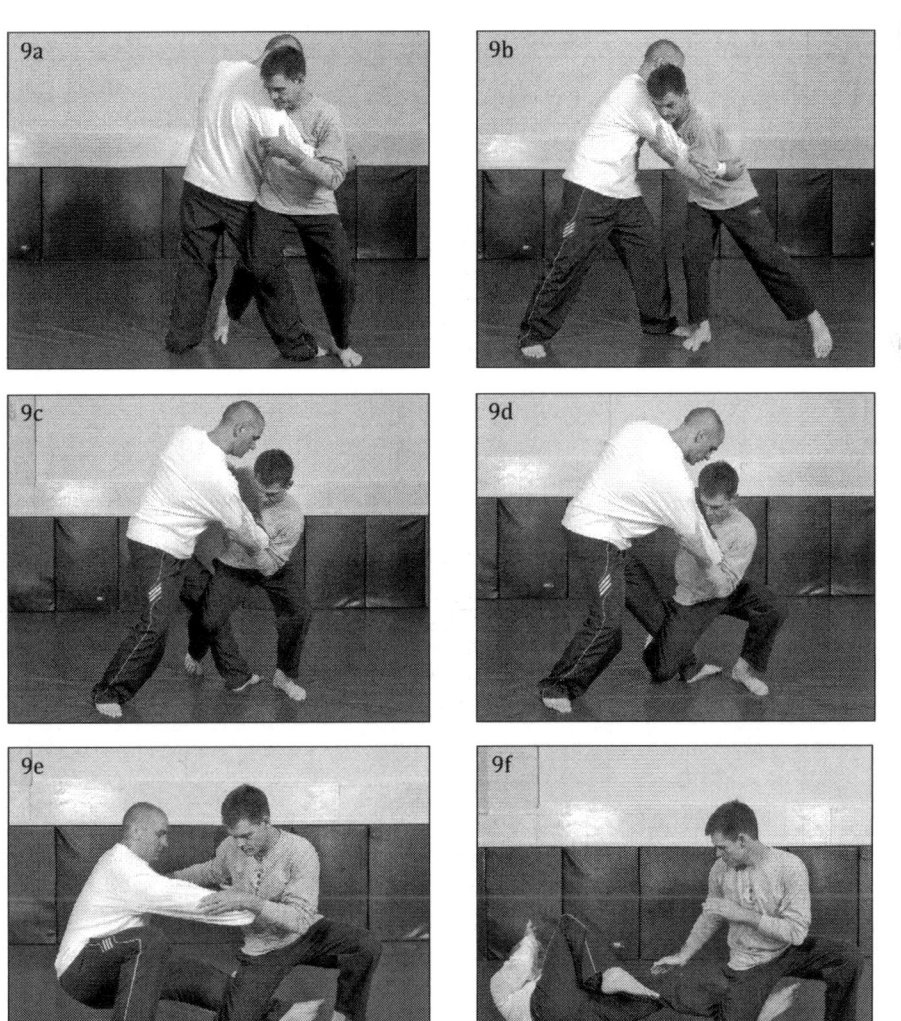

Zhaobao Taijiquan "Jin Gang Pounds the Pestle" Takedown

10a The fighters face off.

10b White attacks with a right straight punch. Grey slips outside the punch and deflects the blow with the rollback movement.

10c Shifting his weight forward, Grey sticks to White's arm and kicks him on the knee with his right foot.

10d The kick causes White to move backward. Following White's motion, Grey steps his right foot down and immediately step his left foot deep behind White's base. As he steps in, Grey simultaneously lowers his weight and uses his body pressure to press White's right arm down into his side. Grey now hooks his left hand around the inside of White's left leg, preventing him from stepping back.

10e Continuing to stick to and follow White, Grey slides his left hand down inside White's right knee and pressures forward into White. Grey displaces White's

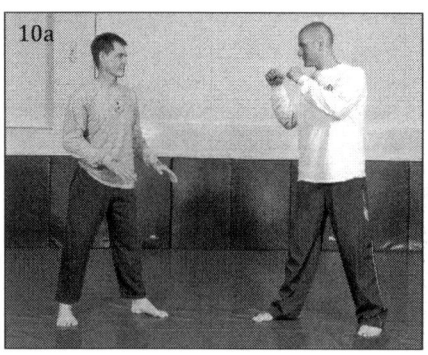
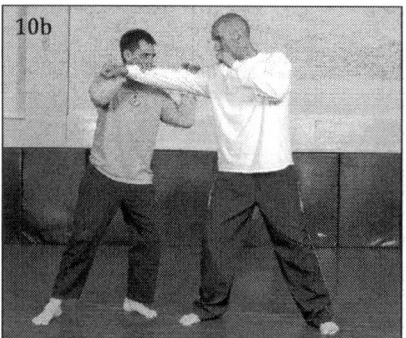
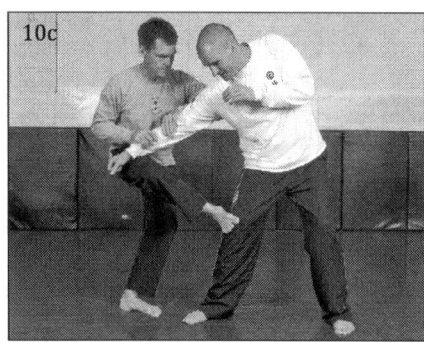
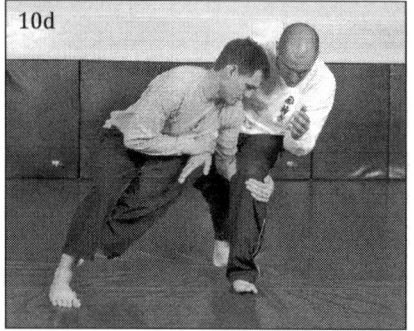
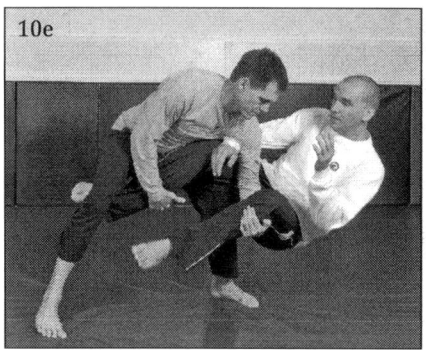
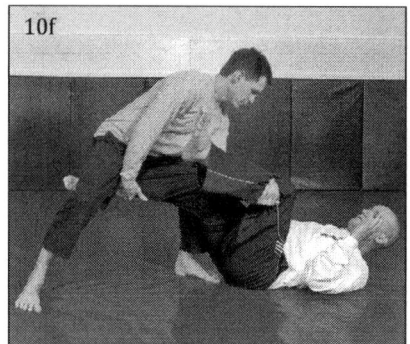

body with his own while fixing his legs in place. White flies off his base.
10f White lands on his back.

Follow-Up Technique: "Brush Knee Angled Walk" Takedown
11a Grey is attempting the "Jin Gang Pounds the Pestle" takedown.
11b White counters the throw by freeing his left leg and stepping away.
11c Following White's motion, Grey adheres to the inside of White's right leg with his left arm.
11d Turning counterclockwise a little, Grey begins to push White's right knee back in a small clockwise circle. The angle of the pressure destabilizes White's posture.
11e Continuing the knee push, Grey drops his right knee inward to the ground, causing him to shift his weight to his left and through White's right leg. White falls onto his back.

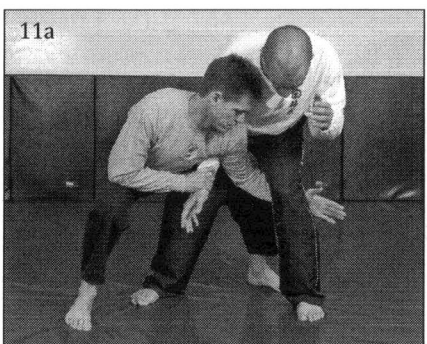
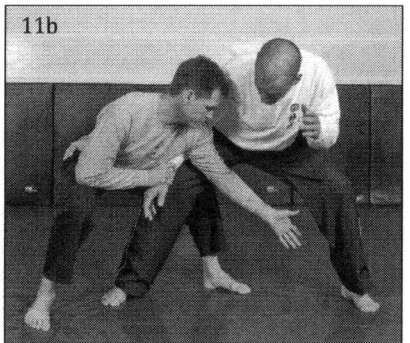
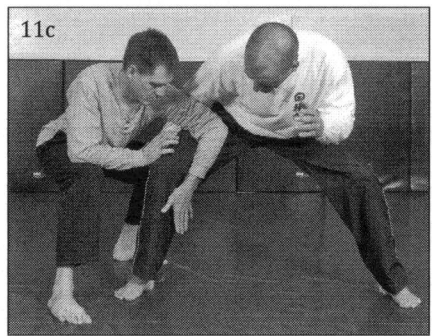
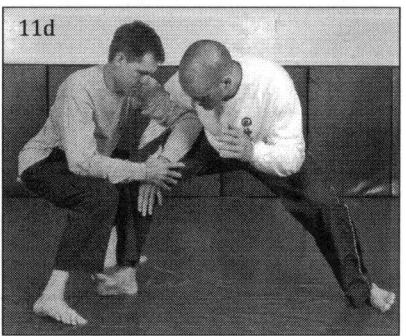
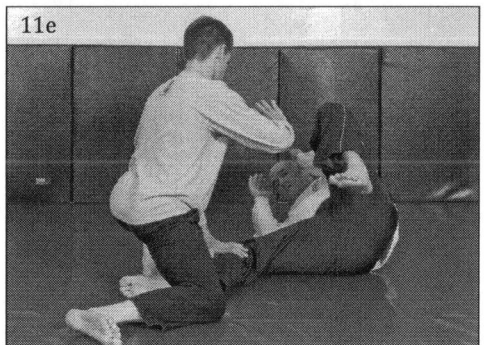

Conclusion

Collections of random techniques without a unifying body method and overall strategy of implementation cannot be considered martial arts. All legitimate martial arts are organized around core principles of force generation, strategy and technique. The so-called Chinese internal martial arts are grouped together into a common "family" precisely because they share a common strategy of application, and by necessity related methods of generating force. From the founding query of how a smaller and weaker man may defeat a larger and stronger man in hand-to-hand combat, the concept of sticking and following was born. Once this concept was realized, it acted as the catalyst for the creation of an overall strategy of technical application, as well as necessitating a particular body method or way of generating force. It is interesting to note that any specific technique or variation thereof that can be applied according to this strategy and conforming to this body method can be adopted into the internal styles. This fact makes possible a certain degree of creativity in technical inclusion without violating the fundamental principles that make CIMA individual arts, in the true sense of the word.

Acknowledgements

I'd like to thank Jake Burroughs for posing with me in the photos. Many thanks to Dana Benjamin for her excellent photography. I'd also like to thank Brian Johnson and the North West Jiu Jitsu Academy for the use of their facility.

Liu Xiheng: Memories of a Taiji Sage

by Benjamin Lo, Xu Yizhong, Yuan Weiming, Xu Zhengmei, and Danny Emerick[1] Compiled by Russ Mason, M.A.

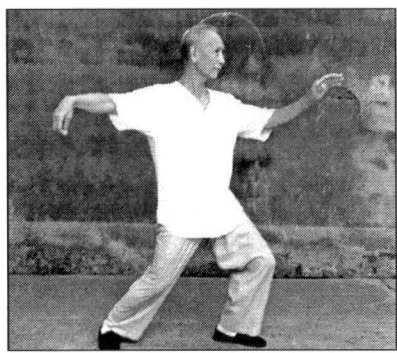

Liu demonstrates the single whip posture. Photo courtesy of Yuan Weiming.

General Introduction

Liu Xiheng's master, the late Professor Zheng Manqing, was a close disciple of Yang Chengfu in the 1930s[2] and was the scribe of Yang's 1934 book, *Essence and Applications of Taijiquan*.[3] Zheng is well known in America as a paragon of traditional Chinese arts and culture and, in particular, as the originator of the thirty-seven-posture short form of Yang Style taijiquan, which became popular here in the early 1960s and is still widely practiced. From the time of his arrival in the US until his passing in 1975, Professor Zheng worked to preserve and research traditional Chinese arts and to teach and interpret these treasures for westerners. In addition to being noted for his soft and effective skill in taijiquan push-hands (*tuishou*) and the use of the double-edged sword (*taiji jian*), Professor Zheng is remembered for his deep commitment to the transmission of the classical principles of taiji and to the practice of taijiquan, not only as a martial art, but also as a Dao of living and personal cultivation.[4]

Liu Xiheng was a living embodiment of this Dao of taijiquan. Left in charge of Zheng's Taibei Shizhong Study Society while "the Professor" was teaching in America (establishing what was known in English as the New York Shr Jung School), Liu did his best to carry forward his master's mission. Later, at the time of Zheng's passing, Liu was officially installed as head of the Taibei school, and he continued to serve in this capacity as head disciple and "gatekeeper" of the Zheng tradition in Taiwan from 1975 until his retirement in 1986.[5] After retirement, Liu settled down to a quiet, contemplative life as a Buddhist layperson, pursuing the practice of meditation and teaching a small, dedicated group of Chinese and international taijiquan students who met for practice first at his home in Taibei and later in parks and various nearby venues.

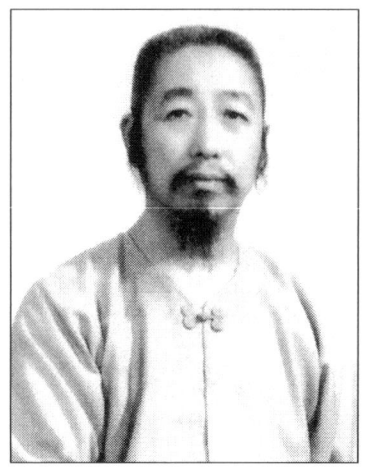 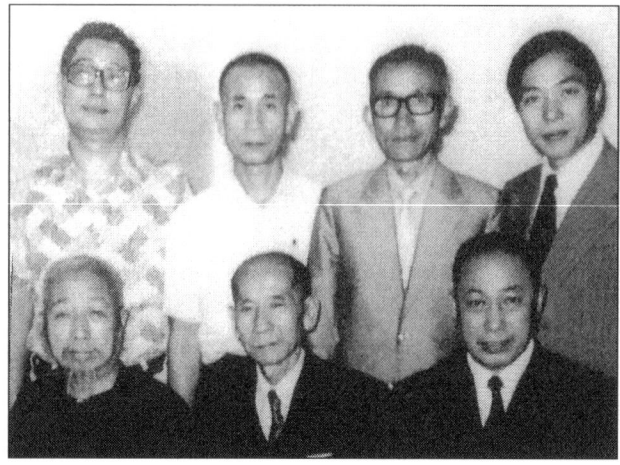

Left: Zheng Manqing. Right, first row, from left: Zheng Manqing, Mr. Hong (friend and legal advisor from Hong Kong), and Wang Yannian. Back row, from left: Mr. Yang (a lawyer friend), Liu Xiheng, Tao Bianxiang, and Xu Yizhong (current association president). Courtesy of Zheng Manqing Jinian Guan.

Although the field of martial arts is sometimes marred by ego and self-promotion, Liu worked quietly and modestly, honoring his master, nurturing students, and caring nothing for the limelight. A shining example of traditional *wude* (martial virtues or morality), Liu's humble character, diligence, and unimpeachable integrity were an inspiration to all who had the privilege of knowing him. Regarding martial applications, Liu's neutralizing and discharging skills in *tuishou* were marvelous to experience. Those who were fortunate enough to cross arms with Liu and to feel his gentle touch often came away shaking their heads in amazement over the apparently effortless ease with which he was able to neutralize and send attackers flying away.

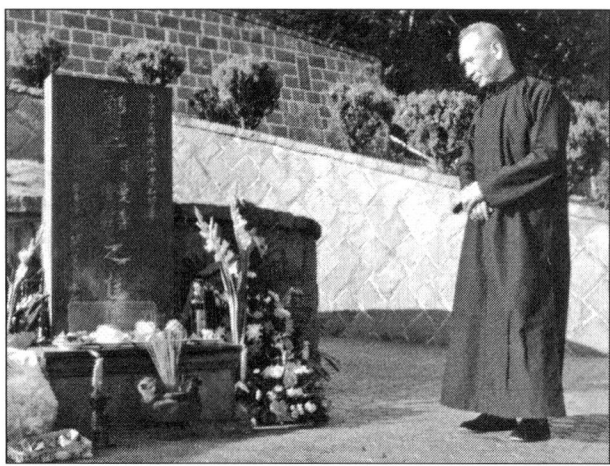 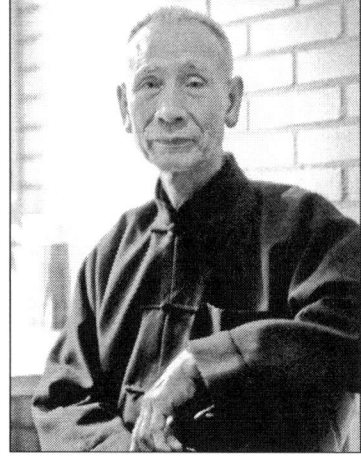

Liu pays his respects at Master Zheng's tomb;
Liu close-up. Photos courtesy of Yuan Weiming.

Liu often said softly and smilingly, "You must relax and eradicate every thought of using force. If you are not relaxed, you are crooked. If you are crooked, you are using force." And again, with twinkling eyes he urged, "We must learn to be tender, soft, and peaceful." Liu seasoned his conversation with frequent quotes from the *Classics* and from Professor Zheng: "The most important factors in taiji are honesty and sincerity, for without these qualities one can't advance."[6] Liu held that the essential thing was to apply the principles of taiji in daily life, to nurture character, and to grow as human beings in our care for others. For those who followed him, he was a living example of the Dao of taiji.

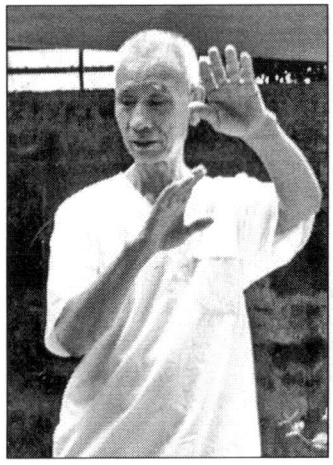
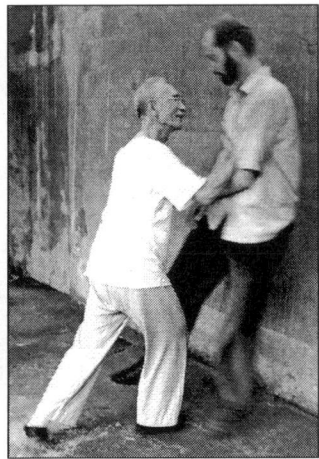
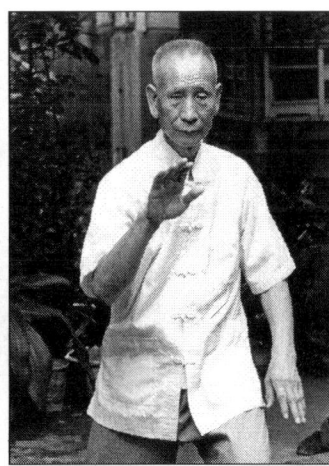

In the courtyard of his Taibei home, Liu demonstrates fair lady works at shuttles (left), brush knee (right), and uproots his student, Bill Tucker. Photos courtesy of Yuan Weiming.

Notes

[1] The first author is commonly known as Ben Lo or as Benjamin Pangjeng Lo. Because the pinyin romanization Luo Bangzhen is unfamiliar to the English-language audience, his pinyin romanization will not be used in this article, except for reference in the glossary. Likewise, the third author became known as "Yuan" Weiming due to a documentation error in the 1970s, when he came to the US for graduate studies. Pinyin spelling of his family name is "Ruan" and is given for reference in the glossary.

[2] A number of Professor Zheng's books and articles have been translated into English and much has been written about him. For more background information and for extensive bibliographies of relevant texts, see numerous *Journal of Asian Martial Arts* back issues (e.g., Davis, 1996; Davis and Mann, 1996; Mason, 2008; Mason, 2001; Smith, 1997; Smith, 1995; etc.), as well as books (e.g., Cheng and Smith, 1967; Cheng, 1950/1985; Lowenthal, 1991; Smith, 1974; Smith, 1999; Wile, 2007, etc.).

[3] See Louis Swaim's English translation of Yang's masterwork (Yang, 1934/2005). See also details of Zheng's collaborative role as Yang's disciple and scribe (e.g.,

Mason, 2008: 36; Mason, 2006: 92; Yang, 1988; Yang, 1993; Yang, 1934/2005: xi; and Yu and Sharp, 1993: 44–46).

4   For an exposition of Zheng's quest for a "unified Dao," see Davis (1996).
5   The sources of this biographical information are the compiler's personal conversations with Liu Xiheng and his disciples, as well as the compiler's own research and study in Taibei during visits to Southeast Asia in 1989–1990, 1998, and 2006. Although disinclined to make public statements, Liu did publish one article in a Kaohsiung periodical and, from time to time, articles and comments were published about him. A few of his lectures have been transcribed. For a fine sample of Liu's own views on taijiquan, see Rick Halstead's English translation of Liu's article, "The concept of central equilibrium in t'ai chi ch'uan," in *T'ai Chi Player* (Liu, 1985) and reprinted in *Taijiquan Journal* (Liu, 1985/2002). For more background information on Liu, see the excellent articles by Lin Farley (1986) and Bill Tucker (2008).
6   See Robert W. Smith's description of Liu (Smith, 1999: 313–314). For more quotations from Liu, see Lin Farley (1986).

Introduction to Benjamin Lo's Memorial Article

Benjamin Lo (Luo Bangzhen) is a well-known proponent of taijiquan and has taught in the United States for many years.[7] He became Zheng Manqing's first taijiquan student in Taiwan soon after Zheng's emigration from the Chinese mainland in 1949. As a teenager, Lo suffered from a serious neurological disorder. After seeking Zheng's services as a doctor of traditional Chinese medicine, he began his study of taijiquan as a part of his treatment. Within a few years, Lo had recovered his health and had made significant strides in taijiquan. In 1974, at Professor Zheng's suggestion, Lo traveled to America, settling in San Francisco, where he has taught taijiquan for thirty-six years.

The long-running and nationally prestigious A Taste of China event, founded in 1983 by Steve Rhodes and Pat Rice and held annually for more than twenty-five years in Winchester, Virginia, honored Lo and his pushing hands skill by naming its highest push-hands competition award (beginning in 1988) the Ben Lo Cup. The award was soon won by Lo's student, Lenzie Williams. For many years Lo has also served as a highly regarded association advisor for the Taibei Shizhong School, as well as for the Master Zheng Taijiquan Study Association, established in Taibei in 1993.

Within a year after Lo began his private taijiquan studies in Taiwan, Professor Zheng began teaching a public class, and Liu Xiheng was among the students in the first formal session. From that day in 1950, Liu and Lo developed a close relationship, not only as classmates and "brothers" in the same martial family, but also as friends. These two disciples greatly respected and faithfully served their teacher, Zheng Manqing,[8] and their warm personal friendship lasted almost six decades, up until Liu's passing in the spring of 2009.

Non-Chinese readers are encouraged to keep in mind that Mr. Lo's remarks (and those of the following three writers) were originally written and published in the context of Chinese culture and for a Chinese audience. This is an environment in which personal modesty is considered a great virtue, and its conventions of speech and writing are quite different from those of Western cultures. Therefore, meanings are sometimes difficult to translate, and subtle cultural implications can easily be lost. The compiler appreciates the reader's sensitivity to this issue in the presentation of the English translation. What follows is Mr. Lo's article.

Notes

[7] For an in-depth interview with Ben Lo exploring his views and personal history, see Davis and Mann (1996). Also see the essay entitled "Ben Lo: Modest man, true taiji" in Smith (1999: 294).

[8] Professor Zheng is reported to have once commented regarding these two outstanding and devoted students that Liu had inherited his "softness," and Lo his "fire." In other words, these two sincere disciples reflected the yin and yang elements of the master's taijiquan style respectively (Smith, 1999: 312).

——— ARTICLE 1 ———
In Memory of Brother Liu Xiheng
by Benjamin Lo • Written on April 30, 2009

On April 8 of this year (2009), I received an international call from Michael Schnapp, one of Brother Liu Xiheng's American students. He told me that Master Liu had passed away. On hearing the news, I was shocked. I had known Brother Liu Xiheng had been bedridden with sickness for some time. His initial condition was up and down, but it gradually went downhill to the point that he had to be cared for by his family because he could no longer take care of himself. However, I did not think it was that critical. I thought his condition was stable and that he would be with us for quite a while, so I was very surprised to hear that he had gone so abruptly. When I heard the bad news, I felt a surge of sorrow. I could not help but reminisce about our good times together, especially our early days in Taibei, and I reflected on our friendship as classmates for over sixty years. Like a movie, all the past seemed to flash through my mind, scene by scene.

I met Brother Liu in 1950, the year Master Zheng Manqing was invited by the mayor of Taibei, Mr. Yu Michien, to teach taiji and to promote traditional culture at Zhongshan Hall in Taibei. Brother Liu was one of the students of the first class. At the time, he was working at the executive office of the provincial food bureau, and I was just a freshman entering the National Taiwan University. There were about forty students in that taiji class. We practiced early every morning. Taiji was for him both a hobby and a means to get exercise. However, I began my study of taijiquan because of my poor health. For over a year, starting in 1948, I had been seeking medical help for my health but to no avail. The fact that I was young and yet in such poor health really worried me. At the end of 1949, when Master Zheng Manqing moved from Hong Kong to Taibei, my father took me to consult him. Master Zheng was an outstanding practitioner of traditional Chinese herbal medicine and had been the chairman of the National Chinese Medical Association in mainland China, in addition to being a professor of painting and other fine arts. His high position bespeaks his excellent medical qualifications. With the aid of his herbal prescription, my health had improved gradually, but Professor Zheng had also advised me to build up the strength of my body. In other words, he felt that I needed to practice taiji to boost my immunity. Motivated to regain my health and at the order of my physician, I plunged passionately into the practice of taijiquan without hesitation. In those early days, before the founding of his official school at Zhongshan Hall in Taibei, I practiced at Professor Zheng's private residence. Naturally, when he began teaching publicly, I also joined that first class to continue my practice and, there, I met Brother Liu Xiheng. After practicing taiji for a time, my health improved, and I have never stopped practicing since. When we had completed the whole session of the first class, some students signed up for the second class and, in addition, routinely met to practice on Sundays at Professor Zheng's house. Brother Liu was among those who never missed a practice session. Under the guidance of Master Zheng we practiced *tuishou* (push-hands). From then on, the Sunday gathering became our tradition no matter where Zheng lived. First, we met at Professor's old house in Xindian City (Hsintien), then at his home on Ren Ai Road, Section 3 in Taibei, and later in Yonghe City. Each and every time we met, we would spend many hours practicing till everyone was drenched with sweat, and then we would happily go our separate ways to our homes. This tradition ended only when Master Zheng moved to the USA. However, whenever Professor Zheng returned to Taiwan for a visit, the tradition would immediately resume.

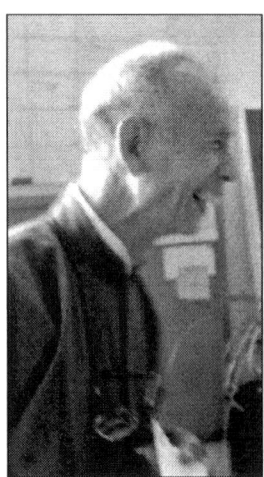 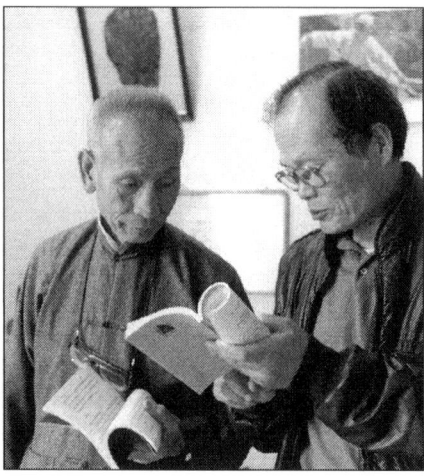 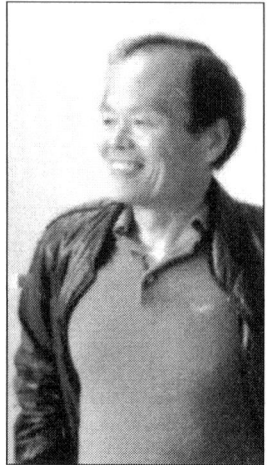

Liu and Lo examine a text under a photo of Professor Zheng and share a lighthearted moment. Photos courtesy of Yuan Weiming.

Time flies, and only a few of the students from that first class still survive today. As I now write these words, I feel a deep sense of the truth of the proverb that "time waits for no man." Although I am now old, I can't escape the feeling that my own efforts have amounted to nothing.

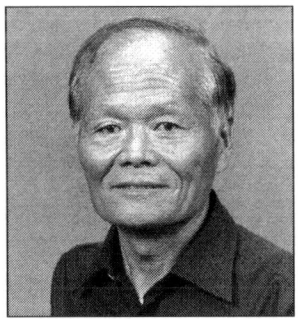

Ben Lo. Courtesy of B. Lo.

In 1953 I graduated from college. When I passed the civil service exam run by the government, I was assigned to work in the provincial government office. Fortunately, the office was located in Taibei, and did not affect my practice routine with Brother Liu. Sometimes after our Sunday practice at Professor's house, a few of us fellow students would lunch together and continue our discussion, sharing our thoughts and describing how we felt when we pushed hands with Professor Zheng. Each time, we ended our discussion with a feeling of happy camaraderie.

Brother Liu was very serious when he practiced taiji. He was extremely hard working and never missed a practice session. He was modest, gracious, and sincere to others. We developed a special relationship beyond that of classmates. He was twelve years older than I, so I respected him as an elder brother. I practiced forms and pushed hands with him a lot. However, the provincial government office where I worked soon moved to Zhong Xing New Village (Xin Cun), Nantou County, in the central part of Taiwan. I had no choice but to part from Master Zheng and all my brothers at the school and, of course, this move also interrupted my routine of practicing with Brother Liu. It was only when Brother Liu took business trips to our provincial government office that we had the occasional chance to get together. At all those meetings, although our time together was short, we were very happy for the chance to talk with each other. One time I suggested that when we retired, we should partner up and set up a school to teach taiji together because of two reasons. First, in both of our cases, our health benefited a lot from the practice of taiji, so we should share this benefit with others. Second, we were both strongly committed to passing on Master Zheng's philosophy of "spreading all goodness to others." Brother Liu totally agreed with my suggestion. What I did not know was that I would move to the USA before my retirement. My dream of teaching taiji in Taiwan did not come true, but Brother Liu's did. He taught taijiquan from the time he retired from his job with the provincial food bureau.

Regarding how I came to America, I had never thought that I would ever immigrate to the USA. My plan was to spend my remaining life in Taiwan, but who can ever know the future? In 1970 my wife was having difficulty adapting to the muggy subtropical weather of Taiwan. She was always troubled by minor health problems, so she dreamed of moving back to the USA for good. By that time, Professor Zheng had set up the US branch of his "Shr Jung" (*Shizhong*) Taijiquan School in New York City. My wife heard this news and was very happy, so he told me that he would love for me to come to America to help him out. I resigned from my regular job in May of 1974 and left Taiwan with my wife and our young child. The three of us moved to San Francisco, California, where I set up a school named the Universal Taijiquan Association. That started my taijiquan teaching career. The dream that I was not able to achieve in Taiwan materialized here in America. Time has passed swiftly, and thirty-five years have already flown by. Except for the first three years that I lived in America, I have traveled back to visit Taiwan almost every year. In Taiwan, I met up with my former school classmates and, of course, with Brother Liu. At every opportunity that we had to meet, he and I always exchanged stories of our personal experience teaching taiji.

In 1975, when Professor Zheng passed away, the Taibei Shizhong Taiji School founded by Master Zheng needed a successor. To ensure Professor Zheng's wishes for the continued promotion of taijiquan, Master Zheng's wife passed the leadership of the school to Brother Liu. Several years passed, and when Brother Liu found himself too old to continue to be in charge of the school, he passed the helm to Brother Xu Yizhong. The Taibei Shizhong School has thus continued operation until today. As one of the school members, I have felt ashamed that I have not been able to make a more substantial contribution. Because of this, I still feel regret.[9]

From the years I was with Brother Liu, there was one incident that I can never forget. It was the year 1950, when Master Zheng completed his book entitled *Thirteen Treatises on Taijiquan*. The manuscript was handwritten in Professor's cursive-style Chinese calligraphy. To avoid any printing errors by the publisher through possible misreading of the master's handwriting, I was asked to recopy the manuscript using standardized "printing-style" characters. When I got to the fourth treatise, "Change of personality," Master Zheng asked me what my opinion was of the article. In it Professor Zheng had written about his idea that a practitioner of the art, after going through taiji's slow, soft movements and peaceful discipline, would eventually change his or her personality. But I said frankly that I disagreed. When Master Zheng asked me why, I quoted a famous Chinese proverb, "Rivers and mountains are easy to change, but one's personality is hard to transform." (This means that, compared to changing a human being's character, it is easier to change the nation's government or the ruling dynasty—an almost impossible task.) Professor Zheng did not agree. After the book was published, Master Zheng still posed the same question to me from time to time. I stuck with my answer, so he called me "stubborn." One day, when Professor Zheng asked me about the issue again, Brother Liu came in. Master was delighted and related the question to Brother Liu for his opinion. Brother Liu said, "Master is right." Professor Zheng smilingly said, "Right, you see!" However, surprisingly, Brother Liu continued and said, "Pangjeng is also correct." At this, I gave a smile. Professor Zheng then said, "No, that can't be. You had better come up with a good explanation for saying this, or you will need to be disciplined by a good spanking!" Brother Liu then explained, saying, "Yes, what Master said is right because it is possible that a practitioner could somehow turn into a better, kinder person, but that does not necessarily mean a complete makeover of his personality. In this sense, Pangjeng is not wrong." I immediately expressed my agreement with this view. Professor Zheng then laughed it off and let the matter be. He never asked me about the issue ever again. When we sauntered out of Professor Zheng's house, I told Brother Liu, "Today, I have seen your ability to handle a delicate issue. I am impressed." I could have never thought of such an answer. This showed Brother Liu's penetrating insight into a matter and my relative stubbornness.[10]

Brother Liu was a lifelong believer in and follower of Buddhism. This may be why he lived to such an old age. He told me that, in his youth, he had lived like a monk but that he had later returned to a lay lifestyle.[11] However, he did practice meditation in considerable depth, and he had not stopped his practice of meditation for several decades. Now, he has passed away. I hope he is reborn in Buddha's paradise. As Chan (Zen) Master Pu Chao, a monk of the Yuan dynasty, once said, "Being released from the mundane world, he has returned to nature; on that day such a one has passed on ahead of us to his next life alone."[12]

(End of Benjamin Lo's article)

Notes

[9] The compiler of this article would like to note that, while Mr. Lo's expression of regret is most certainly sincere, his comment is an example of the virtue of Chinese modesty and humility. Mr. Lo has traveled to Taiwan many times since 1974 and has made important contributions to Professor's school and legacy there, as well as in America. Where a Western writer might focus on his own accomplishments, Mr. Lo chooses not to do so. Instead, he focuses on the lack.

[10] This is yet another case of Mr. Lo exemplifying the virtue of humility. Mr. Lo's purpose here is to praise Mr. Liu and to highlight his wisdom and intelligence, not to praise himself. Mr. Liu was able to skillfully resolve the disagreement between master and disciple by taking the middle path between two extreme positions, stubbornly held, thus upholding both Confucian and Buddhist values and preserving face for both parties.

[11] As a youth, Liu lived for a time in Nanshan Temple in Xiamen (Amoy) with his older cousin, who was a Buddhist monk. Liu was sometimes called upon to read sutras and had frequent interactions and friendships with monks, including the famous Hong Yi (Li Shutong) of Nanputou Temple. After his schooling, he married, raised a family, and pursued a career as a civil servant. However, later in life Liu committed himself deeply to the practice of Buddhist meditation as a

lay practitioner.

[12] Pu Chao was a famous Chan master (Chin., *channa*; Sanskrit, *dhyana*; Jap. *Zen*, after *zazen*, or sitting meditation, i.e., Pu Chao was a master of Buddhist meditation) and monk of the Yuan dynasty (1279–1368 CE). The quotation attributed to him and applied here to Mr. Liu is meant to refer to one who has attained a very high level of insight into "Buddha mind," "original nature," or "fundamental reality." The gist of the quote is that such a person is without peer.

Introduction to Xu Yizhong's Memorial Article

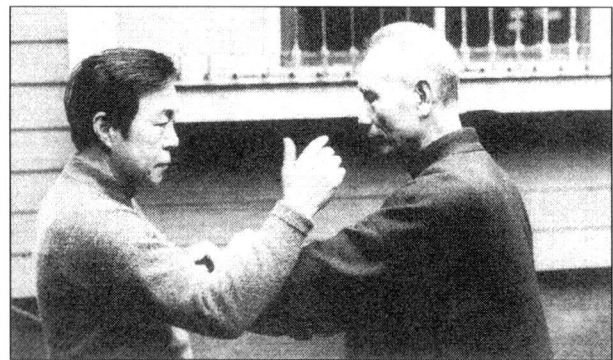

Xu Yizhong (left) and Liu Xiheng (right). Photograph by
Hsiao Peihsien from *Evergreen Magazine*, Issue #14, 1984.

Xu Yizhong is a well-known disciple of Zheng Manqing. He has done much to promote his master's style of taijiquan, especially in Taiwan but also in China. Xu began his studies with Zheng at the same time Liu did, as a member of Zheng's first public class on the island. Xu succeeded his "martial arts brother," Liu, as head of Zheng's Shizhong School (known in Taiwan as the Shizhong Study Society) in Taibei at the time of Liu's retirement from that position in 1986 and continues to head the school today. In 1993 Xu was elected first committee chairman of a new organization, the Master Zheng Taijiquan Study Association. Chairman Xu served the first two consecutive terms of this new post, up until 1999. After brief terms served by Ke Qihua and Ju Hongbin, Xu returned to the post and continued to serve until his retirement in 2008, when he was succeeded by Fu Kunhe.

In addition to holding these important positions and training several generations of students in Zheng's lineage in Taiwan, in 2005 Xu traveled to Nankai University in Tianjin, China, where he had been invited to reintroduce Professor Zheng's thirty-seven-posture Yang Style short form to students on the mainland. More than seven decades prior, Professor Zheng had taught taijiquan at the Central Military Academy (formerly known as Huangpu) in 1933 and at the provincial government's Hunan Martial Arts Academy in 1938 (Davis, 1996: 41). It was at the latter, while given only two months' time to train hundreds of officers, that

Zheng had first experimented with shortening the traditional long Yang form that he had inherited from his teacher, Yang Chengfu (Cheng, 1965/1999: 9; Mason, 2008: 25–26, 37; Wile, 2007: 80, 103–104). Finally, Xu played a major role in the establishment and continued operation of the Zheng Manqing Memorial Hall, located at Zheng's former Taiwan residence in Yonghe City, just south of Taibei City (Mason, 2008: 30). What follows is Mr. Xu's article.

ARTICLE 2
A Salute to Brother Liu Xiheng
by Xu Yizhong • Written in May of 2009

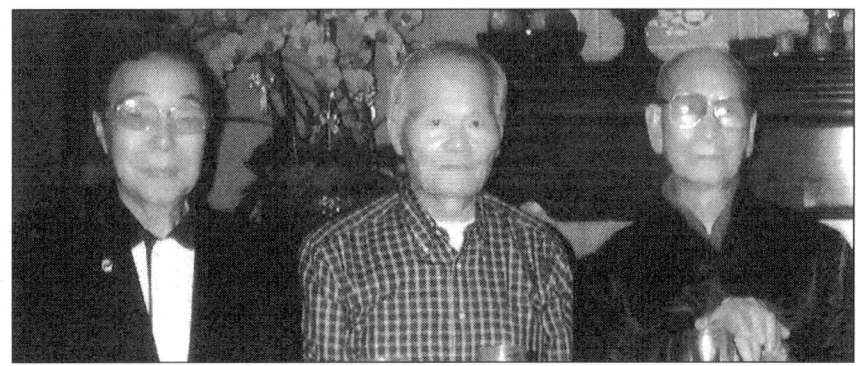

Xu, Lo, and Liu at a banquet in Taibei (December 2004). Photo courtesy of Danny Emerick.

My eldest school brother, Liu Xiheng, was kindhearted and honest. A lifelong believer and practitioner of Buddhism, he also practiced taijiquan diligently and was very healthy. Unfortunately, he passed away in April of 2009. He died in Taiwan University Hospital in Taibei and, at the time of his passing, was ninety-five years of age. He is survived by many children and grandchildren. This is what we call the "fulfillment of life and fortune."

I met Brother Liu in the winter of 1949, when we both attended the first taiji class founded by Master Zheng Manqing after his arrival in Taiwan. The class was held in Zhongshan Hall in the city of Taibei. Although it has been sixty years, I can still recall that our class consisted of about fifty students. Brother Liu often mingled among us and assisted the master with administrative affairs. Due to his warm and modest personality and his enthusiastic attitude toward service, he was well respected by his classmates. Studying together day in and day out, we found each other to have a lot in common. We were very close; we kept no secrets from one another, nor did we ever run out of topics of conversation. His knowledge and experience were way ahead of me, so I benefited a lot from our relationship. Now that he is gone, we can only fall back on our memories of those old times. Here, I would like to share two incidents that may not be known by many people. This will serve as my memorial to my old friend.

(1) There was a book written by Master Zheng Manqing entitled *An Inter-*

pretation of the Analects of Confucius. Brother Liu was assigned to rewrite the text in standard calligraphy in order to prepare it for printing. After the job was completed, Brother Liu saved the original handwritten manuscript and stored it in a box for decades. When Master Zheng passed away, knowing that this could be of value and that it was a precious legacy of the master, he asked how it should be disposed of. He intended to return it to Master's wife, but I suggested that, since she was living in the USA, we should keep it as our heirloom. However, Brother Liu insisted that we should return it to Master Zheng's wife. I am a witness that he did exactly that when she visited Taiwan the next year.

(2) Brother Liu was appointed to work in the provincial food bureau for decades when he moved from mainland China to Taiwan. His position was at the top level of public servants. On his annual job evaluations, he was rated excellent every year. In 1976 the chief minister of the food bureau had to be reappointed to a new position as the general secretariat of the bureau. According to agency policy, Brother Liu should have been able to retain his position; however, as the positions of general secretariat and vice minister were being reappointed, the personnel office had a dilemma as to how to deal with Liu's positioning. Brother Liu heard about the situation and immediately announced his early retirement, thereby resolving the predicament of the newly appointed minister and the personnel office. His courage and willingness to sacrifice himself for the good of others should be a model for all public servants nowadays.

(End of Xu Yizhong's article)

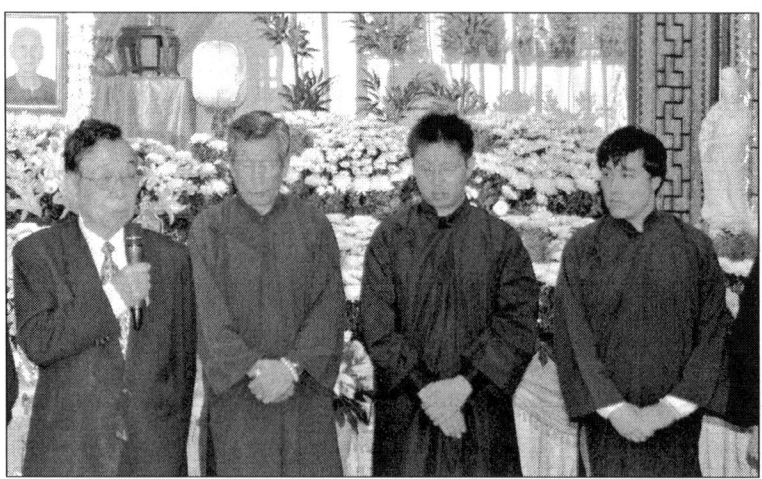

Xu (on left) with mourners at Liu's funeral. Photo courtesy of Yuan Weiming.

Introduction to Yuan Weiming's Memorial Article

The author of the following article, Yuan Weiming, is a disciple of Liu Xiheng, having studied with the master since receiving a formal introduction in 1982. Previously, while pursuing graduate studies in the United States at Washington University, Yuan had studied taijiquan with other senior students of Professor

Zheng Manqing, and he cofounded the St. Louis T'ai Chi Ch'uan Association in 1978. Four years later he returned to Taiwan, became a disciple of Liu, and intensified his training. Yuan subsequently accompanied his master on his overseas trips in the late eighties, serving as his translator and teaching assistant. He has worked for many years as an instructor and coach for the Taibei Shizhong Taijiquan School (a.k.a., the Shizhong Study Society), is a professional photographer, and is a professor of architecture and design at Tunghai University in Taichung, Taiwan. Yuan regularly travels to the US to conduct taijiquan training workshops in the tradition of Professor Zheng and Master Liu. What follows is Yuan Weiming's article.

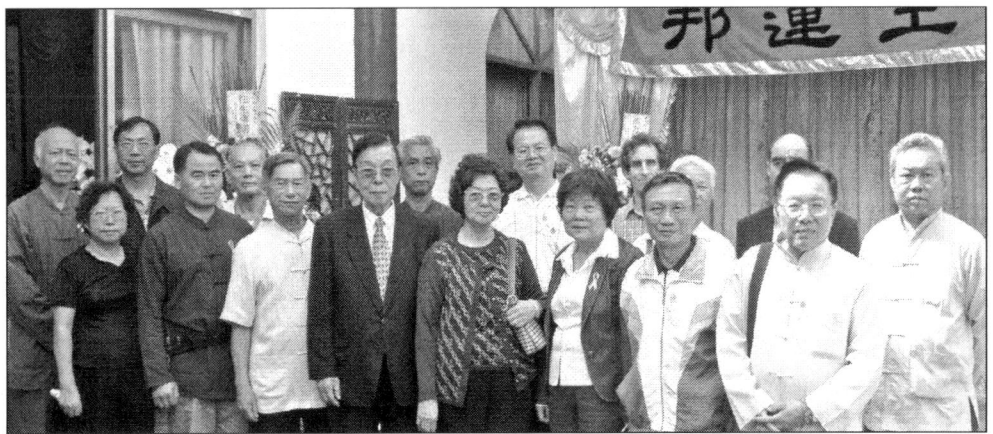

Mourners at Liu's funeral. Standing at far left: Professor Yuan Weiming; seventh from the left in coat and tie: President Xu Yizhong.

―――――――――― ARTICLE 3 ――――――――――
In Memory of Liu Laoshi
by Yuan Weiming • Written on October 8, 2009

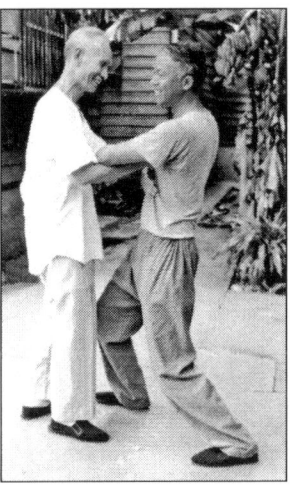

Liu and Yuan push-hands. Photo courtesy of Yuan Weiming.

My respected teacher, Mr. Liu Xiheng (addressed as Laoshi by his students), left us in the spring of 2009 on April 8. He had expected to live only as long as his teacher, Professor Zheng Manqing, but he ended up living twenty years longer. Laoshi's passing brought deep sorrow and a sense of loss to his wife, his family, his taijiquan friends and colleagues, and his students. The regret he felt when he lost his own beloved teacher has now pierced our hearts.

At this time, I think the most meaningful thing I can do to honor the memory of Laoshi is to help people within the taiji community know Mr. Liu better by revealing some of the personal character of this great teacher. It is with this idea in mind that I record these words. In a certain sense, this article has been written by Laoshi himself for, besides some impressions and memories from my personal experience, most of the words used here are his. I have merely reorganized the words of Laoshi's own instructional narrative.

In 1982 I returned to Taiwan after a time of study in the US. Through the recommendation of Mr. Benjamin Pangjeng Lo, I was able to study taijiquan with Mr. Liu. At that time, the classes were held at his personal residence, and this period is also the most memorable time of my studies. The house actually belonged to the Bureau of Provisions, but it was assigned to Laoshi when he worked there as the head secretary of the bureau. It was a walled, Japanese-style bungalow with a red door, located in a quiet alley of Taibei. The little courtyard of the house only allowed space for about ten people to practice taijiquan. In order to be nearby, I also moved into an apartment on the same alley.

I took part in the morning class. The usual three-hour session started with the students and Laoshi performing the taiji form together; then we practiced some basic movements developed by Laoshi and, finally, Laoshi would take turns doing push-hands (*tuishou*) with each student in the class. In between, Laoshi would talk about taiji theory or tell us anecdotes related to taijiquan.

Early in the morning, before the class started, Laoshi always took time to prepare a pot of tea for his students, but I hardly ever saw Laoshi sit down and drink tea; he was the only one in the class who never took a break. There were some fruit trees and flowers planted in the courtyard garden. During the class, Laoshi would sometimes pause to walk aside and smell the jasmine flowers, and he would also invite us to pluck the loquats and bananas from the nearby trees. While practicing, we often saw Laoshi's youngest daughter rushing past on her way to work and his mischievous grandson playing around in the courtyard. From time to time, the class was interrupted by unexpected visitors, most of whom were people from the taijiquan circle. During this morning routine, a joyful mood filled the whole place. Laoshi was always smiling when he pushed hands with his students, as if he were playing a game with great amusement. This childlike character, in my opinion, reflects Laoshi's true nature. It was within this environment that we gradually became better acquainted with the art of taijiquan.

Unfortunately, I was only able to study in this idyllic setting for six years. The house was finally torn down, and an apartment building was erected on the site.

What I missed most was the garage wall where we practiced push-hands. The wall had become soaked with the sweat of many toiling students, and the surface was covered with the words of instruction that Laoshi had written with a fragment of brick while instructing us during class. After he moved from the house, our class subsequently met in several different locations, including a rooftop site and a local park. Finally, we settled in on the grounds of a nearby university campus. Although the class atmosphere never changed, the environment of these later locations was not as moving. Those of us who studied in that tiny courtyard will always remember the inspirational force of this mixture of family life and teaching.

When considering whether to accept a student, the only condition Mr. Liu required was that he (or she) have a respectful attitude. Therefore, he rejected people who just wanted to have a taste of what the class was like and who were not committed to the study of the art. Similarly, he rejected those who came only to test his ability. Sincerity was all that was required; talent was insignificant. The amount of the tuition also depended on a student's personal financial situation. The attitude of sincerity was shown mutually; Mr. Liu also paid the same respect to his students. Laoshi had a theory about this: "Only through sincere teaching and learning can the highest level of taijiquan skill be developed." More often than not, we felt Laoshi offered more sincerity and diligence to his students than we gave him. Once a person had become his student, whether a formal disciple or not, Laoshi would teach without differentiation, and he always taught personally; he never relied on his senior students, even to instruct beginners. The teaching was offered solely in the group-class environment. Laoshi hardly ever gave any private lessons. No matter how much tuition was offered to him, he remained unmoved. Due to his personal example, Laoshi's students were all respectful to one another.

Throughout my years of studying with Mr. Liu, one thing that impressed me greatly was the continuous stream of foreign students visiting from all over the world. Some students stayed weeks, some stayed months, some tried to find jobs and settle down, and some even got married and started families. Perhaps due to the cultural difference, foreign students were particularly fascinated by this special relationship between teacher and students; they respected Laoshi as a mentor and, sometimes, as a father figure. One student even became his foster son. And one of his earliest disciples from America continued to write to Laoshi for about twenty-five years—even though Laoshi did not write him back. Laoshi's only foreign female disciple, Lin Farley, although lacking contact information and not being proficient in the Chinese language, traveled to mainland China, found Laoshi's hometown, and located his relatives. Her efforts to help him reestablish contact with his family pleased Laoshi very much. Later, after Lin left Taiwan and lost contact with her teacher, Laoshi never ceased looking for her.

Mr. Liu's emphasis on loyalty and sincerity was apparently derived from his own loyalty to his teacher, Professor Zheng Manqing. He was among the earliest group of disciples, and, of all Professor Zheng's followers, Mr. Liu spent more time in class with the Professor than any other student. From the time that he first took

Professor's class in 1949, he never stopped learning from him. For example, Professor Zheng taught taiji sword only three times in Taiwan, and Mr. Liu was the only student who was present for all three courses of instruction. Because of Laoshi's honesty, earnestness, and integrity, Professor trusted him very much. He started as a student but gradually became a trusted assistant, helping to handle accounting and proofreading duties. Eventually, he became the senior-most disciple and was asked to lead form practice as a model for the other students from a position at the front of the class.

Laoshi often quoted a sentence from the classical writings of the Daoist philosopher Zhuangzi to express his idea about the proper relationship between a teacher and a student: "When the teacher walks, I follow him walking; when the teacher walks faster, I also walk faster, trying to catch up with him." The loyalty and trust that Laoshi felt toward Professor Zheng were genuine, without the slightest doubt. He said: "Faith is the same as religious belief; the faith that is generated from sincerity can produce wonderful things."

Shortly before his death in 1975, Professor Zheng came back to Taiwan from New York, and the whole class gathered at a banquet in his honor. One student asked Professor: "If you, our master, were not around, who should lead us? Professor pointed to Mr. Liu and said, "Just him." Madame Zheng and the students regarded this event as Professor's appointment of his successor: the "gatekeeper" (*zhang men ren*) of the school, but Laoshi never thought of the matter in this way. His attitude and behavior were as usual, without showing any change or influence from this incident. This reflects his modest demeanor and demonstrates the quality of "no-self" sought by devotees of the Buddhist dharma. After Professor's passing and Mr. Liu's official appointment as head of the Shizhong Society, a position he held from 1975 until 1986, Laoshi continued to exhibit this quality of character.

Mr. Liu always kept a low profile in the public arena. He never brought students with him to perform at public demonstrations, or desired to publish any magazine articles about taijiquan [see footnote #5], and he certainly did not care about things that happened in taijiquan circles. Even in regard to his teaching of taijiquan, he never endeavored to promote it widely; therefore, he had no intention of recruiting a large group of followers and cared nothing about fame. Because of his humble attitude, he remained a somewhat obscure figure in the world of taiji. He only concentrated on teaching a small group of dedicated students. After he resigned from his position as the president of the Shizhong Society, except for an occasional lecture appearance at Shizhong and the teaching of his small class of disciples and students, he had hardly any contact with the outside world. The only thing he concerned himself with was the art of taijiquan itself, and he would accept any theory or idea as long as it was beneficial to the practice of taijiquan.

For Laoshi, taijiquan was a way of self-cultivation and of obtaining wisdom and guidance for life; the martial arts applications were only a minor aspect of the art. For that reason, he did not like to be called "Master" because that conflicted with his beliefs. The best way to exemplify this idea is by describing his attitude toward push-hands. He regarded the push-hands practice as being about learning to be a better human being—in other words, learning to establish good interactions with others. When we practiced push-hands, he instructed us to just calm the mind and to concentrate on "listening to" the movements of the opponent (*ting jin*). Even if a student had developed good listening and neutralization skills and was able to push his partner, he was to resist the temptation to push. Instead, he was to continue to "follow" until his partner had lost all opportunity to advance. In this way, we would not only learn the skill of pushing hands, but we would also cultivate ourselves and develop the qualities of endurance, composedness, and stabilization of the energy (*qi*) and the mind (*yi*). Our focus was to be on cultivating ourselves rather than on overcoming an opponent.

He often repeated the phrase, "Let yourself be untouchable, and don't try to be unmovable." Yielding is always the highest principle. Even when the opponent has committed a fault by using force, one should only pay attention to one's own movements and not try to blame the other person. When he pushed hands with students, Laoshi also followed his own principle. Although he was capable of neutralizing and pushing the student out in every move, he always neutralized several times before he pushed the student away, and even when he did so, it was with a very light touch. The push was just enough to cause the student to lose his balance. He pushed "hard" only when the student was using excessive force or when a student was about to leave the class and travel far away.[13] It seemed that he wanted the student to keep the memory of this feeling of being pushed with correct, clear technique. Only at that moment did we get to witness the tremendous power Laoshi possessed. Mr. Ben Lo once advised him that, at his advanced age, he should not practice push-hands anymore, but Laoshi insisted on continuing to practice with his students. However, as he got older, he sought only to relax and neutralize, not to push.

With this kind of mentality and attitude, I think Mr. Liu had developed a very pure and refined taijiquan art, and only someone who has studied taijiquan for a long time can understand and appreciate the value of this kind of achievement in the art. Several senior students of Professor Zheng in Taiwan (e.g., Xu Yizhong, Ke Qihua, Su Shaoqing, and Chen Youyi) as well as from the US (e.g., Ed Young, Maggie Newman, Robert W. Smith, Carol Yamasaki, and Wolfe Lowenthal) came to Laoshi asking for instruction. Everyone who had pushed hands with Laoshi gave a very high evaluation of his skills. One person said he was like an "agile snake." The late David Chen said trying to push Laoshi felt like pushing with an empty jacket on a hanger. Perhaps the most valuable comments came from several students of Professor from abroad, who claimed that the feeling of pushing with Mr. Liu was the closest to the experience of pushing with Professor Zheng. Laoshi was contented with his regular routine and simple life. Although he was invited many times to teach abroad, he only agreed twice, traveling to Holland and the US in 1987 and 1988, and a good portion of his reason for going on these occasions was to enjoy the experience of traveling abroad with his wife. After Mrs. Liu was unable to travel far, he rejected all sub-sequent invitations to do foreign teaching.

Despite his high achievement in taijiquan, Laoshi insisted that he would not write any books or make any films. When his students asked him to leave us some visual images, he just said: "I am still in progress; do you want me to stop progressing?" Sometimes he would add: "Taijiquan is about the internal and not the external; you should not rely too much on images of the external structure." One time when he was talking about this matter, he said: "I follow Confucius: 'Talk, but do not write.'" The hidden meaning of this statement is that writing is for a luminary, like Professor Zheng, to do. Laoshi considered himself to be just a follower; to propagate the master's teachings was enough for him. Sometimes he would pause in the middle of making a comment about taijiquan. When we asked him why, he would say: "Buddha said, 'It cannot be put into words.'" In profound matters, the more you talk about it, the more confusion will be generated. To extend that idea, in his later days, Laoshi often said that his taijiquan is a "hard but casual" way of practice. Not too many people can comprehend the true meaning of that statement.[14] It is unfortunate that today we only have a few photographs and recordings of lectures to recall Mr. Liu's presence. Most of his teachings existed only immaterially in the form of his oral presentations, and precious images of Laoshi are stored only in the memories of his students.

For Mr. Liu, two essential aspects of taijiquan were to apply the principles of the art to daily life and to join them with the tenets of Buddhism. Many years ago, when Professor Zheng was still in the US, in one of their exchanges of correspondence, Laoshi complained about his heavy workload. Professor replied and upbraided him with these words: "Where is your practice of sinking the qi down to the dantian?" Laoshi suddenly realized that taijiquan had to be practiced in daily life and, from then on, he followed his teacher's admonition and worked hard on that concept. Besides using the principles of push-hands to practice how to deal with other people and to cultivate the virtue of modesty, Laoshi also sometimes quoted a phrase from the taijiquan Classics to respond to the questions students asked concerning the various situations that happen in life. For example, when pursuing a relationship with a girlfriend, one should, "Stick, connect, adhere, and follow; do not detach, do not use force." Again, the way to a happy marriage is to, "Give up your self-will, and follow the other person." These words of advice usually made people smile.

Laoshi had first encountered and practiced Buddhism at a very early age, and he finally committed himself to it at the age of forty-nine. After his retirement, studying Buddhism and taijiquan became his two major tasks. Yet, he considered these two paths to be leading to the same end: peace of mind. He thought that after practicing either "way" and reaching a certain level, one could gain insight into one's own true nature. For this reason, he often used Buddhist doctrines to interpret taijiquan and used taijiquan principles to comprehend Buddhism. He used the Buddhist idea "look through and let go" to describe relaxing (*song*), and the notion "follow fate but remain unchanged" to explain the concept of central equilibrium (*zhong ding*). Moreover, he compared the teaching of taijiquan with "the contribution of the dharma." The words and proverbs of Buddhism were also frequently used to interpret the profound aspects of taijiquan.[15]

Laoshi was not a man of worldly desires; his character was illuminated from inside, and the people who were touched by him were not limited to those in the field of taijiquan. More than twenty years ago, when he accepted his first group of disciples, he wrote a manuscript on the importance of respecting one's teacher and sticking to the Dao. One of the disciples, who is an American and who also studied Buddhism in Taiwan, showed this manuscript to his Buddhist teacher, Master Shengyan (Zhang Baokang, 1930–2009), a very famous Buddhist monk in Taiwan. After looking at the essay, the master said: "Oh, there still is such a person in Taiwan! I want to meet him." He then arranged a dinner appointment with Mr. Liu, but Laoshi was detained by an unforeseen matter, and so they never had the opportunity to meet. After many years had gone by, both Master Shengyan and Laoshi passed away within a two-month interval, and they were both buried in Dharma Drum Mountain. Their fates were connected and so, in this way, they finally "met" each other.

One morning three years ago, my elder classmate, Mr. Jiang, and I went to Laoshi's apartment, which was the last place where classes were held. There Laoshi shared his final state of mind with us. He said that, a few days before, he had not been able to sleep; his mind had been disturbed by the thought that his life was approaching its end. Suddenly, he remembered the words that the famous Buddhist monk, Master Hong Yi [1880–1942], had written down before he died: "Sorrow and joy are mixed together." On thinking of that, he was enlightened, and his mind became clear. We say "sorrow" because life basically is full of suffering and pain, but there is also "joy" as one contemplates his soon approaching departure for the Buddhist paradise. Laoshi has now finally fulfilled his wish. Even though we may not be willing to accept his departure, we should give him our blessing.

(End of Yuan Weiming's article)

Notes

[13] Sometimes it felt to the student that Laoshi "pushed powerfully," but it was only because the student himself was using excessive force (i.e., Laoshi then allowed the student's own force to return to him).

[14] The statement: "*ma ma, hu hu*" usually means "doesn't care much; perfunctory." What Mr. Liu meant more profoundly is, "Your mind should be relaxed; don't care too much about loss and gain; don't try to push others; don't worry about your gongfu achievement . . . ." Laoshi also told the compiler of this article, "If you try to pin it down too definitely, to grasp it tightly with your mind, you will only push it further away. You must relax and use your intuition to grasp the essence with your heart." Also, Danny Emerick remembers Laoshi saying laughingly that taiji was "simple but not easy."

15   Though a number of Master Liu's students had an interest in Buddhism, Laoshi seemed to respect our individual paths and faith traditions and did not push us to follow him in that direction.

Introduction to Xu Zhengmei's Memorial Article
　　The fourth of the memorial articles was written by Xu Zhengmei, a disciple of Liu Xiheng and a retired teacher of mathematics formerly employed by Jianguo High School, Taibei, Taiwan. Xu's primary purpose is to provide some brief biographical material on Liu. He also includes a poem he composed, providing a fitting touch to this memorial project.

──────── ARTICLE 4 ────────
A Brief Biography of Mr. Liu Xiheng
by Xu Zhengmei • Written in 2009

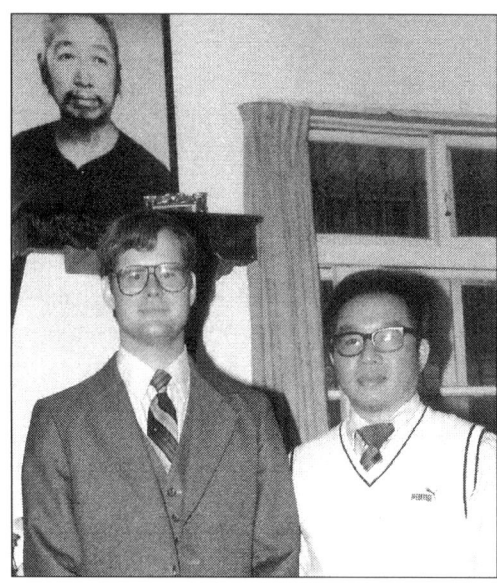

Danny Emerick and Xu Zhengmei at Professor Zheng's home (1984).
Photo courtesy of D. Emerick.

　　Mr. Liu Xiheng was born on December 10, 1915, in Raoping County, Guandong Province. He was the youngest child of his family and, since there were four sisters and five brothers before him, he was the "number ten" child. His father was a fisherman and, although his family was poor, they were happy and contented.
　　In his teens, Liu attended elementary school in Xiamen (Amoy) City with his older cousin, who was a Buddhist monk. Liu lodged and dined in the Nanshan Temple with his cousin. Leading a disciplined life of temple routine, he felt happy. His intellectual giftedness was manifested by his high achievement at school in spite of adversity. However, that was a time of warlords and social upheaval, as

well as the Japanese invasion, so his schooling was interrupted many times. His education proceeded sporadically during his junior high, high school, and college years; however, he never gave up pursuing higher studies, even though he had to continue with self-study during periods when he was not able to attend formal classes. In this way he managed to pass his entrance exams at each and every step, from middle school to college. He was a person of diligence and superb intelligence.

After only a year and a half of high school, he was forced to discontinue his formal studies due to poor health. While recuperating in Nanshan Temple, he bought a book entitled *Taiji: A Scientific Approach*, by Wu Tunan. Through self-study he practiced taijiquan according to the instructions contained in this book. Within a year his health improved. Then he passed the qualifying exam for Amoy University and was enrolled into its Department of Economics. When he had difficulty covering his costs for college, his teacher came to his aid and provided financial assistance. During his college days, he found time to continue his practice of taijiquan in a quiet corner of the campus. One day, the head of the Physical Education Department discovered his ability in taiji and hired him as an assistant to teach the students taijiquan. This was during the Sino-Japanese War, and a majority of the students were suffering from malnutrition and poor health due to inadequate food supplies. Liu was paid for the job, which was a cause of great excitement for him. This small stipend helped him to pay his way through four years of college. During his winter and summer breaks, he also taught Mandarin to the young monks in Nanputouo Temple. There he had the opportunity to befriend Hong Yi Fashi ("Master of the Law," Monk Hong Yi). In 1942 Liu graduated, receiving his degree from Amoy University.

At the end of the war, Taiwan was liberated from Japan. The whole island needed to be rebuilt, and that great task required qualified people from all walks of life. Mr. Liu traveled to Taiwan with his wife and children and was immediately hired by the provincial food bureau. Due to his training in economic theory and his literary proficiency, he was soon appointed the secretariat and was also given a post as a special committee member for the bureau. He worked closely with the minister of the food bureau, serving as his planner. Because of his well-disciplined and no-nonsense attitude and because he could be depended upon to execute his affairs promptly and fairly, he was greatly loved by his coworkers. In 1976 he retired from the bureau.

In the winter of 1949 Professor Zheng Manqing, fourth-generation successor of the Yang Style of taijiquan, was invited by Taibei Mayor Yu Michien to start a teaching program of taijiquan in Zhongshan Hall. The school was officially named the Shizhong Taijiquan School, and Master Zheng became the chairman. At that time Mr. Liu Xiheng enrolled himself as a student in the first class, and he continued to practice Master Zheng's method of taijiquan for the rest of his life, giving him almost six decades of experience in the style. He was well acquainted with all the students of the first class, which included Liang Tongcai, Yin Qitang, Ye Xiuting,

Tao Bingxiang, Ju Hongbin, Benjamin Lo, and Xu Yizhong. Benjamin Lo and Xu Yizhong were two of his best friends. After studying with Professor Zheng Manqing, Liu concluded: "Master Zheng is the real thing; in my past self-study and self-practice at Amoy University, I was using too much force, so I had been wasting the time of others and my own time as well."

Mr. Liu practiced taijiquan diligently during his spare time, and he applied the philosophy of taiji to his life as well. Because of his high intelligence and virtue, Master Zheng valued him highly, and he was appointed as master's first disciple after the founding of the Shizhong Taijiquan School. In the 1960s, while living in the USA, Master Zheng left Mr. Liu in charge of the Taibei school. The master also kept up correspondence with him in regard to the philosophy, theory, and technique of taiji. Master Zheng had high hopes for Mr. Liu.

On March 26, 1975, while visiting Taiwan, Master Zheng Manqing passed away. One year later, Mr. Liu was appointed chairman of the Taibei Shizhong Taijiquan School and was made officially responsible for carrying on the legacy of Master Zheng's Dao. Every Sunday Mr. Liu gathered all the Shizhong School brothers, and they practiced together on the campus of the Taiwan University School of Law, which was located at Xuzhou (Hsu Chou) Road. In March of 1983 he initiated the first session of Master Zheng's Taijiquan Study Class. Each session lasted six months; and thus, the training of a new class of talented students was begun. Mr. Liu was the head coach for each session of form training, as well as the leader of the push-hands group, and Mr. Xu Yizhong served as the general manager. All the coaches were selected from among the top-notch school graduates, and new students were recommended to the program by the previous graduates. This opened the door for the systematic training of a new generation of skilled Shizhong graduates and instructors.

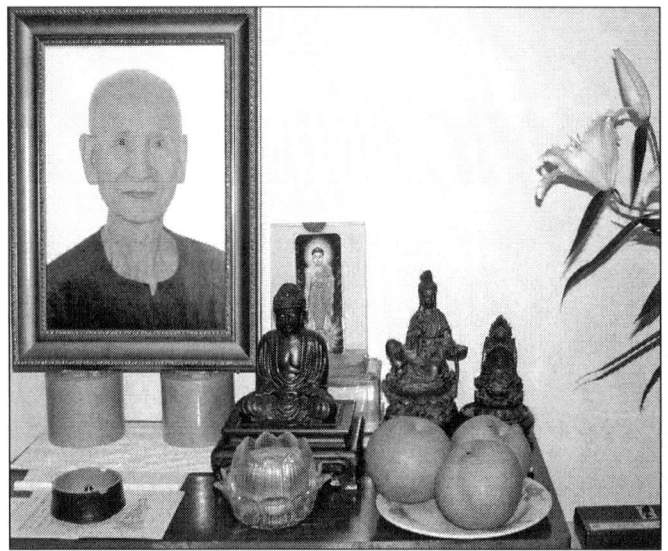
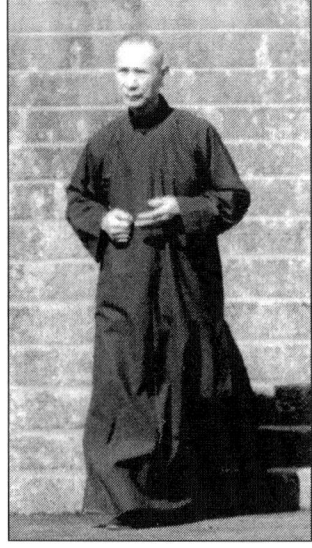

Mr. Liu's funeral portrait with Buddhist imagery and in formal attire at a temple site.

In 1988, at the age of seventy-seven, Mr. Liu retired and passed the school leadership to Xu Yizhong. From that time, Liu led a peaceful life, concentrating on the practice and teaching of taijiquan to a small group of dedicated students and leading a lifestyle of vegetarianism and Buddhist meditation.

In 1987 and 1988 he travelled to Europe and the USA, teaching taijiquan. Mr. Liu's taiji technique was excellent. In particular, his push-hands skills of neutralization and discharge were profound and varied. Hence, he attracted the interest of a number of foreign students. However, Liu picked his students with scrupulous care. His first requirement was that a student be of virtuous character. He taught his students not only taijiquan but also the taiji philosophy of life. He always said, "The true application of taiji is to cultivate a calm spirit, a peaceful heart, and a clear and logical mind. These qualities contribute to a peaceful society."

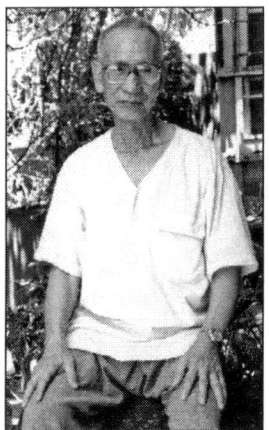 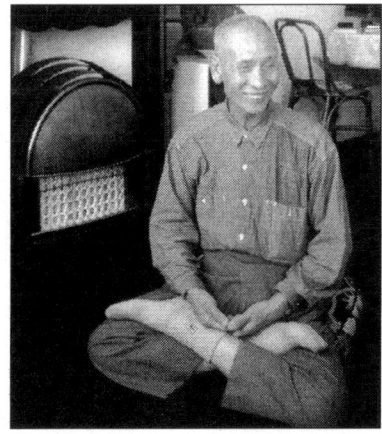 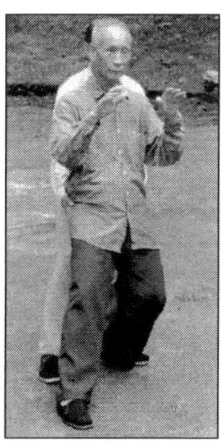

Left: Liu in a restful moment. Center, he prepares for sitting meditation. Right: Liu allows a student to feel the correct position of the hips in rear-loaded posture. Photos courtesy of Yuan Weiming.

Now that Mr. Liu has passed away, his students and associates continue to respect him deeply and to miss him very much. I would like to remember him with the following poem, summing up Mr. Liu's way of life and his achievement in old age.

> A great taiji master of his time.
> For whom had he been working so diligently?
> He passed the torch of Shizhong,
> And he planted a garden full of fragrance.
> Trees he nurtured have grown to become pillars.
> He committed his whole life to
> the principles of honesty, frugality, and simplicity.
> A life that valued dedication and was oblivious to vainglory
> Can also be considered glorious.

(End of Xu Zhengmei's article)

Introduction to Danny Emerick's Memorial Article

The fifth article is an original piece composed in English specifically for this memorial project by an American disciple of Liu Xiheng. Mr. Emerick's knowledge and experience in the Asian martial arts is extensive. He began his study of Zheng's thirty-seven-posture Yang taijiquan short form in the 1970s in the US and moved to Taibei, Taiwan, in 1981 to continue his training under Liu's tutelage. In 1982 Emerick was among the first group of Western students to be accepted as indoor disciples through a traditional *bai shi* ceremony. Today Mr. Emerick is reference librarian at the State Library of Florida in Tallahassee. His memoir brings a Western perspective to the experience of studying with Liu Xiheng. What follows is Danny Emerick's article.

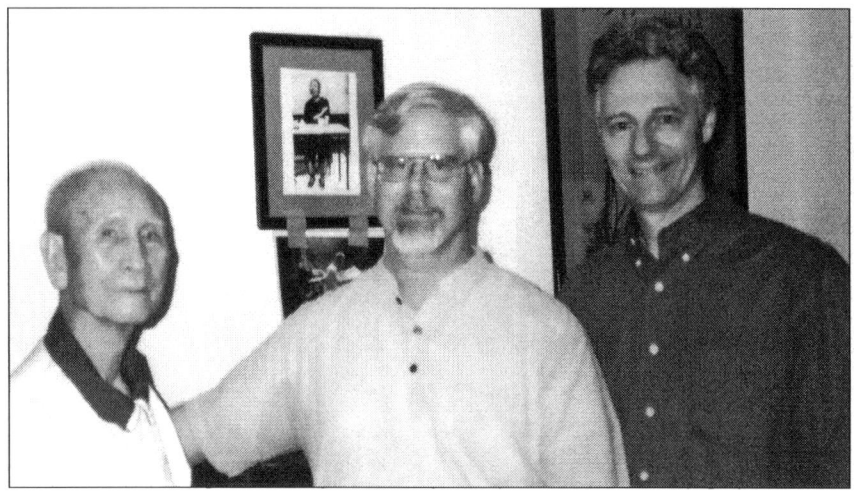

ARTICLE 5

A Garden of Memories
by Danny Emerick • Written on April 11, 2010

I met Mr. Liu in August 1981, but only after an exhausting twenty-four hours of travel on a plane (only my second time on an airplane), a confiscation of contraband items by the ROC customs agent (the "friend" who was to meet me at the airport neglected to tell me that the professional grade walkie-talkies that he asked me to bring from the USA were illegal to "import" under Taiwan's then somewhat strict martial law!), and surviving a car crash (coincidentally driven by that same "friend") ten minutes after leaving the Chiang Kai-shek International Airport. The crash completely totaled the car and could have resulted in an all-too-brief stay for me on Ilha Formosa (not to mention my stay on planet earth), but miraculously left us unscathed!

So, after a few days of recovering from jetlag and jangled nerves (and from a mild case of whiplash) at the International House on Xingyi Road, I figured I was ready to meet Mr. Liu. I asked a Chinese friend (not the driver!) to call the number

I had for Mr. Liu to inquire about class times and was told that there was a class the next morning at 7:30.

Mind you, I didn't know anything about Mr. Liu, only that he was recommended to me by Mr. Ben Lo (Professor Zheng Manqing's senior student) when I asked him about taiji teachers in Taibei, and that Mr. Lo would write a letter of introduction and send it to Mr. Liu so he would be expecting me. Mr. Lo also added that if he did not write this letter of introduction, Mr. Liu would probably not be inclined to teach me.

So the next day at 7:00 a.m., on a warm summer morning typical for that part of the world, I ventured out onto the streets of Taibei, armed with the address (written in Chinese, of course) of Mr. Liu Xiheng.

After consulting a map of the city and walking a few blocks, I realized that I had no idea how to decipher the address that had been given to me and desperately needed help to locate the class. This realization—intensified by the cacophony of street traffic and the bombardment of the senses by the new sights, sounds, smells and general chaos that a newcomer finds in Taibei—stopped me cold. I did what any other foreigner would do in the same situation: I panicked and accosted the next passerby who looked of college age. My Taiwanese friends back in the US told me all college students in Taiwan could speak English. Well, not quite all, I found out.

The unfortunate victim I chose did indeed look like a typical college-age student, but when I thrust the address under his nose and asked, in my best English, for his help in finding the address, instead of hearing, "Sure, no problem," I only got gestures and grins from him. The gestures seemed to be for me to follow him, however, and the grins, I suppose, were meant to be reassuring to me. They weren't. He turned down a little lane off the main road with the address in his hand and with me right behind him!

After walking down the lane for about fifteen or twenty minutes, I was growing more suspicious by the minute as to exactly what my newfound companion was really up to. He stopped in front of a red door imbedded into a seven-foot wall and pointed to the address in his hand and then to the door. Handing the paper back to me, he then turned back to continue the journey I had so rudely interrupted. But as he left, he smiled a real smile, as I tried to stammer out an inadequate "thank you" that did not even begin to repay his genuine kindness to a hopelessly lost foreigner.

Whoever he was, I can only pray that he is well for if it hadn't been for this good Samaritan, I would probably still be wandering around the streets of Taibei! Now, therefore, completely trusting the integrity of my new "friend" to have led me to the correct address, I knocked on the red door. A moment later the door opened, and the kind, smiling face of a Chinese elder looked at me with inquiring eyes. "Are you Mr. Liu?" I asked, again in my best English. "No!" came the unexpected reply from the still-smiling Chinese elder with the kind face and inquiring eyes.

Not knowing what else to do or say, I pointed to the address on the paper in my hand, and the smiling Chinese elder with the ever-so-kind face and impish, inquiring eyes looked at it and said, in his best English, "Are you Danny?" "Yes!" I exclaimed and, to my great relief, he motioned me inside.

I found that behind the red door, and surrounded by the wall, was an old Japanese-style house (Taiwan had been a colony of Japan from 1895 to 1945) that looked as if it had been built sometime in the late Meiji era, but probably wasn't more than fifty years old. The Chinese elder who had so graciously let me inside ignored me completely and began tending to the various plants and flowers in the small and narrow courtyard, obviously being the gardener for Mr. Liu's family.

So, I waited for Mr. Liu to come out of his house, fully expecting him to resemble Professor Zheng in his Chinese robes, or perhaps Master Kan ("Snatch the pebble from my hand") or Master Po ("What do you hear, Grasshopper?").

A minute or so passed, and Mr. Liu was still a no-show when the red door opened behind me and another foreigner entered, greeted the gardener in Chinese, and introduced himself to me.

I told him I had just arrived in Taibei, was here to study with Mr. Liu, and was wondering when he would come out of his house to start class. My new friend just grinned, pointed to the gardener, and gently said, "He is Mr. Liu."

"The gardener is Mr. Liu?"

Before I could continue to verbally express my complete sense of disappointment ("Isn't he supposed to be wearing robes or something?"), the red door opened again, and several Chinese and another foreigner entered and also greeted the gardener with sincere respect.

Then I was somewhat more convinced that the gardener was probably Mr. Liu (especially when he called the class together). He introduced me to my new Chinese classmates and asked me, translated through the new foreign classmate who had just entered, if I would show the form I had learned.

By 1981 I had been seriously studying taiji for two years and figured I knew enough not to completely embarrass my teacher in the US, so I proceeded to do the thirty-seven-posture form of Professor Zheng Manqing.

After I had finished and was feeling rather proud of my "performance," Mr. Liu's first comment was, "Not bad." But then came the gentle admonitions. "However, you need to turn your waist. Don't use your arms independently of your body. Keep the body upright. Don't lean. Move the body as one unit."

Readers who are familiar with taiji will see that these are simply fundamental principles I had neglected to incorporate into my performance of the form. Indeed, I was to learn from Mr. Liu over the next several years not only how to incorporate these principles into the form, but also the importance of internalizing them so that, even in our daily activities, we would also naturally utilize and rely upon the taiji principles.

Despite the glaring deficiencies in my form that day, Mr. Liu never once made me feel embarrassed or inadequate, but rather he revealed to me what he essentially was in his own being: a sincere, caring, and genuinely kind teacher. This first impression I had of him never changed in the twenty-eight years I knew him.

In 1983 Mr. and Mrs. Robert W. Smith visited Mr. Liu for a few days, and I was asked to accompany them around Taibei. After their final meeting, Mr. Smith wrote quite a few notes in a pocket notebook he had, and he shared with me some of what he had written. One particular phrase Mr. Smith used in describing Mr. Liu was "the epitome of taiji." I couldn't agree more!

Indeed, Mr. Liu exemplified the taiji he had learned from Professor Zheng. He was completely unpretentious, utterly simple, and natural in his daily life, and he avoided any publicity as a taiji "master," although he truly was one by anyone's measure.

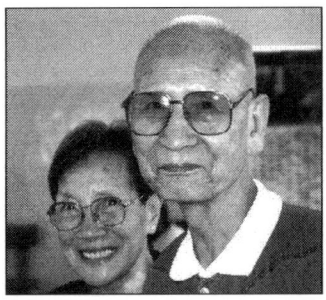

Photo of Mr. and Mrs. Liu by Danny Emerick.

In teaching us push-hands, he emphasized the idea that in our practice we should only concentrate on "feeling" and completely eschew any notion of using the slightest force to push or to resist being pushed. "Don't be against!" (*Bu ding!*) he would admonish us, almost on a daily basis.

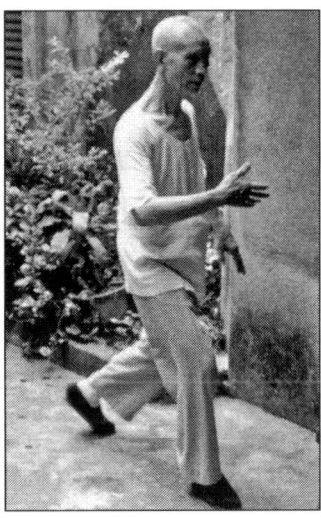

Liu Xiheng in walking ward off. Photo courtesy of Yuan Weiming.

Some other nuggets from Mr. Liu gleaned from class notes include the following:

- I teach the formless form.
- Taiji is simple, but not easy.
- Have a slight, light touch.
- Learn the simple; don't learn the complex.
- Pushing hands is not pushing hands . . . it is "pushing waist" [*tui yao*].
- The hand and body are like a snake, curling and curving and yielding at the slightest touch.
- Study the little curves in the form; they are the most important.
- Don't think of pushing; think only of yielding.
- Taijiquan is *keqiquan*. [*Keqi* means "manners" or "being polite"]
- Yield first!
- Everything comes from the root.
- Remember only two things: straight and relaxed. It is very simple.

And perhaps my favorite piece of advice of all the things I heard Mr. Liu say was in response to a question from my friend and classmate, Russ Mason, when we returned to Taiwan to visit Mr. Liu together in 2006. Russ asked Mr. Liu, "What taiji principles should we use to foster and improve our married life?"

Mr. Liu immediately responded by quoting a phrase in the *Taiji Classics*, "*Bu ding, bu diu.*" Don't resist, and don't let go.

I began this brief memorial to Mr. Liu by telling how I literally mistook him for the gardener. Yet, upon further reflection, I think that he was indeed a "gardener." He never had more than a handful of students at a time, but the ones he had he tended with gentleness and care. He was always attentive to our health and well-being, and he nourished us daily with his words and by his example. This not only improved our understanding of taiji, but it also had a profound effect on our lives.

Mr. Liu has grand-students all over the world now, the result of that "garden" of students he cultivated and tended with sincere care and concern and, most importantly, with love.

May his garden continue to thrive and flourish.

(End of Danny Emerick's article)

Liu Xiheng's Western Disciples

Mr. Liu had scores of students and shared his knowledge with all. His only expectation was that a student should be "sincere" in his study with the teacher. A few wanted to show their complete sincerity to Mr. Liu and his teachings by becoming official students in the discipleship ceremony called bai shi. From 1982 until 2004, Mr. Liu accepted twenty-five disciples. Below is the list of Mr. Liu's Western disciples and the year of their *bai shi*:

- 1982: Mark Lord, Rick Halstead, Mike Moran, Danny Emerick
- 1984: Michael Schnapp, Bill Tucker
- 1986: Lin Farley
- 2004: Alex Makapa, Daniel Altschuler

People Mentioned in the Article		Places and Terms	
Chen Youyi	陳釉藝	dantian	丹田
Fu Kunhe	傅崑鶴	fashi	法師
Hong Yi	弘一	keqi	客氣
Ju Hongbin	鞠鴻賓	Nanputuosi	南普陀寺
Ke Qihua	柯啟華	Nantou	南投
Li Shutong	李叔同	qi	氣
Liang Tongcai	梁棟材	Raoping Xian	饒平縣
Liu Xiheng	劉錫亨	Shizhong Xue She	时中學社
Luo Bangzhen	羅邦楨	taiji jian	太極劍
Ruan Weiming	阮偉明	ting jin	聽勁
Shengyan	聖嚴	taijiquan	太極拳
Su Shaoqing	蘇紹卿	tuishou	推手
Tao Bingxiang	陶炳祥	wude	武德
Wu Tu'nan	吳图南	Xiamen (Amoy)	廈門
Xu Yizhong	徐憶中	Xindian	新店
Xu Zhengmei	徐正梅	Xuzhou	徐州
Yang Chengfu	楊澄甫	yi	意
Ye Xiuting	葉秀挺	Yonghe City	永和市
Yin Qitang	殷啟堂	zhang men ren	掌門人
Zhang Baokang	張寶康	Zheng Manqing Jinian Guan	鄭曼青 紀念 館
Zheng Manqing	鄭曼青	zhong ding	中定
Zhuangzi	莊子	Zhongshan Tang (Hall)	中山堂
		Zhong Xing Xin Cun	興新村

Acknowledgments

The compiler of this article wishes to thank all those who contributed to this project in ways large and small. Professor Yuan Weiming initiated the effort with his request that the Chinese source materials be translated and published for the English-speaking taijiquan community. A bow of deep gratitude is in order to Master Liu Xiheng and to the authors, Benjamin Lo, Xu Yizhong, Yuan Weiming, Xu Zhengmei, and Danny Emerick, as well as to the publishers of the *Tai Chi Journal*, in Kaohsiung, Taiwan. Yuan Weiming and Danny Emerick provided photos and other invaluable assistance, as did Robert W. Smith, Monica Chen, Warren Conner,

Barbara Davis, Lin Farley, Rick Garcia, Jeff Herrod, Mark Lord, Michael Schnapp, Mark Westcott, Carol Yamasaki, and others. A special word of thanks is due Nick Tan (Chen Yuexin) and Professor Maria Tu (Du Zhongmin) for their work with the translation of source materials. Any errors are the responsibility of the compiler, and readers' corrections would be welcomed. This article is dedicated to the memory and spirit of Liu Laoshi and to his devoted family members, classmates, disciples, and students.

Bibliography

Biondi, M. (2006). Interview with grand master Hsu Yee Chung. Published on the Shizhong Study Society webpage at www.37taichi.org.tw

Cheng, M. (1962). *T'ai chi ch'uan: A simplified method of calisthenics for health and self-defense*. Taibei: Shizhong Taijiquan Center.

Cheng, M. (1965/1999). *Master Cheng's new method of taichi ch'uan self-cultivation* (M. Hennessy, Trans.). Berkeley, CA: Frog, Ltd.

Cheng, M., and Smith, R. (1967/2004). *T'ai chi*. Rutland, VT: Charles E. Tuttle.

Cheng, M. (1950/1985). *Cheng Tzu's thirteen treatises on t'ai chi ch'uan* (B. Lo and M. Inn, Trans.). Richmond, CA: North Atlantic Books.

Cheng, M. (1996). T'ai chi ch'uan: A simplified method of calisthenics for health and self-defense. [Video]. Ashville, NC: Cho San.

Chengtu Tai-Chi Chuan Research Association (2007). Zheng Manqing Jinian Guan donors' record. Taibei, Taiwan.

Davis, B. (1996). In search of a unified Dao: Zheng Manqing's life and contributions to taijiquan. *Journal of Asian martial arts, 5*(2), 36–59.

Davis, D., and Mann, L. (1996). Conservator of the Taiji classics: An interview with Benjamin Pang Jeng Lo. *Journal of Asian martial arts, 5*(4), 46–67.

Farley, L. (1986). Master Liu Hsi-heung: We must learn to be tender, soft, and peaceful. *Free China journal, 3*(25). Reprinted in November of the same year in *Full Circle, 1*(4), 22–23.

Lo, B., Inn, M., Amacker, R., and Foe, S. (1979). *The essence of t'ai chi ch'uan: The literary tradition*. Richmond, CA: North Atlantic Books.

Liu, X. (1985). The concept of central equilibrium in taijiquan. (R. Halstead, Trans.) *T'ai chi player*, 3, 7–10.

Liu, X. (1985/2002). The concept of central equilibrium in taijiquan. (R. Halstead, Trans.) *Taijiquan journal, 3*(3), 19–23.

Mason, R. (2001). Fifty years in the fighting arts: An interview with Robert W. Smith. *Journal of Asian martial arts, 10*(1), 36–73.

Mason, R. (2008). Zheng Manqing: The memorial hall and legacy of the master of five excellences in Taiwan. *Journal of Asian Martial Arts, 17*(3), 22–39.

Smith, R. (1974/1990). *Chinese boxing: Masters and methods*. Berkeley, CA: North Atlantic Books.

Smith, R. (1975). A master passes: A tribute to Cheng Man-ch'ing. *Shr Jung newsletter, 1*(1), 2–7.

Smith, R. (1995). Remembering Zheng Manqing: Some sketches from his life. *Journal of Asian martial arts, 4*(3), 46–59.

Smith, R. (1999). *Martial musings: A portrayal of martial arts in the 20th century.* Erie, PA: Via Media Publishing.

Tucker, W. (2008). Liu Hsi-heng: A man of principles. *T'ai chi magazine, 32*(4), 24–30.

Wile, D. (1985). *Cheng Man-Ch'ing's advanced t'ai-chi form instructions.* Brooklyn, NY: Sweet Ch'i Press.

Wile, D. (2007). *Zheng Manqing's uncollected writings on taijiquan, qigong, and health, with new biographical notes.* Milwaukee, WI: Sweet Ch'i Press.

Yang, C. (1934/2005). *Yang Chengfu: The essence and applications of taijiquan* (L. Swaim, Trans.). Berkeley, CA: North Atlantic Books.

Yang, J. (2001). *Tai chi secrets of the Yang style.* Boston, MA: YMAA Publication Center.

Yang, Z. (1988). *Yang style taijiquan.* Hong Kong: Hai Feng Publishing Co. and Beijing, China: Morning Glory Press.

Yang, Z. (1993). *Yang Chengfu shi tai ji quan.* Guangxi Province, China: Guangxi Minzu.

Yu, W., and Sharp, G. (1993 April). Fu Zhongwen: A Yang family legend. *Inside kung-fu*, 44–46.

Tensegrity: Development of Dynamic Balance and Internal Power in Taijiquan

by Michael Rosario Graycar and Rachel Tomlinson, M.Ed.

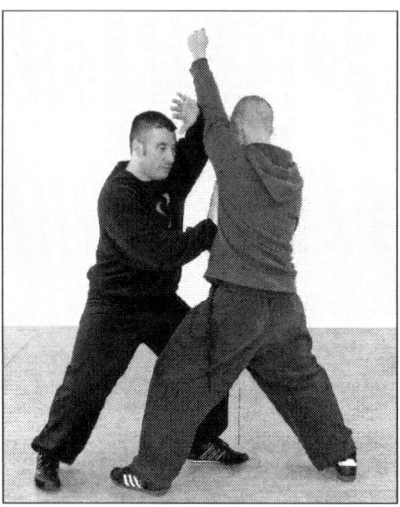

Photographs by Michael Rosario Graycar and Ryan Craig.

The internal martial art of Chen Style taijiquan has been increasing in prominence throughout the United States and the world. Over the years many practitioners have worked with high-level masters, but few have developed the skills demonstrated by these masters. Many of these masters do not possess the English-language skills to impart the "internal feeling" of their given art onto their students. Here's where many Western practitioners run into the biggest issue: rote learning through imitation will not lead to mastery. Only by having a clear understanding of the language of the "internal feeling" of taijiquan can any headway be made.

Languages to Develop "Internal Feeling"

According to Grandmaster Chen Xiaowang (Berwick and Butler, 2003: 36), three languages are necessary to understand taiji:

1) The language of speaking and writing: to explain and theorize
2) The language of the body: to demonstrate and see
3) The language of corrections: to feel (the most important language)

The masters are able to use languages 2 and 3 cited above. However, the English language of speaking and writing has often been deficient in enabling these masters to describe and impart the "internal feeling" of taijiquan to their students.

Therefore, some masters and practitioners have used inappropriate scientific models to describe the static and movement mechanics of the body. Namely, the body has been compared to buildings in which the skeleton is stacked in a compressive state, like a column structure. Modern science tells us that this model is not correct. If bones met other bones under compression, the bones and joints would quickly deteriorate.

The other model used in describing the static body mechanics in taijiquan is the arch, where the tailbone and pelvis act like a keystone. Obviously, the basic mechanics appear to make sense when two feet are on the ground; however, as Grandmaster Chen regularly demonstrates, the ability to root on one foot would not be possible under the arch analogy.

The problem with both of these analogies is that compressive structures can only deal with load force acting directly on them following the pull of gravity. Any shear or torque forces acting on a building structure quickly undermine its structural integrity and can cause the structure to be unstable. Through demonstrations of internal masters, this is simply not the case. These masters can receive both shear and torque forces while maintaining structural integrity.

At the same time, the definition of movement mechanics has also been flawed. Viewing movement like a levering system does not take into account the forces involved in performing the simplest actions, such as picking up a watermelon. As Dr. Stephen Levin notes, "Calculating loads with the body as a lever-beam, linear Newtonian model will create forces that rip muscle, crush bone and exhaust energy" (2002: 375).

We can see from the present paradigm why the human body may be suffering from degenerative diseases, such as carpal tunnel, tendonitis, arthritis, and myofascial disorders, among others. When we treat the body like a stacked column, compressing the structure with the pull of gravity and using our joints in a fixed lever-type manner, we put undue wear and tear on the body as a whole.

So, what model based on science can describe the body mechanics truly experienced in taijiquan and other internal martial arts?

Tensegrity, or tensional integrity, as defined by Wikipedia, is "a property of structures with an integrity based on a balance between tension and compression components." Furthermore, "within the structure, the compression-bearing rigid struts stretch, or tense, the flexible, tension-bearing members, while those tension-bearing members compress the rigid struts. These counteracting forces, which equilibrate throughout the structure, are what enable it to stabilize itself" (Ingber, 1998: 49). So, a structure formed under the principles of tensegrity is under a state of prestress even before an external force can be applied.

This scientific model can be applied to both the static and movement mechanics of the human body. According to Dr. Donald Ingber, "in other words, in the complex tensegrity structure inside every one of us, bones are the compression struts, and muscles, tendons and ligaments are the tension-bearing members" (1998: 50).

This type of structure is stable through the constant interplay of its tension (*yang*) and compressive (*yin*) parts. This prestress (*wuji*, "without ridgepole") balances the body regardless of its shape or orientation. The practitioner has the ability to stand on one or both legs, or on the hands, while still maintaining whole-body equilibrium. The body is no longer bound to stacking or bracing the force into the ground; it can move freely while dissipating any force that acts on it throughout the entire structure such that each part takes up a fraction of the force.

One of the interesting qualities of tensegrity is its ability to shape change, particularly when the structure is made of both flexible-tensile material and compressive-rigid structural parts, as seen in Figure 1. A tensegrity object can expand or compact, or turn and move, in relationship to forces acting upon it without becoming slack or pulled apart. As soon as a force acts on it, all parts adjust to maintain the integrity of the structure. When the force is released, the structure springs back to its original shape. The faster the external force compacts the structure, the faster it springs back, unleashing its stored force (*fajing*: "explosive power discharge").

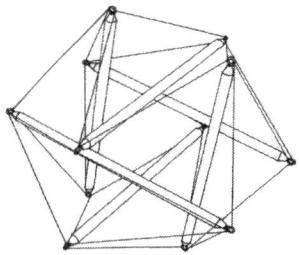

Figure 1

Consequently, the only way to destroy a tensegrity structure is to know the inherent weakness in the materials in the structure and exploit that weakness. For example, in a structure comprised of wood and rubber bands, fire or a saw could quickly destroy the structure. And while overextension would eventually rip the rubber bands, any compacting force would not destroy the structure. In theory, we physically start with our body parts as strong as wood and rubber bands and transform them into hardened steel beams and flexible steel cables.

Using the above tensegrity model, we can interpret and possibly understand the archaic language of the *Taiji Classics*. We will use three stanzas from the classics and the foundation-training exercises of Chen taijiquan to further discuss this model and develop a clear language to describe and understand the "internal feeling."

According to the *Taiji Classics*, "Stand like a balanced scale, (move) lively like a cartwheel" (Yang, 1991: 220).

Under tensegrity principles and mechanics, the body can "stand like a balanced scale," whether it is on one foot or two, since the fundamental principle of tensegrity is that the compressive and tension elements balance out, creating a sense of *wuji* in the body.

Although this analogy uses the term cartwheel, this type of wheel is a rigid structure, under constant compression. When a cartwheel is in motion, only the spokes in line with the pull of gravity are sustaining loads at any one time.

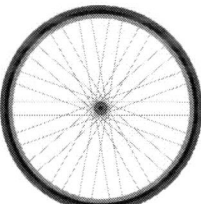

Figure 2

A bicycle wheel with wire spokes (Figure 2), on the other hand, is an example of a tensegrity structure. The forces are divided evenly across all of the spokes and the compression of the rim, while the hub floats in the tension network of the spokes, allowing it to turn freely under the load force acting around it. So, using the bicycle wheel instead of the cartwheel, the *dantian* ("cinnabar or red field"; body center) is the hub with the ability to freely turn, while the limbs act as the rim and the soft tissue connecting them to the dantian acts like the spokes. When any outside forces act on the limbs, the compressive aspect of the limbs themselves and the tensional aspect of the soft tissue connecting the limbs through the torso to the dantian zeros out the force so that the dantian is not inhibited from freely rotating.

The cartwheel is really the analogy of our present, untrained state. Before intensive internal training, we tend to lack tensegrity, so that any force acting on our body instantly invades our dantian center, stutters it, and destroys our centralized equilibrium. It will then force us to overtly tense localized areas of the body to maintain upright balance, which creates the column or stacked structure.

To develop tensegrity, we need to understand that it works from the cellular level to the tissue level, to the whole body structure. "Thus, from the molecules to the bones and muscles and tendons of the human body, tensegrity is clearly nature's preferred building system. Only tensegrity, for example, can explain how every time you move your arm, your skin stretches, your extracellular matrix extends, your cells distort, and the interconnected molecules that form the internal framework of the cell feel the pull-all without any breakage or discontinuity" (Ingber, 1998: 56).

Fundamental Taijiquan Practices to Enhance Tensegrity Mechanics

In Chen taijiquan the fundamental methods of developing these principles are harnessed through the practice of post standing (*zhanzhuang*) and silk reeling exercises (*chansigong*). These methods enable the practitioner to develop both static and movement tensegrity mechanics.

Through post standing practice with direct corrections by a master, the practitioner can develop the feeling of a tensegrity body structure in which all parts are neither too tense nor too relaxed, producing the central equilibrium state. The overall goal of standing is to produce natural and effortless action (*wu wei*).

When the practitioner begins standing, many aspects of the body are out of alignment with the pull of gravity. This causes excess localized tension in parts of the body. This can be seen in Figure 3a. The shoulders, hips, and ankles are not in alignment. The shoulders and chest are lifted, causing excess stress in the upper torso. The diagonal line on the body shows the body mass lifting forward, up, and away from the pull of gravity. The line at the lower back demonstrates the excessive curvature of the lumbar spine, causing the dantian to shift out and forward, which lifts the hips and tailbone up and back, decreasing the angle between lumbar and tailbone. The upper line illustrates the forward curvature of the neck, lifting the jaw and head up and out. As a result of these unbalanced forces, any external force acting directly on the torso would cause the structure to be rendered unstable.

In Figure 3b, Master Ren Guangyi corrects Michael's alignment, bringing his body into a state of equilibrium.

In Figure 3c, Michael demonstrates a balanced state. His shoulders, hips, and ankles form a line. The dantian creates an equalized force from front to back and top to bottom, which causes the angle from the tailbone to the lower back to increase, releasing the localized tension in the lumbar region. With the neck and the lower back opening up and the jaw and chest relaxing down, the body balances out all of the opposing forces, which exhibits the principles of tensegrity.

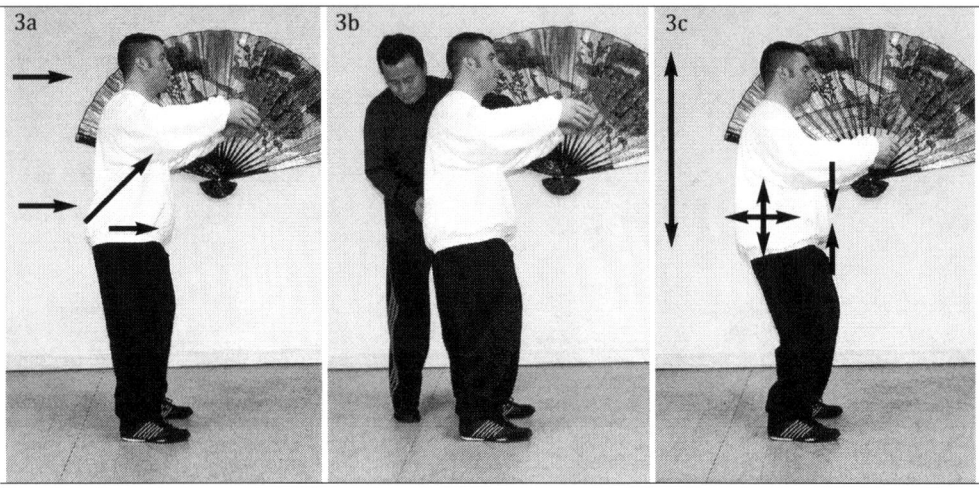

The ability to sense these changes in the body's structure from unstable to a balanced tensegrity structure relates to the body's proprioceptive sense. According to www.bio-medicine.com, "proprioception" (from Latin *proprius*, meaning "one's own") is the sense of the position of parts of the body, relative to other neighboring parts of the body."

What Does the Proprioceptive Sense Mean within Our Taijiquan Practice?

This sense of the body is partially responsible for how the body creates an unconscious balanced state. Therefore, this sense helps to develop a habit that's hard to break, since it causes a feeling of comfort in how the body relates to its environment. Post-standing practice can be an intensely painful experience for the beginner. By causing a complete structural change, muscles are stressed in different ways than the normal state of the body. The more we resist the pain, the harder it will be for the body to recalibrate the proprioceptive sense to the more efficiently balanced state.

When our body experiences intense pain, we tend to internally run away from the corrections and unconsciously seek out our old ways of standing and holding our body. On the other hand, if we grit our teeth and force ourselves to hold the posture, we end up developing excessive strength tensions, which again negates our body's tensegrity. Therefore, we need to reprogram our motor movements so that we can maintain a balance of tension and compression throughout the body.

Only by driving oneself consistently and developing the practice into a meditation so that the mental and physical state can become comfortable and relaxed will the proprioceptive sense change to the new demands. By connecting a deep sense of respiration causing micromovements to occur in the lumbar spine, the practice of this helps bring the practitioner's consciousness into this meditative state.

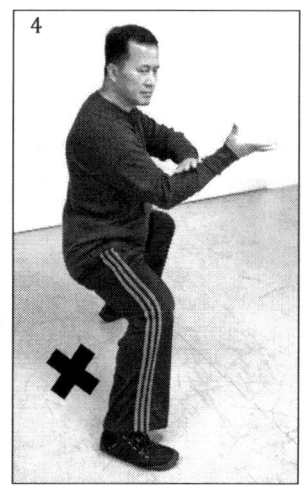

Once the proprioceptive sense has been reprogrammed, the biggest obstacle has been overcome and the *wuji* stance has become our unconscious balanced state. Unlike many other martial arts where the taking of a balanced stance is a conscious effort, in taijiquan, wuji is the natural state of the body. Hence, our bodies are always ready to act and react to any external force.

The practitioner can further develop wuji and extend the tensegrity state of the body's structure by holding various postures from the taijiquan forms. In Figure 4, Master Ren demonstrates the entrance into the "White Crane" posture from new frame first routine (*xinjia yilu*). When the hip is sunk and the knee-to-foot line is perpendicular, the body appears to be unstable due to the mass of the torso being sunken behind the feet. The location of his center of gravity in relationship to the ground is marked with an X.

In the stacking method, without a chair—or a tail—it is virtually impossible to lower the body behind the feet and maintain balance on all sides. The structure should only be stable and strong from right to left, where either foot can act as the support to offset the pressure. Any force forward or backward should destroy the structure, and send him on his back or chest, respectively.

For the average practitioner, the knees typically pass over the toes and the heels start to rise off the floor, creating a stacked structure and putting excessive load force on the knees and ankles in an angle that cannot be supported with balanced integrity.

However, in reality, the tensegrity of Master Ren's structure allows for him to maintain a relaxed, balanced state with no excessive forces building at the knee and ankle. The quadriceps and hamstrings both work together like tension steel cables to balance out the load forces, while his femurs, shins, and hips create the compressive stability of his structure with every other part of his body acting in concert.

Mastering Wuji

The *Taiji Classics* state, "First look to expanding, then look to compacting, then you approach perfection" (Yang, 1991: 227).

The above statement can be very misleading. In a literal tone, we could say to stretch out your moves as far as you can, and then make them tight—and you're a master. We all know that it's not this simple.

If we return to the tensegrity model, we can see the truth in this statement. The larger the structure, the more stable it will be, due to the amount of prestress internally acting on it. When it is compacted by an external force, the body will store the force within the structure. In effect, the force is being concentrated as the structure is compacted. Consequently, when the force is suddenly released and the structure is able to resume its original shape, it does so with an explosive release of force in three-dimensional space.

In Chen Style taijiquan, we call this aspect of the curriculum "large frame training." After we learn to expand within the structure of basic wuji standing and the form postures, we begin to increase the range of motion of the joints and space within the joints, which in turn increases the synovial fluids in the joints, as well as the fluids in the spine, sacrum, hips, the whole abdominal region, and the fascia lining of the entire body.

As we all know, humans are comprised mostly of water. The fascia serves as a flexible membrane that forms intricate layers, similar to plastic wrap, which holds the water. These layers of connective tissue hold us together; the tissue is the most abundant component that makes up the human body. Due to the compressive element of the fascia, it maintains a constant pressure in the body, known as hydrostatic pressure (*peng jin*, "ward off/universal inflation force"). We see this in the plant world as well: since a plant has no skeleton, it is the work of hydrostatic pressure (*peng*) that makes it stand up.

Masters regularly tell us that we need to develop this peng energy. Through the tensegrity model, we now have a systematic method from which to develop this elusive energy. Now we can see why typical practitioners cannot replicate the feats of high-level masters, such as bouncing the opponent away on first contact.

They do not have enough hydrostatic pressure and cannot maintain the tensegrity of their structures.

Through the changing of our somatic balance state, from stacking to tensegrity, we start to increase the fluids in the body. Since a tensegrity structure always moves with the force direction, the structure provides the mechanical advantage of automatically having the ability to balance out any force the opponent tries to apply to our body. With the structure maintaining the integrity of the body center (*dantian*) to react, the body can efficiently balance or compact the force without creating direct resistance.

After the practitioner is able to develop and maintain tensegrity while the structure is static (*wuji* state), the quest is to effectively compact and expand the body in a balanced state through rotation and movement. Silk reeling is the primary method for developing this ability.

Circles, Spirals, and Folding: The Way Tensegrity Moves

As stated in the *Taiji Classics*, "Once in motion, everything in motion. Once at rest, everything at rest. Tugged into motion, back and forth. The breath-energy [*qi*] adheres to the back, and is absorbed into the spine" (Wells, 2005: 237).

Tensegrity theory teaches us that once an external force is applied to the structure, the entire structure simultaneously changes its shape. There is no sequential linking, like a domino effect; rather all parts change and reorient to the force to maintain the structure. Obviously, when the structure is put in motion, every part moves. Once the force stops, the structure stops and returns to its normal prestress state (*wuji*).

Again, the tensegrity theory proves the above line from the *Taiji Classics*. When the tensegrity body is tugged or pressed, everything goes into motion through expansion and contraction, hidden within movement and rotation.

With regard to the last stanza of this quote, we are not here to prove or disprove the existence of bioenergy (*qi*). If we look at the life energy as related to respiration and our hydrostatic state, we can see some truth in this statement. By suspending the spine, utilizing the theory of the tensegrity truss, such as the Kurilpa Bridge in Brisbane, Australia, we can effectively create this expanded tensile shape with the spine serving as the powerful connector between the body's center (*dantian*) and the rest of the body. Just as the Kurilpa Bridge works, the spine can move force in either direction while maintaining its own centralized balance, even though the spinal shape will subtly change in relationship to the stress forces.

Now the body has a pathway to move our own force and our opponents force without any part developing any localized resistance or excessive tension. When hydrostatic pressure (spinal fluid) increases in the spine, it creates suspension between the vertebrae, maintaining the compressive aspects of each vertebra within itself while the intervertebral discs serve as the tensional parts.

If post standing is a method to develop static tensegrity, silk reeling is a method to develop movement tensegrity. The parts of the body expand and contract in coordination with the movement of the spine, as described above. Silk reeling provides a repetitive pattern of body movements that, when developed with a calm and controlled mind, can further develop the proprioceptive sense. If this pattern is forced, it is not yet the natural state of the body, and the correct "internal feelings" will never be realized.

In the following illustrations, Master Ren depicts the four main points of the silk reeling movements, as taught by Grandmaster Chen Xiaowang. This slow, focused, repetitive pattern training provides the setting for the practitioner to allow the proprioceptive information to be sent to the brain, which will stimulate an intense dynamic and internal awareness to further enhance the mind/body integration.

Numerous authors have written on the fundamentals of silk reeling; consequently, we will only provide a brief outline, along with a description of the "internal feeling" of the movements, which is the most important.

The silk reeling being demonstrated by Master Ren is considered the one-handed positive circle silk reeling movement. He is demonstrating the left side only. This movement can also be done with the right hand, or with both hands coordinating together or alternating the pattern.

Grandmaster Chen teaches four important energy qualities within the silk reeling pattern:

1) qi descending to the waist
2) qi gathering at dantian center
3) qi filling the back
4) qi filling out to the fingertips

These four energy qualities are the root of silk reeling. Just shifting the weight and tracing the circle in the air with the arm will not develop anything but stamina and muscle tone. Without the correct "internal feeling" developed within silk reeling, the exercise is practically useless.

Master Ren demonstrates these energies of silk reeling. Through the reeling movement, the qi travels through the entire system, unobstructed. Starting with energy in the hand (Figure 5a), Master Ren is at a stable point to start moving the qi from the extremities toward the waist.

In Figure 5b, Master Ren demonstrates "qi descending to the waist." The correct feeling under tensegrity rules will be a uniform compacting of the structure, three dimensionally, from the fingertips inward toward the torso. At this point there is no weight shift, and the body is still resting mainly on the left leg.

In Figure 5c, we see Master Ren has now shifted his weight to the right and has reached his limit of the compacting side of the equation. Here he has achieved "qi gathering at dantian center." Now the left side of the body, through the compacting from outside to in and left to right, has prepared a path for an external force to follow without resistance.

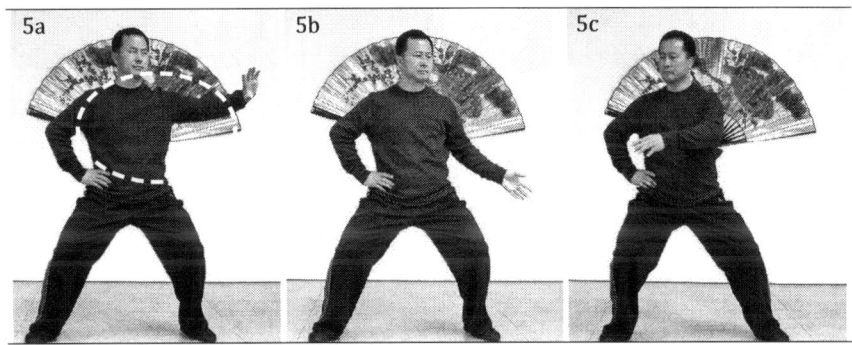

In Figure 5d, his weight is focused on the right foot while the torso has rotated, effectively releasing a load stress that would be acting on his left side if an opponent were there. As we know from tensegrity theory, once a force isn't directly acting on it, the structure seeks to move from a compacted state to an expanded state. Here, we have "qi filling the back" with the feeling of a slow, steady expansion through the left side of the back up through the shoulder.

As Master Ren completes the reeling cycle, he expands and extends into the "qi filling out to the fingertips" position in Figure 5e. The weight has shifted back to the left foot from the slow, steady expansion from the back shoulder area to the fingertips. The feeling of a three-dimensional expansion on the left side of the body includes both the left side of the back and chest/ribcage area as well as the entire left arm expanding uniformly out to the palm and fingertips.

The cycle returns to Figure 5b in a continuous, repetitive pattern.

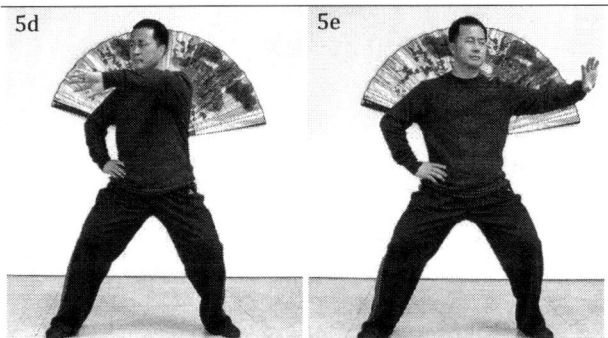

The Need for Fangsong to Fajing

For anyone who trains with any of the Chen taijiquan masters, a commonly repeated term is *fangsong*. This term is commonly translated as "relaxation." Nevertheless, Grandmaster Chen Zhenglei describes fangsong within taijiquan as a relaxed, extended, expanded, pliable, stable structure, which is another way to describe tensegrity in certain states. As we see from the above information, relaxation is only one component of *fangsong*. In tensegrity structures, through the constant state of tension/compression on the microscale, you will observe the subtle "relaxing" of some tensional components as others increase strength to maintain a balanced state under any pressure. The tensegrity theory offers a mechanical understanding of how the body and mind can achieve this fangsong state, both physically and mentally.

When we can develop this fangsong state, all the requirements to explosively release a tremendous amount of force on our opponent are realized, and Chen taijiquan "explosive power discharge" (*fajing*), with its apparently relaxed, effortless expression, can impact the opponent without a loss of our tensegrity. In figure 6a, the opponent's force enables Master Ren to compact into the center of his structure. In figure 6b, once the opponent's force is released off the center, Master Ren explosively expands from his center through his opponent, which violently launches his opponent off the ground without a loss of his structural integrity.

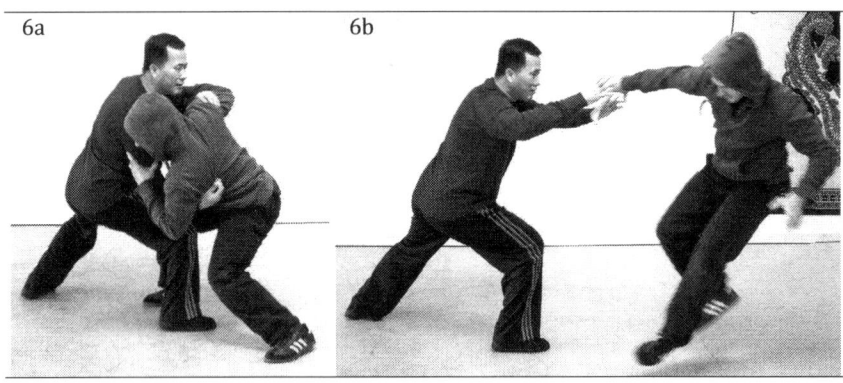

Tensegrity: Defining a New View of Body Maintenance and Development

The tensegrity model and the biology of hydrostatic pressure provide the language to describe both static and movement mechanics in the human body, particularly relating to Chen taijiquan and internal martial arts practice. The connective tissue, bones, and spine work in coordination to provide a stable structure from the inside out for the body. We can apply these ideas into almost every facet of internal martial arts curricula, as well as anything that we do in life.

When applied to the martial arts, the tremendous power exhibited by high-level practitioners is fully explainable. On the internal side, you have the compacting and concentrating of power and relaxed, explosive, expansive release, combined with the external power of speed and mass in motion.

When we look toward the healing side of internal martial arts, we can see why these arts can be enjoyed by the elderly and injured and provide the environment for sometimes seemingly miraculous healings to occur. Since the body is being reprogrammed to move with the least amount of resistance and expenditure of energy, it now has the energy to do what it is intended to do: maintain itself.

Furthermore, some orthopedic doctors, chiropractors, and bodywork practitioners have started using tensegrity as a basis of their practice. Therefore, the implications for body development and enhancement are far reaching, particularly in terms of repetitive strain injuries and personal physical growth.

Taiji Applications: Tensegrity in Motion

According to Dr. Donald Ingber, "A local force can change the shape of an entire tensegrity structure," while maintaining the integrity of the entire structure. In applications, the taiji practitioner employs wuji to maintain the tensegrity structure. Then the opponent's forces can be compacted or expanded while the practitioner utilizes postural fluid shape changing through folding and turning actions to maintain his or her own balanced state such that no localized resistance or excessive tension is experienced throughout the movement.

The following series of applications will demonstrate a few possible ways the body can maintain tensegrity while under resistive pressure from an attacker and effectively maintain a relaxed, fluid body action, utilizing silk reeling and folding methods.

Protect the Heart
1. The attacker (on left) is violently pushing both of the defender's arms down at the elbows. This causes the defender's body to compact toward the center, with the weight on the left foot.
2. The defender splits the forces by raising his right fist straight up and lowering his left fist.
3. The defender folds both of his fists/arms over the attacker's arms, towards his own center. This brings him into a fully compacted state.
4. From this compacting, the defender starts explosively expanding his structure, and extends his fists, with the right fist higher than the left, into his attacker's chest. The fists end level with his heart region, while his body relaxes back into the wuji position.

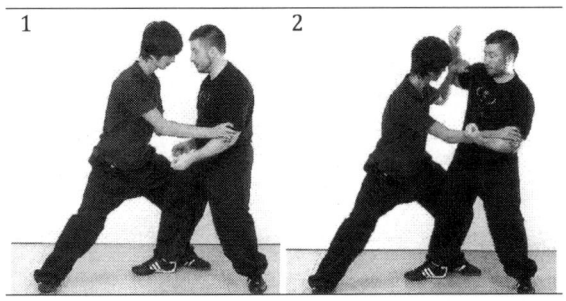

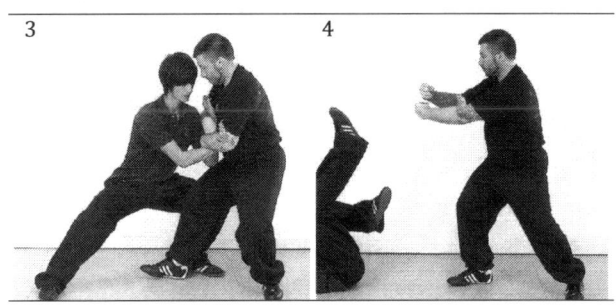

Single Whip
1. When the attacker attempts to lock his right arm, the defender maintains his compacted, balanced state (*wuji*).
2. The defender then folds his right elbow, raising it above his attacker's arm while preparing to sink down on his right leg.
3. The defender continues to fold his elbow/arm on top of his attacker's arm, sinking his weight down on his right leg. At the same time, he uses his left hand to grab his attacker's wrist.
4. The defender continues to grab, torque, and lock his attacker's right wrist to control him. As his body explosively rises, he uses his right hook hand to strike at the attacker's head, which naturally returns the defender to a balanced wuji position.

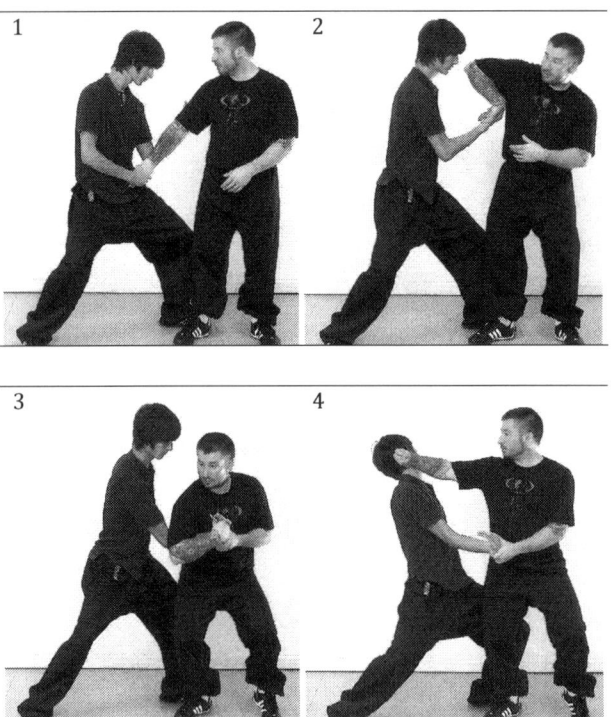

Six Sealing, Four Closing
1. When the attacker attempts to suddenly pull down then upward on the defender's right arm, he maintains his compacted, balanced stance.
2. The defender transfers his weight to the left side and lifts his right leg. At the same time, utilizing ward off (*peng*), his right hand lifts his attacker's right arm, as he grabs the attacker's left wrist with his left hand.
3. The defender steps behind the attacker with his right foot, keeping his weight on the left side, and proceeds to fold and twist both of the attacker's arms toward his left side, while the defender's body rotates and diverts the attacker's power away from his center as he coils into his left leg.

4. The defender starts to explosively unwind and expand his structure as he transfers his weight right. His body then descends onto his right leg as he strikes both hands toward his attacker's center. The defender's attack ends with his hands at a 45-degree angle from his center, while his weight is relaxing down on his right foot, returning his body to its natural wuji state.

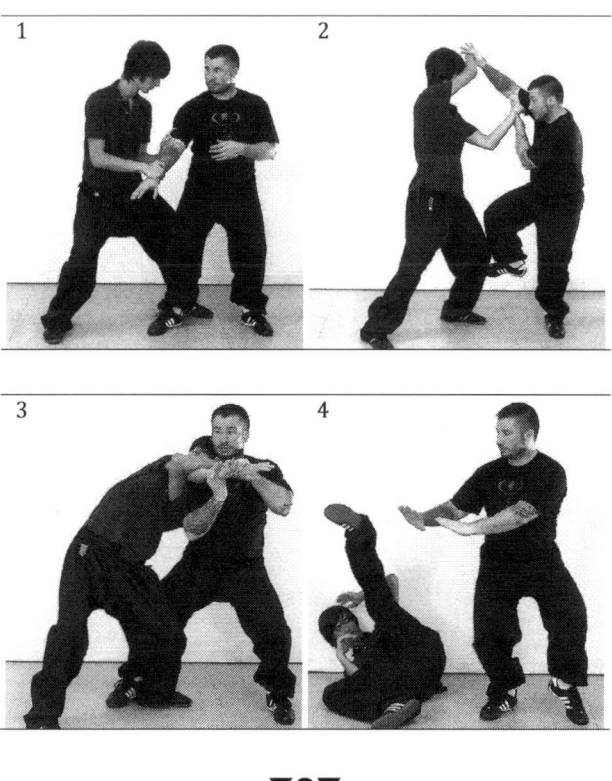

▼●▼

Glossary

- 纏絲功 *chansigong*: silk reeling exercises
- 丹田 *dantian*: "elixir field" or physical center of gravity, located in the abdomen
- 發勁 *fajing*: explosive power discharge
- 放松 *fang-song*: relaxation; or, a relaxed, extended, expanded, pliable state
- 掤勁 *peng jin*: "ward off/universal inflation force"
- 氣 *qi*: bioenergy
- 無極 *wuji*: without ultimate; ultimateless
- 站樁 *zhanzhuang* : standing like a post; or, a method of training in many Chinese martial arts in which static postures are used for physical training, to develop efficiency of movement, perfection of structural alignment, and hence maximal strength, for martial applications

- *proprioception*: the sense of the position of parts of the body, relative to other neighboring parts of the body
- *tensegrity*: a property of structures with an integrity based on a balance between tension and compression components

Acknowledgment

A special thanks goes to Master Ren Guangyi for his high standard of teaching, support, and collaborating on this article. Also, thanks to Ryan Craig and Aaron Ocker for being great attackers.

Bibliography

Berwick, S. and Butler, D. (2003). Comments on selections from Chen Xin's Illustrated Explanations of Chen taijiquan. *Journal of Asian Martial Arts, 12*(4): 34–47.

Ingber, D. (1998). The architecture of life. *Scientific American, 278*(1): 48–57.

Levin, S. (2002). The tensegrity-truss as a model for spine mechanics: Biotensegrity. *Journal of Mechanics in Medicine and Biology, 2*(3–4), 375–388.

Proprioception. (n.d.). Retrieved February 13, 2010, from Bio-Medicine.org website: http://www.bio-medicine.org/biology-definition/Proprioception/.

Tensegrity. (2010). In *Wikipedia*. Retrieved February 13, 2010, from http://en.wikipedia.org/wiki/Tensegrity#Basic_Tensegrity_structures.

Wells, M. (2005). *Scholar boxer: Chang Naizhou's theory of internal martial arts and the evolution of taijiquan*. Berkeley, CA: North Atlantic Books.

Yang, J. (1991). *Advanced Yang style tai chi chuan: Volume one: Tai chi theory and tai chi jing*. Jamaica Plains, MA: YMAA Publication Center.

Form and Function: Why Push-Hands is Essential to the Practice of Taijiquan

by Hal Mosher, B.A.

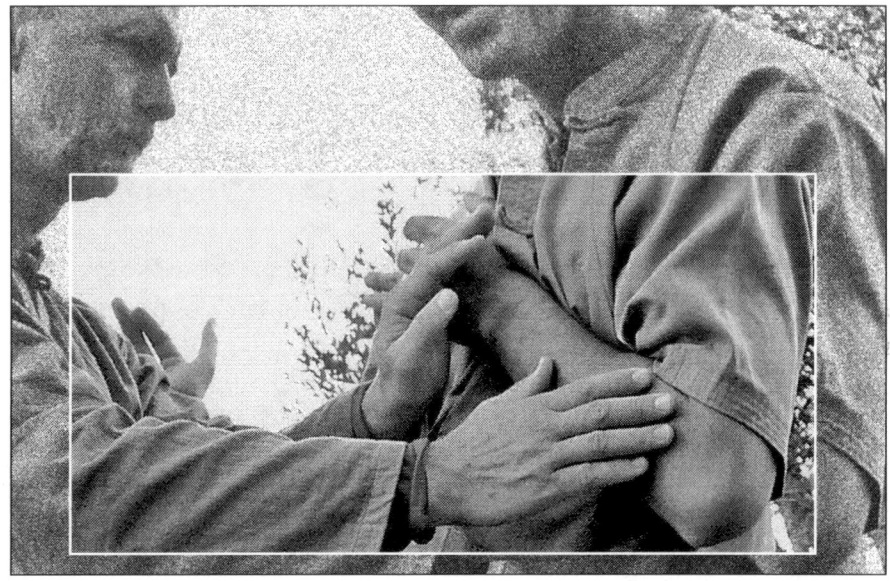

Allen Pittman (left) and Hal Mosher pushing-hands.

Introduction

Push-hands practice is often overlooked or misunderstood by taiji practitioners. Many allow the exercise to devolve into a mere shoving contest, missing the nuance and multilayered complexity of this vehicle for researching yielding, the heart of taijiquan. The great importance of push-hands lies in the use of yielding against an attack without using force, following the movements of one's opponent with acute sensitivity, and remaining firmly rooted and balanced in the process. When push-hands is practiced correctly with a partner, one may quickly discover problem areas, such as a lack of responsive shifting, the use of force, holding unnecessary tension in the body, the use of too much upper-body strength ("double heaviness" in taiji), and the lack of root or strength in the legs ("double lightness").

Immediate and valuable feedback is experienced when one is pushed off balance as a result of committing one or more of these errors. These problem areas may also be present in one's solo taiji form, and they can become easily ingrained through repetition if not corrected. Thus, push-hands helps to test the degree of embodiment of the taiji principles in one's solo form. It highlights the faults in one's postures. The process of identifying and correcting these faults will greatly improve the quality of one's form and application.

One of the main focuses of taijiquan training is to clearly differentiate substantial (representing an aspect of *yang*) and insubstantial (representing an aspect of *yin*). The goal is to embody the yin and yang symbol by keeping substantial and insubstantial elements in balance throughout all movements. While practicing push-hands, a dynamic exchange of yin and yang is created between the two partners. If one person uses too much force (*yang*), then the other must yield to that force (*yin*) and bring the mutual dynamic back into balance. As this practice becomes more refined, one will develop the ability to feel one's partner become imbalanced even before he commits to an attack. At this level, one may learn to yield in a more timely and complete fashion. If one person is imbalanced, then the partner must bring yin and yang back into balance, which often results in the overextended partner being "pushed out" or thrown off balance in an apparently effortless way.

Push-hands helps one develop very specific martial skills—primarily the ability to quickly recognize the weight distribution of one's opponent. It uses the postures of the taiji form to create weakness in an opponent through imbalance and allows for the conversion of the opponent's force into a counterattack. This practice is especially effective against a throw. The weight shift required for the throw to be executed will become obvious to the push-hands practitioner, even before it fully occurs, thereby allowing one to respond swiftly with a countermeasure, all while remaining firmly rooted. The opponent will give away the game plan without even knowing it.

The Basic Principles of Push-Hands

When beginning push-hands practice, both partners face one another with only a few inches of separation and both palms touching the creases of the other partner's elbows. The legs are bent and shoulder width apart; one foot is positioned ahead of the other. Both partners begin shifting forward and back until one partner goes off balance.

This close contact interaction tests one's ability to stay centered when an opponent is in very close proximity. This spatial disadvantage can be turned into an advantage through the over extension and ultimate "pushing out" of one's opponent while remaining balanced and centered. Response training of this kind is not common in most other systems of martial arts, where the emphasis is placed on strength to overcome an opponent. Push-hands uses relaxation and waist flexibility to respond to an attack, not force. This flexibility and slow turning of the waist at close range gives one the ability to easily absorb and redirect the weight and movement of one's opponent instead of struggling to counter it with arm strength.

The movements of solo practice in taijiquan must be fine, continuous, slow, and even. When applying this to push-hands, the goal is to feel this kind of continuous movement throughout the body while pushing with a partner. The response to a push should be as above: slow, continuous, soft, and even. If a person's push-hands partner moves hard and fast, one will be able to meet this speed with agility and softness to bring that mutual dynamic of yin and yang back into balance.

The absorption of a partner's weight is accomplished by taking that energy and transferring it into one's hands, letting it then travel through the body until it reaches the "full" weighted foot (containing all of, or the majority of, one's weight). Once it reaches the "full" foot, it is transferred again through the body and returned to the partner. This is much like pushing down on the coil of a spring—the energy given is returned with the same force. This is how yielding and pushing work together as a single technique. There should be softness in the upper body while the lower body is strong and heavy. This upper-body softness is what allows yielding, while the strong lower body stays rooted, resulting in the unbalancing of one's partner.

Yielding, Not Forcing

After a while, the push-hands practitioner will start to notice that a minimal amount of physical strength is needed to push a partner. As advised in the *Taiji Classics*, each partner should put forth only four ounces of force. Four ounces is, of course, impossible to actually measure when pushing, but is used more as a reminder of how little force is necessary. As mentioned above, the idea in push-hands is to avoid using the strength of the arms to push. For this to happen, all previous knowledge about pushing must be transformed into movement that is generated by the shifting of one's weight and the turning of one's waist. The taijiquan classics state, "If there is a problem in responding to an attack, look for the source of the problem and the antidote in the waist and legs." When yielding is done properly, the result will be the redirection of the partner's energy.

Every push has a source, and the push-hands practitioner is constantly attuned to this. If the opponent pushes by using only one side of the body, then the push originates on the opposite side. Most of the time, the upper body of one's partner is moving well ahead of the lower body, so one only needs to push the lower body to cause an imbalance. For example, when the partner's left shoulder leads during the push, one can yield by turning one's waist to the right and pushing on the partner's right hip to cause the upset (the partner's energy continues to flow in a circular motion and is only being helped along that path.) A person should only move in response to one's partner, no more and no less. Practicing push-hands this way will greatly increase one's ability to sense and follow the movements of a pushing partner.

Absorbing the Push

When one's partner pushes, the push must be followed and absorbed into the sacrum in order to remain centered. One can think of the energy going into the sacrum like catching a ball. Once the weight enters the sacrum, it is pulled down and tucked slightly forward in a "rolling under" type of movement. The energy then goes down one's "full" leg and comes out through the opposite hand. As in the coiled spring description, when moving only in proportion to the partner's movement, one can take the energy that is coming forward in the push, absorb it, and then redirect the energy safely away. As long as a yield—not force—is used to deflect an attack, then the cycle of yin and yang in the push and yield process will be successfully completed.

Double Heaviness and Double Lightness

These are both faults that occur in push-hands practice. Double heaviness (too much tension in both the upper and lower body) makes the form too hard or limp. Double lightness (not being firmly rooted in the legs and a collapsed upper body) creates floating and makes the form dysfunctional while pushing. The right combination of lightness (empty, without tension) and heaviness (sinking) in one's practice is what creates the ability to yield and respond with the proper amount of force. The lower body should be thought of as "heavy" while, in contrast, the upper body is "light." This is done by bending one's knees deeply and remaining upright and centered. The most common error in push-hands practice is heaviness in the upper body and lightness in the lower body. Each time the weight shifts onto one leg, there is heaviness going down the outside of the leg while lightness comes up the inside of the leg. This sinking is very active and quite subtle at the same time and requires relaxation while practicing, especially during push-hands. If one's upper body remains soft and light, then the push coming from the partner is easily absorbed as the waist turns and the legs remain firmly rooted. Essentially, the partner has nothing to "push"—no hardness to stop the momentum of the energy that will continue to move forward, resulting in overextension and imbalance. By contrast, if one's upper body is tense and the lower body is heavy, one is then "double heavy" and can be easily toppled by an effective push.

Every part of the body has its "full" and "empty" aspect, depending on the posture, in solo taiji practice and in push-hands. While practicing with a partner, if both hands are equally hard, they are double weighted. To avoid this, one hand must be light (empty, or relaxed) and the other heavy (full, or dynamic). The hand that is heavy, or full, is the opposite one of the leg that is full (for example, if the right leg is full, then the left hand is full). This sensitivity to yin and yang in one's partner will become honed into different ways of dealing with the angle of an attack. If one can yield by relaxing the side of the body that is being pushed, then the push will drop into the waist. As the waist turns, the push will be transferred to one's opposite side. This will help in the distinguishing of full and empty in the left and right sides of the body and will become clear in the upper and lower body over time through practice.

The Four Directions of Yielding

There are four ways to deal with an attack in push-hands, or four directions in which to yield. The first way is by using "the square." This is when a partner pushes on the side of a person's body (left or right), one returns the push using one's opposite side. The points of the square are the shoulders and hips. This is the most basic way of yielding by turning off the centerline and is used in most other martial arts systems. The second way is using "the circle," also called ward off. The arms are used as a shield that turns horizontally to protect the centerline. When the attack comes in, one would rotate on the circle of the attack. The circle will always defeat the square. The third way is "the sphere," which uses the circle in three dimensions. When an opponent attacks on the surface of the sphere, then the attack is returned. This way is unique to taiji and is equated with the down/up turn and left/right turn together. The sphere can defeat both the circle and the square. The fourth is "the point." The point combines all three techniques in one indistinct posture. The yielding and attacking happen simultaneously and effortlessly. The point can overcome any of the first three attacks.

Guide to Practicing Push-hands

There are some general guidelines that a push-hands practitioner should follow during practice:

- The arms should never be disconnected from the waist and root. Instead, allow the whole body to be used to absorb an attack. The arms and hips move together with one turn.
- A circular approach should be used to aid in yielding and pushing. If one's partner pushes straight ahead, then one can turn the waist and make the attack circular.
- One should not make the mistake of overextending, creating holes, gaps, or discontinuity. A hole is created when one is pulling on a partner. Gaps are formed when one's hands are too far apart. And, discontinuity happens when not all body parts are connected to the turn or weight shift.
- One should not try to win, but just listen and feel. Push-hands is not sumo wrestling. Partners must agree not to use too much force and instead learn to yield. If one's partner uses excessive force, the attack should be side-stepped and not confronted. Excessive force always results in the bigger person being victorious, and no skills are acquired that way. The skill one is trying to attain is yielding, not punching or kicking. This is why the concept of using four ounces is so important when practicing push-hands.

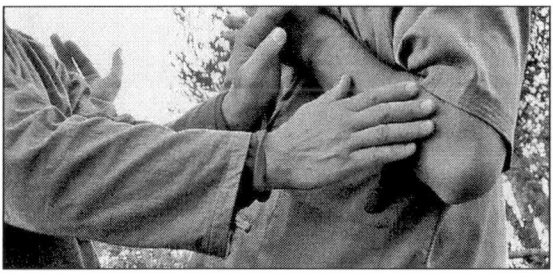

PUSH AND ROLLBACK TRAINING EXERCISES

Sensitivity Training

All two-person taiji practices highlight sensitivity to movement and the shifting of weight. The following exercises are to be done very slowly in the beginning, with an emphasis on softness to help develop awareness of the whole body.

1) Playing the Piano One Finger at a Time

This is the simplest way to develop "listening skills."

a) *A* puts one hand on *B's* chest at sternum level. *B* stands upright with all weight on one leg. *A* gently pushes one finger into his chest while *B* turns away from that finger. *B* should only move in response to *A's* push and keep contact with *A's* finger, even as it retreats (this technique is called "following" or "sticking").

b-c-d) *A* then chooses the next finger and repeats the process. *A* repeats the same exercise with the ring and then the pinky fingers. It is important for person *A* to go slowly and to choose only one finger at a time until *B* becomes used to responding.

B is receiving the real practice of listening while at the same time strengthening his leg, so both partners should play the roles of *A* and *B*. This exercise will teach the different angles that one must be aware of when yielding to a push.

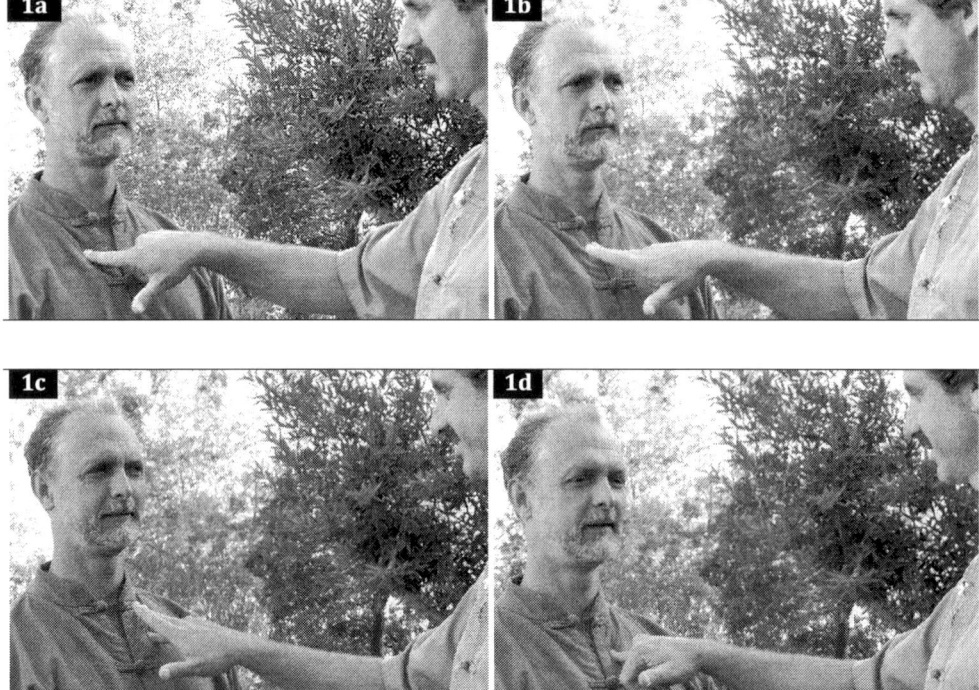

2) Pushing Four Corners

This exercise is like the previous exercise, but instead involves pushing on the four corners with one hand (two shoulders and two hips). In this case, 1) person *A* pushes on *B's* right shoulder, then 2) left shoulder, 3) right hip, and then 4) left hip.

During all of this, *B* has all weight on one leg with both hands relaxed at his sides. *B* yields to person *A* by turning with the push and not resisting it. As above, after yielding to the push, *B* will "follow" person *A's* hand and keep contact with it as it retreats. This same process is repeated with the other three corners. Switch roles with person *A*. This practice is used to learn how to yield and follow.

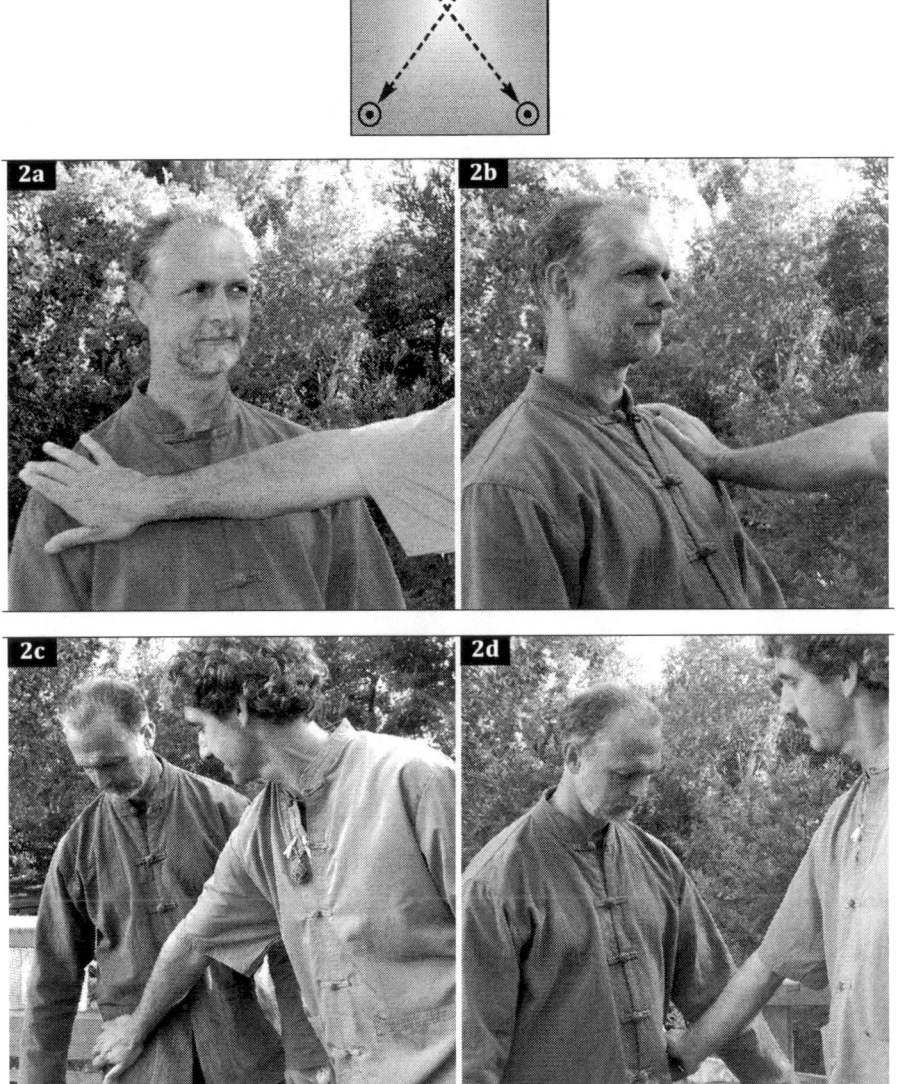

Single-Hand Push, Weighted on One Leg

This is a modified version of a one-handed push-hands practice as taught by Zheng Manqing. In this practice, both *A* and *B* have full weight on one leg throughout the practice.

1) Both *A* and *B* stand with their right legs at front.
   A pushes with his right palm toward *B's* right shoulder.
2) *B* starts turning to the right.
3) As B's hand comes close to *A's* shoulder, *A* turns further to the right.
4-5-6) The roles are then reversed, starting with *B* pushing and
   A turning his waist in order to yield to the incoming force.
7) The cycle is continued with *A* pushing and *B* neutralizing.
8-9) Now *B* is pushing and *A* is neutralizing.

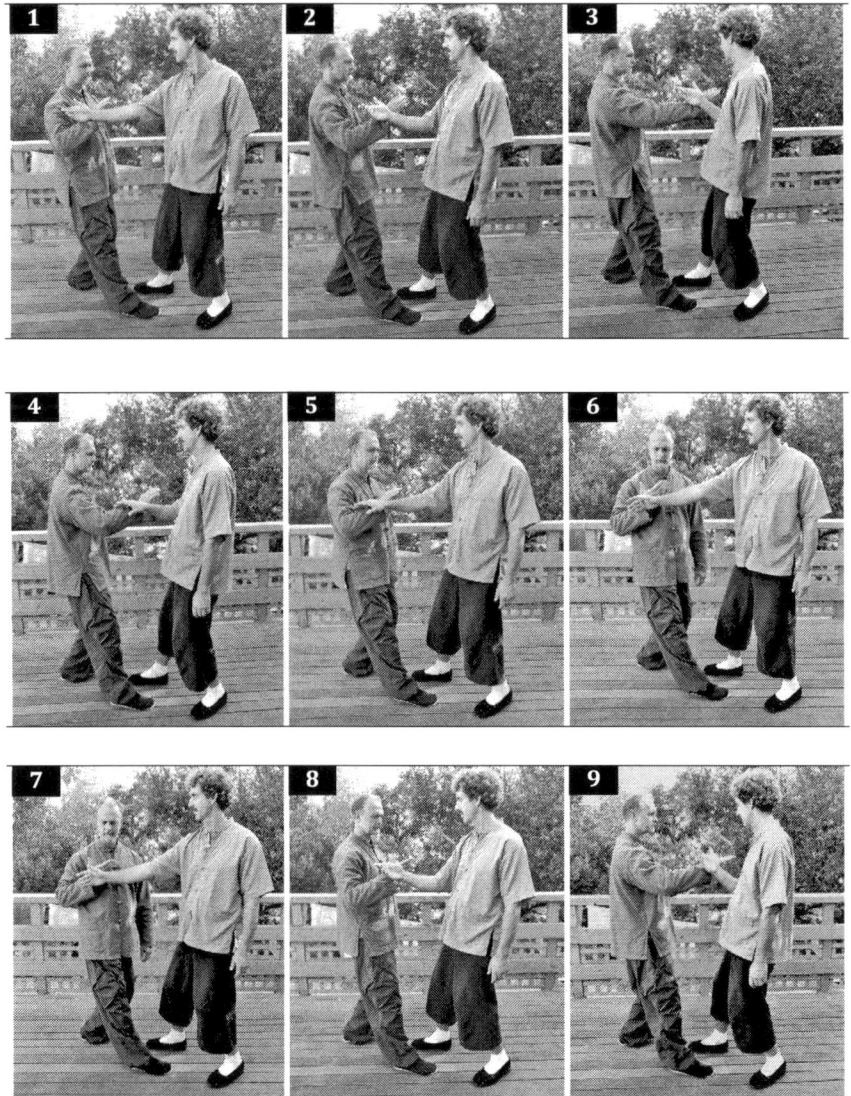

Partners should both switch legs and hands to practice both sides. This exercise is done to emphasize moving the arm with the waist and eventually the whole body as a unit. It also helps the two participants learn to be connected, in this case at the wrists. Here, movement is generated by the waist via rotation of the thighs. As one's thighs rotate, the arms must move in direct proportion to them. In order to practice central equilibrium, the sacrum must be vertical and lined up with one's feet.

One Person Pushing

This training exercise only uses the two-hand push technique, where one person pushes while the other receives the push.

1) *B* has all the weight on one leg while *A* stands in front of *B* with the same foot forward in a 70–30% stance. If there is a wall nearby, *B* should get pushed with his back to the wall so he can gently fall against it. (Having a surface close by helps one relax and let go of the fear of falling.) *A* then pushes on *B's* left arm resting on his body.

2) *A* pushes slowly and gently until *B's* front foot lifts off the ground. *A* then backs off his push to let *B's* foot down. This is done to show that even in push there is an element of yielding. Repeat three times to person *B*.

3) The third time, *A* pushes *B* gently against the wall as *B's* body comes back into *A's* hands. *B* is not completely passive, however; he tries to hide his center while being pushed, and to stick to person *A*. More important, *B* tries to relax his natural tendency to tense up when being pushed. *A* is trying to make the gap between *B's* rising up and his foot dropping imperceptible. *B* should not feel *A* go back at all and should just feel him relax.

4) If this sequence is done correctly, *B* will bounce like a ball before hitting the wall. This happens because lifting *B's* foot and then letting him come back uproots him. After three pushes on each side, the roles are switched.

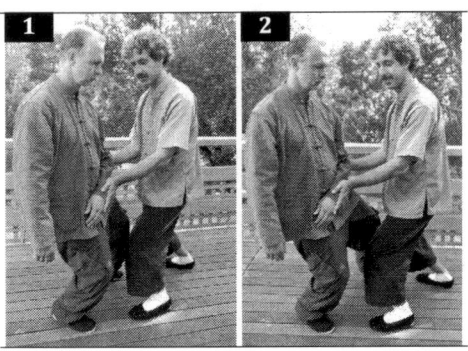

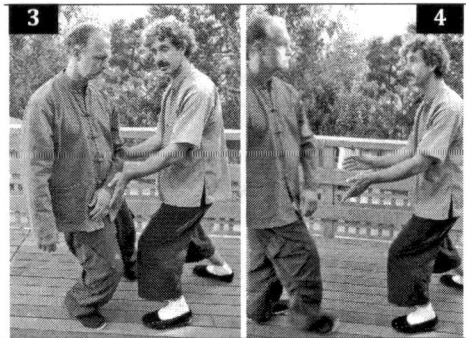

In the beginning, A might feel resistance in B; he may resist putting all his weight on one leg. Most people resist being pushed. The antidote is to shift back and forth until both partners relax into the momentum and movement. The goal of this practice is to yield completely when being pushed. A should be trying to push at different angles and notice the quality of push each time. The less force used to push, the better the quality of the push.

One Person Rollback
1) A and B are facing each other in a 70–30% stance, with B pushing and A doing rollback.
2) B fully commits to his push and over-extends into A's rollback. A then sits on his back leg, taking all of B's weight into it.
3) When the weight is fully received, A does rollback by turning his waist.
4) This should push person B off diagonally if done correctly. This technique reinforces the need to yield completely before rollback can be done effectively.
5) Once A has all of his weight on his back leg, he needs to find more "space" in his foot for partner B's weight—so, essentially, going as far into the yield as possible without falling back, and then yielding just a little more. A does this by continuing to move the rear thigh forward, creating the circle needed to move the opposite arm in rollback. This practice combines using central equilibrium to remain upright, and the absorption of the push.

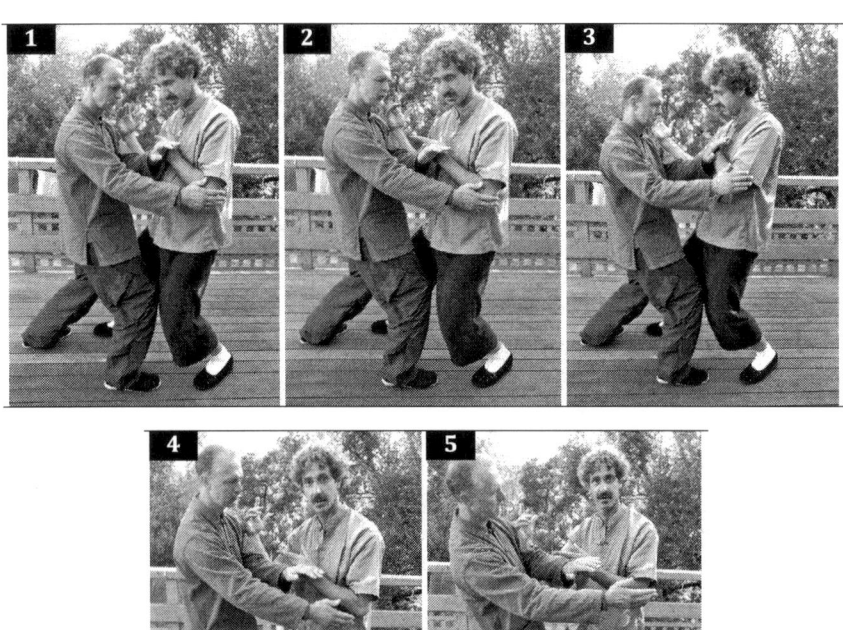

Push and Rollback Together

This last exercise combines push and rollback together as one unit of movement with both partners equally engaged in each activity. One person will push or rollback, depending on the situation.

1-2) If person A overextends, then B does rollback.
3-4) Person A will push and B will respond with rollback; then person B will respond with a push while person A does rollback. The movements should be light, with both partners following one another while shifting back and forth together, like a pendulum. This exercise is spontaneous and without set limits, so partners must not use force. It is recommended that the first four exercises be mastered before moving on to this practice. When done with softness, this practice becomes an easy way to develop listening skills and an ability to follow one's opponent completely to anticipate his movements. This is the pinnacle of push-hands practice.

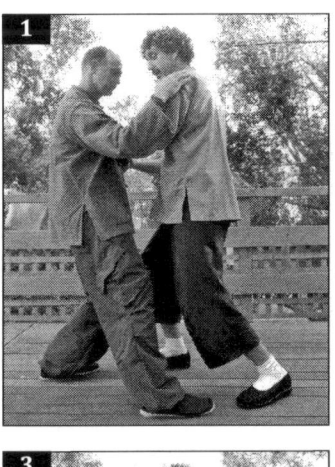
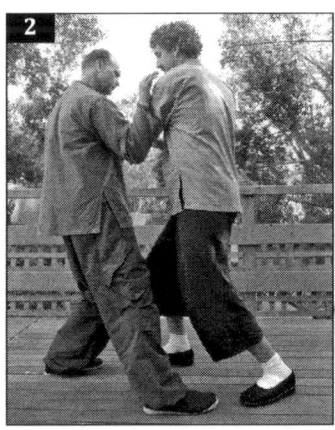
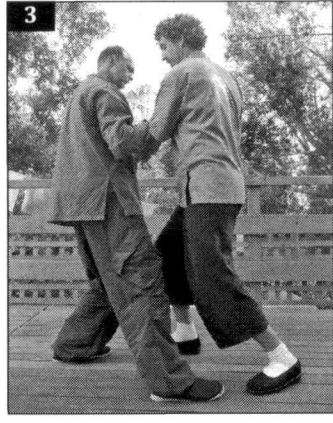
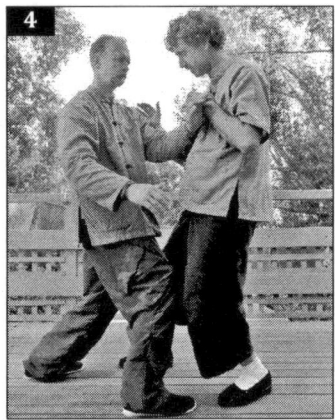

Conclusion

As a taijiquan practitioner, one can use the skills of acute sensitivity to an opponent's movements along with the ability to read and follow those movements effectively as the basis for understanding and redirecting an attack. A major goal is to overextend an opponent by yielding to his or her own momentum. Once this is accomplished, then any attack (a pull, strike, or throw) can be easily applied while one's opponent is off-balance. Shifting and turning the waist allow more response time and directional flexibility when yielding, and sinking will allow one to remain balanced and centered. This is where the proper embodiment of the taiji form becomes essential to push-hands; thus the solo form and the partner drills become important symbiotic practices.

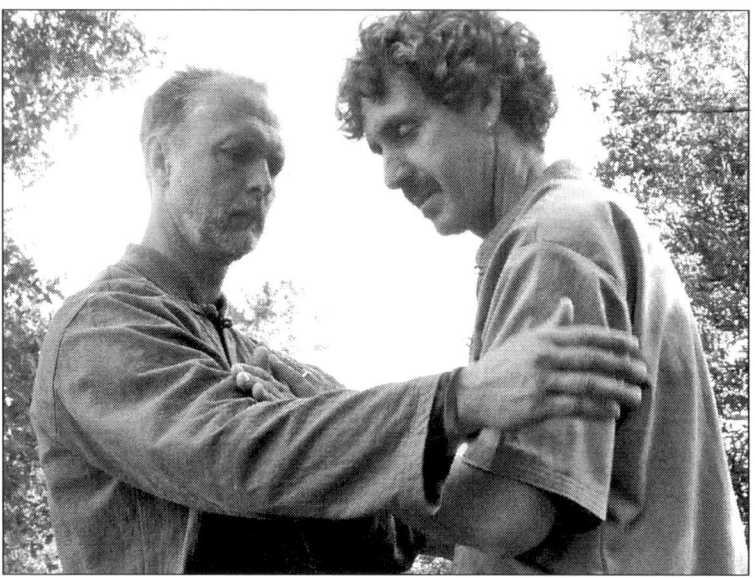

▼●▼

Acknowledgment
This chapter is dedicated to my push-hands teacher, Mr. Liu Xiheng (a senior student of Zhang Manqing). Thanks goes to Allen Pittman for his good-natured participation in the photographs for the technical section, and a very heartfelt thank you to Laura Ballard—her hard work, dedication, and encouragement are what made this chapter possible.

• 58 •

Multiple Intelligences in the Process of Learning Martial Arts Using Taijiquan as an Example
by S. Dale Brown, M.A.

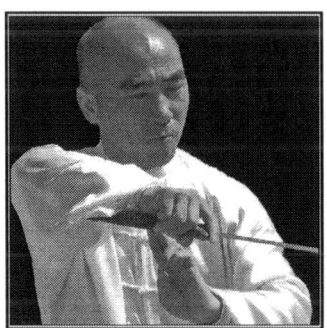

Dr. Zibin Guo teaching taiji sword. Photography courtesy of Dr. Zibin Guo, Chattanooga Tai Ji Community, and Applied Tai Ji, except where noted.

Abstract

Taiji practice makes an ideal vehicle for the discovery and examination of multiple intelligences. The purpose of this paper is to illustrate various taiji teaching strategies that engage multiple intelligences to help facilitate learning and retention. The multiple intelligences strategies offered are synthesized from the following sources: the appropriate literature, informal interviews with practicing professional taiji teachers, and the author's personal experience. Taiji practitioners can benefit from these strategies for a more comprehensive learning experience.

Introduction

The exceptional art of taijiquan (taiji) is a mind-body exercise/martial art that is practiced all over the world by millions of people. Taiji is constructed from a variety of diverse Chinese disciplines, specifically: philosophy, medicine, and martial arts. This unique conglomeration makes the practice of taiji an ideal vehicle for the discovery and examination of multiple intelligences.

In 1983, Dr. Howard Gardner, a professor of cognition and education at Harvard Graduate School of Education, proposed a new theory of intelligence. Gardner's theory of Multiple Intelligences (MI theory) provided a framework for identifying and classifying a multitude of possible intelligences, as opposed to a single general intelligence. According to Gardner, MI theory is about the intellectual and cognitive features of the human mind.

Human intelligence manifests in many different ways. People learn and retain information through a variety of styles and methods. The question is not "How smart are you?" but "How are you smart?" Taiji provides us with a means to explore and discover how you are smart.

Development of Multiple Intelligences Theory

After years of research, Gardner proposed a new theory and definition of intelligence in his 1983 book entitled *Frames of Mind: The Theory of Multiple Intelligences*. Gardner believed that the human mind is better thought of as a series of relatively separate faculties. The basic question Gardner sought to answer was: Is intelligence a general, single entity, or various independent intellectual abilities (multiple intelligences)?

According to Gardner, intelligence is much more than standardized intelligence quotient (IQ) scores. Gardner argued, "Intelligence is a bio-psychological potential to process information that can be activated in a cultural setting to solve problems or create products that are of value in a culture" (1999: 34). Consequently, Gardner endeavored to define intelligence in a broader context.

Gardner concluded that strength in one area of performance did not reliably predict comparable strength in another area. He studied intelligence in a multidisciplinary and scientific manner, drawing from psychology, biology, neurology, sociology, anthropology, the humanities, and the arts. This resulted in the emergence of his theory of Multiple Intelligences. Gardner and other researchers have continued to research MI theory and its implications, specifically in the educational field.

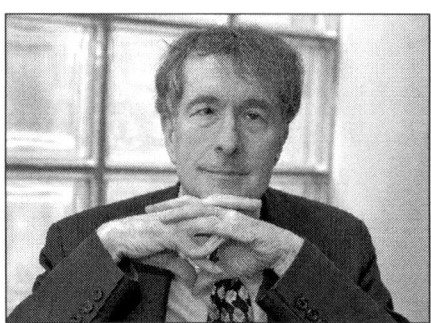

Dr. Howard Gardner, Hobbs Professor of Cognition and Education, Harvard University. Photograph courtesy of Jay Gardner.

To be considered an "intelligence," the ability under consideration had to meet several criteria, rather than rest on the outcomes of a narrow psychometric approach (Gardner, 1983, 1999). The particular intelligence under study was considered from a variety of perspectives consisting of eight specific criteria drawn from the biological sciences, logical analysis, developmental psychology, experimental psychology, and psychometrics. Gardner's eight criteria for identifying intelligences are as follows:

1. Potential for Brain Isolation Due to Brain Damage
2. Existence of Prodigies, Savants, and Exceptional Individuals
3. Presence of Core Operations

4. Developmental History and Progression
5. Its Place in Evolutionary History
6. Supported from Experimental Psychology
7. Supported Psychometric Findings
8. Susceptibility to Encoding

From the preceding eight criteria, Gardner defined the following eight multiple intelligences: Logical/Mathematical, Linguistic/Verbal, Spatial/Visual, Kinesthetic, Rhythmic/Musical, Intrapersonal, Interpersonal, and Naturalist.

Multiple Intelligences

Taiji is diversified in its training construct. It touches on each of the intelligences identified by Gardner. Resourceful taiji teachers should be able to incorporate strategies and methods into their training programs that cater to multiple intelligences, thus making learning more comprehensive and inclusive. Pedagogy that addresses multiple intelligences benefits everyone and exposes practitioners to the appropriate means to capitalize on intellectual strengths and enhance underutilized intelligences.

A person's intellectual disposition will affect how he or she learns. No two people learn exactly the same way, and strategies that work well for one may not work well for another. Practitioners who are conscious of their dominant intelligences can embrace teaching strategies that are effective and relative to their given learning styles. Several MI theory assessments exist online to help determine one's intellectual aptitude.

The key to teaching taiji effectively is to instruct in ways that facilitate multiple intelligences. There are no right or wrong learning styles, but some people may respond more favorably to one learning style as opposed to another. Most people are a mixture of learning styles with certain intelligences being more prevalent than others (Lam, 2007).

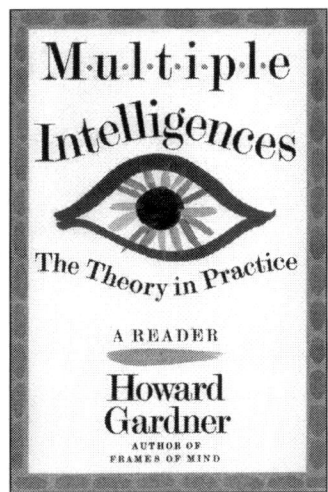
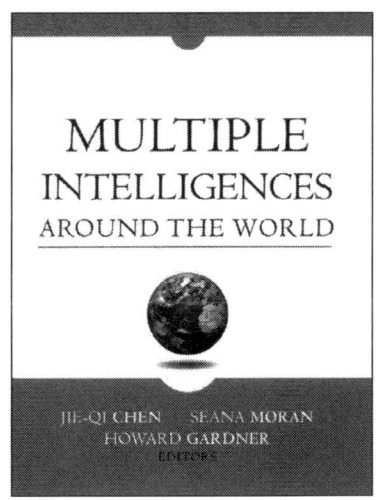

Many of the taiji teaching strategies presented engage both specific and multiple learning styles. The multiple intelligences strategies offered are synthesized from the following sources: the appropriate literature, informal interviews with practicing professional taiji teachers, and the author's personal experience.

Logical/Mathematical Intelligence

Logical/mathematical learners are considered "reasoning smart," which means they have the capacity to discern and solve logical sequences or numerical patterns, the ability to inductively and deductively reason, and they can investigate issues scientifically.

Logical learners have an aptitude for sequencing, so they learn best by doing things in a logical progression. They prefer detailed training instructions and approach new tasks one step at a time, learning as they go. Teachers can instruct logical learners by breaking postures down to a numerical count. Using a numerical count can help in learning the sequence, mechanics, and flow of each posture. The complexity of the taiji form can be simplified for logical learners by linking postures into small sequences, small sequences into sections, and finally the combination of sections into the whole routine. Flowcharts and diagrams can also be particularly useful teaching tools.

Teachers can illustrate the martial applications of each posture to help logical learners get a more comprehensive understanding of what they are doing. Logical learners may take interest in the scientific aspects of taiji training relating to anatomy, kinesiology, and physics.

Push-hands practice (*tuishou*) provides logical learners the opportunity to engage in pattern-recognition exercises. Push-hands relies on strategies and tactics employed by players through a process of sensitivity and action/reaction. Through constant practice, taiji players become sensitize to the patterns and can play within given perimeters. Taiji requires a logical, incremental learning process.

Linguistic/Verbal Intelligence

Linguistic/verbal learners are considered "word smart," which means they have sensitivity to sounds, structure, meanings, and functions of words and language. They demonstrate strengths in speaking, writing, reading, and listening.

Teachers can aid linguistic learners by verbalizing the instructions step by step. They can also use vocalized imagery as they go through the movements, such as "hold the ball" and "embrace the moon." Students can later use the same vocal prompts to recall the postures. Also, teachers can use analogies and metaphors to help communicate the various principles and concepts of taiji to their students. Conversations, lectures, and group discussions are also particularly effective communication tools to engage linguistic learners.

Linguistic learners may keep journals or notes about class, instruction, and their reactions. Reading, writing, and explaining to others help them remember what they were taught and process the information. Also, some linguistic learners may be compelled to learn the Chinese language or calligraphy to enrich their taiji experience.

Communication is fundamental in learning and teaching taiji.

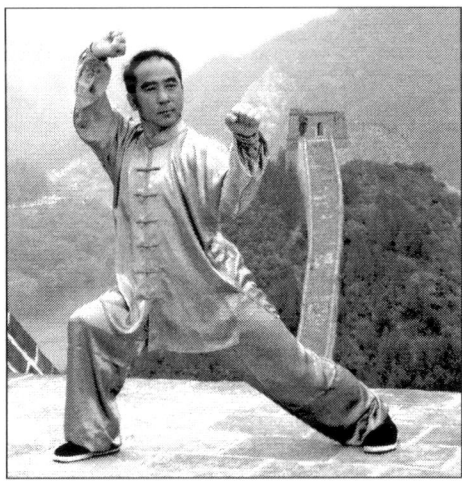

Dr. Zibin Guo on the Great Wall.

Spatial/Visual Intelligence

Spatial/visual learners are considered "picture smart," which means they have the capacity to perceive the visual world accurately and are able to perform transformations on their perceptions.

Spatial learners learn best by seeing how it's done. Spatial intelligence is an important element in interpreting the movements and replicating the intricate postures, subtleties, and aesthetics of taiji. Students must be able to visually follow the teacher from various angles for a large part of the training process and eventually be able to perform independently. In essence, the teacher becomes a three-dimensional model of structure and movement.

Teachers can utilize a four-step modeling process to visually instruct various postures or movements. The process is as follows: 1) Teacher does it (demonstration and explanation of content). 2) Teacher does it; students follow (students follow the teacher's movements). 3) Students do it; teacher helps (teacher observes students and gives feedback for improvement). 4) Students do it (acceptable execution of movements and principles).

Spatial learners can utilize illustrated books, charts, pictures, diagrams, and other visual media to aid in their taiji training. Flowcharts showing each movement step by step are helpful to them in remembering the sequence and direction of the form. Also, the use of visualization techniques and mental imagery to engrain movement and sequence can be of great use to spatial learners. Multimedia tools may appeal to them to learn new material or to record practice sessions for review.

Spatial intelligence also comes into play during push-hands, group practice, and weapons training. Spatial learners may learn the taiji movements more quickly and naturally than others. Taiji movement is a wonderful challenge for spatial learners.

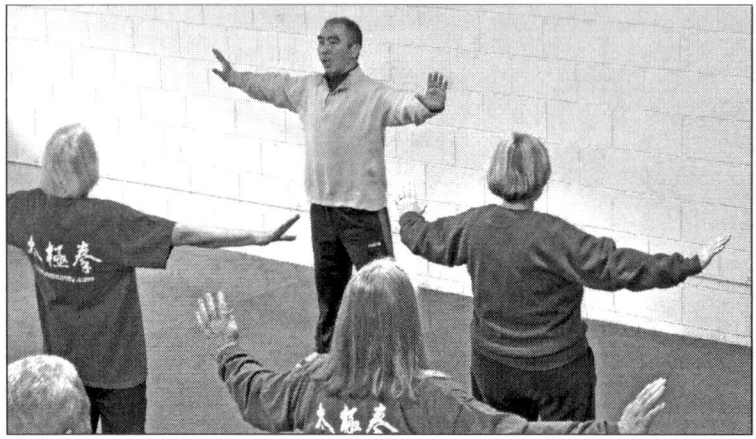
Dr. Zibin Guo teaching at the University of Tennessee at Chattanogoga.

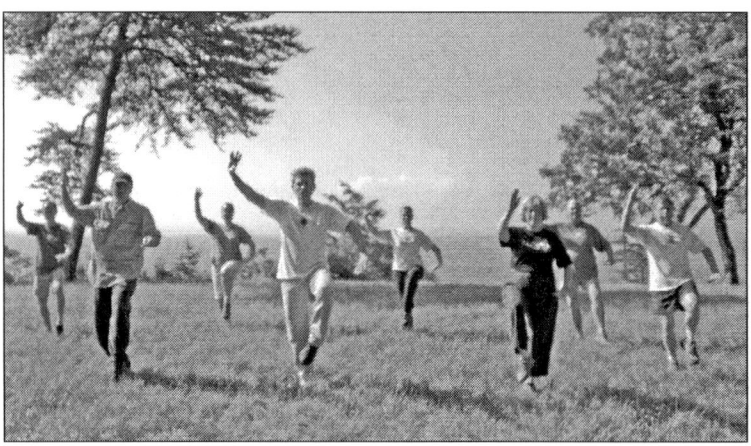

Kinesthetic Intelligence

Kinesthetic learners are considered "body and movement smart," which means they have the capacity to coordinate their body movements and handle objects skillfully. They learn more easily when movement is involved.

Kinesthetic learners take a hands-on approach to learning and learn best through physical experiences and activities. Teachers can connect with kinesthetic learners by physically modeling the taiji principles and concepts through their body language and structure. Also, teachers can demonstrate the layers of meaning within the movements: philosophically (open/close), martially (applications), and biomechanically (*jing*—trained force) to enhance their understanding. Kinesthetic learners want to experience the taiji applications applied on them and prefer manual correction from their teacher. They may have an aptitude for competitive or cooperative games. Push-hands and taiji competitions may be of particular interest to them.

Kinesthetic learners enjoy the coordinated movement of the body, the dexterity of manipulating weapons, the physical interplay of push-hands, and the overall athleticism of taiji. The emphasis on controlled movement and self-awareness makes taiji an exceptional mind-body exercise and sophisticated means of physical expression. Taiji training is ideal for kinesthetic learners.

Rhythmic/Musical Intelligence

Rhythmic/musical learners are considered "music smart," which means they have skill in recognition, performance, composition, and appreciation for musical patterns.

Rhythmic learners can recognize and utilize music as a training aid in their taiji practice. Many standardized forms have accompanying music that correlates to the movements. Rhythmic learners can use the music as an audible cue for specific moves, and to help set the cadence of the form. Then they can recall the same piece of music to perform specific movements in sequence. Teachers can also use hand clapping and vocal prompts to initiate movement and help establish the proper tempo.

Typically, music is a component of a taiji class to assist in calming the mind and relaxing the body. The practice of taiji is often likened to a symphony of flowing movement consisting of inner spiraling rhythms manifested in harmony and balance throughout the body. Rhythmic learners may respond affectively to the peaceful combination of music and movement, thus helping reduce stress and anxiety. Music is a wonderful addition to any taiji class.

Intrapersonal Intelligence

Intrapersonal learners are considered "self smart," which means they have access to their own emotions, values, and ideas. They have the ability to discriminate among their strengths, weaknesses, and limitations.

Intrapersonal learners tend to be introverts by nature and are self-reflective about their experiences. They are intuitive about what they learn and how it relates to them. Intrapersonal learners learn best independently and may favor personalized instruction or private lessons. Teachers can embrace intrapersonal learners through individual practices, such as meditation, solo forms practice, and internal skills (*neigong*) training. Discussions relating to psychological issues such as metacognition, active reflection, self-development, and sports performance may be of interest to intrapersonal learners.

Intrapersonal learners may become engrossed in their taiji practice and experience a sense of being "here and now." Noted psychologist Mihaly Csikszentmihalyi refers to this phenomenon as being in a state of "flow." Flow occurs when a person is totally absorbed or so fully engaged in an activity that he or she loses all sense of time, often associated as a joyful experience (Csikszentmihalyi, 1991). Many athletes refer to this experience as being "in the zone." Taiji as a moving meditation is perfect for intrapersonal learners.

Interpersonal Intelligence

Interpersonal learners are considered "people smart." They have the capacity to discern and respond appropriately to the moods, temperaments, motivations, and desires of other people.

Interpersonal learners are extroverts by nature and they learn best in groups or with a partner. Teachers can engage interpersonal learners through effective communication via personal conversations, class instructions, individual mentoring, body language, and group discussions. Interpersonal learners prefer group dynamics and learn best through cooperative learning strategies, group training, peer tutoring, and other interactive exercises.

The ability to get along with all sorts of people is a very important skill, and a taiji class provides a great opportunity to extend our interpersonal intelligence. Often, a taiji class will be used for social gatherings and may become a social network or a community of friends. Many students are motivated by these activities, which help them enjoy their taiji practice even more. A taiji class is a great environment for interpersonal learners.

Naturalist Intelligence

Naturalist learners are considered "nature smart." They respond to the outdoors, animals, and field experiences. They have innate fondness, responsiveness, and sensitivity to the features of the natural world and prefer to spend their time outside.

Naturalist learners may be inherently drawn to taiji since it is often practiced outside. Taiji is practiced outdoors as a means of drawing energy from, and connecting oneself with, nature. Practicing in the park, sunrise classes, and outdoor retreats are great ways for teachers to engage and motivate naturalist learners.

Naturalist learners may enjoy several of the natural themes associated with taiji. The characteristics of taiji are often spoken of in naturalistic terms, such as "flowing like a river" or "rooted like a tree." Also, many of the taiji postures take their names from the natural world and help give a sense of the proper aesthetic, such as wave hands like clouds or white crane opens its wings. Daoist philosophy's influence on taiji and its emphasis on longevity and how one should live in balance and harmony with nature may also be appealing to naturalist learners. Naturalness is fundamental to taiji practice and theory.

Currently, other possible intelligences are being observed and evaluated, such as existential and humoristic intelligences. Presently, they do not live up to the scrutiny of all of Gardner's eight criteria. However, they still provide valuable insight into human intelligence, MI theory, and taiji instruction and training.

Existential Intelligence

Existential learners are considered "philosophically smart," which means they have the capacity for pondering profound questions relating to philosophy, religion, and human nature.

Teachers can engage existential learners by examining the concepts and philosophies of *yin-yang* (open-close), *wuxing* (five elements), and *bagua* (eight trigrams) as they relate to taiji training and theory. Discussions on self-development and spirituality may be meaningful to existential learners.

Existential learners enjoy wondering and have the capacity to see how things relate to the big picture. They have a firm understanding of their own personal beliefs, preferences, and convictions. Discussions on Daoist philosophy, Confucian morals, and martial ethics in comparison to other world-views may be of significant interest to them. Existential learners are more inclined to see taiji as a healthy and meaningful way of life. Taiji is philosophically rich and meaningful.

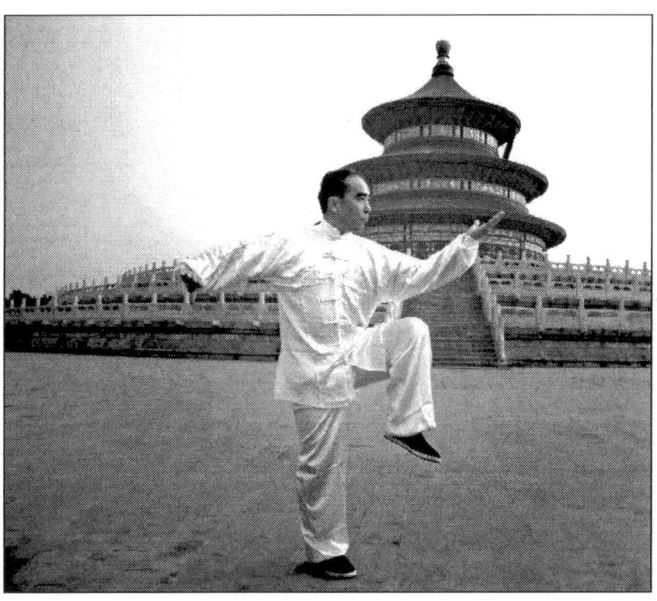

Dr. Zibin Guo practicing at the Temple of Heaven, Beijing.

Humoristic Intelligence

Humoristic learners are considered "witty smart," which means they could apply humor to various aspects of life and have the capacity to laugh at themselves and others.

The amazing power of humor can be used to set a peaceful tone even in an intense training environment. Teachers can use humor to break any possible tension in a class and make people feel comfortable and at ease. During push-hands practice, having a playful and kind spirit is very important. Players must "invest in loss" for a period before progress is made, and having the proper temperament is fundamental. Having a good sense of humor is important for all participants.

Teachers should include humor thoughtfully in the learning dynamic. Taiji practice should be fun and enjoyable.

Conclusion

Taiji provides a wealth of knowledge for lifelong learning and discovery. Students learn in a variety of ways and the challenge is for taiji teachers to create effective strategies that engage multiple intelligences. Teachers also need to be aware that they are more inclined to teach to their own learning preferences. Therefore, teachers must be vigilant in understanding their own learning styles and be diversified in their teaching methods to cater to the multiple intelligences of their students. The goal for taiji teachers is to provide systematic pedagogical skills that facilitate comprehension and retention in their students' taiji education.

As with all good theories, Multiple Intelligences theory is not without its critics. The theory has been criticized on theoretical, conceptual, empirical, and pedagogical grounds. Regardless, MI theory provides a fascinating window into the dynamics of human intelligence. The theory provides a profound framework for diversified instruction and enhanced learning. Practically, taiji practitioners can benefit from this framework for a more comprehensive, meaningful, and engaging learning experience.

Bibliography

Csikszentmihalyi, M. (1991). *Flow: The psychology of optimal experience.* New York: Harper Perennial.

DeMarco, M. (1997). Taijiquan as an experimental way for discovering Daoism. *Journal of Asian Martial Arts, 6*(3), 48–59.

Gardner, H. (1999). Intelligence reframed: Multiple intelligences for the 21st century. New York: Basic Books.

Gardner, H. (1995). Reflections on multiple intelligences. *Phi Delta Kappan, 77*(3), 200–208.

Gardner, H. (1993). *Multiple intelligences: The theory in practice.* New York: Basic Books.

Gardner, H. (1983). *Frames of mind: The theory of multiple intelligences.* New York: Basic Books.

Lam, P. (2006). *Teaching tai chi effectively.* Australia: Tai Chi Productions.

Li, D. (2008). *Taijiquan.* London: Singing Dragon.

Loupos, J. (2003). *Exploring tai chi: Contemporary views on an ancient art.* Boston: YMAA Publication Center.

Waitzkin, J. (2007). *The art of learning: An inner journey to optimal performance.* New York: Free Press.

Yang, Y. (2005). *Taijiquan: The art of nurturing, the science of power.* Champaign, IL: Zhenwu Publications.

• 59 •
Three Techniques of Dantian Rotation in Chen Taiji:
Internal Energy Techniques and Their Relationship with the Body's Meridians
by Bosco Seung-Chul Baek (白承哲), B.S.

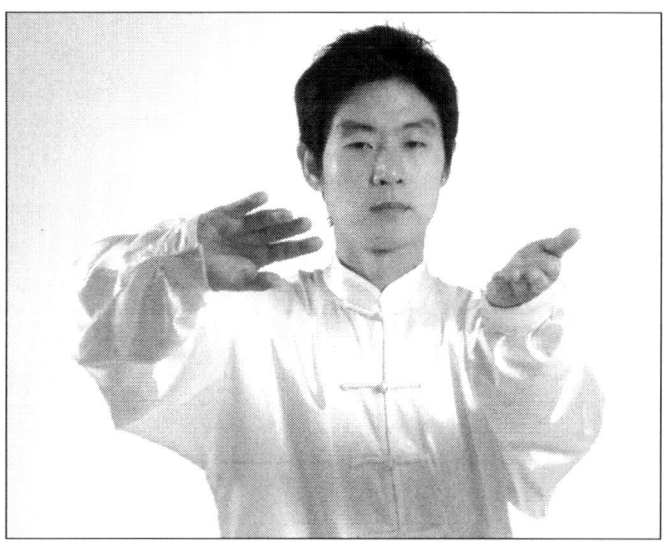

Photography and graphics by Chris Soule.

Introduction

Chen family taijiquan is the original system from which all other taiji styles are ultimately derived. The ninth-generation representative, Chen Wangting (1580–1660), created taijiquan from boxing heritages of past generations. Unlike other taijiquan styles, the Chen Style still utilizes explosive power (*fajing*), as expressed in the practice routine called "cannon fist." Authentic taijiquan requires harmony of four characteristics: sturdiness, softness, fastness, and slowness. It is impossible to master Chen taiji without these characteristics. To become relaxed and grounded, exercises and routines are practiced slowly, including the old frame first routine, since it helps one to deeply relax the muscles, joints, and spine while breathing naturally.

Training with speed, such as in the old frame second routine, helps a practitioner understand the use of the fast energy exchange between the positive and negative forces within the body and thus increase the power from one's dantian, which is the physical center of balance and energy. If a practitioner trains under a qualified Chen Style instructor, he or she should be able to get familiar with the dantian and learn to internally control its rotational movements (*neizhuan*) and utilize its function as a source of movement and power.

Before attempting any complex practice, it is a prerequisite to open one's energy pathways so that the dantian circulates qi powerfully. In other words, anywhere energy is blocked in the body should be unblocked by circulating energy (*qi*) through the energy meridians. For instance, if a practitioner has an injury or ailment, qi will not flow smoothly through that impaired area. However, the practitioner may remove foul energy caused by the ailment by silk reeling practice to circulate qi through the area.

Silk reeling is defined as a spiral movement that initiates from the dantian and leads the rest of one's body movement. All taiji movements must originate from the dantian to be done properly—this is the key concept in the silk reeling method. In order to circulate and cultivate powerful energy by silk reeling practice, one should know how to mentally direct energy flow through certain internal pathways. These pathways, called meridians, circulate energy throughout the body. A correct understanding of the meridians helps one to direct energy through the meridians naturally. With time and practice, the relationship between taijiquan and the meridian system will become progressively closer.

In order to maximize the use of meridians, it is important to acquire certain techniques of dantian internal rotation. In Chen taijiquan, silk reeling energy is activated due to these dantian rotations, and with consistent practice, it eventually interpenetrates through the meridians. The following descriptions are authentic training methods of Chen taijiquan's silk reeling and dantian internal rotations.

Silk Reeling Energy

Silk reeling is the key practice in Chen taiji that focuses on moving spiral energy from the dantian throughout the entire body. When the dantian rotates, all related joints and muscles follow its direction. From a dantian's movement, silk reeling energy will penetrate through the hips, knees, ankles, waist, back, shoulders, elbows, wrists, and fingertips. In this way, a practitioner can circulate qi through the entire body and sink energy into the dantian area. Eventually, a practitioner can learn to harmonize energy between the body and mind by stimulating meridian energy pathways. After becoming familiar with the basic silk reeling exercises, practicing the old frame first routine instills profound knowledge of the various expressions of silk reeling energy found within its different postures. If the basic silk reeling practice is not deep, old frame practice will fail to embody the guiding principles of the art.

Understanding the Eight Extraordinary Meridians

To circulate energy effectively, it is important to know basic meridian pathways for silk reeling exercises. It is believed that Chen Wangting created taijiquan by synthesizing yin-yang theory and breathing exercises that nourish *qi* (*daoyin tuna*) with twenty-nine postures found in General Qi Jiguang's (1528–1588) book on military tactics (*New Book Recording Effective Techniques*), and Chinese medical meridian theory. Understanding how meridians function is important for making progress with silk reeling exercises, breathing exercises, and related forms of inner cultivation.

It is easy to observe that many taijiquan practitioners lack knowledge of meridians theory. Any practice without this understanding would not seize the essence of taijiquan and could easily become a "taiji-like dance." Chen taijiquan aims to involve the use of meridians through the practice of standing post (*zhanzhuang*), silk reeling exercises, and the practice routines. Without these progressive steps, it is inauthentic. During this process hands-on correction from a teacher is mandatory to acquire genuine taijiquan skills.

In Chinese medicine, the eight extraordinary meridians are considered the root of energy pathways, while the twelve standard meridians would be considered branches. Even more sophisticated meridians cannot exist without the eight extraordinary and twelve standard meridians. The terms "vessel" and "course" are also commonly used to denote an energy pathway. Diagrams are included below for reference, showing only the main meridians from the complete list of eight extraordinary and twelve standard meridians. For more detailed information, please refer to meridian diagrams in Chinese medical textbooks.

The most important meridians in the body are called the eight extraordinary meridians, which we will discuss in the following paragraphs:

| 1) directing | 3) penetrating | 5) yin linking | 7) yin heel |
| 2) governing | 4) girdle | 6) yang linking | 8) yang heel |

Simplified Diagrams of Four Extraordinary Meridians

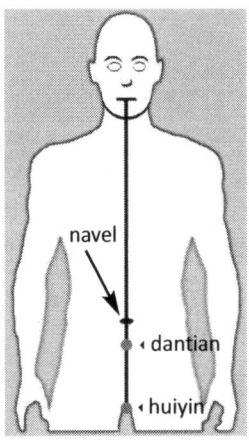 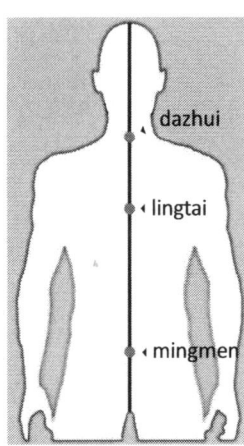

Left, directing meridian: Dantian exists approximately 1.79 inches below the navel. Huiyin is the perineum. **Right, governing meridian:** Mingmen exists between lumbar 2 and lumbar 3 on the spinal column. Lingtai exists at thoracic 6 on the spinal column. Dazhui exists at cervical 7 on the spinal column.

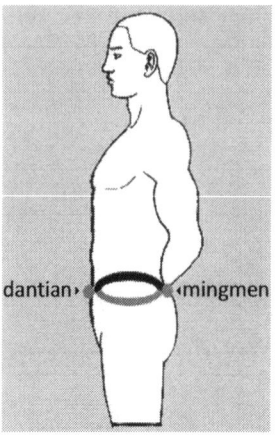 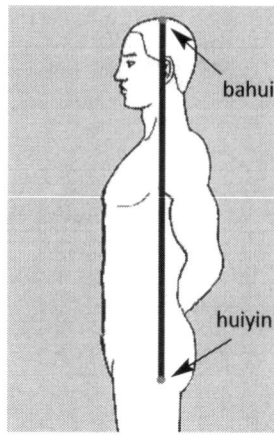

Left, girdle meridian: Dantian exists approximately 1.79 inches below the navel. Mingmen exists between lumbar 2 and lumbar 3 on the spinal column. **Right, penetrating meridian (back):** Huiyin is the perineum. Baihui is 8.33 inches above the midpoint of the posterior hairline and 5.95 inches above the midpoint of the anterior hairline.

Extraordinary meridians are powerfully independent regardless of the sequence of energy circulation in the pathways. For example, it is possible to activate the girdle vessel before the meridians in the legs and still maximize the effectiveness of each meridian. In other words, it is possible to take advantage of part of these extraordinary meridians individually or in unison. This is why they are considered extraordinary. However, the goal is to synchronize these meridians. If there is a blockage due to an ailment, the meridians cannot be combined. In order to lessen this type of error, Chen taijiquan aims to develop four extraordinary meridians in the lower body at the start of training. These are located in the *calcaneus* (heel bone: the yang heel and yin heel vessels) and in the *talus* (ankle bone: the yang linking and yin linking vessels).

The standing post and silk reeling practices both vigorously stimulate the four extraordinary meridians that pass through the legs due to the dantian's central place in these exercises and the effects of gravity on the thighs. It is not necessary to try to sense the energy in these meridians because it brings a very physical and direct stimulation of the legs. This is the reason the four meridians in the lower body are omitted in the diagram of the eight extraordinary meridians. For instance, the thighs feel burning and shaking because the upper body's energy is condensed into the dantian, and the lower body makes full spiraling movements when executing silk reeling movements. The hip, knee, ankle, and all related muscles, joints, and nerves are used to make the spiraling and coiling movements from the dantian internal rotations, which produce silk reeling energy. These meridians are linked throughout the entire body. Unless the meridians are fully opened, there is normally physical pain while practicing, but this is how a practitioner is able to dissipate any blockage in the meridians. A few indications of powerful energy cultivation and dissipating a blockage in the meridians are a burning sensation in the thighs, shaking legs, and warmness throughout the body.

The girdle vessel is directly related to opening the dantian because its meridian pathway passes through the lower abdominals and the waist area. In other words, it controls the internal organs that exist in the lower abdominal area. There is a specific technique to use this meridian in Chen taijiquan. The key is conditioning the upper body and lumbar to allow a practitioner to breathe naturally. In this way, a practitioner is able to activate the girdle vessel by natural breathing. This specific technique requires physical movements of the lower abdominal muscles and lumbar with inhalation and exhalation. In order to execute this, the dantian and mingmen should have horizontal alignment to be stabilized. The technique for the girdle vessel will be explained later in this article.

The penetrating vessel is considered the most difficult energy pathway to acquire because it passes through an internal spinal course. If the seven vessels of the eight extraordinary meridians are truly open, then it satisfies a prerequisite to train this vessel. The use of this vessel should only be taught after clearly mastering the "small heavenly circle" and the "big heavenly circle" (established when the directing and governing vessels are connected). A master can test a student's success in circulating energy through these pathways by confirming it through subtly sensing it with his own hands.

Direct lineage masters and grandmasters of Chen taijiquan—such as Chen Xiaowang, Chen Xiaoxing, Chen Yu, and Chen Bing—still possess all dantian internal-rotation techniques for opening all of the eight extraordinary and twelve standard meridians. This instruction is only open to their disciples.

Understanding the Twelve Standard Meridians

In addition to the eight extraordinary meridians, there are the twelve standard meridians that are directly derived from internal organs. For silk reeling and dantian-rotation practices, only three of the standard meridians are usually used with two of the eight extraordinary meridians. Therefore, nine of the twelve standard meridians are omitted for simplification.

The Twelve Standard Meridians
- lung meridian of the hand (*taiyin*)
- heart meridian of the hand (*shaoyin*)
- pericardium meridian of the hand (*jueyin*)
- *sanjiao* meridian of the hand (*shaoyang*)
- small-intestine meridian of the hand (*taiyang*)
- large-intestine meridian of the hand (*yangming*)
- spleen meridian of the foot (*taiyin*)
- kidney meridian of the foot (*shaoyin*)
- liver meridian of the foot (*jueyin*)
- gallbladder meridian of the foot (*shaoyang*)

- bladder meridian of the foot (*taiyang*)
- stomach meridian of the foot (*yangming*)

The Three Standard Meridians
- pericardium meridian of the hand (*jueyin*)
- spleen meridian of the foot (*taiyin*)
- small-intestine meridian of the hand (*taiyang*)

The Two Extraordinary Meridians
- directing
- governing

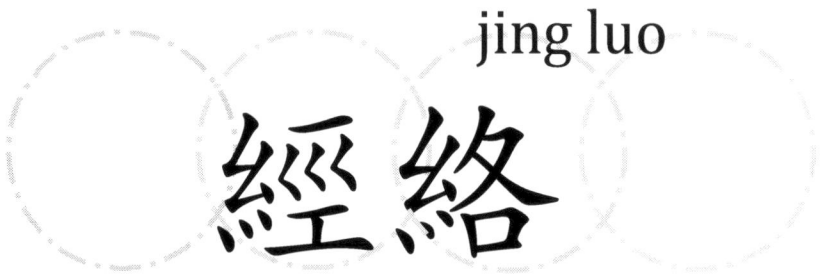

jing luo

Since the eight extraordinary meridians are the true source of all energy pathways, it is not required to use all of the twelve meridians for dantian-rotation exercises. In silk reeling exercises, the directing and governing vessels are combined because together they synergistically employ the eight extraordinary and twelve standard meridians at the same time. The primary meridians utilized in practice are the pericardium meridian of the hand, the spleen meridian of the foot, and the small-intestine meridian of the hand.

Simplified Diagrams of Three Standard Meridians

Pericardium Meridian of the Hand
- *Zhongchong* is in the center of the middle finger.
- *Laogong* is between the second and third metacarpal bones.
- *Quze* is at the ulnar side of the biceps brachii tendon.
- *Tianchi* is about 1.19 inches lateral to the nipple in the fourth intercostal space.

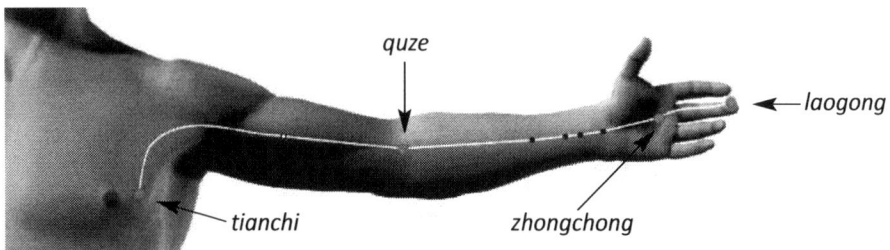

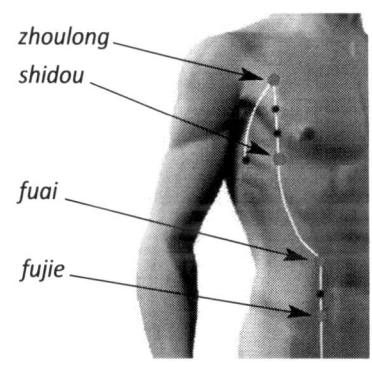
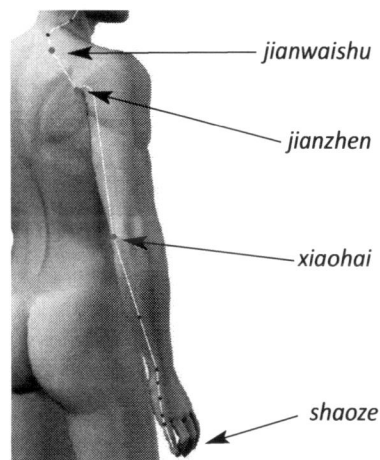

Left: Spleen Meridian of the Foot
- *Zhourong* is 7.14 inches lateral to the anterior midline in the second intercostal space.
- *Shidou* is 7.14 inches lateral to the anterior midline in the fifth intercostal space.
- *Fuai* is 4.76 inches lateral to the anterior midline at the directing vessel.
- *Fujie* is 4.76 inches lateral to the anterior midline, on the lateral side of the rectus abdominal muscle.

Right: Small-Intestine Meridian of the Hand
- *Jianwaishu* is 3.57 inches lateral to the lower border of the spinal column of T1.
- *Jianzhen* is 1.19 inches above the posterior and inferior to the shoulder joint.
- *Xiaohai* is in a depression between the elbow and the ulna with elbow flexion.
- *Shaoze* is 0.119 inch posterior to the corner of the nail on the ulnar side of the little finger.

In the actual silk reeling practice, two extraordinary meridians (the directing and governing vessels) are used with three standard meridians (the pericardium, spleen, and small-intestine vessels). Practitioners should become acquainted with the following guide, which provides an order for circulating energy in the meridians by visualizing the flow from point to point:

1) **Meridians:** Pericardium Meridian of the Hand + Spleen Meridian of the Foot
   Points: zhongchong ▸ laogong ▸ quze ▸ tianchi ▸ zhourong ▸ shidou ▸ fuai ▸ fujie
2) **Meridians:** Spleen Meridian of the Foot + Directing Meridian
   Points: fujie ▸ dantian
3) **Meridians:** Directing + Governing Meridians
   Points: huiyin ▸ mingmen ▸ lingtai ▸ dazhui
4) **Meridians:** Governing Meridian + the Small-Intestine Meridian of the Hand
   Points: dazhui ▸ jianwaishu ▸ jianzhen ▸ xiaohai ▸ shaoze

Whenever practicing silk reeling exercises, one should visualize the progressive energy flow from point to point as outlined above. The intention must be very natural. If the level is unnatural and creates too much tension in the body, it is hard to maintain correct postures and circulate energy. The feeling should be maintained midway between consciousness and unconsciousness. If this kind of mental awareness can be maintained, it will open the energy pathways even if a practitioner has a serious ailment. All he or she needs is a strong desire and determined effort for regular practice.

Locating the Dantian

In order to maximize use of the meridians in the legs, it is necessary to know where the dantian exists and to learn what is known as "abdominal breathing." The dantian is located three fingers downward from the navel, or approximately 1.79 inches below the navel. Since the dantian location varies due to different body shapes, this will vary slightly for each practitioner.

If you are not clear in understanding the concept, it is fine to think of the dantian as the central area of lower abdominals that controls the whole body. However, it is not just a muscular group or singular body part. It is like an antenna that senses and is connected to all of the big and small changes in the body. For instance, the dantian will feel uncomfortable and imbalanced if a practitioner has a physical error in body alignment or if the energy is not sunken. On the contrary, it will feel full, and a sensation of heaviness is apparent, and should be very relaxed during silk reeling exercises, or during any taijiquan practice for that matter. Additionally, the mind is able to be clear, calm, and peaceful. There should always be a deep sense of stability and sensitivity in the dantian at all times during practice.

Opening the Dantian

In classical Chen taijiquan practice, one's quality of motion and use of internal energy is dependent upon the dantian. At a beginner's level, it is not easy to sense or feel the existence of the dantian because the body and mind are not yet experienced in taijiquan's fundamentals. There is a methodical way to open one's dantian, and this specific training method is called the standing post (*zhanzhuang*). To practice, the entire spine should be relaxed, and a practitioner must utilize all of the taijiquan principles to sink energy into the dantian. Since taijiquan's principles are very well known, let us focus on specific techniques used to open one's dantian.

The first principle is to have the upper chest relaxed with a sunken diaphragm, while keeping the upper back slightly rounded. There is a common misunderstanding about this, as a lot of practitioners create tension in the upper body by making the upper chest too hollow. This and all other requirements should be done naturally. The second principle is to have the lower back (lumbar) relaxed so there is no convex or concave shape to it. If done correctly, the coccyx will be naturally rolled up so that a practitioner feels a physical expansion from the lumbar to the coccyx. With the chin in proper position and the neck muscles relaxed, a practitioner is able to expand the entire spine to sense it as "one big stick."

If the spine is truly relaxed, the energy point called mingmen will be ready to cultivate powerful energy. *Mingmen* is translated as the "door of life." The mingmen is located at the spine's protuberance between lumbar 2 and 3. In a correct standing post posture, a horizontal line can be visualized between the dantian and mingmen, which interpenetrate each other energetically. It is the main energy spot used for refreshing the entire spine while training in standing post and is the key practice to making the internal alchemy of taijiquan.

This horizontal alignment line of the dantian and mingmen is called *damai*, which is noted as the girdle meridian and activates the dantian (Note: This meridian is quite different from Chinese medicine's girdle meridian). It is important that this alignment be always kept during taijiquan practice because within these two energy points is where the dantian exists. Opening the girdle vessel is the seed to making the dantian truly open. In order to stimulate the dantian to be active, it is necessary to visualize breathing through it and the mingmen while in the standing post posture. The dantian and mingmen points expand naturally while inhaling, as a balloon is expanded when air is inserted in it. They contract while exhaling. Without proper instruction, there are health risks with this practice. It is important that a practitioner be taken care of by an authentic instructor with hands-on corrections. A clear sign of this technique done properly is warmness in the lower abdominals. A sensation of coldness in the dantian area is an indication of improper practice.

The mind's intention during this breathing practice must be natural while still physically engaging the lower abdominals and back—ultimately executed with the same intent used in combative applications. Done properly, one should experience expansion and contraction of both the front and back of the waist while breathing. In this way, a practitioner will develop the dantian core and cultivate powerful energy with standing post practice. This is the stage of energy cultivation called "dantian breathing." In later stages of practice, the dantian and the mingmen should expand and retract by themselves. Delicate instruction from qualified instructors to properly learn this process of breathing is a necessity. If not, side effects may occur due to incorrect instruction or relaxation technique.

THREE TECHNIQUES OF DANTIAN INTERNAL ROTATION

After accomplishing the previous requirements of energy cultivation, it is important to contemplate how to circulate energy by silk reeling from the dantian. According to the theory of dantian internal rotation, the dantian articulates in three-dimensional movements congruent with taijiquan's fundamental principles and requirements, such as "sink energy to the dantian," "loosen the waist," and "maintain a dantian base."

Standing-post practice cultivates energy in the dantian through the girdle meridian (*damai*). In a common standing posture, the dantian is blocked because it and the mingmen are not facing each other on a parallel line. Unlike Chinese medicine's meridians around the skin, the damai line in taijiquan internally penetrates directly through the dantian. This interpenetrating line required by standing post practice does not access the dantian for internal rotation, but if the dantian moves, there is silk reeling energy. If the dantian does not initiate and control movement in the body, there will be no silk reeling energy. The three physical techniques of dantian rotation consist of horizontal, vertical, and multidirectional internal rotations. Without this understanding, any form practice will be a dance-like taiji performance and will be ineffective in application.

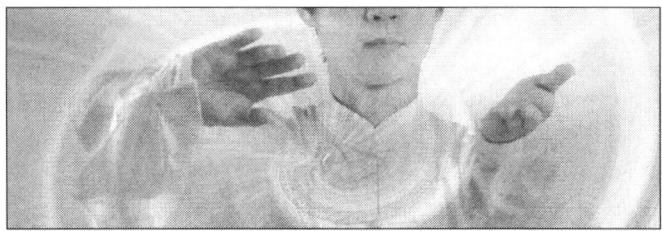

FIRST TECHNIQUE: Horizontal Dantian Rotation
For a novice, the first technique is easy to sense and acquire because it only moves horizontally in two directions, to the left or the right. Building upon the principles of standing post practice, a practitioner now must rotate the dantian horizontally. Practiced to the front, this silk reeling exercise is designed to familiarize the horizontal dantian internal rotation.

Preparation: Standing with Feet Together (Fig. 1)
This is not just a boring stationary position. It requires relaxing the whole body from head to toe. Wait until everything becomes calm and breathe deeply three or five times for deep relaxation. Do not start to practice unless you feel relaxed enough. When one is truly relaxed (*fangsong*), the body feels like jelly or pudding. It is a good sign to have a higher level of relaxation.

STEP 1: Lowering the Hand (Figs. 1a-b)
Slowly bring down the hand with the intention of activating meridians 1 and 2. To effectively lead the energy, focusing on the thumb and pinky finger is helpful. When the energy comes into the negative vessels, the pinky leads the arm movement. The thumb is a standard point of focus when the energy comes through the positive vessels. In this step, the energy goes down from the middle finger to meridians 1 and 2 when the joints are rotating. Step 1 requires a natural vertical dantian internal rotation so the upper chest can relax to condense the energy. Please be sure to relax the back and "dangle" the coccyx. When the hand is near the level of the dantian, energy will arrive around the ribs.

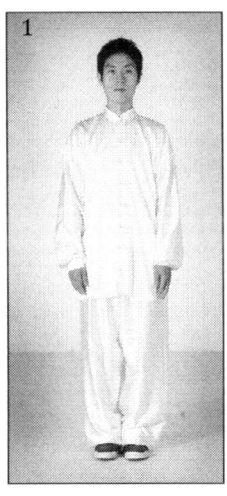
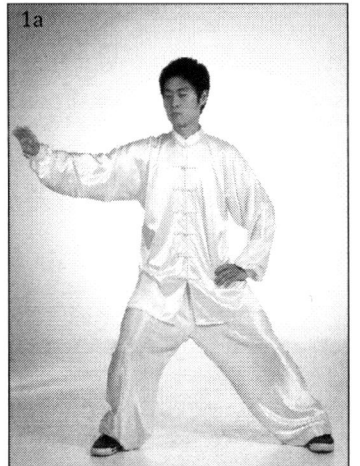
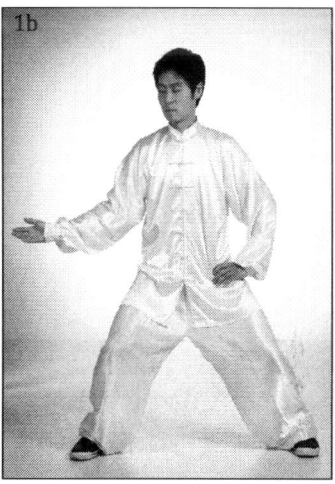

STEP 2: Moving the Dantian Horizontally;
Directing Energy to the Dantian (Figs. 1c-d)
Softly shift the weight and turn the dantian to the left. Energy will come back to the dantian area due to the horizontal dantian's internal rotation. The hip's level should be parallel to the ground so the dantian has central stability.

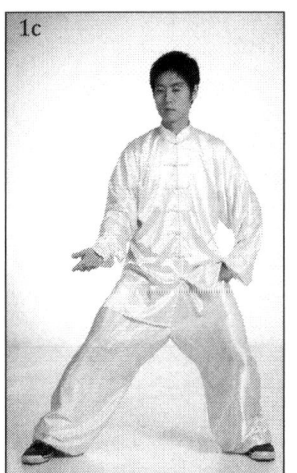
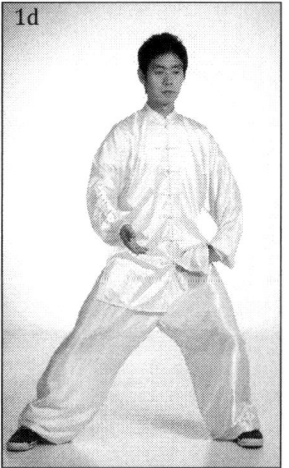

STEP 3: Sending Energy Down to the Perineum (Figs. 1e-f)
This requires delicate instruction. Upon finishing the previous steps, the dantian begins to rotate in an oblique circle. When the hand reaches the shoulder level, the energy rises to cervical 7 (*dazhui*). In this step, the directing and governing vessels are used. Although the weight stays on the left foot, the right foot should be rooted.

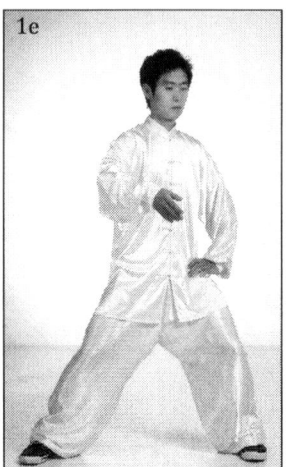
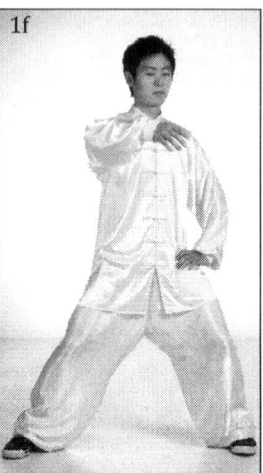

STEP 4: Sending Energy to the Pinky Finger, Meridian 4 (Figs. 1g-h)
Smoothly shift the weight to the right foot and slowly turn the dantian to the right side without turning the right knee outward. After rotating the dantian, the arm should be moved afterward. If the elbow is lifted too much, the energy will not flow through the arm.

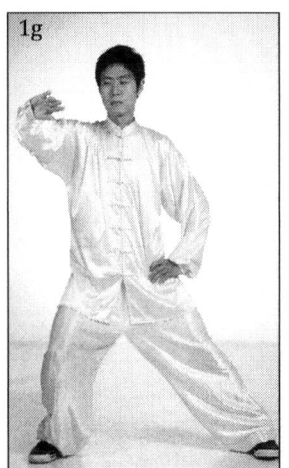
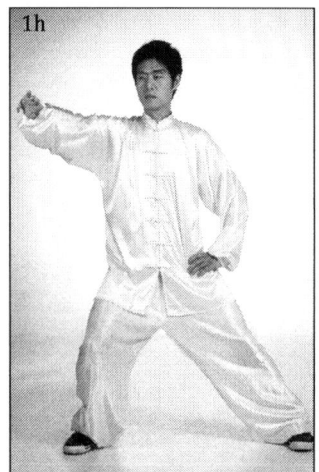

SECOND TECHNIQUE: Vertical Dantian Rotation

This second technique of dantian internal rotation is not simple to acquire; however, this small silk reeling exercise helps one's understanding of the physical requirements and sensation of proper silk reeling execution. Here the dantian rotates vertically, forward and backward, with the upper chest, diaphragm, and lower back. This rotation connects the force of the dantian when raising and lowering hands in practice. For example, to capitalize on properly generated energy with correct alignment while doing jumping kicks, one must use vertical dantian rotation. In this way, the energy flows through the back to the fingertips.

Preparation: Same as previous technique (Fig. 2)

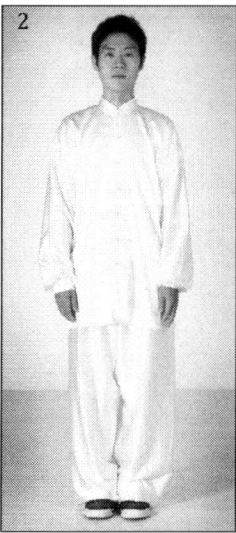

STEP 1: Vertical Forward Rotation: Directing and Governing Meridians
(Microcosmic Orbit) (Figs. 2a-g)

When the thumb goes outward from the dantian, energy circulates from the governing vessel to the directing vessel. This is a vertical forward rotation of the dantian, which needs close awareness to keep from hollowing the upper chest too much. The upper chest makes a natural curve during this type of dantian rotation. In this exercise, the height of the body makes downward and upward adjustments by rotating the dantian and the hands. The wrist, elbow, and shoulder joints have to make a big circle with relaxation. When the body is lowered, the energy circulates from the *dantian* ▸ *huiyin* (perineum) ▸ *mingmen* ▸ *lingtai* ▸ *baihui* ▸ *renzhong* ▸ *shanzhong* ▸ *dantian*. This is the small heavenly circle, or microcosmic orbit. You'll sense less energy in the hands as energy circulates in the microcosmic orbit.

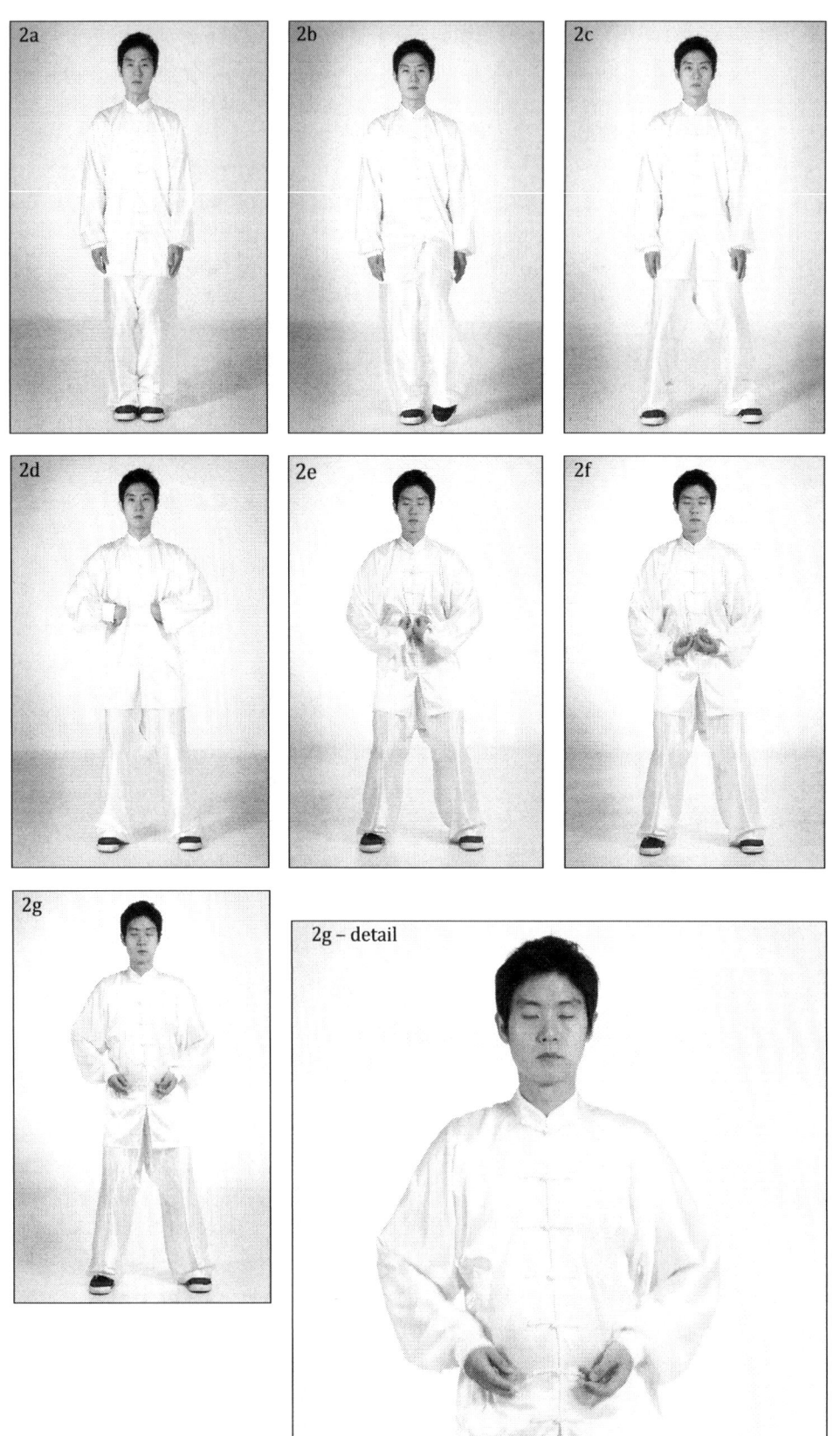

STEP 2: Reversal of Microcosmic Orbit (Figs. 2h-l)

For the vertical backward rotation of the dantian, one simply directs the thumb inward toward the dantian. With this movement, the energy circulates from the directing vessel to the governing vessel. This type of energy circulation is rare to find in Chinese medicine and qigong because it conflicts with the traditional meridians. However, Chen taijiquan masters have held this concept for a long time, basing it on a practical heritage and the principle of contradiction between yin and yang. When the thumb comes toward the dantian, the energy circulates from *dantian* ▸ *baihun* ▸ *dazhui* ▸ *lingtai* ▸ *mingmen* ▸ *huiyin* ▸ *dantian*. It reverses the direction of the energy flow in the small heavenly circle. With this practice, severe neck and shoulder pain can be relieved and arms will increase physical flexibility. The lungs should not be used too much in order to avoid making the shoulder tense. It is because the lower abdominals and dantian are mainly used instead of using the lungs.

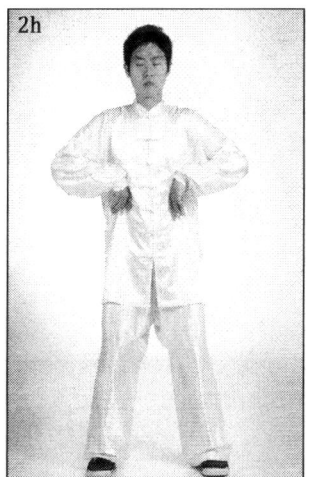
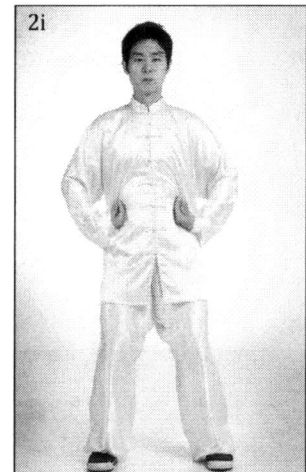
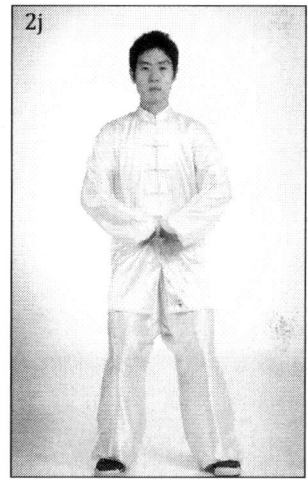
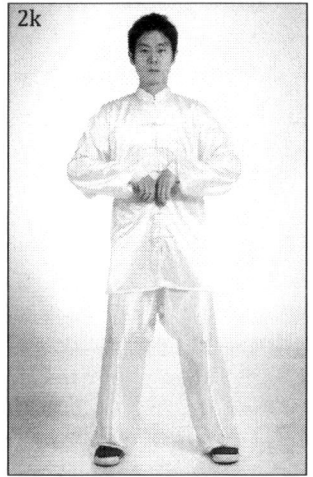
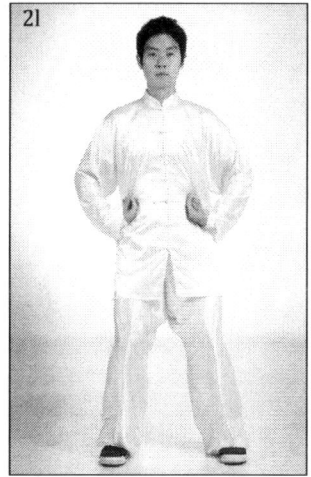

THIRD TECHNIQUE: Mixed Dantian Rotation

A third type of rotation is a combination of the first and second techniques presented previously. The double-hand silk reeling maximizes all three techniques of dantian internal rotation. It can be defined as the combination of the first type of lateral and second type of vertical rotations while practicing silk reeling movements within the old frame forms. This mixed type of dantian internal rotation is not fixed, with unique paths throughout each movement to adhere to correct posture. To acquire this type of dantian rotation, it is crucial to be very familiar with the previous techniques. Since the classical Chen taijiquan practice forms are based on the theory of dantian rotation, their movements include many mixed dantian rotations. This concept should be kept simple, and if there is anything unclear or ambiguous about this mixed rotation, one should go back to mastering the previous exercises.

Use of the meridians becomes more complicated than in the previous exercises, since one begins to use both hands to activate the left and right sides of meridians simultaneously. However, with correct guidance and proper training of the first and second techniques, there will be no problem in applying this third technique.

Preparation: Same as previous technique (Fig. 3)

STEP 1: Simultaneously Activating Two Meridians (Fig. 3a)
If the two previous practices are properly learned, it is comfortable to activate two meridians at the same time with this third technique. As shown in the picture, the left hand activates meridian 1 while the right hand activates meridian 3. However, do not be overly concerned with trying to sense the simultaneous energy flow in these two meridians because the centralized dantian position will circulate the energy itself by a practitioner's correct movement. For example, if the dantian is centered, one will feel both feet are rooted and then the mind will become calm and peaceful. If the practitioner is not confident in using these meridians, meditating on the dantian's internal rotation would be an alternative way to acquire this exercise. Please keep the hip (*kua*) parallel to the ground. Hands and feet feel swelling or tingling if the energy is circulating correctly. If not, the whole body will become cold. Please be advised by your instructor, for that is a bad sign while doing this practice.

In this step, the weight is on the left foot and both hands are raised. Open the *laogong* point while relaxing the shoulders and lowering the elbows. The left knee does not go beyond the toe line, and the back has no concave or convex shape.

STEP 2: Rotate the Dantian Horizontally to the Right Side (Fig. 3b)
Slowly shift the weight onto the right foot with the first dantian-rotation technique, which is a horizontal rotation. The dantian leads the movement of the arms. The hips are parallel to the ground. Because meridian 2 for the left hand and meridian

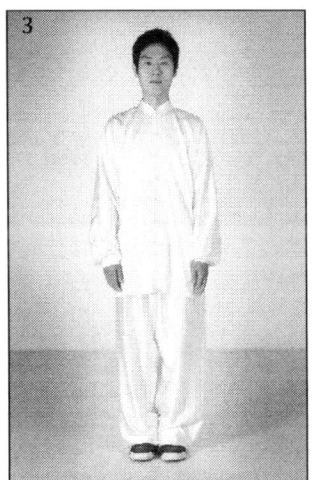
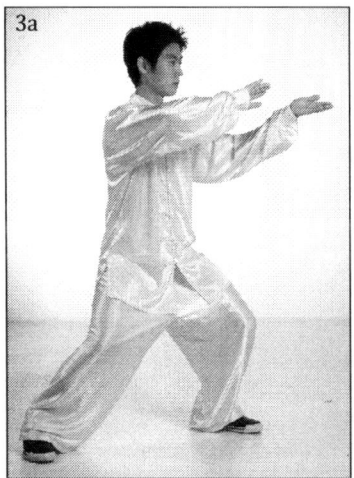

4 for the right hand are being used, the dantian forms the core axis that combines these two meridians, and the lower body becomes very full of energy. One's intention must stay on the dantian for the meridians to circulate energy well. If there is an error, energy will be stuck in the upper chest, and the area around the dantian will become tense. If this movement is done incorrectly, the body and hands will feel cold. This type of error should be corrected.

Step 3: Mixed Rotation of the Dantian (Figs. 3c-d)
There is no weight change, but a third technique of dantian internal rotation is being activated in this step. After the first dantian rotation is made in the previous step, the dantian makes a vertical and a horizontal rotation at the same time the energy sinks downward. Although the dantian internal rotations of the first and second techniques can be clearly felt, other dantian internal rotations can be complex and multidirectional. In this step, the yongquan meridian point feels very soft and supple due to sinking energy. Meridian 3 for the left hand and meridian 1 for the right hand are activated.

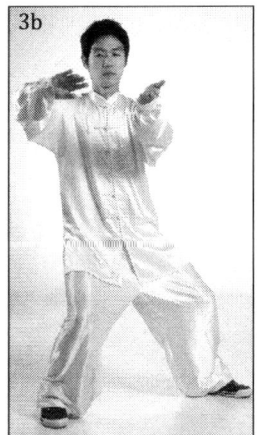
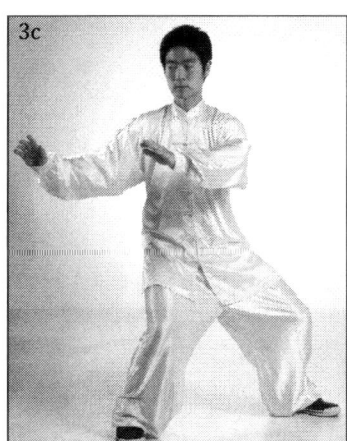
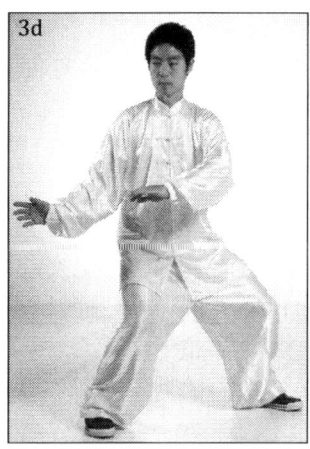

STEP 4: Horizontal Dantian Internal Rotation (Figs. 3e-h)
After the previous step, slowly change the weight to the left foot and smoothly execute a horizontal dantian internal rotation. The dantian should have a horizontal circular movement, and both hands should be around the level of dantian. If the body structure is correct, you will sense a powerful amount of energy in the governing vessel's mingmen and lingtai points. It is a common mistake for the upper body to lean, and a practitioner will not be able to sense this energy. Meridian 4 for the left hand and meridian 2 for the right hand are activated simultaneously. Using two different meridians at once is the balance and zest of yin and yang.

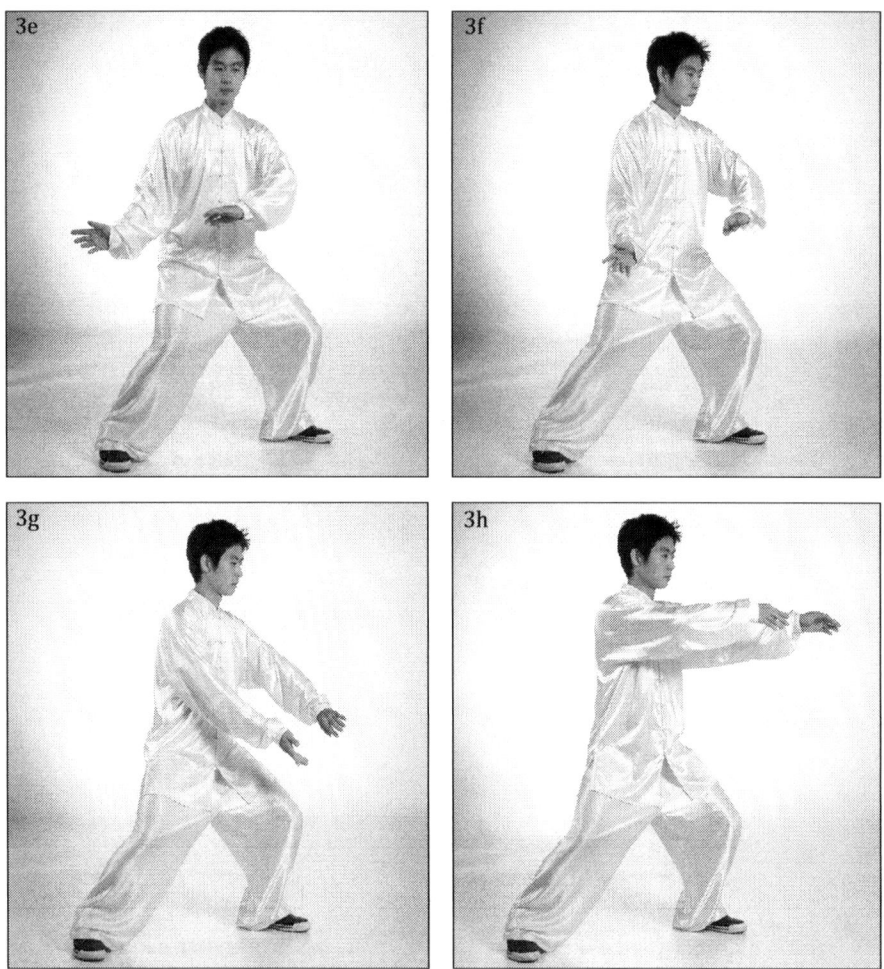

Double-hand silk reeling exercises may provide some relief or cure ailments because they stimulate meridians on both sides of a practitioner's body, resulting in good energy circulation. For example, the pericardium meridian of the left arm is used while the small-intestine meridian of the right arm is activated. This method embodies Chen taijiquan's two characteristics of "using the waist as an axle" and "folding the chest and waist" while silk reeling.

Practicing silk reeling and forms are considered methods of energy circulation in which the dantian is the core center axis that directs all movements. The theory of dantian internal rotation is the essence of Chen taijiquan and practicing the three practical techniques as described in this article will gradually develop one's taijiquan level. As time passes, one will experience the penetration of all joints by silk reeling energy, while physical ailments are significantly lessened by fully cultivating energy from the dantian. It is known that the form practiced does not matter after achieving the highest taijiquan level because the dantian controls internal energy and external motions by itself, thus allowing one's martial application to become free of form. This explains why different taijiquan styles exist.

Internal Alchemy of Chen Family Taijiquan

After a certain amount of time practicing taijiquan, one must confirm his or her level with push-hands practices. These are hands-on exercises by two people with direct applications of the above exercises. The practice includes various exchanges of sturdiness, softness, fastness, and slowness. Chen taijiquan has five kinds of push-hands that require the third type of dantian internal rotation. In other words, push-hands practices are not helpful for those who do not have a base study of dantian internal rotation. Just practicing silk reeling exercises is not enough to study all various changes and techniques of taijiquan. While the second routine (cannon fist) is helpful in developing explosive energy (*fajing*) with fast applications of dantian internal rotations, the first routine is able to train the dantian rotations for developing deep relaxation (*fangsong*) with slow applications of dantian internal rotations. If practicing the two characteristics of slowness and softness alone, one will not seize all the requirements of authentic taijiquan; therefore, one must express power through proper expression of explosive energy, all while employing correct dantian usage. The three types of dantian rotation are crucial for correct silk reeling exercises and the key to understanding and practicing taijiquan forms and push-hands practice.

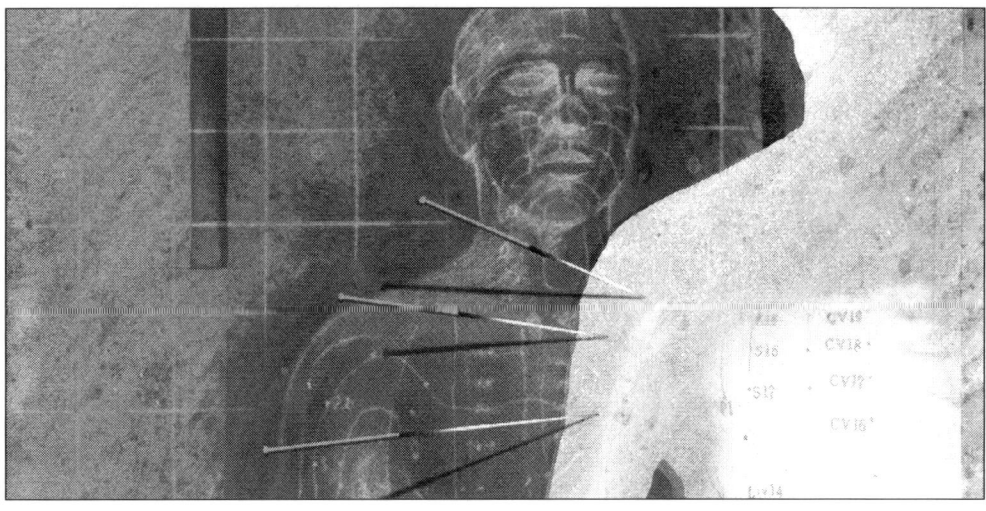

With permission from a master, a practitioner should learn the microcosmic and macrocosmic orbit techniques (small and big heavenly circle) for the internal alchemy of Chen taijiquan. If the dantian possesses powerful energy within, it should eventually circulate through the directing (*renmai*) and governing (*dumai*) meridians. This is called the microcosmic orbit, or small heavenly circle. In later stages of development, energy interpenetrates through the entire spine directly from the *huiyin* to the *bahui* point. This later level of energy interpenetration is called the macrocosmic orbit, or big heavenly circle.

As described previously, dantian breathing through the damai meridian is the impetus of dantian internal alchemy necessary before executing the microcosmic and macrocosmic orbits. The meridian orbits require the energy flow from the dantian to enable continued circulation. Including the direct and governing vessels, all other meridians are controlled smoothly by the full energy supplied by the dantian. By repeating correct authentic methods, one's dantian will continue to develop until the practice stops.

Historically, the three dantian internal-rotation techniques have been what the direct lineage of Chen family taijiquan masters used to develop and maintain a "golden internal alchemy." This tradition will surely continue. Please be simple and clear about these concepts, as practical application of taijiquan is not mysterious. If there is doubt or an unclear concept of taijiquan practice, it may be the case that one's instruction or understanding of this practice lacks depth. This is why authentic taijiquan lineages exist and why the techniques remain as sound in application as they were when first developed. In this day and age, taijiquan has been practiced and exists in various forms, but as a true martial practitioner, one must release form and appearance and truly contemplate the essence of taijiquan.

Chinese Glossary

chansijing	纏絲勁
chen jian zhui zhou	沈肩墜肘
Chen shi taijiquan	陳氏太極拳
chongmai	衝脈
daimai	帶脈
dantian	丹田
dantian gen	丹田根
dantian neizhuan	丹田內轉
daoyin tuna	導引吐納
dumai	督脈
fajin/fajing	發勁
han xiong ba bei	含胸拔背
jiejie guanchuan	節節貫串
Ji Xiao Xin Shu	紀效新書
pericardium meridian of the hand	手厥陰心包經
laojia yilu	老架一路
laojia erlu	老架二路
mingmen	命門
neidan	內丹
qi	氣
Qi Jiguang	戚繼光
qi jing ba mai	奇經八脈
renmai	任脈
shi er zheng jing	十二正經
ta yao	塌腰
small-intestine meridian of the hand	手太陽小腸經
spleen meridian of the foot	足太陰脾經
wei lu zhong zheng	尾閭中正
xiong yao zhe die	胸腰折疊
yang qiao mai	陽蹻脈
yang wei mai	陽維脈
yi yao wei zhou	以腰為軸
Yijing	易經
yin qiao mai	陰蹻脈
yin wei mai	陰維脈
yongquan	湧泉
zhen tou xuan	貞頭懸

Taiji and Qigong Health Benefits: How and Why They Work

by C.J. Rhoads, D.Ed., M.Ed., Duane Crider, Ph.D., and Dina Hayduk, D.Ed., M.Ed.

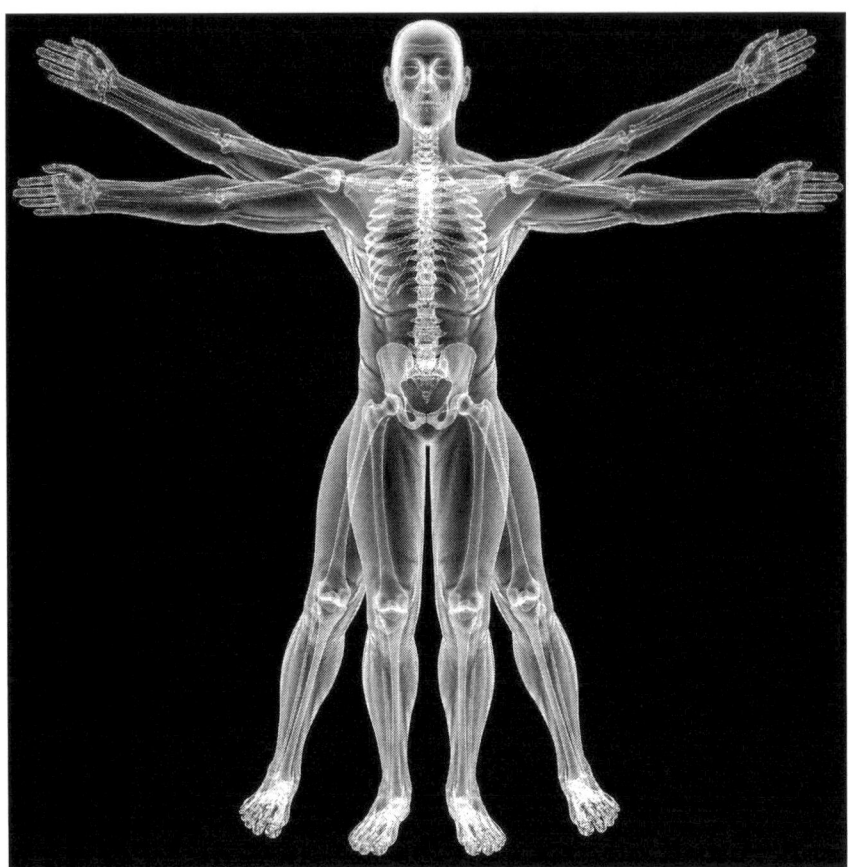

Image © Dmytro Demianenko—123RF.com

Introduction

Decades ago there were not very many health studies on taijiquan (taiji) and qigong.[1] Those that did exist were not highly controlled or validated. But slowly this has begun to change. In the last six years there have been hundreds of studies that explored the health benefits of taiji and qigong.

Two recent events were conspicuous in drawing attention to the difference: the International Taijiquan Forum held at Lakehead University in Thunder Bay, Canada, in 2006, and the International Taijiquan Symposium held in 2009 at Vanderbilt University in Nashville, Tennessee. These two academic events forever changed our understanding of taiji and qigong by revealing the improved amount and quality of research in this field. By including both practitioners and medical researchers, they bridged the gap between the anecdotal stories of improved health (which have been around for centuries), and the peer-reviewed scientific studies available just recently that demonstrate well-supported evidence that qigong and taiji work.

Purpose: Document and Explain

The purpose of this chapter is to discuss not only the academic medical evidence for taiji and qigong and their impact on health, but also a proposed description of how and why taiji and qigong work so well. This paper will attempt to describe the research in laymen's terms (though in some cases, more specific descriptions are necessary to clarify the physiological and psychological effects on the body).

Taijiquan vs Qigong

To achieve the goal of demonstrating clear evidence of the impact on the health and well-being of human beings from taiji and qigong, first we must define what we mean by those terms. Qigong is an "integrative health exercise," and is generally comprised of a series of repetitive movements practiced in combination with proper body alignment, coordinated deep breathing, and focused attention (i.e. "intention"). Staying relaxed and moving in ways that are aligned while being able to enhance strength and flexibility are very much central to the practice. The "focused attention," or "intention," is generally using either external imagery (i.e. raising the sun, gazing at the moon, bring heaven to earth, etc.) or internal imagery (i.e., imagine the light flowing down through your body, pull energy into the *dantian* [lower abdomen area], etc.)[2]

Taiji is often considered a specific type of qigong. Taiji is a practice that involves memorizing specific postures in sequence, known as a form, which was originally developed as a practice for self-defense moves. In order to achieve an advantage over an opponent, the practitioner must remain balanced and in alignment at all times, breathing optimally, and remaining calm and clear headed. The taiji practitioner must be able to "sense" or "listen" to the intention of the opponent. He or she must then be able to move with intention, while remaining completely relaxed, in such a way that whatever the opponent tries to do is neutralized. Movements require both strength and flexibility, and imagery is focused on the self-defense aspect of what an opponent is doing.

Figures 1 through 3 show typical qigong postures (the first one is annotated with some of the essential points). Figures 4 through 6 show typical taiji postures (again, the first one is annotated with some essential points). In general, taiji requires much more leg development than qigong exercises tend to require, as the stances have the knee bending a bit more in some styles (Sun Style being the exception, as Sun Style tends to keep the legs straighter and includes a follow-up step). Furthermore, the postures have martial applications; blocks, punches, and kicks (as can be seen in Figure 6) are generally part of taiji forms.

Figure 1 Typical qigong.

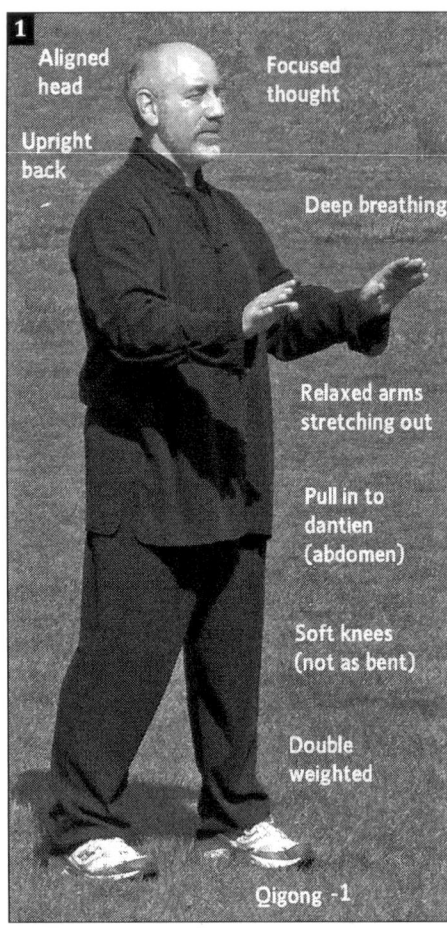

Figure 2
Qigong with more movement.

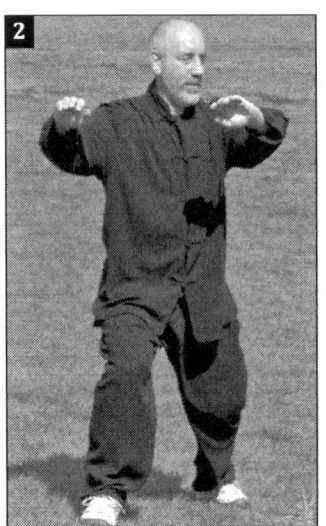

Figure 3 More advanced qigong.

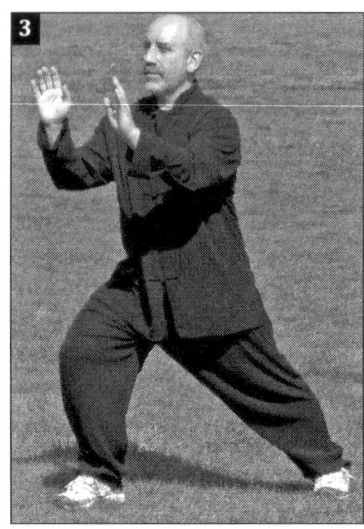

Figure 4
Yang Style Part Wild Horses Mane.

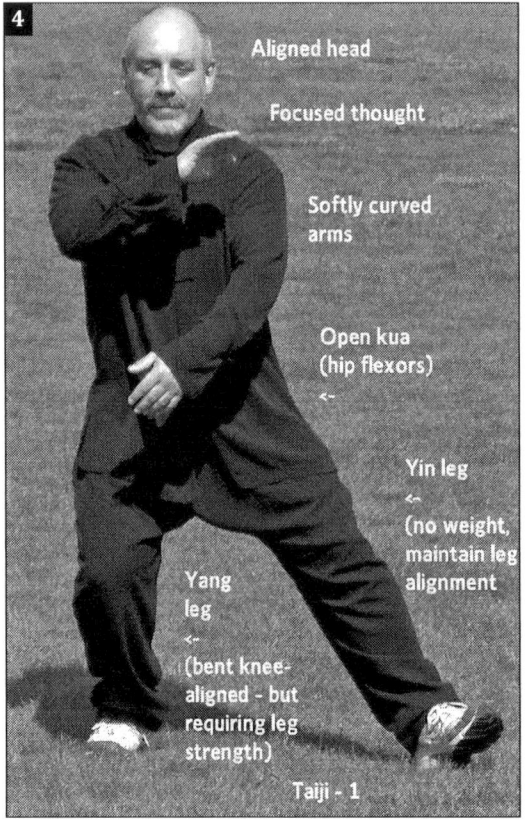

Check list for Figure 1:
Aligned head, upright back, focused thought, deep breathing, relaxed arms stretching out, pull into *dantian* (abdomen), soft knees (not as bent), double-weighted.

All exercises use prescribed inhalation and exhalation (focused intention), and some movements stretch to range of motion. Movements are generally not memorized; imagery (heaven, earth, animals, air, etc.) is used to calm the mind.

Check list for Figure 4:
Aligned head, focused thought, soft curved arms, open *kua* (hip flexors), Yin leg (no weight, maintain leg alignment), Yang leg (bent knee aligned, but requiring leg strength).

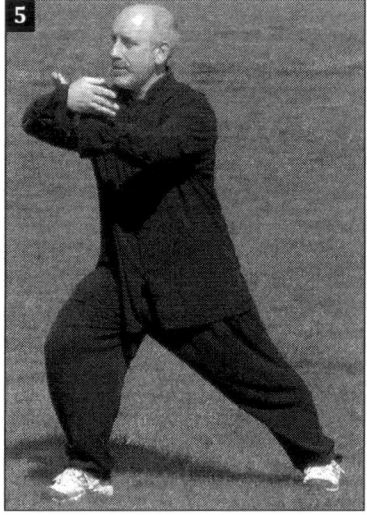 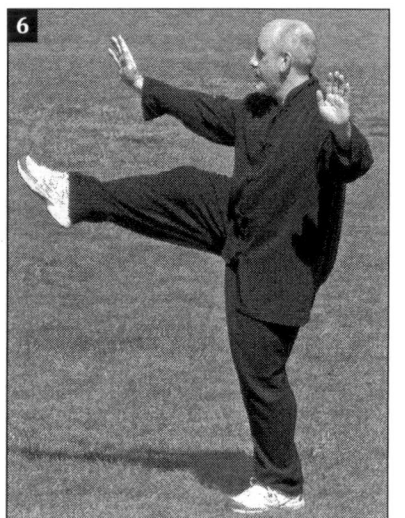

Figure 5 Yang Style press. **Figure 6** Yang Style right kick.

Focused intention is on an opponent's imagined attack and defensive moves in response. There is no range of motion (it is harder to defend stretched or straightened joints), and breathing (though deep) is not prescribed. Generally, the weight shifts from one leg to the other rather than remain equal (double weighted) on both legs.

The model is Jan Gyomber.
Photographs by C.J. Rhoads.

Current Research

Since 2004 there have been several meta-analyses of studies of the health benefits of taiji and qigong (Klein, 2004; Klein, van Hooydonk and Kutlesa, 2010; Kuramota, 2006; Rogers, Lareky and Keller, 2009; Verhagen, Immink, vander Meulen and Bierma-Zienstra, 2004).

Specifically, Ospina et al. (2007) did an exhaustive literature search in order to compare mantra meditation, mindfulness meditation, yoga, taiji, and qigong. The initial 11,030 studies were reduced to the 2,285 studies that followed standard scientific guidelines. After applying even more meticulous scientific rigor criteria, the authors further reduced the number to 813 studies described in 803 articles. The articles that were included were primary research utilizing a control group and measurable, clearly defined health-related outcomes with a sample size greater than ten subjects. Of these articles the authors did a "deep dive" to ascertain the characteristics and benefits of each of the meditative health practices. For example, one finding focused on the impact of the different alternative health treatments on blood pressure. Taiji was a highly effective method for lowering systolic blood pressure (though the evidence pointed to yoga as being slightly more effective for reducing diastolic blood pressure). The resulting tables (see Tables 1 and 2, adapted from Ospina et al. 2007: 145–6) show the probability of each treatment being the best intervention.

The specific findings of the meta-analysis were extremely enlightening, but there was still not enough clear, unequivocal evidence that meditative health practices, as whole, were effective treatments (Ospina, et al. 2007) when compared to current standard-of-care practices. To quote from the abstract:

> Firm conclusions on the effects of meditation practices in healthcare cannot be drawn based on the available evidence. Future research on meditation practices must be more rigorous in the design and execution of studies and in the analysis and reporting of results.

KEY to Tables 1 and 2
BF = biofeedback
CMBT = contemplative meditation plus breathing techniques
DBP = diaostolic blood pressure
HE = health education
NA = non applicable
NS = not specified
NT = no treatment
PMR = progressive muscle relaxation
RR = relaxation response
SBP = systolic blood pressure
TM = Trancendental Meditation
WL = waiting list

TABLE 1: Mixed treatment comparisons of SBP (mm Hg) reductions compared to NT

Intervention	Point estimate	95% credible interval		Probability of being "best" intervention (%)
Taijiquan	-21.9	-37.9,	-5.7	32.0
Yoga + BF	-20.1	-36.7,	-3.1	23.8
Qigong	-18.4	-47.4,	10.7	27.2
CNBT	-14.9	-30.6,	0.9	8.1
Biofeedback	-13.2	-35.9,	9.4	5.1
Yoga	-13.1	-21.7,	-4.4	0.6
RR	-10.8	-30.5,	8.9	0.9
Zen Buddhist meditation	-7.3	-22.1,	7.6	0.9
Rest/Relaxation	-5.9	-22.4,	11.0	0.3
Mantra meditation (NS)	-5.6	-21.8,	10.5	1.0
TM®	-2.5	-14.0,	8.7	0.0
PMR	-2.4	-15.0,	9.6	0.0
HE	-0.5	-11.8,	10.6	0.0
WL	-0.3	-26.9,	26.3	0.0
NT	0.0	NA		0.0

TABLE 2: Mixed treatment comparisons of SBP (mm Hg) reductions compared to NT

Intervention	Point estimate	95% credible interval		Probability of being "best" intervention (%)
Yoga + Biofeedback	-17.1	-30.9,	-3.0	34.0
Qigong	-15.2	-40.4,	-9.3	30.6
Taijiquan	-12.1	-25.8,	-1.5	12.5
Zen Buddhist meditation	-12.0	-24.4,	-0.2	9.1
Yoga	-11.8	-19.1,	-4.6	1.8
BF	-11.4	-32.1,	8.5	9.2
Rest/Relaxation	-8.5	-22.0,	5.0	1.3
RR	-7.4	-24.2,	8.6	0.8
TM	-3.4	-13.3,	5.9	0.1
WL	-3.3	-26.4,	19.3	0.0
PMR	-2.2	-12.8,	7.7	0.1
HE	-1.9	-11.8,	7.3	0.0
Mantra meditation (NS)	-1.0	-14.4,	12.4	0.6
NT	-0.0	NA		0.0

Difficulties of Scientific Research

The health benefits associated with mediative practices have been difficult to quantify. As shown by the meta-analysis by Ospina et al., for the scientific/medical community, the real evidence is in well-designed double-blind research and practice trials. Predictably, research studies on health practices associated with taiji and qigong are rare—for many reasons.

First, who would pay for such studies? Most medical research is supported by pharmaceutical companies, which typically get a return on their investment for drugs when they are successful (i.e., profitable enough to also cover the costs of the unsuccessful trials). Getting an investment return is much more difficult within the fragmented organizations that deliver physical treatments such as taiji, qigong, or other exercise classes.

Funding is not an insignificant obstacle, and it often determines which treatment will be more prevalent (regardless of effectiveness). For example, imagine that there were two equally effective treatments for high blood pressure. Treatment 1 will provide $12 billion in revenues to a single company (the typical revenues on a blockbuster drug such as Lipitor, according to Berenson [2005]). Treatment 2 will provide several million dollars in revenue to several thousand unrelated disconnected health providers (integrative health centers and martial arts schools). Furthermore, treatment 1 is covered by health insurance. Treatment 2 must be covered directly out of the patient's pocket. Which treatment do you think might garner research funding, and from whom? Which treatment would be utilized more often? Even if treatment 2 is demonstrably more effective at a quarter of the cost without the side effects of treatment 1, the number of people who would choose treatment 2 over treatment 1 will be very limited simply because of who is paying the bill. Funding sources will not be abundant without a clear path to return on investment.

Second, the requirements of a scientific study are often at odds with the treatment itself. How do you keep the daily practice of taiji "blind"? In a drug trial you can give sugar pills that look the same as the treatment, so the subjects can't tell if they are getting the treatment or not. (In a "double-blind" study, the doctors and researchers don't know which subjects are getting the treatment either.) With a daily practice treatment, it is more difficult to "hide" who's getting the treatment. People usually can tell if they are doing taiji or qigong or yoga or just plain exercise. Bias for or against the treatment can interfere with the results.

Third, to complicate matters, as noted earlier, taiji is not easily defined and can mean different things to different people. Taiji might mean daily practice of a form such as the Yang, Sun, Chen, Wu, or Wu-Hao forms. Taiji might mean living a philosophy that is based upon the *Daodejing*, a quintessential book of ancient Chinese wisdom. Taiji might mean doing a type of wushu—competitive taiji practiced as a sport rather than a health activity. Taiji might mean doing gongfu—using the term gongfu as "skill" or the focus and intent on being the best that is the essence of this art. Taiji might include those who constantly challenge and test their bodies and skills against others—a more martial aspect of taiji as a fighting art. Or taiji might mean the healthful ability to monitor, control, and direct the bioelectrical energy in the body that is often called qi—the same healing energy[3] that is attributed to the success of acupuncture and reiki (Lai and Tong, 2010). Even worse, the problem of defining taiji is dwarfed by the problems of defining qigong. There are probably hundreds of thousands of different activities and behaviors that fall under the umbrella term of qigong.

Despite thousands of studies on the impact of various components of taiji and qigong, few specified exactly what was meant by "taiji" or "qigong." For example, one study that showed a significant improvement in insulin resistance in diabetes described the qigong simply as KaiMai Style (Liu, 2011). Further investigation reveals that the qigong was developed by one of the authors and is not documented either as part of the study or in a public forum. Additionally, the intensity of the exercise varied among participants. No further description was available.

With additional focus on research, more standardized practices may become more prevalent. For example, one study was done on the impact of taiji and qigong on the body's immune response to the influenza virus (Yang, et al., 2007). The form taught was based upon the Evidence-Based Taijiquan (EBT) Form.[4] While further investigation would reveal that this form was also developed by the lead author, there is a major difference: the specific movements and training methods were fully documented as part of the study, and the form and the accompanying qigong practices were done exactly the same way by all participants, with the same movement (broken down by arm, waist, footwork), direction, energy/intention, and weight shift. The duration and intensity of the exercise remains equalized throughout the study.

Despite progress in this area, the lack of a common definition makes finding clear and unadulterated evidence extremely difficult. One method to overcome this problem may be to avoid the terminology typically used and instead focus purely on the specific movements and behaviors. Ospina et al. (2007) discussed the "effect modifiers" (dose, duration, direction of attention, rhythmic pattern, and individual variables) that should be described in every research article. Even more simply, researchers could describe the movement/breath/intention sequence. Defining taiji and qigong through the sum of their parts (movement, breath, and intention), rather than the specific terms and practices commonly called taiji or qigong, we may be able to identify the specific underlying stimulus and response of the practice. By doing so the distinguishing features of the practice can be identified to determine if there is a difference in therapeutic value between them. Most studies, for example, completely ignore the imagery or martial applications in their description of the movements, yet it may be important to maintain the focus of attention or imagery for these practices to work.[5] Furthermore, the three components can be broken down into different aspects of their development:

1) movement: strength development.
2) movement: flexibility development.
3) intention: focused attention.
4) breathing: deep (either natural or reverse breathing).
5) repetition.

Using nontraditional descriptions for the movements, breath, and intention would "defrock" taiji and qigong practices from their mystical foundations without losing the essential nature of the exercises. Adopting this method of description would make it much easier to conduct research and would enable the researchers to conduct double-blind studies that could provide stronger (or weaker) evidence of the efficacy and effectiveness of taiji and qigong for health. For example, a researcher might establish that treatment 1 is movement/ breath/intention sequence A plus movement/breath/intention sequence B plus (etc.). Treatment 2 would be movement/breath/intention sequence P plus movement/breath/intention sequence Q (etc.), and treatment 3 would be movement/breath/intention sequence X, Y (etc.). In actuality, the sequences of treatment 1 may be the same as a particular taijiquan form, whereas the sequences of treatment 2 might be the same as a particular yoga style, and the sequences of treatment 3 might be classic qigong. As long as the terminology is only treatment (i.e. the subjects are not told if they are following treatment 1 or treatment 2 or treatment 3, and they are definitely not told which each treatment is based upon), subjects would be blind to which group they are in. Of course, another group, treatment 4, would be required. This group might do nothing at all; perform movements that are unrelated to taiji, qigong, or yoga; or perhaps just sit in a room as a control.

Additionally, when the outcomes are measured (whether it be blood pressure, immune response, pain levels, etc.) the researcher measuring the outcome should be unaware of which treatment the subject is in. This study design would result in double-blind, reproducible, verifiable research that would further the agenda of establishing practices based upon clear evidence.

Furthermore, when we start using the framework of movement, breath, and intention, we start quantifying items in such a way that they could eventually be prescribed. "Go do taiji," or "Go do yoga" is not a prescription. "Perform these specific movement sequences with accompanying intention and breath practices three times a day for ten minutes, seven days a week" is a prescription. If the goal is to improve people's health, being able to quantify exactly how much they need to do, with what intensity, and how often, is critical. Yet this information is sadly lacking in our current state of research (Ospina et al. 2007). Only when therapeutic levels of the practice/sequence can be verified and replicated can taiji and qigong take a place among the prescriptions and medical advice coming from primary physicians.

Another step toward scientific inquiry would be to hypothesize why taiji and qigong work. The traditional explanations regarding qi and energy channels are insufficient in order to establish and test hypotheses. In order to find supporting evidence, we need to look at a molecular, measurable level. It is not essential to establish how taiji and qigong work in order to use them. Indeed, the mechanism behind why aspirin reduces pain was only established in 1971, yet physicians have been prescribing aspirin since Felix Hoffman synthesized the compound in 1897 (Warner and Mitchell, 2002).[6] But starting with a potential framework might help identify the most promising avenues for research. To that end, the next section will propose some potential frameworks for how and why taiji and qigong work.

Muscle Mechanisms—Fast-Twitch versus Slow-Twitch

One difference between taiji/qigong and many other forms of exercise such as running, walking, or basketball is that the movements are performed slowly. It would make sense to thoroughly understand the muscle mechanisms for building strength and flexibility using slow movements, which might lead to one aspect of how and why taiji and qigong work.

Strength training on the muscle fibers (collections of myofibrils) is clearly documented. Roig, MacIntyre, Eng, Narici, Maganaris, and Reid (2010) outlined the mechanisms in their research on how to preserve strength in the elderly. Frontera and Bigard (2002) provided an in-depth explanation in their description of the benefits of strength training in the elderly. Westerblad, Allen, and Lännergren (2002) furthered the work in 2002 by publishing an article that changed the current medical thinking on what causes muscle fatigue.

When a muscle is given the signal by the brain to move, actin and myosin (the protein filaments) slide across one another and the muscle fiber shortens, which contracts the muscle (sliding filament theory). Repeating the contracting and adding tension (by holding a weight, for example) slowly increases the number of myofibrils, so the muscle gets larger and stronger. Preventing the movement (as would happen if the muscle were in a cast) causes the amount of actin and myosin to decrease so there is less to slide across one another. The muscle cannot contract as much, and the number of myofibrils decreases. The muscle atrophies, getting smaller and weaker (supporting the concept of "use it or lose it"). As the myofibril bundles contract, they use up energy and must replenish it.

There are three types of energy sources used by the myofibril bundles: immediate, short term, and long term. To produce energy each of these energy sources involves a chemical reaction. The long-term energy source is the only one that requires oxygen to be present in the chemical reaction in order to produce energy.

For immediate use, within the muscle itself is a high-energy molecule (creatine phosphate, or CP). CP donates one of its phosphate molecules to combine with adenosine diphosphate (ADP) to produce adenosine triphosphate (ATP). This process is only applied to fast muscle contractions that last no longer than a few seconds. After that, the ATP runs out.

For short-term energy the muscle fibers must use an alternative source:

glucose. To produce ATP, glucose combines with a phosphate and that makes it split into two molecules of pyruvic acid, which then combine with two ADP molecules to form two ATP molecules. This process too has a limited application in terms of time and can only allow the body to perform muscle contractions for approximately two minutes.

The long-term source of energy is aerobic because it requires oxygen in the formula for energy production. Carbohydrates or fat (triacylglycerol) and oxygen combine to form ATP. This production of ATP through this aerobic process is slower than the anaerobic due to the need for oxygen. But the amount of energy that is released, especially through converting triacylglycerol to ATP, is many times the amount that is available through the immediate or short-term process.

Using long-term sources of energy has a major impact on the myofibril bundles. The fibers that replenish their energy with oxygen (the long-term source) are called slow-twitch fibers. They develop more blood capillaries, increase the amount of mitochondria (which contain the enzymes needed to break down the oxygen) and myoglobin (which contain a protein similar to red blood cells), and adopt a deep red color. Fast-twitch fibers use the anaerobic metabolic mechanisms (immediate and short-term sources). They are much lighter in color (often called white fibers) and have fewer blood capillaries, fewer mitochondria, and less myoglobin.[7] In Figure 7, the illustration shows a cross-section of a predominantly slow-twitch myofibril bundle on the left and a predominantly fast-twitch myofibril bundle on the right.

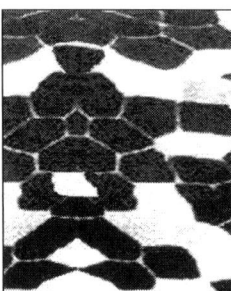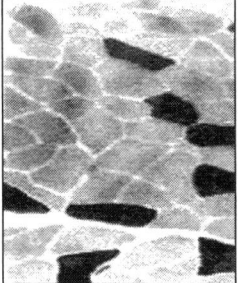

Figure 7 Slow-twitch fiber bundle (left)
and fast-twitch fiber bundle (right).

As the glucose and the glycogen break down, the process releases lactic acid, which creates lactate. Lactate is an important fuel that our muscles can be trained to use and is the preferred fuel for the heart muscle and the brain itself. There is also recent evidence that lactic acid can increase endurance and decrease muscle fatigue (Westerblad et al., 2002).

This may be where the rubber meets the road in terms of why taiji works more effectively as an exercise for improving the health and well-being of the body. Using this information, we can contrast taiji and qigong with other exercises, such as walking, swimming, and biking, or other more active external martial arts such as judo, karate, or taekwondo. In an external martial art, the body moves quickly, kicking and punching. The fast-twitch fibers predominate, and the source of fuel is glucose and glycogen. This would apply to any sport that requires the muscles to contract quickly. That movement, again, is dominated by fast-twitch fiber.

Biking, walking, and swimming typically use a more mixed combination of fast- and slow-twitch fibers. The typical movements of taiji and qigong do something more, however. The movements are slow, not fast. The focus on alignment and relaxation further encourages the body to utilize slow-twitch fibers in the muscles. Slow-twitch fibers cause the body to use fat, rather than glucose, as the fuel. Fat provides much more energy and using it up decreases the fat deposits in the body. Excess fat deposits can increase inflammation and release adipokines into the body, which increase insulin resistance and contribute to metabolic syndrome and diabetes, so utilizing that excess fat as an energy source for exercise is a double benefit.

Slow-twitch fiber use also puts more pressure on the aerobic system, which is why taiji players may find themselves breathing deeply (or huffing and puffing if they are not fit) despite moving very easily and slowly. Breathing more deeply (as opposed to breathing faster and more shallowly) invigorates the entire system. It increases the oxygen in the blood, which then supplies the organs and muscles, including the heart and the brain. The heart can beat more slowly and deeply, energizing the circulatory system and improving its ability to distribute nutrition to the muscles and organs. The brain also gets energized, enabling the synapses to work more effectively. Memory and the ability to think clearly and learn new things are enhanced.

Muscle Mechanisms—Motor Units and Nerves

Muscles move based upon the nerve connected to them. Nerve bundles with muscle fibers are called motor units. The number of muscles connected to each nerve can vary from two to hundreds or thousands. When the motor unit sends out the signal for the muscles to move, the amount of demand (a small weight versus a heavy weight, for example) determines how many motor units respond. Each motor unit contracts to maximum capacity. When a motor unit is repetitively called upon, it increases the number of muscle fibers under its control. When a number of motor units are called upon together, it increases the body's ability to recruit and utilize more motor units. Strength and coordination improve without sacrificing flexibility because the increased capability comes without a corresponding increase in muscle size (as would happen if we increase capability by lifting weights). Bigger muscles have the potential to interfere with flexibility in two ways. First, larger muscles may be made up of more fast-twitch muscle fibers than slow-twitch fibers. That means they will fatigue more quickly and increase hydrogen ions, which traditionally has been thought to cause acidosis, which causes muscle fatigue.[8] Additionally, larger muscles, being physically bigger, will make it more difficult to engage the motor units, making it more difficult for the actin and myosin protein filaments to slide across each other. This may be why, even though slow-twitch fibers dominate in taiji players, they can often move faster in a relaxed state than someone who has more fast-twitch fibers. The smaller muscles have less of an obstacle to overcome to contract, making them faster than larger muscles, enabling a taiji player to "start later but arrive earlier."[9]

In summary, the slow repetitive movements of taiji and qigong are more likely than quick-moving activities (such as running or external martial arts) to:

1) develop fat-burning slow-twitch muscles,
2) increase the number of muscles within each muscle unit,
3) enhance the coordination between muscle units,
4) improve the cardiovascular system and increase the number of neurotransmitters in the brain because of the elevated oxygen levels in the bloodstream and the availability of a preferred fuel source for the heart and brain.

Brain and Metabolic Mechanisms

There is more to the improved brain and metabolic functions than improved fuel supply and increased oxygen. To understand the impact of taiji and qigong on the brain, it will be helpful to first consider the feedback loop connecting the muscles, the nerves, the brain, and the metabolic system controlled by the brain. One of the easiest ways to see this feedback loop is how pain is "felt." The physical manifestation of pain occurs when the muscle tenses or is damaged and the nerves send the signal to the dorsal horn (a spot at the base of the spine), which then sends the signal to the thalamus region of the brain (Willis, 1985). One influence of the amount of pain we feel is the sensitivity of the dorsal horn. With repeated use, the dorsal horn becomes very sensitive, dialing up the amount of pain (Price, 1999). People who experience chronic pain have a dorsal horn that acts like a loaded gun with a tricky trigger finger: it is tensed up to fire a pain sensation at the least provocation. The pain sensation then causes the nerves to tell the muscles to contract, which causes tension, which is felt by the dorsal horn (danger, danger!), which sends the message to the brain that there is pain, which causes the tense–pain–tense–pain feedback loop.

To break this loop, it is necessary to reduce or completely eliminate the muscular tension, making the muscles so relaxed that they do not alarm the dorsal horn and wake the dragon of pain. When a person is in pain, his or her brain is in a constant state of attention, what one researcher calls "narrow focus," which releases a constant stream of stress hormones such as cortisol and adrenaline. Blood pressure and heart rate go up. Respiration becomes shallow and the rate increases. The capillaries contract. Over a long term, these hormones begin to cause damage, inhibiting the digestive system, restricting nutritional absorption, causing muscle fatigue, and increasing pain.

Open-focus attention, on the other hand, is the opposite. Open focus is a relaxed state of attention associated with enhanced critical thinking, complemented by ultra-awareness of the environment (Fehmi and Robbins, 2010). This open focus has also been called being "in the zone" or "flow" within the realm of sports medicine (Payne, Jackson and Noh, 2011). Meditation and stress-reducing activities (including taiji and qigong) can shut down narrow focus and lead to open focus.

Biofeedback is the medical treatment's name for meditation. When a person is connected to a biofeedback machine, a visual illustration of tension appears on the computer screen. In order to "lower" the amount of tension, the person must breathe deeply and relax his or her muscles. Relaxing the muscles sends a signal to the brain that there is no danger. Stress hormones such as cortisol and adrenalin are reduced or stopped. Blood pressure and heart rate go down. Respiration becomes deep and the rate decreases. Capillaries expand. Digestive systems resume normal processes, increasing nutritional absorption, increasing muscle endurance, and decreasing pain.

Simply put, practice of taiji and qigong, as well as biofeedback and meditation, cause chemical changes in the brain. Because of these chemical changes, the brain switches from narrow focus to open focus. Focus (either narrow or open) is measured using brain waves. Narrow focus is characterized by beta waves, whereas open focus tends toward alpha waves and gamma waves.

There have been others who noted the profound impact of meditation on the brain. Research shows that Buddhist monks who are regular meditative practitioners have different brain-wave patterns (Lutz, Greischar and Rawlings, 2008), typically an increase in alpha and gamma, and a decrease in beta waves. Bradley (2010) proposed that the pineal gland is affected by chanting meditation and visualization techniques in martial artists to release dimethyltryptamine (DMT). DMT is a hallucinogenic compound formed by the combination of the neurotransmitter serotonin and the amino acid tryptophan. Bradley conjectures that DMT enables martial artists to change the perception of time (making time appear to slow down when defending and speed up when attacking), as well as help them deal effectively with stress, overcome spiritual blocks, or reach another level of training.[10]

The existence of certain types of brainwaves has a domino effect on the body. When the brain exhibits alpha and gamma waves, neurotransmitters such as dopamine, serotonin, noradrenaline, acetylcholine, GABA, and endorphins are released into the bloodstream. These are often called the "feel good" hormones because they cause a feeling of contentment and well-being. They do more than make people feel good, however. The increased neurotransmitters prompt the vagus nerve to activate, which lowers the heart rate and blood pressure. (The vagus nerve is one of the largest, and wanders around the body from the brain stem to the colon, as can be seen in Figure 8.) When the heart rate and blood pressure are lowered, that prompts the lungs to expand more fully and breathe more deeply, which activates the digestive system. A smooth-working digestive system improves nutritional absorption (Healy, 2011) (when combined with nutritional food, of course).

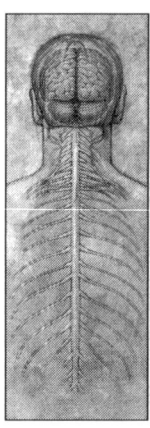
Figure 8

While these changes are healthy for the body in the long term, they also have an impact in the short term—an impact that can modify pain sensations. This process indirectly causes the body to decrease the amount of pain felt by overriding the body's response to pain. Instead of allowing the body to go into hyper drive, increasing tension and stress hormones (which actually increase the pain by getting the individual into the pain-escalating feedback loop), the response is short-circuited, and the brain is convinced of the reality—there is no danger, no tension, no reason to elicit the stress response. Over time the override becomes the norm and the stress response decreases. The doral horn becomes less sensitive to perceived threats of pain, and the pain dissipates.

Similar to the way taiji and qigong can decrease the amount of pain felt, the metabolic changes in the body can also decrease the impact of illness, especially metabolic dysfunctions such as diabetes and obesity; autoimmune disorders such as Graves disease, rheumatoid arthritis, celiac disease, and multiple sclerosis; and blood disorders such as porphyria and leukemia. All of these chronic problems are exacerbated by the stress response of the body and tempering that response can not only alleviate symptoms but cause them to disappear entirely.

Muscle/Intention/Breath Combination is Recommended

The combination of the physical impact of long, slow movements, the open-focused attention of the brain (i.e., intention), and the resulting deep breathing of typical qigong, taiji, and even yoga is highly effective as a health booster.[11] These same metabolic influences may prevent or slow down the onset of viruses, flus, and cancers, as well as metabolic dysfunctions, autoimmune disorders, and blood diseases.

Unfortunately, until recently, in medical school few doctors learned about integrative health practices. The effects were thought to be merely the placebo effect (Katz, 2008) and were, for the most part, not considered to be part of established standard-of-care practices. The most influential medical schools have revised their thinking on that point, however, in face of the growing evidence to the contrary.

Mayo Clinic doctors recommend taiji (Mayo Clinic, 2009). As stated on their website:

> Preliminary evidence suggests that [taiji] may offer numerous benefits beyond stress reduction, including:
>
> - Reducing anxiety and depression
> - Improving balance, flexibility and muscle strength
> - Reducing falls in older adults
> - Improving sleep quality
> - Lowering blood pressure
> - Improving cardiovascular fitness in older adults
> - Relieving chronic pain
> - Increasing energy, endurance and agility
> - Improving overall feelings of well-being

Harvard Medical School doctors also recommend taiji (Brown, 2010). Peter M. Wayne, assistant professor of medicine at Harvard Medical School and director of the Tai Chi and Mind-Body Research Program at Harvard Medical School's Osher Research Center, has stated:

> A growing body of carefully conducted research is building a compelling case for taiji as an adjunct[12] to standard medical treatment for the prevention and rehabilitation of many conditions commonly associated with age.

Harvard Women's Health Watch (Harvard Medical School, 2009), says:

> This gentle form of exercise can prevent or ease many ills of aging and could be the perfect activity for the rest of your life. Taiji is often described as "meditation in motion," but it might well be called "medication in motion."

WebMD (2011) also recommends taiji. The website states:

> Some people believe that taiji improves the flow of energy through the body, leading to better wellness and a wide range of potential benefits. Those benefits include:
> - Improved strength, conditioning, coordination, and flexibility
> - Reduced pain and stiffness
> - Better balance and lower risk of falls
> - Enhanced sleep
> - Greater awareness, calmness, and overall sense of well-being

MedicalNet (2011), also recommends taiji. They state on their website:

> In China, it is believed that taiji can delay aging and prolong life, increase flexibility and strengthen muscles and tendons, and aid in the treatment of heart disease, high blood pressure, arthritis, digestive disorders, skin diseases, depression, cancer, and many other illnesses.

Summary

In summary, the medical community in the past has dismissed as anecdotal any effectiveness taiji and qigong might have as a treatment for many chronic health problems. However, there is now growing evidence that it does work, and works very effectively. It may even be that taiji and qigong work better than some medication and other treatments, with fewer negative side effects.

Further research is needed. More double-blind controlled studies are necessary. By focusing on specific sequences of movement/intention/breath we can document what works and what doesn't, and we can develop a prescription model that can provide a more specific description of integration health treatments that work.

By creating a hypothesis about how taijiquan and qigong work in terms of bio-mechanisms, we can begin to isolate the essential components. This paper introduced the concept that taiji and qigong work by affecting the metabolic processes of the body, starting with the muscles, but also influencing the circulatory system, the digestive system, the metabolic system, and the nervous system. When practiced frequently (daily) and consistently (for months or years) taiji and qigong may bring about the benefits as listed below.

Potential Benefits from Regular Taiji and Qigong Practice

- Development of slow-twitch muscles (rather than fast-twitch muscles)
- Increased number of muscle fibers controlled by each motor unit
- Increased coordination among increasingly larger numbers of motor units
- Increased muscle strength and flexibility
- Decreased muscle tension
- Increased lung capacity and deeper breathing
- Lowered sensitivity of the dorsal horn to pain
- Increased levels of neurotransmitters such as dopamine, serotonin, noradrenaline, acetylcholine, GABA, and endorphins
- Decreased levels of stress hormones, such as cortisol and adrenaline
- Smooth-running digestive system
- Increased nutrition absorption
- Decreased insulin resistance
- Decreased visceral body fat
- More balanced immune response (more properly

identifying whether components are truly dangerous, thereby improving both immune deficiencies and autoimmune disorders)
- Lower blood pressure
- Slower heartbeat
- Increased alpha and gamma brain waves
- Decreased beta brain waves

The time for this type of research is now. Healthcare costs are skyrocketing, the population is aging, and chronic disease rates are exploding. The lifestyle of the modern world is not necessarily the best for human bodies, and general ill-health and incidents of obesity reflect this. Everyone is looking for answers—and some in the medical community are now willing to look at alternative, complementary, and integrative health practices if they can be proven to work.

One way to jump-start the effort would be if researchers could conduct some in-depth financial analysis and compare the treatment costs of the most common chronic health dysfunctions using traditional drugs/surgery/rehab to the cost of treating the same chronic health dysfunctions using integrative health practices. If integrative health practices become economically feasible, it would decrease the health costs for insurance companies and government agencies. That could be the source of funding for further refinements and research.

The goal must be to develop proof, using double-blind statistical studies, beyond a shadow of a doubt, of the efficacy, efficiency, and effectiveness of integrative health practices such as taiji and qigong.

Notes

1. *Taijiquan* (or simply *taiji*) is also known as *t'ai chi ch'uan*. These are just different romanizations of the same Chinese characters (coming from either the Wade-Giles transliteration method or the pinyin transliteration method). *Qigong* is also known as *chi kung*, or *ch'i gung*. We could have just said "qigong" since taiji is a type of qigong, but more people are familiar with the name taiji, and though qigong is becoming more well known in medical circles, it is not always recognized as the umbrella term for taiji and other healthful exercises. Often, in practice, the two terms are used interchangeably.
2. "Intention" or the "image" or "thought pattern" is an essential component of taijiquan and qigong practices. For further information, see Chen and Chan (2009).
3. The word "energy" is a poor translation for the word "qi" or "chi." Note that the Chinese character "chi" in "tai chi" (taiji) is not the same character as the "chi" in "chi kung" (qigong). A more in-depth description can be found in an editorial by Tsung O. Cheng (2006: 119).
4. EBT form is a short seven-posture form based on Chen Style, but it is easy enough

for elderly and infirm subjects to perform while still maintaining the essential components central to all taijiquan forms.

5 The focus of attention may be an essential ingredient in why taiji and qigong work, which may be why research studies produce varied results; not all practitioners include the "mind-thought" control as part of the exercise.

6 Of course, since the early Greeks prescribed willow bark in 400 BCE, one could say we've been using aspirin for over two thousand years.

7 There are several muscle types. Type I, slow-twitch, is a slow oxidative. Fast-twitch have multiple types: Type IIb or glycolytic produce most of their ATP through creatine phosphate breakdown and glycolysis. Type IIa fibers are "fast oxidative glycolytic" and produce the greatest force when stimulated and are resistant to fatigue because of the large numbers of mitochondria and capillaries involved. They are sort of like a hybrid between slow-twitch and fast-twitch. Type IIx is yet another type, a hybrid between Type IIa and Type IIb. These are all skeletal muscles. There are also smooth muscles such as found in the stomach and cardiac muscles found in the heart.

8 More recent research suggests that it is inorganic phosphates or potassium ions that cause the fatigue rather than acidosis, but regardless of the source, fast-twitch fibers fatigue more quickly than slow-twitch fibers. See Westerblad, Allen and Lännergren (2002).

9 Another interpretation of this principle is that taiji players, because they can sense more effectively and think more clearly, move with a super-efficient path, allowing them to arrive at the proper location with the proper alignment before the opponent can finish the move he was planning.

10 Bradley also postulates that the pineal gland enables taiji and qigong practitioners to "experience qi," because it is a "vehicle to consciously experience the movement of our life-force in its most extreme manifestations" (to quote Rick Strassman, the lead medical doctor involved in DMT research).

11 Keep in mind that often the term taiji, because it is better known, is used as a synonym for qigong. Most research points to the common elements of both taiji and qigong (the magic combination of deep breathing, slow, aligned, movements, and open-focused thought/intention) rather than any specific form or style.

12 An adjunct therapy is one that is used together with primary medical treatments, either to address a disease itself or its primary symptoms, or, more generally, to improve a patient's functioning and quality of life. Taiji or qigong will not overcome the impact of an unhealthy lifestyle. In order to be effective, taiji or qigong must be combined with nutritional food, quality sleep, and high-intensity cardiovascular exercise that lasts more than fifteen minutes or so, at a relatively high heart rate (i.e. 80% of maximum heart rate). Additionally, taiji and qigong work more effectively as a preventative activity than a treatment for injury or acute disease.

References

Berenson, A. (2005, Oct. 15). Lipitor or generic? Billion-dollar battle looms. *New York Times.* Also found at http://www.nytimes.com/2005/10/15/business/15statin.html?pagewanted=all

Bradley, S. (2010). The pineal gland's biochemical function in the fighting and meditative arts, Exemplified in Korean Sinmoo Hapkido. *Journal of Asian Martial Arts, 19*(2), 22–33.

Brown, N. (2010, Jan.–Feb.). Easing ills through tai chi, *Harvard Magazine.* Found at http://harvardmagazine.com/2010/01/researchers-study-tai-chi-benefits

Chen, W., and Chan, C. (2009). The role of imagery in practice of tai chi. *Hong Kong Journal of Occupational Therapy, 19*(2), A5.

Cheng, T. (2006). Chi in tai chi does not mean energy. *International Journal of Cardiology, 107*(1), 119.

Cohen, J. (2007, Jan.–April). Pushing high-dose Lipitor: Medical science or slick marketing? *Medication Sense.* Also found at http://medicationsense.com/articles/jan_apr_07/pushinglipitor_020607.html

Fehmi, L., and Robbins, J. (2010). *Dissolving pain: Simple brain-training exercises for overcoming chronic pain.* Boston: Trumpeter.

Frontera, W., and Bigard, X. (2002). The benefits of strength training in the elderly. *Science and Sports, 17*(3), 109–116.

Gray, H. (1918). Anatomy of the human body, IX. *Neurology.*

Harvard Medical School (2009, May). The health benefits of tai chi. Harvard Women's Health Watch, published by Harvard Health Publications. Retrieved September 15, 2011, from: http://www.health.harvard.edu/newsletters/Harvard_Womens_Health_Watch/2009/May/The-health-benefits-of-tai-chi

Healy, K. (2011). Knowledge of brain development and mental functioning opens up a fresh perspective on therapeutic interventions in psychotherapy. *Advances in Psychiatric Treatment,* 17, 240–242. DOI: 10.1192/apt.bp.110.008870

Howley, E., and Franks, D. (2003). *Health fitness instructor's handbook.* 4th edition. Champaign, IL: Human Kinetics.

Katz, A. (2008). Reduced falls in the elderly: Tai chi or placebo or hawthorne effect? *Journal of the American Geriatrics Society, 56*(4), 776–777. DOI: 10.1111/j.1532-5415.2008.01651.x

Klein, P., and Adams, W. (2004, September). Comprehensive therapeutic benefits of taiji: A critical review. *American Journal of Physical Medicine and Rehabilitation 83*(9), 735–745.

Klein, P., van Hooydonk, K., and Kutlesa, M. (2010, October 14). Therapeutic benefits of tai chi/qigong: An overview and critical review. January 1990 through January 2010. Working paper available from the author: kleinpj@chitime.info

Kuramoto, A. (2006). Therapeutic benefits of tai chi exercise: Research review. *Wisconsin Medical Journal, 105*(7), 42–46.

Lai, X., and Tong, Z. (2010). Study on the classification and the 'catching' of the 'arrived qi' in acupuncture. *Journal of Traditional Chinese Medicine, 30*(1), 3–8.

Liu, X., Miller, Y., Burton, N. Chang, J., and Brown, W. (2011). Qi-gong mind-body therapy and diabetes control: A randomized controlled trial. *American Journal of Preventive Medicine, 41*(2), 152–158.

Lutz, A., Greischar, L., Rawlings, N., and Ricard, M. (2008). Long-term meditators self-induce high-amplitude gamma synchrony during mental practice. *Proceedings of the National Academy of Science, 101*(46), 16369–16373.

Payne, B., Jackson, J., Noh, S., and Stine-Morrow, E. (2011). In the zone: Flow state and cognition in older adults. *Psychology and Aging, 26*(3), 738–743. DOI: 10.1037/a0022359

Roig, M., MacIntyre, D., Eng, J., Narici, M., Maganaris, C., and Reid, D. (2010). Preservation of eccentric strength in older adults: Evidence, mechanisms and implications for training and rehabilitation. *Experimental Gerontology, 45*(6), 400–409.

Ospina, M., Bond, T., Karkhaneh, M., Tjosvold, L., Vandermeer, B., Liang, Y., Bialy, L., Hooton, N., Buscemi, N., Dryden, D., and Klassen, T. (2007). *Meditation practices for health: State of the research*. Edmonton, Canada: Evidence-based Practice Center, University of Alberta.

Price, D. (1999). *Psychological mechanisms of pain and analgesia*. Seattle: IASP Press.

Qigong Institute (2011). Differences between tai chi and qigong. Retrieved March 13, 2011, from: http://www.qigonginstitute.org/html/taichihealth.php.

Rogers, C., Larkey, L., and Keller, C. (2009, March). A review of clinical trials of tai chi and qigong in older adults. *Western Journal of Nursing Research, 31*(2), 245–279.

Mayo Clinic (2009, November 14). Tai chi: Discover the many possible health benefits. Mayo Clinic, Published by Mayo Foundation for Medical Education and Research. Retrieved September 15, 2010, from: http://www.mayoclinic.com/health/tai-chi/SA00087

Warner, T., and Mitchell, J. (2002, October 8). Cyclooxygenase-3 (COX-3): Filling in the gaps toward a COX continuum? Proceedings from the National Academy of Sciences, doi: 10.1073/pnas.222543099

Yang, Y., Verkuilen, J., Rosengren, K., Mariani, R., Reed, M., Grubisich, S., and Woods, J. (2007). Effects of a taiji and qigong intervention on the antibody response to influenza vaccine in older adults. *American Journal of Chinese Medicine, 35*(4), 597–607.

Verhagen, A., Immink, M., van der Meulen, A., and Bierma-Zeinstra, S. (2004). The efficacy of tai chi chuan in older adults: A systematic review. *Family Practice, 21*(1), 107–113.

Westerblad, H., Allen, D., and Lännergren, J. (2002). Muscle fatigue: Lactic acid or inorganic phosphate the major cause? *News in Physiological Sciences*, 17, 17–21.

Willis, W. (1985). The pain system: The neural basis of nociceptive transmission in the mammalian nervous system. *Pain Headache,* 8, 1–346.

• 61 •

Yoga Alchemy in Taijiquan
by Greg Brodsky, Lic. Ac.

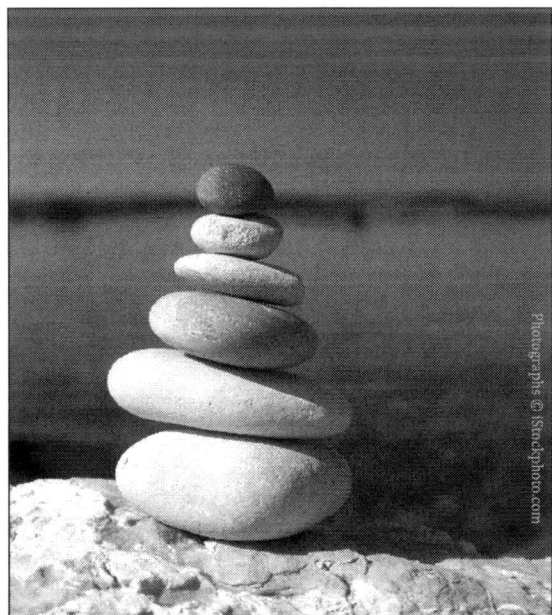
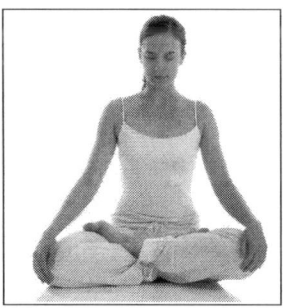
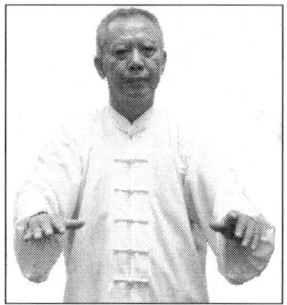

Balance

I always ask beginning students what they want from their investment in taijiquan. Without hesitation, the great majority of them talk about "balance." They don't mean physical balance, although that, much to the appreciation of our older students, is guaranteed to improve with practice over time. They are looking for a way to *inner* balance—a method for increasing their ability to weather the storms in their lives without being knocked around too much, without losing their emotional footing so often and paying such tremendous costs for their mistakes, or perhaps a way to avoid draining all their reserves of energy and optimism into endeavors or obsessions that consume them then disappear like last night's fleeting dream.

This is the kind of balance you need when your love seems betrayed, or your career collapses, or you realize that your religion was an exploitive hoax. Our beginning students hope that something in taijiquan will teach them how to develop the skill, strength, and resilience with which they can meet the rest of their days with greater wisdom.

"No problem," I tell them with a wry smile. But they usually recognize the irony behind my smile.

Yes, this is a tall order. Such inner development, achieving a state of internal balance, does not come naturally to most people. It follows years upon years of admitting mistakes, facing the consequences of our actions, cultivating consciousness, giving unqualified forgiveness, and softening... all the time softening our stance. When the time comes for each of us to find out what we are made of, the difference between drawing it all together or missing the opportunity as if it were not there comes from the degree to which we have tuned our inner resources to be prepared for a transformation we cannot predict. If we meet such a moment in balance, we transcend something we no longer need, embrace something we once feared, and emerge as our greatest self.

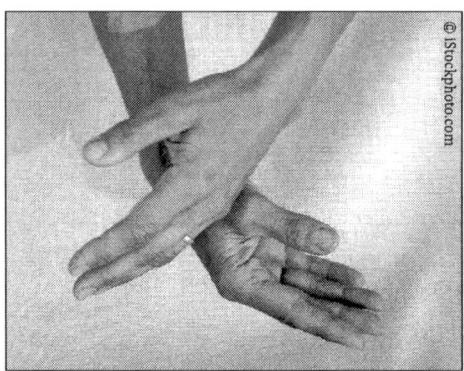

Self-Tuning

In any arena of human endeavor, those of us who can tune ourselves while in motion, who can learn to relax, to listen, to become hypersensitive to early warning signs and navigational signals of many kinds, and to make critical course corrections without having to stop or pause when the heat is on will have a better chance of prevailing than those who invested themselves in a single skill, or method, or technique. It is not too much to say that the better we can be at tuning ourselves, the better will be our entire experience of being.

This critical element becomes increasingly important as we mature, especially as we approach our later years. Maturing toward mastery, self-tuning enables us to continue dissolving unhealthy tensions in our bodies and rigidity in our minds. Relaxing more deeply year after year, we can enjoy finding a little more space in our aging joints, space that gains value with every passing day. Having learned to enhance our *gaze* (I address this below) and quiet our emotions, we can see more clearly, even as our eyes grow older. We feel with greater sensitivity, respond more appropriately, and waste less energy on nonsense. These enhancements come to us because we tune ourselves like a musician tunes her instrument, day after day after day.

Eventually, if our practice touches the whole of our lives, we learn how to experience inner peace. The *gongfu* (martial arts effectiveness) in our art gives us a unique kind of pleasure, but the result of years of practice is the state of mind/body that we bring to our families, colleagues, and communities. We are tuning our very *state of being*. In this sense, for us, taijiquan is a yoga as well as a martial art.

This chapter began because I wanted to improve my ability to tune my aging body/mind, to keep my balance during unusually difficult times, and to help our students do the same. Since 1964, taijiquan has humbled me, confounded me, and challenged every instinct with which I grew up. Now seeking to better understand my blind spots, I sat back from my typical approach to training (do more) and took a long look at several of my colleagues whom I admired. These weren't people who never fell out of balance, nor were they taiji purists who counted on this one art to have given them everything they needed to know. We shared the realization that, while our chosen art might have *all* the answers, we weren't necessarily able to assimilate them. For us, an occasional look through another lens could be useful. One close friend, a farmer, a great boxer, and an accomplished musician, found his most profound respite and reflection in music. Another, whose push-hands skills always amazed me, also took hatha yoga classes several times a week. We agreed that sometimes the best way to see inward is to look through a completely different set of principles. I decided that comparing the principles of taijiquan and hatha yoga would be interesting. Several taiji teachers told me later that, for them, taijiquan and yoga had blended into a single discipline.

In examining that "single discipline," I had to separate these two schools of thought and then compare their components, their principles, and their methods. To be fair minded, I put the gongfu aspect aside to focus on the straightforward benefits to body, mind, and spirit—but I could not put it far. Among the great treasures hidden within taijiquan, there are those that can only be realized by "tasting bitter," "investing in loss," and "listening to and following one's opponent," gifts that come in ways one cannot imagine until something goes still and silent inside. I touch on these below.

But first, I had to ask the question: how does taijiquan measure up as a yoga?

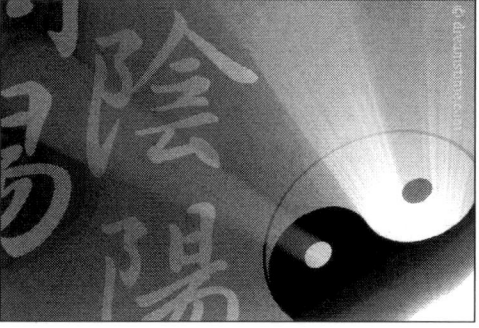

Hatha Is Yang-Yin

The word *yoga* means "union" (Devereux, 1998: 5). The practice of hatha yoga attempts to create the union of polar opposites in the way that taijiquan seeks to establish a dynamic balance between yin and yang. *Ha* means "sun" (*yang*) and *tha* means "moon" (*yin*), so "sun-moon union" loosely translates to "yang-yin reconciliation."

Both philosophies have articulated the characteristics of each end of the polarity in great detail. Distinctions such as hot-cold, male-female, aggressive-passive, strong-weak, hard-soft, to name a few, build a picture of opposites that could form a bipolar, tripolar, or multiple-polar matrix. In some cases, the poles could represent the tendency to do good, the tendency to do evil, and the tendency to transcend both good and evil. In another example, every being lives with the simultaneous urge toward agency (coming into being) and dissolution (going out of being), while equally being driven toward progressing and regressing. The key point is that each individual can manifest relatively more of one pole than another and, in so doing, be out of balance.

Both philosophies consider the reconciliation of these grand cosmological opposites to be essential milestones in a person's development. According to yogic philosophy, for example, until we achieve this reconciliation, we exist in a state of inner conflict. Perceiving an "either–or" world, we cling to one end of an eternal polarity and reject the other, it's opposite. Unable to experience the greater whole, we feel exposed, isolated, and unsafe. The very act of being makes us anxious because we try to fit in (to be "good") while desperately separating ourselves from essential parts of our true selves (that which we consider "bad") and the world in which we live.

Both the Chinese and Indian philosophies consider the dynamic balance of their polarity to be essential for life, but at some point, the idea of balancing energies that one considers positive (sun, yang) and negative (moon, yin) loses its moral attribution. Positive does not mean "good," with negative being "bad." They are simply describing characteristics, such as a positive electrical charge, for example, or negative (empty) space. In a balanced system, they complement each other, support each other, and become each other. Too much of either destabilizes that balance, giving the practitioner the task of finding ways to restore it, just as does the natural universe in its incomprehensibly dynamic ways.

After years of pattern-challenging and consciousness-raising practices, we can realize that our separation is an illusion. Through this awakening, we achieve union within ourselves, and with it, union with the world. Through personal reflection and practice over time, dualism becomes oneness. The yogi surrenders to the whole and realizes Brahman. The Daoist resonates with the very movement of the universe. The "Way that cannot be named" can be lived, and so we live it.

The taiji practitioner learns to become quiet enough to "hear" the intentions of others, sensitive enough to feel forces previously unknown to us, and still within ourselves, whether our bodies are in motion or not. Our practice settles and expands our sphere of thought until we experience both the polarity and the unity of yin and yang. The words of the great sage, Laozi, inspire us: "To the mind that is still, the whole universe surrenders."

Both yoga and taijiquan offer breathing and movement exercises, meditative processes, behavioral injunctions, and other disciplines that propose to cultivate such expansive stillness; both seek to prolong the life and enhance the health of the practitioner. For adepts of these systems, the path is one of inner transformation that eventually leads to outer transformation.

Compatible Elements

Looking into the cosmologies that support these concepts, our scope expands beyond the specific disciplines of yoga and taijiquan. The five-element models described below form the bedrock of Chinese and Indian cultures, for example, most importantly where their systems of medicine are concerned.

Within, and perhaps as products of this balancing process, both cultures also discern the emergence of five essential elements. The Chinese model identifies wood, fire, earth, metal, and water (Veith, 2002); the Indian model identifies, respectively: ether, fire, earth, air, and water (Devereux, 1998: 6). Exploring the comparative depths of these elements is beyond the scope of this chapter, but understanding how the yogic use of them can apply to taiji practice proves handy. The names and foci of the yogic elements are as follows (Devereux, 1998: 5–7):

Drushti (space, ether)
Asana (structure, alignment, earth)
Vinyasa (quality of movement, water)
Pranayama (quality of breathing, air)
Bandha (energetic transformation, fire).

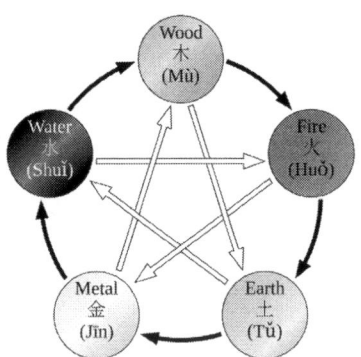

And here we gain a useful tool: the yogic blueprint for a balanced practice. With this blueprint in mind, let's look at how one organizes and approaches the work we do. I invite you to examine your own practice to identify comparable, conflicting, and perhaps missing elements. If you find something missing in your practice, or you see the opportunity to refine a part of it, please note that the only requirement is that you make your enhancements responsibly.

Drushti: The Mind's Eye

Drushti, the element of ether, determines the context in which one lives. In the Chinese medical model, it is loosely analogous to wood, which governs an individual's capacity for planning and decision making. Drushti describes a person's attention, intention, or awareness. Your drushti determines the "gaze" through which you perceive your situation and your purpose in it.

When playing taijiquan through the yogic gaze, one can find oneself easing into a growing awareness of previously unknown paths to self-realization. For those who have strong instincts about martial arts, and who require of themselves the achievement of extraordinary levels of skill and awareness, such achievement might define the completion of the path. Still others, as has been the case for me, can find themselves drawn to the inner and outer game of metaphorical combat and disciplined playfulness that martial arts provide. We interact in the spirit of bear cubs rolling on a grassy hillside, enthusiastically locked in each other's jaws while never intending to cause real harm. Like other natural animals, we want to develop our innate survival tools and abilities; as culturally conscious and moral animals, we wish to never need to use these tools in earnest.

If, as a student, one's mind's eye focuses on cultivating playfulness and mutual well-being, he is already practicing taijiquan as a yoga, an exercise of union. This drushti creates agility in the body/mind and, because you take yourself lightly, enables you to move lightly on your feet.

I find that in taiji form practice, a yogic frame of mind enables a person to learn while simultaneously enjoying a healthy sense of self-acceptance. One must begin with what is, and this acceptance or recognition of that which already is provides a foothold for learning. Rather than complacency, such a willing acceptance can promote exquisite attention to what you are doing as you become aware of your body's position in space—head, hands, feet, hips, shoulders, knees, elbows—as well as spinal alignment, quality of movement, breathing, thinking, and in time, the intrinsic energies moving through your body. The demands you place on yourself, while dedicated to drawing out the best in you, are gentle, even loving. Such is the nature of most yogic drushti.

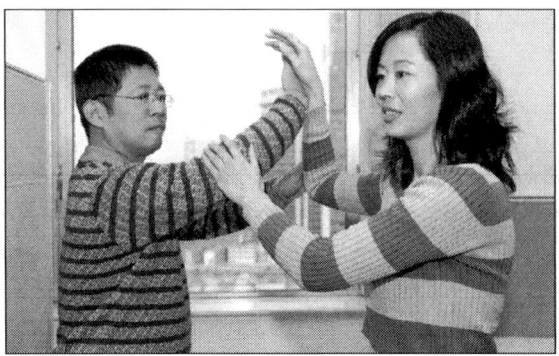

Push-hands becomes play. © iStockphoto.com

By contrast, one might approach yoga or taijiquan or any other practice as a performance art. The competitor in us wants to win; the insatiable ego wants to be recognized, to outdo others while insisting that we continually surpass our previous performances. We expect to "get it" quickly, and are dismayed—instead of intrigued—to find that our chosen path might confound us for years, maybe forever. We bring pressure into our practice that, while generally useful in excellence-oriented contexts like sports, can be the very opposite of our long-term purpose in choosing taijiquan over other paths.

As students, excellence demands that we walk a thin line between driving ourselves and cultivating ourselves. The compulsively driving mindset, a psychological characteristic of many educational and cultural traditions, assumes that the student is lazy or mediocre by nature and must be whipped into shape, driven to develop, forced out of the comfort zone. The teacher has to push, even humiliate, each student into stepping beyond his limitations, and as students we sustain the harsh voices of our most vociferous teachers in our heads long after they are gone. Instead of union, we try to learn through constantly self-evaluating pressure.

In this state of mind, our mistakes embarrass us. We try learning while feeling self-conscious about not knowing what we don't yet know. Our practice is never good enough, and the eye of our teacher makes us feel vulnerable and inadequate.

SIDEBAR

Imagine yourself at taiji camp for the next five days on the Big Island of Hawaii (circa mid-1990s). The hot, tropically aromatic air melts your very bones as you find yourself among fifty or so practitioners of various ages and skill levels coming from different parts of the world to dedicate six hours a day to practice taijiquan. Some are just beginning. For others, this is their fifteenth camp and a chance to mix it up with some good boxers.

The teacher is Grandmaster William C. C. Chen, who is showing the group how to throw a punch. An astonishing boxer, he demonstrates a straight right several times with explanations, then asks the students to try it themselves. Surveying the group for a few moments, he picks a fifty-something woman who clearly has no martial arts background and asks her to show what she can do.

"We're looking at Shirley" (not her real name), he says. "Go ahead."

Shirley punches, appropriately looking like she's never done this before.

"Yes!" Chen exclaims with enthusiasm. "That's great. Now, just do it again and drop your shoulder."

Shirley punches again, dropping her shoulder.

"Yes!" he exclaims again, with enough enthusiasm to get her grinning. "Now, just bend your knee."

She punches; he acknowledges and corrects her. She punches again; he encourages her more and makes additional corrections. By the time she has thrown a dozen punches, she is starting to get the idea. He never tells her no.

Chen is not telling her that she is doing it right. He is saying yes to her effort. It takes courage for her to try in front of this group, to learn something foreign to her background, to listen to feedback and apply it. He knows what he is doing: he is building her spirit, expanding the space in which she can learn, cultivating drushti.

Many ancient schools fostered this approach with the intent of toughening and enabling students to overcome their weaknesses. In their most philosophical contexts, they taught that real victory was "victory over the self." In their more misguided moments, they simply taught ways to brutalize self and others under the rubric of learning.

After thirty or forty years of training, I find, one comes to realize that victory over the self is an illusion. We might develop tremendous discipline, but we conquer nothing within. Real maturity means discovering what we are, coming to peace with it, and thus ending the war with ourselves. Inner peace enables us to cultivate better habits and prune away our worst ones in sustainable, low-maintenance ways. Instead of fighting with ourselves, we learn how to genuinely update our ideas and behaviors. In the process, we reconcile with our inner demons, and when we do, they can become allies, willing participants in our continued evolution as human beings.

Cultivation is the operant word here. Inner cultivation occurs as a slow, nurturing, loving, fearlessly honest process of realizing how we think and behave, responding more sensitively to the world around us, recognizing the feelings that attune us to our true nature and purpose in life, trusting these feelings, optimizing them, and acting on them. The mind that watches and directs this process is our drushti.

Asana: Sound Structure

Asana means "alignment" (Devereux, 2006: 7–8), and all the postures that yogis practice are called *asanas*. These are not static poses, but instead dynamic combinations of opposing and balancing forces that send spirals of energy through the body to awaken its cellular intelligence.

In the yoga of taiji, we find cellular intelligence in the *jin* (intrinsic strength) (Zhang, 2006: 14–20), which is the very nature of our cells expressing their collective power. We become adept at sensing and cultivating this natural power when we relax, focus our minds on a single action, and take that action in ways that *passively* compress our bones and tissues along a line that starts in our foot or feet, runs through our legs and spine, and ends in one hand, both hands, or the other foot—when kicking, for example.

The line being compressed is the line of *jin*, the internal hardness hidden within an envelope of softness. Our *jin* is the intrinsic strength of our cells. Compare this to untrained *extrinsic* effort, or *li* (raw force), which is not part our cells' essential nature and so demands actively exerted force.

We find our *jin* by becoming mentally quiet and physically relaxed enough to feel the strength that is already there, then moving in ways that optimize that strength. This means we let our *jin* influence our movements in the way that the heft of a sword influences how we wield it. In this state of attentiveness, we "listen" to the *jin*.

Walking, standing, and jumping provide straightforward ways to understand this idea. Your body knows just how much you need to tense your muscles to stand. If you jump, you don't have to think about how much to tense and which muscles to tense when you land. Your body already knows (personal communications with William C. C. Chen).

This is somatic intelligence, *jin* in action. Translating the body's wisdom from these mundane actions into the elegant movements of taijiquan marks the beginning of cultivating internal power. Recognizing that the practitioner doesn't move by magic, but by physiology and kinetics in which muscles contract to pull bones into place, we can pay attention to what happens in our bodies when we move with coordinated ease and power. Our attentiveness enables us to blend metaphor (what we are thinking) and mechanics (what we are doing) in ways that make us move more competently. While for years we might focus primarily on relaxing, we don't relax completely; if we did, we would fall to the floor in a heap. We relax selectively so unnecessary tensions dissolve and necessary ones occur, giving us essential hardness with no sense of effort.

You can't cultivate this hardness—internal *jin*—by trying to be strong.[1] Effort and force lead to excessive tension that masks the very power you are trying to discover. Instead, you cultivate internal *jin* by aligning your body—guided by gravity—so that in each moment you can feel the force vector that extends from your substantial foot through your *dantian* (lower abdomen) and spine to your hands, relaxing everything that is not on this vector, and activating it through thought.[2]

Your interpretation of a movement—a push, for example—defines the line of force being delivered; your *qi* (energy) then gets your body parts in place to deliver it. But qi, being directed by your conscious mind, is distinct from the *jin* you discover.

In this sense of discovery, you cultivate *jin* by getting out of its way. As you align the firm line from foot to hand in each taiji movement, you think of the line being passively compressed as it joins its real or imaginary target. Instead of feeling effort when you apply a move, you have the sensation of letting go. This sensation occurs whether you are uprooting a training partner or practicing form on your own.

To sense this in solo practice, students are advised to imagine applying the moves to an actual person; your intention to "apply" the move will define a line of firmness between your root and your virtual opponent. Don't tense this line; just visualize it connecting your foot to your contact point—your hand, for example—in a way that compresses you into your foot. Relax, and let the firmness reveal itself to you.

To find the same sensation in push-hands, which requires seriously tempering your ego, imagine your partner to be a mirror of yourself: your beneficent twin. Instead of trying to uproot an opponent, imagine letting your beneficent twin compress you from time to time—no effort, no winning, just joining your twin and aligning yourself between him and the earth so his mass compresses you into the earth. When your twin gets uprooted, it's not because you try to do anything; you just happen to be there when he gets overly ambitious and uproots himself.

Zheng Manqing taught, "Play form as if you were with an opponent; play push-hands as if you were alone" (Lowenthal, 1993: 109). While this practice takes imagination and can prove psychologically challenging, it awakens your awareness of the *jin* that embodies your somatic intelligence. The hard within the soft awakens the bright within you where your brightness might have been clouded by social conditioning.

Alone or with others, you cultivate *jin*—as well as qi—by practicing congruency in your thoughts and actions. This means you do one thing at a time and pay attention to what you are doing. Practicing congruency reduces habitual, chronic tensions and extends through your taiji forms, interactive exercises, everyday societal encounters, personal behaviors, and even meditations. As you learn to calm your busy thoughts, you can develop single-mindedness. As you learn to move with gravity-aligned balance, you can discover the power waiting in your cells. In time, you find that single-minded—unconflicted—*jin* is intelligent in the sense that it keeps you from doing stupid things to yourself; it is always economical, simple, respectful of physical reality, and present, if you can become mentally and emotionally still enough in yourself to feel it.

Yoga calls this stillness "dying in the posture" (Devereaux, 1998: 16). Yogis put themselves into shapes that challenge their chronic tension patterns, then stay there for a specified time based on the body's needs and capacity to respond. When the body/mind has let go, one has "died" in the posture. Waiting for this moment takes tremendous discipline and loving, noncompetitive, unambitious patience. The taiji version occurs during standing-posture practices and in the moment of release that happens in form practice each time you reach the peak or energized part of a movement (Brodsky, 2005).

While much of yoga's somatic opening occurs on a mat, yogis also rely on standing postures to bring the body back together. Master practitioner Godfrey Devereux (1998: 27) declares, "Of all the yoga postures the most important for awakening somatic intelligence are the standing postures." The yogic idea of alignment in these postures is opened, connected, engaged, energized, and balanced.

Vinyasa: The Quality of Movement

Most people think of yoga practice as "stretching." This superficial idea misses the point in the same way as interpreting taijiquan's goal to be "relaxing." While we relax to release and open our joints (*sung*), we do so to enliven and empower our movement. In the way that yoga seeks to awaken the body/mind, taiji seeks to generate extraordinarily powerful, effortless action that leads to the same awakening: the awakening of our inner power and the cultivation of the spirit that gives us life.

Yogis can hurt themselves by forcing themselves to stretch, and taiji players hurt themselves by forcing themselves into stances that are too low for them, tucking the tailbone too far forward, forcing or resisting during push-hands, and a myriad of creatively destructive ways of holding knees, necks, and shoulders in unnatural positions. Over time, practicing your forms with some yogic consciousness can change those habits and bring about therapeutic changes.

Vinyasa means "to place [the body] in a special way" (Devereaux, 1998: 44–45). It refers to the order in which one practices asanas and the quality of movement and breathing with which the practitioner goes from posture to posture. Here yoga more resembles qigong than taijiquan, because rather than just gaining the outcome of enhancing qi, the "quan" part also seeks to develop martial arts effectiveness and the personal equanimity that comes from dealing with one's ego in relationship to others, friendly or otherwise.

Neither yoga nor taiji is about posing. In the same way that the asanas are dynamic states of balanced forces, the taiji "postures" are snapshots of moments in a continuum, conveniently named so we can talk about them. No two pushes are alike, just as no two situations are alike. We just think we are doing the same movement over and over again, when in fact we are setting up a series of actions and "launching" them without knowing precisely where and how they will complete themselves by connecting with each other. When you are present in your practice, despite the fact that you have done a move a thousand times, each time is unique.

Nor is taiji form about moving slowly, but rather about operating in such a way that we optimize our most powerful natural energies: life force, intrinsic strength, spirit. We learn to sense and cultivate those energies when we develop a state of mind that approaches mindfulness meditation. This could involve fast or slow or no movement, but it just happens that we find it easier to cultivate this state when we move slowly. Once awakened, our mindfulness can be exercised no matter what we are doing.

With these different intentions noted, the principles of movement are similar: relax and open the joints; elongate your spine from the top of your head downward; surrender to gravity in both your vertical alignment and in your movements; link your movements together in such a way that each movement creates the one that follows; breathe freely; focus; be present.

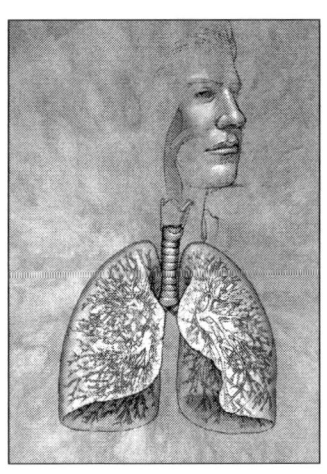

Pranayama: The Quality of Breathing

Pranayama is the practice of energetic regulation through the breath (Devereux, 1998: 56–59). *Prana* is essentially qi, and *ayama* loosely translates to "extension." Practices for personal transformation through energetic regulation date back thousands of years, and all consider breathing to be a primary tool.

Some yoga employs audible breathing (*ujjayi*), which, because of the throat tension it requires, is not recommended when practicing taijiquan. According to classical instructions, taijiquan calls for slow, silent, long, and thin breathing during form practice, and, often, the use of compressive sound during fast movement or qigong. Exceptions abound to this statement, so it appears here as a rule of thumb. Whatever the practice, students are advised to breathe freely.

In applying yogic principles to taiji practice, we confront the chicken/egg question: which comes first, the breath or the movement? If we momentarily set aside the schools that say, "Don't worry about the breathing; it will come naturally," or "Just breathe naturally," we can ask what, precisely, the relationship is between breath and movement in taiji.

Conscious "compression breathing" provides each movement with a pneumatic boost (Brodsky, 2004: 37–44). William Chen taught me about compression breathing, but my personal conviction about it comes from studying breathing when doing physical work (gaining added power), when my spine became injured (bracing the spine), with older people (helping them move), when we are surprised or excited (we inhale), when passively relaxing (even my dog lets out a sigh when he is done running around), and when decompressing and compressing my body in practicing taiji form.

With compression and decompression in mind, I contend that the chicken—that is, the movement—comes first and dictates how one should breathe. My favorite test is to ask a person to go from a seated to a standing position and experiment with different ways of breathing: inhaling, exhaling, or holding. The reader is invited to try these and see which way feels most natural and powerful.

But let's ask the opposite question: if you were standing and suddenly your knees caved in as if you were passing out, what would happen to the air in your body? Would your lungs fill with air? Or would the air in your lungs be expelled without your trying to exhale? Then, if you caught yourself halfway down, how would you breathe to regain yourself?

I propose that you would lose air as you fell and inhale as you recovered, catching your breath as you caught yourself from further falling. By testing breathing in a wide variety of situations, experimental and practical, I have concluded that natural breathing in the slow practice of taiji form means inhaling when you extend your body and exhaling when you flex it (Brodsky, 2004).

Zheng Manqing's instructions on the matter of breathing during form practice consist of inhaling when the arms move up and away from the body and exhaling when the arms move down and close to the body (Cheng and Smith, 1966: 11). William Chen is much more explicit about using the breath, instructing his students to exhale just before each energized move (the "applied" part) in the form, and to gently inhale to compress the dantian as the move is energized ("applied"). When demonstrating fast punches, he almost always lets out a sound, releasing compressed air, but not simply exhaling.

Along with compression breathing, one can practice a useful technique that we'll call here "expansion" breathing. I discovered this method while doing standing/rooting practices. As do many schools, we often hold postures for a few minutes while we adjust our form and settle into the substantial foot to deepen our root. Periodically, I notice some people cringing instead of sinking. It is as if they are trying to get shorter, smaller, to occupy less space in the room. Once noticing this cringing and making sure it wasn't just from burning thighs or other pain, I began to spot the same pattern in their form and push-hands practice as well.

This cringing is especially noticeable in tall people, who might have developed the habit while trying to fit in while growing up in a shorter world. Others, with the idea of "sinking the elbows" or "depressing the chest" (Liao, 1990) sometimes pinch their armpits inward, which contracts their torsos across the line of the clavicles. The corrective response is to "smile" across the clavicles, widening them to take their full, allotted space.

This gentle clavicular smile remedies the armpit pinch and relieves the upper torso and neck of much of their tension. Instead of depressing the chest, one empties the chest of its grip on itself and lets the clavicles roll back into the chest and the scapulae drop until the whole shoulder girdle finds its natural angle of repose. This enables the idea of suspending the head from above to extend into the upper torso. Long spine, wide frame, released chest.

Expansion breathing adds to this relief and extends the mental space that a person occupies. To practice it, I suggest playing a round of your form and stopping at each posture for three full breaths. Imagine that each inhalation expands your entire body in all directions, as if you were filling up like a balloon, becoming one or two sizes larger. Then imagine that each exhalation emanates from your pores, so you "exhale through your skin" as you let gravity relax you. Expand on each inhalation and release on each exhalation. Stay in each posture for three breaths, adjusting into your most satisfying alignment; then move on. As you breathe, affirm to yourself that you are taking all the space to which your body/mind is entitled.

Esoterically described, we might call this practice "expanding your field of qi." In simpler terms, I think of it as just a wholesome exercise that changes how you see and feel your body.

Bandha: Energetic Transformation

Bandha means "seal" or "lock" (Devereaux, 1998: 48–51), and, like the gates and internal channels of taijiquan and Daoist meditation, the bandhas of yoga are thought to open certain energetic doors in the body while closing others. Daoist alchemists and yogis consider these to be spiritual openings through which one can enter a dimension of the self that can't be accessed by ordinary means. Because traditional explanations can prove arcane, we are best served here by comparing only a few generalized commonalities of yogic and Daoist models and keeping our terms as anatomical as possible.

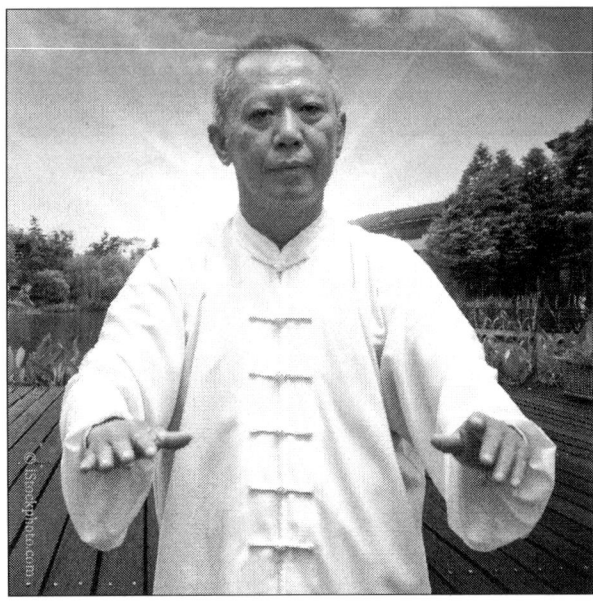

Also, a disclaimer: Esoteric schools sometimes offer promises that few, if any, fulfill. Immortality is hard to come by; tantric transmutation into pure white light might require batteries; astonishing stories of physics-defying qi rarely pass the test of public scrutiny. When delving into the transformative aspects of taijiquan, the less magical is often more reliable.

With that caveat in mind, exercising the bandhas in your taiji practice can liberate considerable energy. One can introduce oneself to this practice by standing comfortably with feet parallel to each other and wide enough apart that they could be hanging off your hips. Too wide will create unnecessary tension, and too narrow might feel unstable. Bend your knees.

Begin by thinking about the highest point of the top of your head. This is the area from which you "suspend your head from above," the crown chakra in yoga, the upper dantian (*ni wan*) in Daoist yoga, and associated with the *bai hui* point (hundred meetings) of the energetic governing vessel that runs up the back of your body in Chinese medicine (Lu, 1970: 124). Here you maintain part of your attention, a sense of lightness, as if you were being pulled upward and gently reaching upward at the same time.

Building on this light feeling, gently expand the space between the base of your skull and the back of your neck. When you "empty the chest and raise the back," a sense of fullness and softness begins here. At the same time, imagine your whole head floating upward, away from your shoulders, which gently drop to your sides. Think, "Long spine, wide frame."

Extending your attention downward to the seventh cervical vertebra, which is known as the "great hammer" in Chinese medicine, relax the base of your neck. This is the posterior portion of the yogic throat chakra, which is thought to be the seat of your personality. Here the forward curve of your neck starts to become the backward curve of your torso, and so presents a stress point, a gate that closes with tension and that you can open through gentle elongation. Preparing to yawn without actually yawning is a simple way to open this point.

The backward curve of your torso switches to a forward curve at the twelfth thoracic vertebra, the last one that has ribs attached to it, and the backdrop to your heart chakra and middle dantian. If you think of the space between this vertebra and the one below it, the first lumbar, gently expanding, the curve naturally flattens an appropriate amount and this gate opens. Do this without effort by breathing into your heart. A good sigh goes a long way here.

The lumbar spine meets your sacrum around the level of your hips. By continuing to think about elongation, you can align this juncture a little more vertically. As implied earlier, you don't need to tuck your sacrum as much as to drop it so you feel like you are sitting. This promotes the release of your *kua* (hip crease) and flattens your low back.

Now hang there, sensing your lower dantian and thinking, "Long spine, wide frame." The only work you should feel is in your thighs, depending on how much your knees are bent. Your spine is elongated, and its gates are open: minimal tension, optimal alignment with gravity, and the energy can flow.

From here continue to widen your frame. This occurs at your shoulders and hips. Imagine your shoulders falling to the sides as you "smile" across the clavicles. Simultaneously rotate your clavicles back toward your shoulder blades as you gently release those blades to fall toward your posterior ribs. "Plucking up the back" (Liao, 1990) doesn't mean becoming slightly hunchback; it means filling the back with qi by thinking about the energy that runs up the back as you align and relax. Lengthening your spine and smiling into your shoulders as just described facilitates this movement of energy.

Regarding the pelvis, some schools advocate contracting the perineum. I find this unnecessary, being an appropriately neurotic product of Western culture, and prefer to smile across the pelvis instead. This pelvic smile automatically causes the pelvic floor to raise a little, gently engages the abdominal muscles, and supports the lumbar spine better than trying to contract the perineum. To find the smiling muscle, which is the *transversus abdominus*, just bend forward a tiny bit and press your thumbs into your abdomen at a point halfway between your navel and pubic bone, about two inches to each side. Press firmly, then cough. The muscle you feel contracting when you cough is the *transversus*.

Now smile across the clavicles and pelvis, and you have a "wide frame."

"Long spine, wide frame" provides the basis of taiji's bandha, or transformational energy work. The next step is in the spirals and gates in your arms and legs.

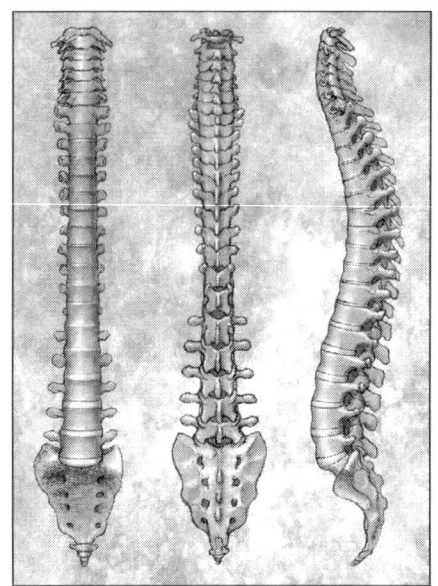
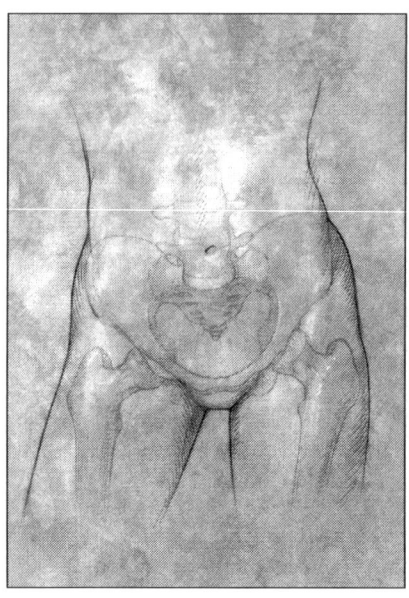

Bandhas and Gates

Taiji literature describes the "nine pearls" namely: the wrist, elbow, shoulder, ankle, knee, hip, and the three major curves of the spine (Wile, 1983: 107). These are the gates that open to release qi and close to contain it. When open, the gates decompress, elongate, and loosen as we have just done. When closed, the gates compress and express the firmness of *jin*. In taiji practice, your task is to align your skeleton so the force vector that passes through your body travels easily and naturally from foot to hand, connecting the gates in between. Peter Ralston describes it as "lining up the billiard balls."

Having long been confused by the descriptions in the classics—e.g., what do I do with "When the outer gate opens, the inner gate closes?"—I have often found myself experimenting with the gates. Once I realized that *jin* felt different from qi, statements like "Where there is no qi, there is pure hardness" started to make sense. Distinguishing more sensitively between substantial and insubstantial helped as well, as did a deeper surrender to gravity. Bottom line: relax everything that is not working, direct your qi with thought instead of effort, and listen to the *jin*.

Once your spine is aligned and elongated, next come the spirals that move through your arms and legs as you energize your moves. The task is to feel the lines through which *jin* and qi operate.

To sense these lines, take any comfortable stance and focus your mind on one leg. As you feel that foot pressing into the floor, *imagine* that you are gently rotating your lower leg inward (toward the center of your body) along the axis of your bones while rotating your upper leg outward to the sides. Don't move anything, most notably your knees; just add a little tone to the lower leg one way (inward) and to the upper leg the other way (outward). Gently tense the tiniest bit with these rotations in mind.

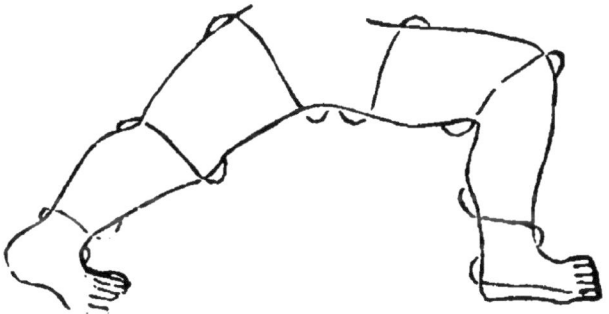

Spirals indicate energy flow through the legs, depicted in Chen Xin's book, *Illustrated Explanation of Chen Family Taijiquan*, from the 1920's.

It will feel like you are creating dynamic tension in your leg, and you are. This engages the bandha of the leg, exciting your qi more than you would by just standing there. Try it in one leg, then the other, then both. Then try it in different stances.

You can easily overdo it, so make it more of an attitude than an effort. Stand still and feel what energetics these rotations produce; then see if you can feel those energetics as they extend up your spine to the top of your head. Take your time; relax your torso as much as possible so you can feel the soft flow of qi that passes through your sinews and the hard line of *jin* that passes through your bones.

While maintaining "long spine, wide frame," extend your awareness into your arms. Taking any posture that you typically practice, gently rotate the upper arm outward as you torque the lower arm in toward your thumb. No movement is necessary, just the very subtle tension that comes with intention. The energetics of this intention end up in your thumb, index finger, and middle finger.

Now, connect your feet to your hands. Feeling the pressure of your feet on the floor, the spiral inward of your lower legs, the spiral outward of your upper legs, the feeling of firmness (*jin*) that signals the connective power of your legs, pelvis, and spine, your long spine and wide frame that reaches to the top of your head, the outward spiral of your upper arms, and inward spiral of your lower arms, you are connected.

Breathe deeply and enjoy this feeling. You are experiencing the yoga of taijiquan. When practicing form, one can concentrate on any aspect of this experience or none of it, since the natural spirals and alignments will come in time.

As we have seen, these yogic ideas—drushti, asana, vinyasa, pranayama, and bandha—can become embedded into your skill set as gentle enhancing nuances. Your gaze can be gentle and clear, your alignment sound, movement fluid, and breathing easy as you cultivate transformative energies throughout your body, preparing pathways for your spirit to rise. And rise, it will.

Notes

1. This refers to *nei jin*, the subtler internal strength. *Wai jin*, which is related to physical power, can be developed through muscle-oriented training.
2. According to taiji principles, one leg is always more weighted and in higher tonus, therefore more "substantial" than the other. Power emanates from the substantial leg as the practitioner visualizes the intended move being applied.

References

Brodsky, G. (August 2004). "Compression breathing," *Tai Chi Magazine, 28*(4): 37–44.

Cheng, M. and Smith, R. (1966). *T'ai Chi: The "supreme ultimate" exercise for health, sport, and self-defense.* Boston: Charles Tuttle Publishing.

Devereux, G. (1998). *Dynamic yoga.* Toronto, ON: HarperCollins/Thorsons Publishing.

Liao, W. (1990). *Tai chi classics.* Boston: Shambhala Publishing.

Lowenthal, W. (1993). *There are no secrets: Professor Cheng Man-ch'ing and his tai chi chuan.* Berkeley, CA: North Atlantic Books.

Lu K'uan Yu (1970). *Taoist yoga.* London: Rider and Co.

Veith, I. (2002). *The yellow emperor's classic of internal medicine.* Berkeley, CA: University of California Press.

Wile, D. (1983). *T'ai chi touchstones: Yang family secret transmissions.* Brooklyn, NY: Sweet Ch'i Press.

Yang, J. (1999). *Taijiquan: Classical Yang style.* Boston: YMAA Publication Center.

Zhang, Y. (April 2006). "Zhang Yun on the use and development of jin in taiji, Part II." *T'ai Chi Magazine, 30*(3): 14–20.

Ward Off, Diagonal Flying from Zheng Style Taijiquan
by Russ Mason, M.A.

Practical Applications of Taiji's Ward Off and Diagonal Flying Postures

Ward off is one of the fundamental postures of Yang Style taijiquan. The Chinese character for ward off is *peng* (掤), an obscure pictogram containing elements representing "hand" and "twin moons" reflecting each other as "friends." Another theory posits that the origin of *peng* may be a primitive character for the tail of the legendary phoenix, a bird symbolic of natural harmony and yin-yang balance. Both images present a good metaphor for the principles of sticking and following, which are essential to the application of taiji boxing. As a signature technique of the art, ward off employs *peng jin* (掤勁), an outwardly expanding energy that is further developed in the diagonal flying posture. Applications of the ward-off left and diagonal flying postures will be illustrated here.

Zheng Manqing was a disciple of Yang Chengfu and the creator of the thirty-seven-posture Yang short form, which he taught to my instructors who, in turn, passed the art to me. Zheng taught that the ultimate principle of taijiquan resides in the application of neutralization and the substance of central equilibrium (*zhong ding*). Attacking energy is received and, through yielding and neutralizing, redirected around one's constant central axis. Therefore, the principles of neutralization, sticking, and following permeate every application of taijiquan. Accordingly, the ward off posture is primarily soft, receptive, and perceptive (like a cricket's antenna); however, ward off energy (an expanding energy that rises upward and outward) can be used to issue energy as well as to sense it.

While learning the solo form as a beginning taijiquan student, my first encounter with ward off left me puzzled. Since I had heard that taijiquan eschews blocking, the use of this posture seemed mysterious until I experienced its application at the hands of Zheng Manqing's senior student, Benjamin Pang Jeng Lo. At a workshop hosted by Robert W. Smith in the 1970s, I had a chance to cross arms with Mr. Lo. As soon as he touched me, to my astonishment, I felt completely vulnerable, as if through that contact he could perceive my intentions. His eyes dancing with amusement, Mr. Lo used his soft ward off arm to totally control me, literally wiping the floor with my sprawling body. Two decades later, my understanding of the function deepened as Liu Xiheng, head of Zheng's Taipei school, used his profoundly relaxed ward off arm and an almost imperceptible whole-body movement to effortlessly receive my attack and send me flying several meters away.

In applying ward off, one must remain soft, alert, and sensitive. The body is relaxed, rooted, and balanced, always maintaining central equilibrium. First, one must receive and yield to the opponent's attack, perceiving its force and direction and following the attacker's intention. After the attack has been neutralized and controlled, the attacker's body will be disordered and unbalanced, leaving an opportunity for counterattack. One must be careful not to resist force with force. By joining with rather than blocking the attacking limb, the energy of the attack can be stored and returned.

The diagonal flying posture appears in only a right-handed version in Professor Zheng's system. It consists of a more complex series of transitional movements culminating in a flamboyant extended attack that extrapolates the ideas introduced by ward off. I vividly remember the moment of stunned terror I felt when Robert W. Smith applied this technique with a lightning fast thrust to my throat, gripping my trachea expertly and inextricably between his thumb and index finger. His firm but gentle grasp did not injure me but left no doubt in my mind of the potential lethality of the technique.

The diagonal flying posture includes a deep, 135-degree step and turn, suggesting a wide range of movement, and the hands move through splitting, tearing, and piercing actions. Finally, the articulation of the right arm and the waist suggests a "folding" technique in which the downward energy of an arm grab above the elbow is converted circularly to a thrusting attack by folding the elbow down and extending the hand forward.

The final piercing extension of the upturned palm in diagonal flying can be used to attack the throat by spearing, grasping, or striking. The "V" created by the right thumb and index finger of the upturned right hand can grasp the cricoid cartilage surrounding the opponent's larynx and thyroid, or slightly below that, where the trachea meets the larynx. The first joint of the index finger can apply pressure to the common carotid artery as the thumb presses into the windpipe or internal jugular vein. Alternatively, the posture may be used to lock the opponent's right arm, or, with an outward rotation of the palm, forearm, and waist, the technique can be modified to create an unbalancing deflection or a throw using the knife edge of the downturned hand against the side of the neck.

Like ward off, diagonal flying can be an effective counter to a right or left punch, or a front kick. The essence of the application is in yielding and following, so the exact articulation of the counterattack depends on the situation and the opponent's responses.

Technique 1: Ward Off
1a) Russ Mason neutralizes Erik Flannigan's left punch, controlling the arm with ward off's transitional "hold the ball" stance.
1b) After blending with and sticking to the attack, Mason shifts and follows Flannigan's retreat, stepping in and controlling his balance with ward off.
1c) Mason sits deeply into ward off to uproot and discharge Flannigan.
1d) Alternatively, Mason neutralizes Flannigan's right punch.
1e) Mason unbalances Flannigan and shifts weight to the right foot while pivoting left, throwing him.

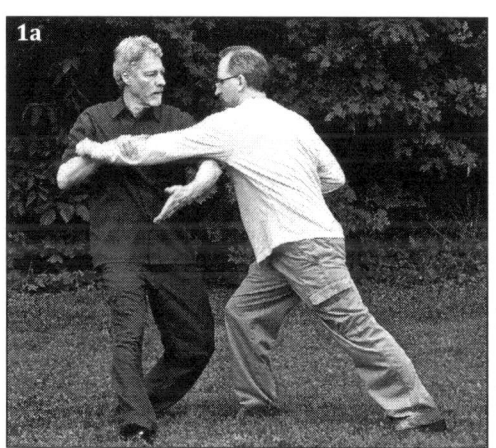
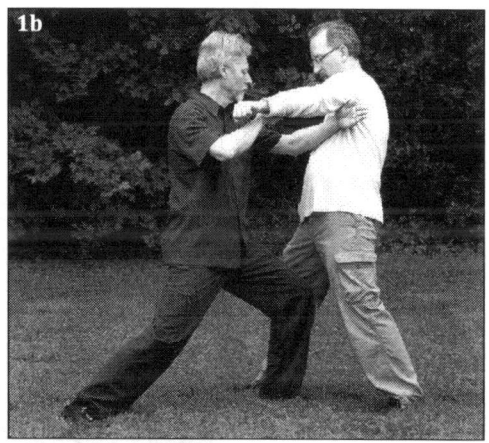
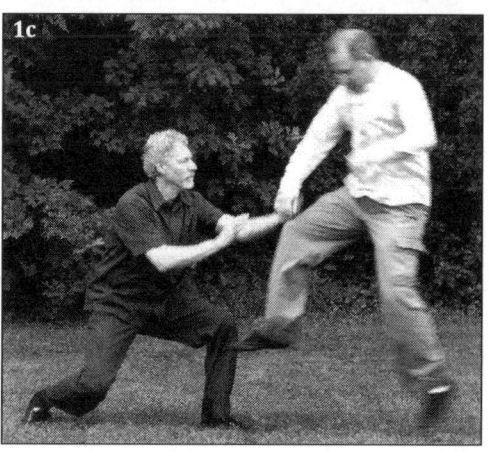
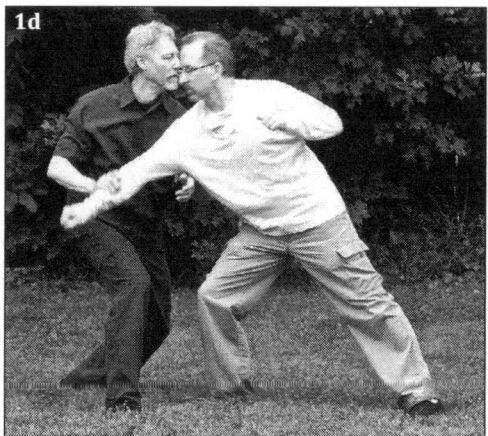
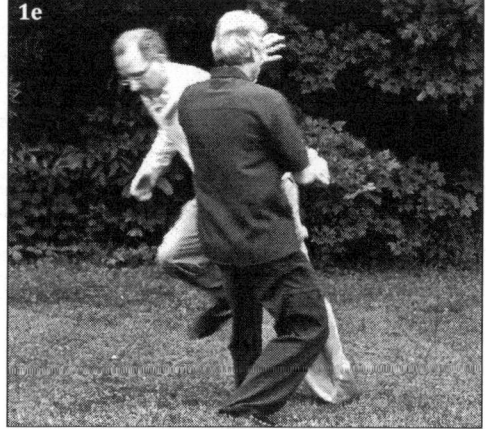

Thanks to colleague Erik Flannigan (3rd dan TKD) for assistance with the demonstrations and to Laurie Fuhrmann for the photography.

Technique 2: Diagonal Flying

2a) Mason neutralizes Flannigan's right front kick, capturing the leg.
2b) He uses diagonal flying to attack Flannigan's throat, immobilizing his right leg and controlling his balance.
2c) Mason uses a throat attack to unbalance and throw Flannigan.
2d) Alternatively, Mason uses diagonal flying against his right punch to lock Flannigan's arm and break his root.
2e) Mason uses a knife-edge hand and whole-body power against Flannigan's neck to unbalance and throw him.

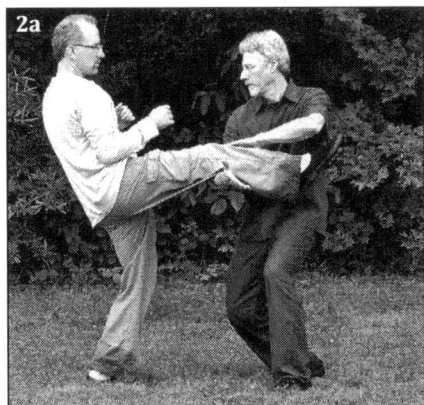
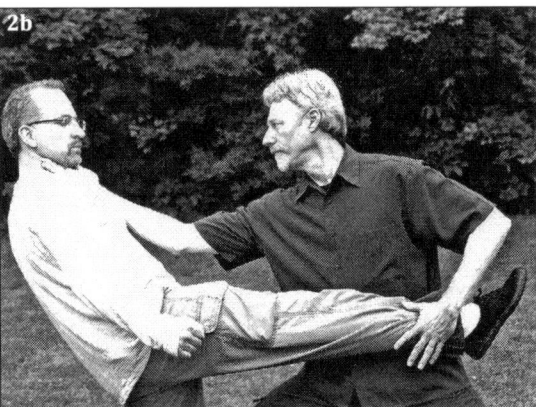
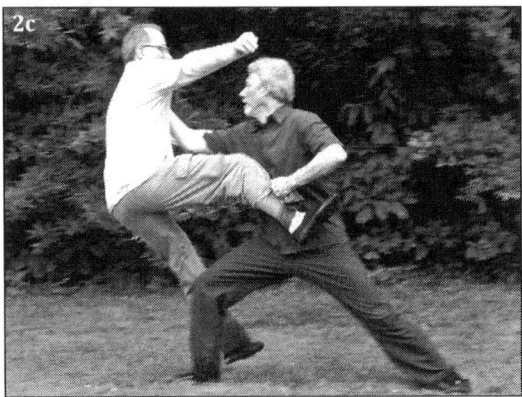
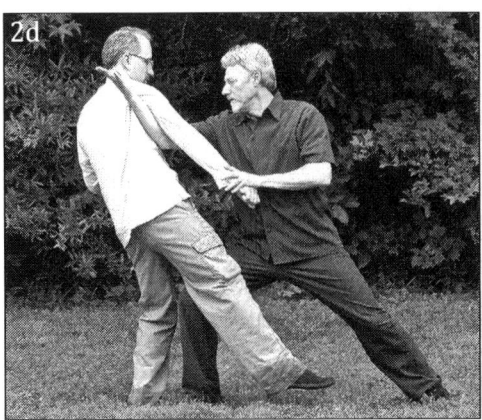
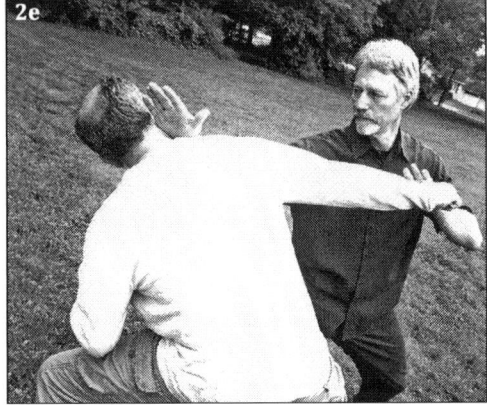

• 63 •

Chen Taijiquan: The Master's Touch
David Gaffney, B.A.

Chen Village Style: Using Soft to Neutralize and Hard to Emit

Chen Wangting created a new kind of martial art almost four hundred years ago in Chen Village. Chen Taijiquan has been refined and passed on through generations of village boxers up to the present day. An important concept lying at the heart of its devastating fighting skills is the use of softness to change and neutralize an attack, followed by hardness to emit force at the point when an opponent's position has become compromised. Since the mid-1990s—training with Chen Xiaowang and with his younger brother, Chen Xiaoxing—I've come to realize the breadth of this principle.

In the school, training is intense and physically very demanding, as befits one of China's most traditional martial arts. While Chen Taijiquan includes many kicks and strikes within its arsenal, in essence it is a close-range throwing and grappling system. The realities of combat necessitate that a practitioner be well versed and comfortable during close-quarter fighting. The system is renowned for its joint locking, throwing, and takedowns—all built upon its unique use of spiraling energy. It is this silk reeling quality that enables a skilled practitioner to use the strength of an antagonist against himself.

Chen Xiaowang (2011) explains: "When somebody comes with force we use the soft neutralizing method to change the direction of the incoming force. The opponent attacks our centerline and we change the direction and take the momentum out of his force. That is what is called *rou hua* (pliant neutralizing). At the moment that the opponent loses his balance we use our gang jin [hard power] to attack the most appropriate part of his body and that is what is called *rou hua gang fa*."

Chen Zhaochi Defeats a Bandit

Training applications with Chen Xiaowang is a painful experience. He is adamant that you must experience the real technique if you are to really understand it and have confidence in the method. This confidence is vital if a taijiquan practitioner is to meet a true attack with softness and without hesitation. Chen Xiaowang recounted the story of how Chen Zhaochi (1928–1981) used the principle of "neutralizing before returning force" to deadly effect when he was suddenly ambushed on a remote mountain path: "A bandit was hiding in a tree with a stick with the intention of attacking him when he passed. Before the stick could make contact, Zhaochi instinctively reacted by intercepting and then returning the weapon, striking the bandit on the head and killing him" (2008: 43). To his way of thinking, kicking and punching represent a relatively low level of martial skill compared to the internalized ability to instantaneously blend with a sudden violent and unexpected attack, in the process turning it back upon the person who launched the attack.

Practice Tips

• As an opponent attacks, it is crucial to remain balanced and centered. In the instant that contact is made, one must be able to assess the attack's speed, direction, strength, and quality. This is referred to as "listening" and "discerning" energy. During this process, one must make constant subtle changes to the body's posture, maintaining the center while following the direction of the incoming force.

• Don't neutralize and only then think of what to do next. In the process of neutralizing, one should be storing energy to instantly attack once the incoming force is dissipated. Chen Xiaowang (2011) says, "This is very effective because as he is losing his balance, I am storing my strength." While you are neutralizing, the aim of the practitioner is not to think of hitting the opponent; first defuse the incoming force. Placing too much emphasis on hardness during push-hands is a common error and represents a loss of principle.

• Following and exploiting an opponent's strength is the skill of spotting the right opportunity to take advantage of his position when it is compromised. As an opponent executes his attack, the aim is to follow the direction of his movement and, at the point when he is uncomfortable and in a disadvantageous position, to then enter and attack. As the opponent realizes his technique is not going to work, he naturally tries to change his movement. As he begins to go back after failing with an attack, a person with good push-hands ability just adds a little of his own strength to take advantage of the situation. In Taijiquan parlance this is known as borrowing strength.

Technique 1

1a)   Chen Xiaowang and the author practicing forward and backward-stepping push-hands.

1b)   As Chen pushes forward, David follows the movement and neutralizes the attack with diverting force.

1c-d)   When the force is dissipated, Chen returns in a smooth circular motion to apply a forceful joint-locking technique.

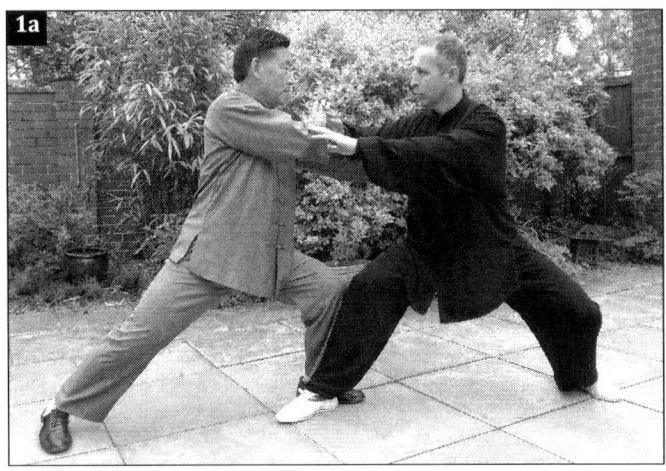

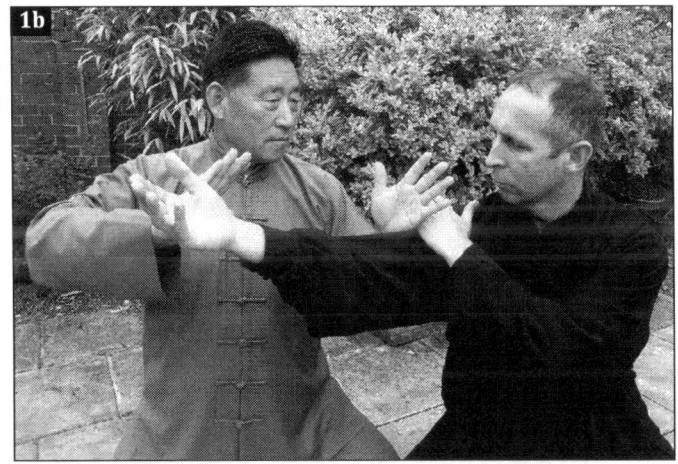

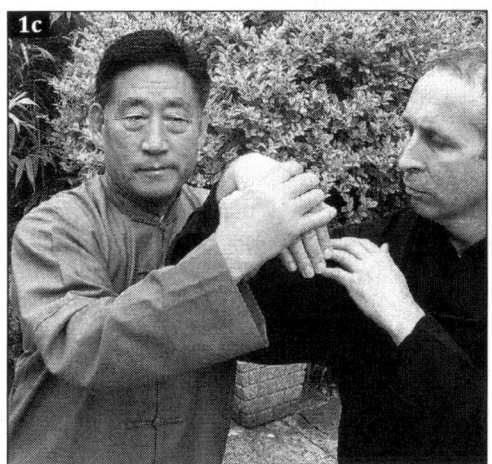
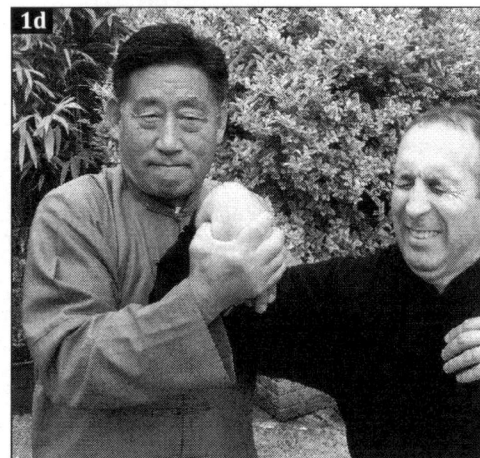

Technique 2

2a-b) Andrew Hesketh punches toward the author, who diverts the attack.

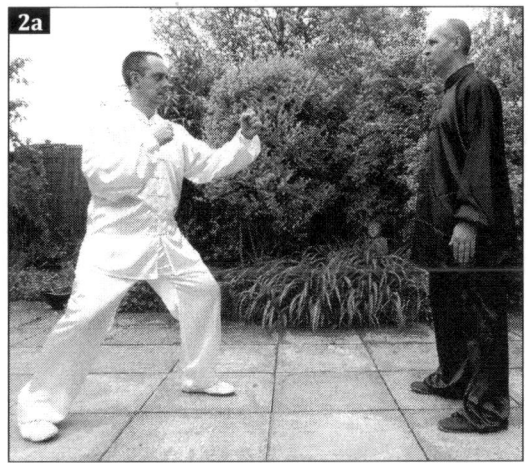
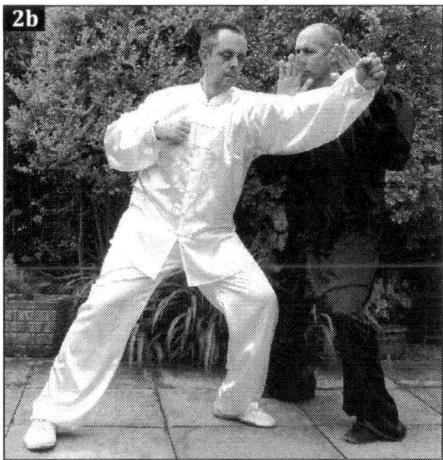

2c) Immediately after the force of Andrew's punch is spent, David attacks with an elbow, pulling Andrew's arm in the opposite direction to increase the effect of the technique.

2d-e) Without any stop, David extends his right arm while controlling Andrew's left arm. Finally David applies a tight neck lock, at the same time stepping in close to control Andrew's ability to respond.

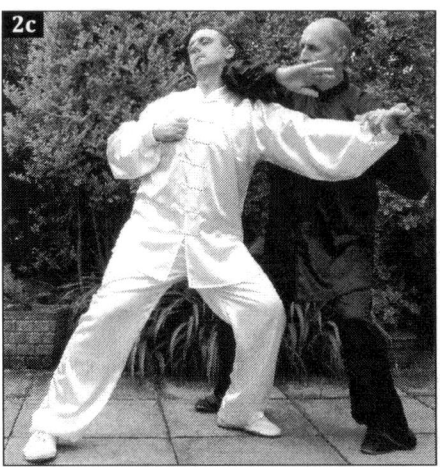

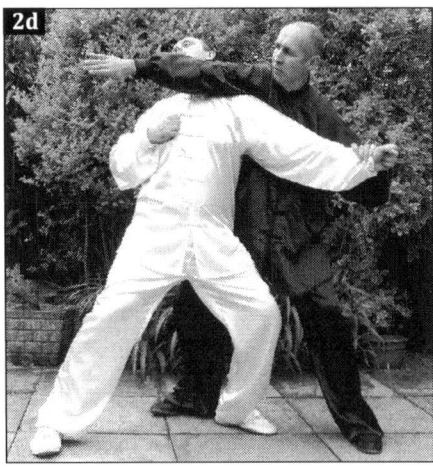   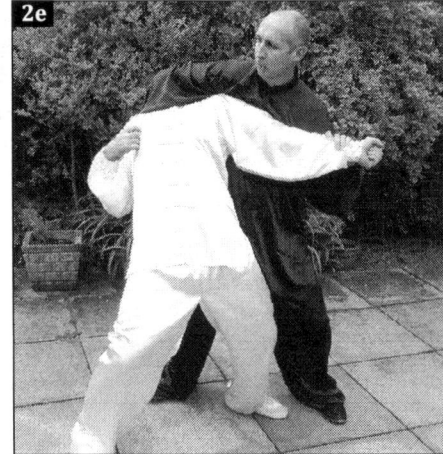

References
Chen X.W. (2008). *Chen Family Taijiquan*. Henan: People's Sports Publishing Co.
Chen X.W. (2011). *Secrets of Taiji: Taijiquan tuishou* (episode 8). Beijing: China Central Television, CTV5, Sports Channel.

• 64 •

The Yang Style Taiji Spear Lineage
Zhang Yun, M.S.

A famous Chinese martial arts classic said, "Spear is the king of all weapons." The spear was one of the most common and important weapons in ancient times. Compared with other kinds of weapons in its time, the spear was considered powerful because of its length, which made possible faster and more dynamic attacks than any other weapon. On the other hand, when considering spear-on-spear conflict, high level skills are very difficult to master. In the Ming dynasty, traditional spear skills were developed to a high level. In his book *Hands and Arms Journal*, Wu Shu (1610–1695) compared the skills from the most famous spear schools and summarized the features among traditional spear skills. Most of the principles elaborated in Wu's book are still applied in many martial arts groups today.

To learn the spear, the first order of business is to build a solid foundation. In his book, Wu Shu told a story about the importance of basic skills as follows:

> When Wu's teacher Shi Jingyan was young, he and his spear master, Shaolin monk Hongji, the best spear master in the Shaolin Temple at that time, traveled a great deal in order to challenge many masters. They were very confident in their skills and won all of their challenges until one day they met Liu Dechang in Zhending County. When Hongji and Liu fought, after only one touch of their weapons, Liu made Hongji's spear fly from his hands. The experience left Hongji and Shi shaken. The two became Liu's disciples immediately and Liu taught them a few foundation skills. Liu told them that they must practice these skills very hard and carefully for two years.
>
> Hongji and Shi practiced day by day according to Liu's instruction. After two years, they went back to meet Liu again. Liu was satisfied with their skills and said, "Good. You are done." Hongji and Shi were surprised because they supposed that Liu would teach them more application techniques. But Liu explained to them. "You have already learned many useful techniques before you met me. But your basic skills were not good enough. So this is why I easily won when we fought. Now that your foundation is improved, I do not need to teach you any further techniques; right now you can use all of the techniques which you knew before, but now at a higher level. Just as if you built a house on a poor base, the building cannot stand well in a hard storm. So I simply rebuilt the base. I do not need to add other materials on other parts of the house. The integrity of the house will now be solid."

Later, both Hongji and Shi became great spear masters. This story tells us the importance of a solid foundation in basic skills, especially for advanced study. It is said that the level you achieve depends on the quality of your foundation. What is a foundation skill? There is a classic poem in answer to this question:

> A warrior holds a golden spear,
> Only uses nine inches' length,
> Draw a circle day by day,
> He can send a good master
> to meet the king of hell.

Here two technical terms express the meaning of the basic skills of the spear. One is "Only use[s] nine inches' length," which alludes to the skill of thrusting. The other is "Draw a circle day by day," which describes classic spear circling practice. Basic thrusting skill pertains to offense, which should be fast, powerful, and accurate. Circling skill is defense. All blocking and changing techniques come from circles. It is said that even for a successful master, these foundation skills should still be practiced daily throughout life.

Taiji spear inherits all of the principles and skills of traditional spear, as well as employing taiji philosophy, principles, and skills. Taiji spear employs these principles in order to develop highly efficient abilities and to apply the basic skills of taijiquan, such as sticking, adhering, following, linking, and so on. These principles and skills make taiji spear different from other types of spear.

It is said that taiji empty-hand and spear practice were taught at the Qianzai Temple (千載寺) in the Ming dynasty. Later when Yang Luchan (1799–1872) taught taiji in Beijing, he passed his spear skills to Wu Quanyou (1834–1902). Then Quanyou taught these skills to Wang Maozhai (1862–1940). Wang also got instruction from a mysterious master Li. Wang Peisheng (1919–2004) learned taiji with Wang Maozhai from the age of thirteen. Wang Peisheng won a great reputation as a fighter, especially in spear fighting. I was lucky enough to learn taiji spear with Wang Peisheng starting in 1980.

In the following section, we introduce two techniques of taiji spear. Both are based on the foundation skill of circling. One is a variation of the foundation skills. The other is based on well-known traditional spear skills with the addition of taiji features.

TECHNIQUE 1 Golden Rooster Pecking—Circling and Pecking
If your opponent attacks you with his spear at midlevel, drop your spearhead downward slightly (1a). When the tip of his spear is close to you, turn your spear up in a circle from the right side of his spear (1b). As soon as your spear is higher than his, turn your spear down in a circle and make the tip of your spear peck his front hand. It is a hard downward strike. If it hits on his hand directly, it will hurt badly. If he dodges his hand, your spear will still hit the shaft. Both can easily knock

his spear from his front hand (1c). At this time, the only thing your opponent can do is jump backward to escape, so immediately following this strike, you should step forward to chase and thrust toward him (1d). Here the key is that your spear is controlled and moved in a circle from your waist. The spear should be moved smoothly and in a relaxed way. The circle should be as small as possible in order to make your internally trained force reach the tip of the spear.

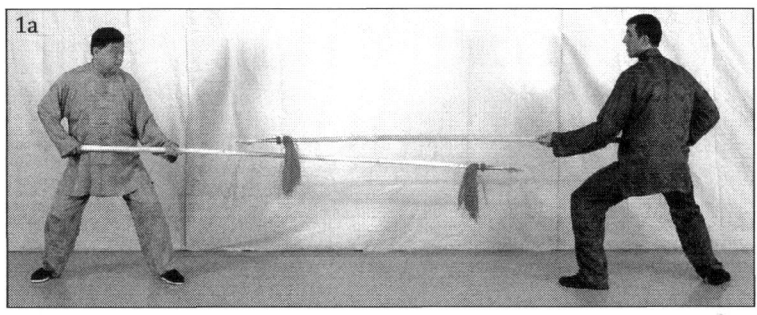

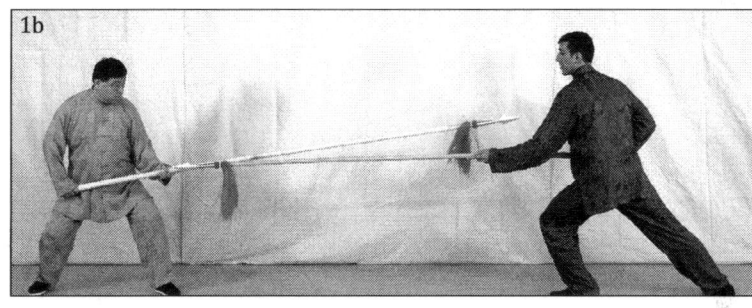

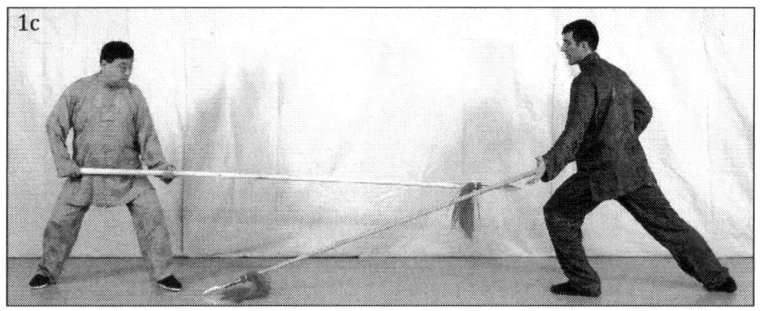

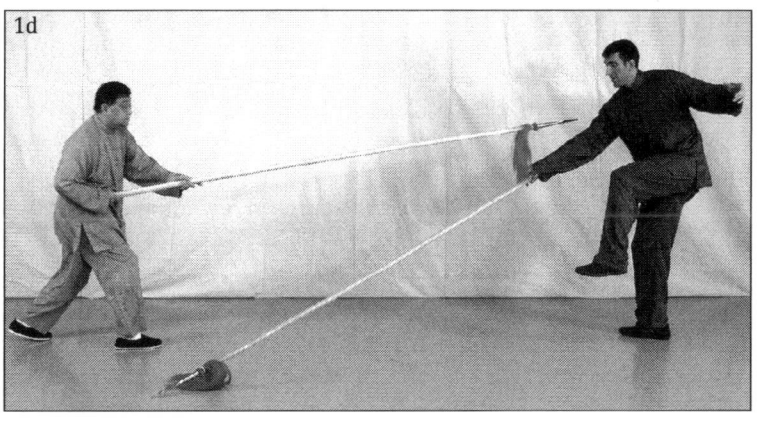

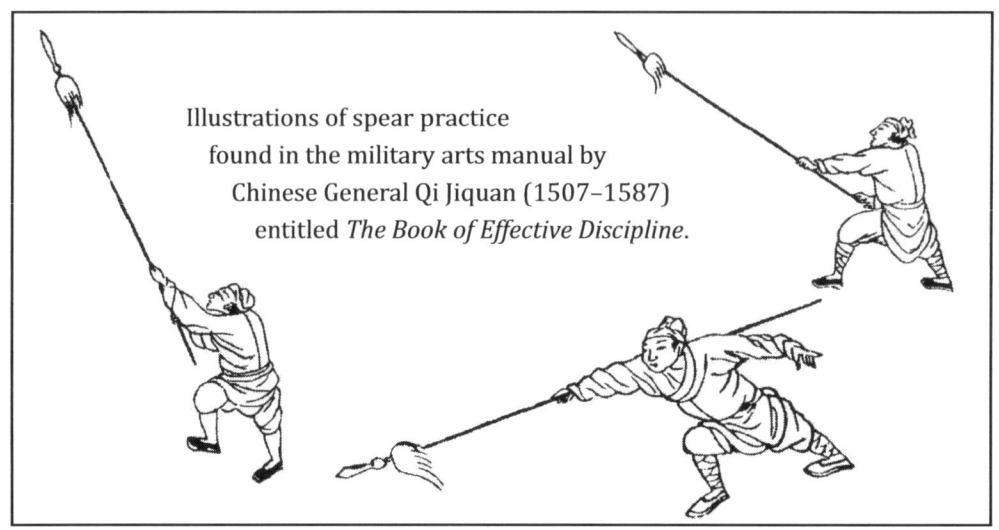

Illustrations of spear practice found in the military arts manual by Chinese General Qi Jiquan (1507–1587) entitled *The Book of Effective Discipline*.

TECHNIQUE 2 Breeze Shakes Lotus—Circling and Cutting

If your opponent attacks your head with his spear, raise your spear to cross his, and stick and follow his spear. Your body may need to move back slightly (2a). Turn your shaft outward and slightly press down, which should move your opponent's spear off the centerline. Keep sticking to your opponent's spear (2b). Keep your spear in the center and point to his head. Then step forward with your rear foot quickly in order to continue sticking and controlling his spear (2c). If you can get close to your opponent, rotate your spear, and use the tip to attack your opponent (2d). If your opponent moves back, you can step forward to chase and thrust him (2e). Here the key is to use the taijiquan skills or linking, following, and sticking to control your opponent's spear at all times.

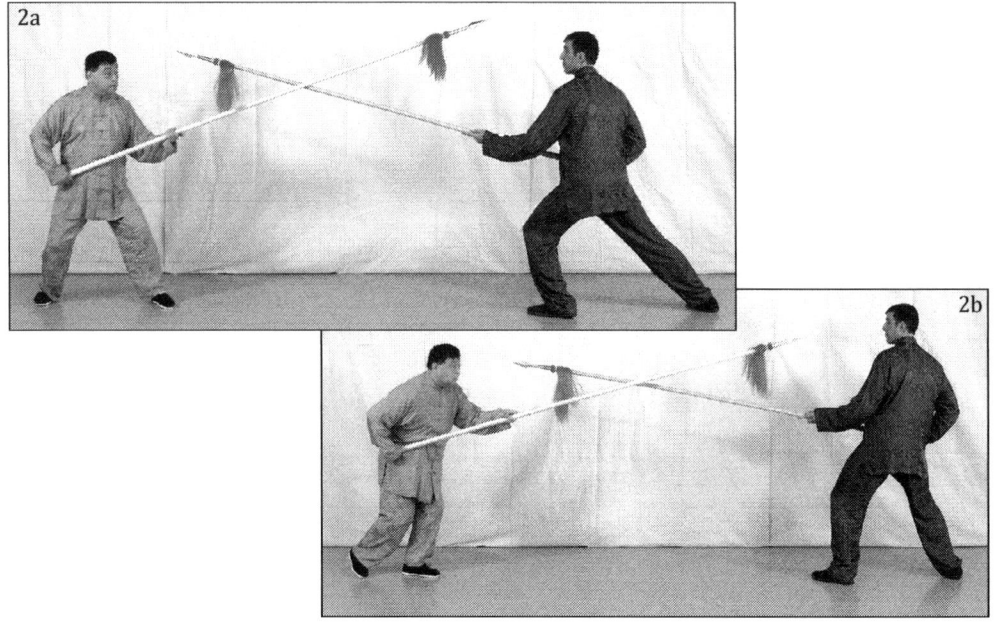

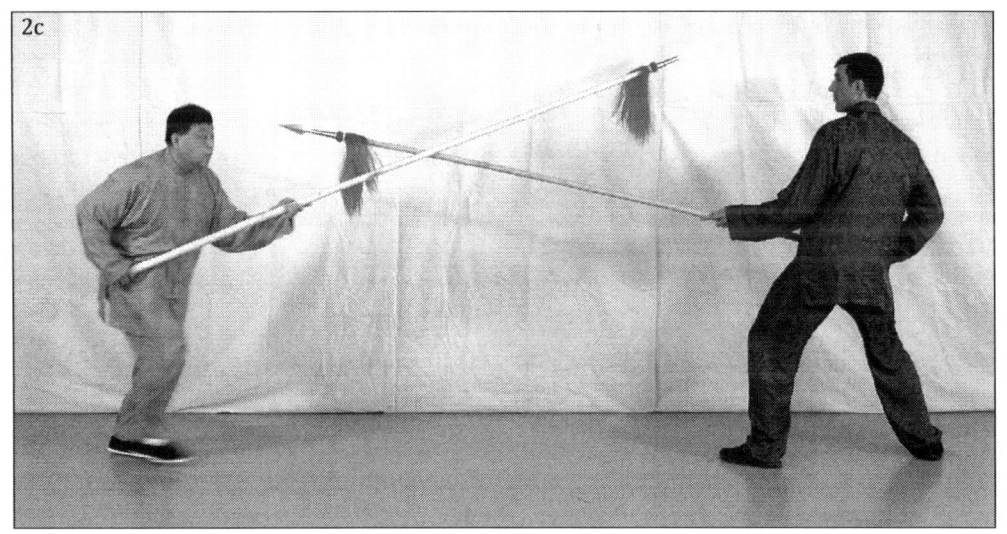

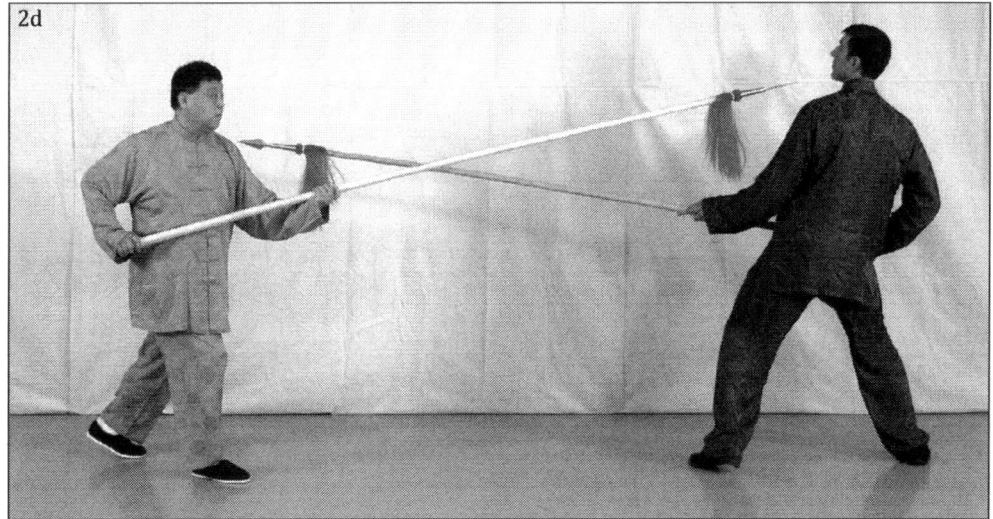

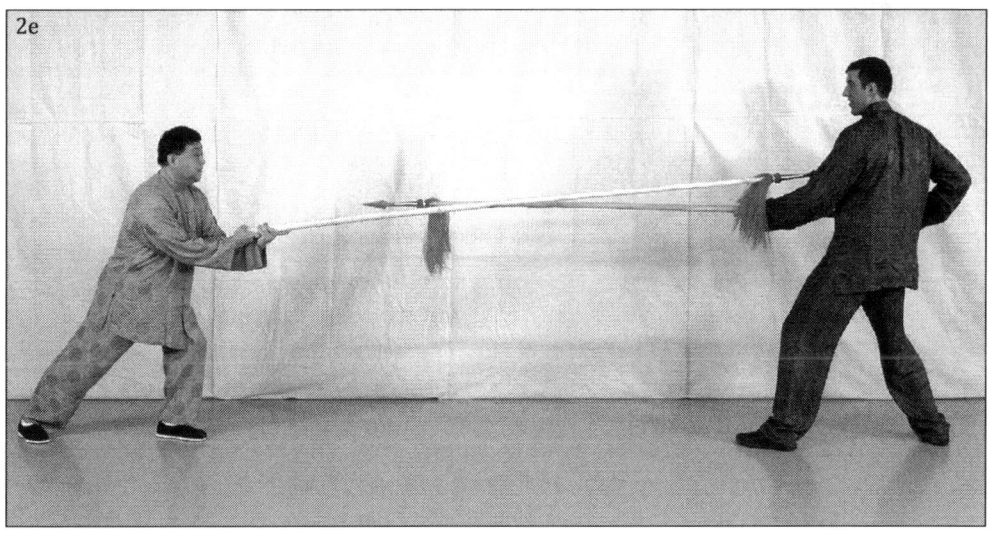

937

Sources of Original Publication

Articles in this anthology were originally published in Via Media Publishing's *Journal of Asian Martial Arts,* and from the book titled *Asian Marital Arts: Constructive Thoughts and Practical Applications.* Listed according to the table of contents for this anthology:

Author (Year)	Source
DeMarco, M. (1992)	Vol. 1 No. 1, pp. 8–25
Wong J./DeMarco, M. (1992)	Vol. 1 No. 1, pp. 26–35
Delza, S. (1992)	Vol. 1 No. 4, pp. 80–89
Holcombe, C. (1993)	Vol. 2 No. 1, pp. 10–25
Lerhaupt, L. (1993)	Vol. 2 No. 1, pp. 60–69
Derrickson, C. (1993)	Vol. 2 No. 3, pp. 64–75
Sutton, N. (1994)	Vol. 3 No. 1, pp. 56–71
Stubenbaum, D. (1994)	Vol. 3 No. 1, pp. 90–99
DeMarco, M. (1994)	Vol. 3 No. 3, pp. 92–103
Smith, R. (1995)	Vol. 4 No. 1, pp. 50–65
Lim, T.K. (1995)	Vol. 4 No. 2, pp. 64–73
Kohler, S. (1995)	Vol. 4 No. 2, pp. 74–85
Smith, R. (1995)	Vol. 4 No. 3, pp. 46–59
Davis, B. (1996)	Vol. 5 No. 2, pp. 36–59
Tyrey, B., and Brinkman, M. (1996)	Vol. 5 No. 2, pp. 74–79
Lim, T.K. (1996)	Vol. 5 No. 3, pp. 90–99
Smith, R. (1997)	Vol. 5 No. 4, pp. 20–45
Davis, D. and Mann, L. (1996)	Vol. 5 No. 4, pp. 46–67
Willmont, D. (1997)	Vol. 6 No. 1, pp. 10–29
Smith, R. (1997)	Vol. 6 No. 1, pp. 50–61
Smith, R. (1997)	Vol. 6 No. 2, pp. 56–69
DeMarco, M. (1997)	Vol. 6 No. 3, pp. 8–17
Wallace, A. (1998)	Vol. 7 No. 1, pp. 58–89
Breslow, A. (1998)	Vol. 7 No. 2, pp. 10–25
Mainfort, D. (1998)	Vol. 7 No. 3, pp. 56–71
O'Conner, M. (1998)	Vol. 7 No. 4, pp. 10–21
DeMarco, M. (1998)	Vol. 7 No. 4, pp. 22–35
Kohler, S. (1999)	Vol. 8 No. 1, pp. 91–101
Peck, A. (1999)	Vol. 8 No. 3, pp. 76–83
Hawthorne, M. (2000)	Vol. 9 No. 1, pp. 70–81
DeMarco, M. and Matthews, A. (2000)	Vol. 9 No. 2, pp. 48–79
Berwick, S. (2001)	Vol. 10 No. 2, pp. 88–97

Berwick, S. (2001)	Vol. 10 No. 2, pp. 98–101
Seidman, A. (2001)	Vol. 10 No. 3, pp. 76–83
Stein, J. (2002)	Vol. 11 No. 1, pp. 58–67
Cordes, A. (2002)	Vol. 11 No. 2, pp. 64–79
DeMarco, M. (2002)	Vol. 11 No. 4, pp. 30–53
Berwick, S. (2003)	Vol. 12 No. 4, pp. 34–47
Gaffney, D. (2004)	Vol. 13 No. 2, pp. 32–43
Loupos, J. (2004),	Vol. 13 No. 4, pp. 52–55
Wong, Y.M. (2005)	Vol. 14 No. 2, pp. 44–51
Gaffney, D. (2005)	Vol. 14 No. 4, pp. 32–47
Cai, N. (2006)	Vol. 15 No. 1, pp. 76–85
Kucher, S., et al. (2007)	Vol. 16 No. 1, pp. 36–45
Wolfson, G. (2007)	Vol. 16 No. 2, pp. 34–47
Henning, S. (2007)	Vol. 16 No. 3, pp. 22–25
Kauz, H. (2007)	Vol. 16 No. 3, pp. 60–63
Wile, D. (2007)	Vol. 16 No. 4, pp. 8–45
Cohen, R. (2001)	Vol. 17 No. 1, pp. 8–27
Gaffney, D. (2008)	Vol. 17 No. 2, pp. 56–67
Mason, R. (2008)	Vol. 17 No. 3, pp. 22–39
Burroughs, J. (2008)	Vol. 17 No. 4, pp. 42–55
DeMarco, M. (2009)	Vol. 18 No. 3, pp. 18–39
Cartmell, T. (2009)	Vol. 18 No. 4, pp. 46–63
Mason, R. et al. (2010)	Vol. 19 No. 2, pp. 72–107
Graycar, M. and Tomlinson, R. (2010)	Vol. 19 No. 3, pp. 78–95
Mosher, H. (2011)	Vol. 20 No. 1, pp. 94–109
Brown, D. (2011)	Vol. 20 No. 2, pp. 8–21
Baek, S. (2011)	Vol. 20 No. 3, pp. 62–85
Rhoads, C.J. et al, M. (2011)	Vol. 21 No. 1, pp. 8–31
Brodsky, G. (2012)	Vol. 21 No. 1, pp. 82–101
Gaffney, D. (2012)	*Asian Martial Arts*, pp. 66–69
Mason, R. (2012)	*Asian Martial Arts*, pp. 106–109
Yun Zhang (2012)	*Asian Martial Arts*, pp. 148–153

INDEX

A

acupuncture, 50, 96, 270, 315, 329, 373, 383, 588, 644, 658, 679, 683, 686, 893
adhering, 677, 934
alchemy, 225, 258, 265, 269-270, 272, 274 note 6, 350, 617, 628, 635, 642, 645, 647, 654, 657, 659, 672, 675, 873, 883-884, 907
An Exposition of the Principles of Taijiquan, 650
Analects, 1, 174, 180, 718, 808
Anglo-Chinese War, 757
anxiety, 32, 363, 597-598, 861, 901
arm movement, 9, 106-108, 110-114, 147-148
awareness, 32, 60, 96, 388, 392, 547, 557-558, 571, 575, 607, 613-614, 621-623, 644-645
Art of Taijiquan, 278-279, 283, 287 note 1, 631, 637
Art of the Internal School's Boxing Methods, 628, 634, 643, 645
Art of War (Sunzi), 180, 356 note 6, 648
Attaining Softness Taijiquan Society (*zhi rou*), 169
automatic writing, 162

B

baguachang, 51
baguazhang, 314, 562, 678
bajiquan, 733
baihui acupoint, 328, 868, 877
balance, 32-33, 104-106, 303, 319, 324-325, 327, 398, 408, 525, 571
Baopuzi, 45, 49, 265, 348, 617-618
beginning posture, 147, 302-303, 765
Beijing, 2, 10-13, 15, 20, 278, 280-281, 287 notes 1 and 2, 359-360, 407, 419, 422, 427-428, 463, 560-561, 606, 635, 648, 652, 660, 673, 703, 709, 713, 734, 754, 759, 763, 863, 934
Beijing Physical Education Research Institute, 287 note 1, 631, 755, 757
Beijing Martial Arts Research Society, 679
Beijing University, 713-714, 720
Bian, Renjie, 636
blood pressure, 218, 232 note 12, 314, 389, 407, 660, 678, 890, 892, 894, 898-899, 901-903

Bodde, Derk, 42
Bodhidharma, 3, 213, 220, 252, 254 note 8, 628, 630, 632-633, 655
Book of Changes (*Yijing, I Ching*), 69, 79, 91, 169, 174, 176, 180, 192-194, 248, 259-264, 269, 325, 374-378, 528, 627, 633, 637-638, 640-641, 659, 672, 675, 718
Book of Odes, 308
bow stance, 263, 402-404, 613
Boxer Uprising, 10, 660, 757
breathing, 318-319, 349-350, 362, 414, 416, 548, 642, 644, 682, 692 note 8, 866-867, 869, 872-873, 884, 887-888, 894, 897
breathing "pre-natal" or "reverse," 134, 210, 215, 217-218, 223, 227, 230, 231 note 10, 353, 894
broadsword (*dao*), 89, 154, 486, 579-582, 606, 618, 770
bubbling spring accupoint, 683, 397-404
Buddhism, 45-46, 52 note 24, 157, 220, 342, 350, 637, 639-640, 661, 708, 805, 807, 814-815, 816 note 15, 818-819, 899

C

Cai, Yuanpei, 168, 713
cannon fist (*paochui*), 8, 26, 98, 240, 313, 316, 318, 325, 475, 544, 573, 575, 698, 700, 856, 883
Cao, Delin, 24, 28
cardio-respiratory, 390, 599
cardiovascular system, 389, 751, 898, 901, 904
cat stance, 403
central equilibrium, 611, 736-737, 800, 814, 832, 851-852, 925
Central Military Academy (Huangpu, Whampoa), 169, 716, 806
Cernuschi Museum of Chinese Art, 127, 172, 718
Chan, Bun-Piac, 673, 691
Chan, Hak Fu, 594
Chang, Naizhou, 627, 640, 643, 645, 653
Chen, Bing, 709, 869
Chen, Bu, 634, 695-697
Chen, Changxing, 9-10, 12, 26, 193, 313, 316-317, 375, 380 note 7, 385, 454-455, 457, 537, 542, 544, 561, 572-573, 576, 583, 630-632, 635-636, 660, 691 note 3, 700-701, 706, 754-755, 759
Chen, Chunyuan, 11
Chen, Fadou, 703

940

Chen, Fake, 10–11, 24, 97–99, 315, 407, 427, 454, 457, 463, 483, 542–543, 569, 573, 583, 633, 673–674, 679, 703, 708
Chen family biographies, 312, 648, 656
Chen, Gene, 11
Chen, Gengyun, 10, 759
Chen, "Tacky" Hanqiang, 153–154
Chen, Kesen, 704, 707
Chen, Liqing, 360, 703
Chen, Panling, 216–217, 717
Chen, Pengfei, 456
Chen, Qingping, 11–12, 122, 314, 630, 653–654
Chen Village (Chenjiagou), 5–7, 10, 23–27, 98, 122, 312, 315, 328, 423, 427, 453, 455, 457–460, 481, 527, 560, 566, 569–573, 577, 579, 581, 583, 633–636, 643, 647–648, 650, 660, 695–709, 754, 756, 759
Chen, Wangting, 7–9, 11, 253 note 2, 312–313, 316, 318–321, 325–326, 384, 456, 539, 542, 544, 751, 573, 575, 579, 581–583, 634, 648, 659–660, 691 note 3, 697–700, 705–706, 865–866, 929
Chen, Weiming, 118, 120, 123–125, 160, 169–170, 177, 179, 183 notes 17 and 20, 193–194, 214–215, 239, 242, 252 note 2, 253 note 5, 277–279, 287 note 5, 281–286, 287 note 1, 288 note 11, 631, 637, 659, 715, 722, 729 note 9, 730 note 11, 761
Chen, Xiaowang, 11, 93–102, 313–318, 322, 324, 337, 427, 433, 452, 454, 456–457, 462–465, 481, 507, 524
Chen, Xiaoxing, 452–460, 574, 576, 696, 704–705, 828, 836, 869, 929–931
Chen, Xin, 372–380, 397, 464, 508, 527–540, 569–570, 633–634, 636–637, 643, 646, 648, 650, 703, 923
Chen, Xiufeng, 13–14, 281
Chen, Xiyi, 640, 660, 672, 675–676, 680–681, 692 note 5
Chen, Yanxi, 10, 24, 26, 94, 703
Chen, Yu, 869
Chen, Yuben, 11–12
Chen, Yuheng, 11
Chen, Zhangxing, 192, 238, 241, 280
Chen, Zhaokui, 99, 426–427, 433, 454, 457, 463, 481, 483, 547, 551, 553, 578, 708
Chen, Zhaopei, 453–454, 456–457, 463, 481–483, 488, 703–705, 707
Chen, Zhaoquai, 11

Chen, Zhaoxu, 99, 462
Chen, Zhenglei, 452, 481, 545–456, 550, 579–580
Chen, Zhongshen, 374, 539, 702
Chen, Zichen (William C.C. Chen), 20, 80, 119, 214–116, 221, 229 note 3, 232 note 10, 719–720, 915, 918
Chen, Ziming, 11
Cheng, Jincai, 482, 484
Cheng, Man-ch'ing (see Zheng, Manjing)
Cheng, Tinghua, 733–734, 739
Chenjiagou (see Chen Village)
Chenjiagou Taijiquan School, 573, 706–707
Chiang, Kai-shek, 714, 716, 718, 758, 763–764
Chiang, Kai-shek, Madam, 80, 731 note 17
Chongqing, 151, 153, 155, 159, 163 note 3, 169, 285, 632
Choi, Wai Lun, 416–417
Choy, Hokpeng, 15
Choy, Kamman, 15
Chu, Gin Soon, 476
Chu, Vincent, 475
cinnabar, 47–48, 185 note 39, 348, 831
Classic of Taijiquan, 65–66
coiling energy, 143, 326, 338, 544, 674, 868
cold energy, 203, 435
College of Chinese Culture, 171, 255 note 12
Commentaries on Taijiquan, 633, 640
Complete Form and Practice of Taijiquan, 606
Complete Principles and Practices of Taijiquan, 631
Communist Party, 169–170, 413, 418, 758
Confucianism, 166, 184 note 28, 242, 258, 261–262, 270, 342, 348, 350, 617, 626, 639–640
Confucius, 122, 128, 162, 164 note 6, 166, 173–174, 176, 180, 185 note 42, 260, 262, 271, 296, 347–349, 376, 378, 640, 654, 711, 808, 814
contact, 42, 63, 133–134, 137, 204–205, 247, 319, 321, 326, 554, 605, 608, 613–614, 700, 771, 777–796, 925
Cultural Revolution, 173–174, 482–484

D

Dai, Peisu, 358–360, 363
dalü (see large rollback)
damai meridian, 873–874, 884
Danjiangkou Wudang Martial Arts Research Association, 652–653

dantian, 95–96, 133–134, 175, 185 note 39, 211–213, 216, 219, 223, 229 note 2, 232 note 10, 249, 255 note 21, 274 note 4, 318, 324, 326–334, 336, 353, 404, 435, 464, 467, 531, 548–550, 553, 572, 583, 611
dantian rotation, 553, 686, 865–884
Daoism, 2–3, 6–8, 29, 41–56, 67, 74, 98, 103, 116, 119–120, 125, 155, 166, 173, 176, 180, 185 note 43, 192, 218–220, 224–225, 232 note 14, 233 note 17, 234 notes 21 and 23, 238, 248, 252, 254 note 8, 355, 361, 363, 378, 380 note 12, 412, 418, 625–662, 672–673, 691 note 2, 708
Daodejing, 79, 169, 173, 180, 219, 248, 415, 688, 718, 892
daoyin, 44–45, 47, 50, 116, 219, 318, 414, 642, 672
"dead spot", 143, 146
Delza, Sophia, 14, 66
Deng, Huijian, 590
Despeux, Catherine, 373, 376
diabetes, 315, 389, 893, 897, 900
diagonal flying, 123, 284, 364, 925–926, 928
Ding, Yidu, 169, 714
dianxue (see vital points)
A Discussion of Taijiquan, 66
dispersing hands (see *sanshou*)
Dong, Haichuan, 248, 562, 658
Dong, Huling, 15
Dong, Yingjie, 15, 119, 121, 157, 163 note 4, 177, 286–287, 288 note 10, 299, 631–632, 637, 762
Dongtuhe Village, 696
Du, Yuanhua, 644, 653
Du, Yuze, 10, 23–31, 94
dumai meridian, 884
Dun Prince Palace, 561–562

E
educational institutes, 546
effort, 59, 63, 70, 137, 569, 739, 779–780, 798, 844, 847, 872, 915–916
eight gates, 565
Eight Harmonies Boxing, 761
Eight Immortals, 351, 353
eight methods/energies (*bafa*), 316, 328, 417, 490, 554, 576, 681, 736
eight techniques, 563–564, 605
eight trigrams (*bagua*), 51, 261, 325, 380 note 12, 638
elixir field (see *dantian*)

elixir of immortality, 265, 344, 349–350, 355
Emerick, Danny, 151, 721, 727
emitting energy (*fajing*), 209, 316-317, 321, 323, 325, 328, 360–362, 400, 464–465, 475, 485, 535, 544, 547, 575–576, 578, 583, 703, 830, 837–838, 865, 883
energy cultivation (see *qigong*)
energy flow, 142, 145, 148, 200, 208, 866, 872, 877, 879–880, 884, 923
Epitath for Wang Zhengnan, 628, 630, 633
essence (*jing*), 74, 193, 213, 265, 267–273, 350–351, 574, 646, 684, 687
Essence and Applications of Taijiquan, 714–715, 729 note 6, 797
The Essential Principles and Practice of Taijiquan, 632
Evidence-Based Taijiquan (EBT), 893
Explanation of the Taiji Diagram, 660
external school (*weijia*), 280, 416, 418, 485
extraordinary meridians, 866–871
eye function, 32–40, 267, 305, 575

F
falling split, 537–539
falls, 595–603, 901
Falun Gong, 661
famine, 586, 618, 696, 702, 756
fangshi (magicians), 46–49, 53 note 26, 261, 344
fangsong, 609–610, 614, 837–838, 874, 883
Farber, Dan, 673
fascia attacking, 207–208, 255 note 17
fast-twitch muscle, 895–898, 902, 902 notes 7 and 8
FAR Gallery, 127, 718
feet, 109, 132–133, 147–148, 263, 398–401, 506, 621, 683
Feng, Yuxiang (General), 154, 758
Feng, Zhiqiang, 422, 427, 481, 646, 671, 673–674, 679–680, 685–688, 692 note 5
first routine (*yilu*), 8, 30, 98, 314, 316–317, 322, 325, 374, 424–425, 437–439, 441, 484, 489, 543–544, 551, 572–575, 578, 700, 703, 833, 865–866, 883
five animal frolics, 414, 673, 678, 764, 768
five phases/elements (*wuxing*), 42, 68, 265–266, 271, 304–306, 308–309, 374, 380 note 12, 863
five steps (*wubu*), 563–565, 647
Fong Ha, 40, 673
force (*li*), 73–74, 120, 124–125, 136, 138,

151, 248, 283, 383, 914
four corners, 290, 296, 302, 736, 849
four directions, 306, 387–388, 513, 736, 846
four frames, 135
Four Important Points of Solo Practice, 564
Fu, Zhongwen, 215, 287, 299, 427, 716
Fu, Zhongquan, 561, 568 note 5
Fundamentals of Tai Chi Chuan, 650

G

gait, 337, 400, 596, 598
Gan, Fengchi, 630, 633, 761
Gao, Fu, 671, 674
Ge Hong, 46, 265, 341, 348–349, 353, 617–619, 642
Gibbs, Tam, 91 note 1, 124–125, 130 note 7, 150, 161, 162 note 1, 176, 185 note 41, 254 note 8, 255 note 11, 297–298, 355 note 3, 725
glucose, 896–897
God of War (see also Guan Gong, Xuanwu), 3
great rollback (see large rollback),
group practice, 386, 393, 556–559, 768–769
Gu, Liuxin, 407, 427, 433, 581, 634, 648–649, 629 note 7
Gu, Luxin, 372
Guan Gong, 655
Guangzhou city, 15, 287 note 3, 585–586, 619
Guo, Lianying, 763
Guo, Qinfang, 151–152, 154, 156–157, 162–163
Guo, Shaojiong, 587
Guo, Tiefeng, 644
Guo, Tingxian, 764, 768
Guo, Yunshen, 216, 733

H

halberd (*guandao*), 97, 579, 581–582, 618, 619 note 2
Hall of Happiness, 724–725
Han, Qingtang, 717
Hangzhou, 46, 65, 71, 132, 138, 167, 198, 207, 272, 287 note 3, 349, 352, 354, 358–360, 362, 388, 625, 713
Hangzhou Wushan Taijiquan Society, 358, 362
Hao, Weizhen, 11–12, 122, 630, 734, 736
Hao, Weizheng, 11–12
Hao, Yuehju, 12
hatha yoga, 218, 909
He, Hongming, 635

health, 314–315, 318, 320, 327, 351, 363, 383–386, 389–394, 886–903
Hebei Province, 2, 12, 15, 116, 278–279, 281, 560, 651, 733, 754
Henan Form, 563
Henan Province, 3–7, 10, 12, 14, 26–27, 80, 102, 122, 220, 238, 278, 280, 312, 379 note 3, 384, 453, 463, 483, 488, 691 note 4, 562, 631, 634, 659, 695–697, 702, 754, 759, 762, 764
herbology, 206, 268, 270, 355, 642, 643, 712, 714, 716–717, 734, 802
Hong, Junshen, 360
Hong Kong, 14–15, 123, 128 note 2, 158, 247, 585–586, 588, 590, 594 note 1, 650, 673, 802
Hong Kong Jin Wu Sports Association, 586
Hong Kong Taiji Main Association, 594 note 1
Hong Kong YMCA, 586
Hong, Shihao, 158
horizontal dantian rotation, 874–876
horse stance, 263, 402, 404
Hu, Puan, 636, 761–762, 771
Hu, Yaozhen, 231 note 7, 673–674, 678–679
Hua Tuo, 414, 630, 678, 764
Huainanzi, 260, 266–267, 377
Huaiqing Prefecture, 26, 649, 696–698, 701–702
Huang, Baijia, 628, 631, 634, 640–641, 645
Huang, Feihong, 82, 586
Huang-Lao, 46, 345
Huang, Wenshan, 650
Huang, Xingxian, 83–85, 91, 118–119, 124
Huang, Zhaohan, 655
Huang, Zongxi, 625, 628, 634, 640, 651, 654
Hudson River Museum, 127, 718
huiyin acupoint, 328, 867–868, 871, 877, 879, 884
Hunan Martial Arts Academy, 716, 806
Hundun myth, 260, 263
Hunyuan Gong, 438
Hunyuan Taiji, 674
Huo, Chengguang, 673

I

Illustrated Explanation of Chen Taijiquan, 569, 703
Illustration of Taijiquan, 397
immortal (*xian*), 3, 218, 341, 343–344, 348–349, 351, 353–355, 356 notes 10 and 11

943

immortal pounds mortar, 318
immortality, 46–50, 53 note 38, note 54 note 45, 225, 232 note 14, 261, 265, 270, 341–357, 378, 617, 619, 627–628, 630, 637, 642–644, 647, 649, 651, 654–655
in vivo exposure therapy, 595, 598–599, 602
incense, 47
inner circle training, 144, 146–147, 149
inner elixir (*neidan*), 48–49, 54 note 43, 265, 348, 350–352, 638, 643, 656
intention, 67–68, 72, 75, 374, 388, 400, 472, 530, 548, 554, 575, 579, 610, 613, 645, 887, 894, 900, 903 note 2, 904 note 11, 910, 925
internal school (*neijia*), 249, 252, 279, 387, 412, 415–420, 627–629, 631–632, 642, 645, 648, 652, 655
Internal School's Boxing Methods, 628, 634, 643, 645
internal strength (*jin, neigong*), 78–79, 248–249, 255 note 20, 286, 322, 338, 546
International Taijiquan Forum, 886
Introduction to Chen Family Taijiquan, 634, 636, 646
Brief Introduction to Chinese Martial Arts, 633
Introduction to Original Taijiquan, 653
Isle of Immortals, 344
issuing energy (*fajing*), 202, 316, 321, 323, 325, 328, 360–362, 400, 464–465, 475, 485, 535, 544, 575–576, 578, 583, 703, 830, 837–838, 865, 883

J
jade, 43–44, 219
jade lady at shuttles, 78, 80, 126
Japan, 14, 26, 52 note 24, 124, 151, 168–169, 177–178, 210, 221–123, 232 note 10, 234 note 22, 242, 285, 344, 463, 483, 488, 577, 585–586, 634, 637, 639, 641, 646, 698, 713, 716, 734, 756, 758, 810, 817, 822
Jiang Fa, 630, 632–633, 654, 660, 702
Jiangsu Province, 2, 12, 169, 183 note 19, 239, 760–761, 763
Jianquan Taiji Association, 586, 588
Jin Yong, 640
Jiu Hao, 193, 197
Jou, Tsung Hwa, 66
Ju, Hongbin, 720, 730 note 16, 806, 818
judo, 222, 225–226, 503–504, 636, 639, 734, 897
Jung, Carl, 308

K
KaiMai acupuncture style, 893
Kan, Guixiang, 11
Ke, Qihua, 720, 806, 813
kinship, 629, 695–696
knight-errant (*xia*), 628, 630, 641, 657
Koh, Ahtee, 87, 91 notes 6 and 9

L
lactate, 896
Lai, Zhide, 376, 378
lance, 193–196,
laogong accupoint, 679, 870–871, 880
Laozi, 46, 164, 173, 213, 219, 240, 273, 301, 377, 393, 415, 627, 631–632, 637–640, 644, 653–654, 656, 661–662, 672, 684, 688, 728 note 2, 729 note 9, 910
large frame (*dajia*), 314, 360, 473–480, 482, 834
large rollback (*dalü*), 137, 283, 290–296, 388, 395
Le, Huanzhi, 761–762
Leaning on a Board (*kao ban*), 681
li (see force)
Li, Houcheng, 24, 28
Li, Jiying, 562
Li, Kuiyuan, 733
Li, Pinfu, 14
Li, Ruidong, 561–565
Li, Shirong, 636, 659–660
Li, Shoujian, 291, 298, 300
Li, Shudong, 482, 487
Li, Xiheng, 117–118, 128 note 2, 151, 717–718, 721, 727, 797–825, 925
Li, Xiyue, 642, 655
Li, Yaxuan, 288 note 11, 635, 714–715, 730 note 10
Li, Yiyu, 299 note 1, 630, 645, 653–654, 659
Li, Zhaosheng, 649, 656–658
Liang (T.T.) Dongcai, (Liang, Tongcai), 20, 66, 74, 78, 291–292, 297, 763
Ling Shan, 561
listening energy (*ting jin*), 127, 134, 137, 200, 204, 319, 553, 605, 613, 813
Liu He, 761
liuhebafa, 416–417, 672
"Lively Pace" Style, 12, 299
Lo, Benjamin Pangjeng, 238–257, 284, 291, 300 note 4, 716–717, 720, 727, 729 notes 3 and 8, 730 note 12, 800, 802–803, 813, 821

local defense, 756
locking techniques (*qinna*), 9, 97, 207, 246, 312, 316–317, 319, 321, 338, 361, 417, 422–423, 445–446, 451, 461, 467, 469, 471, 484, 487, 490–495, 544, 573, 578, 583, 781
long energy, 202
Long Fist (Changquan), 7, 316
longevity, 21, 47, 219, 248, 255 note 19, 261, 270, 273, 314, 320, 345, 383, 475, 644, 646, 654, 676, 678, 684, 773, 862
Lowenthal, Wolfe, 63–64, 124, 184 note 26, 247, 509, 813
Lu, Botang, 588, 591
Lu, Dimin, 635, 659
Lu, Dongpin, 672
Lu, Tongbao, 83–84, 86–87, 89, 91, 120, 124
Luo, Banzhen (see Lo, Benjamin)
Luoyang city, 5–6

M
Ma, Hong, 553
Ma, Jiangxiong, 589
Ma, Yuehliang, 14
Ma, Yueliang, 427, 589, 633, 637
magic, 2, 42, 50, 86, 193, 195, 349, 354
magical practitioners (*fangshi*), 46–49, 53 note 26, 261, 344
Malaysia, 77–92, 115, 118, 124
Manran San Lun, 77, 167, 174, 184 note 23, 286
Mao, Zedong, 173–174, 413, 705, 758
Master Zheng Taijiquan Study Association, 719, 728, 800, 806
Master of Five Excellences, 166, 242, 711–712, 719
Mayer, Michael, 673
Medium Frame, 473–480
Mencius, 42, 166, 180, 637
mental focus, 139
meridians, 96, 139, 186 note 56, 208, 255 note 15, 373–374, 437, 548, 671, 682, 686–687, 865–884
Ming Dynasty, 3, 6, 66, 177, 312, 376–377
mingmen acupoint, 327, 867–869, 871, 873
Mongkok School, 591, 594 notes 1 and 2
monkey/repulse-retreats, 114, 298, 510, 736, 738

N
Nanjing, 2, 15, 43, 116, 162, 170, 287 note 3

National Association for Practitioners of Traditional Chinese Medicine, 243
National Chinese Medical Association, 169, 714, 802
National Martial Arts Exhibition, 652
National Palace Museum, 176, 185 note 36, 720, 731 note 17
National Physical Education Committee, 652
National Zhinan University, 168
Nationalist Party, 14, 169–171, 174, 176, 763
Needham, Joseph, 41, 219–220, 225, 232 note 14
neigong (internal work), 79, 84, 116–117, 119–120, 124, 546, 673
Ng, Kionghing, 82
Neo-Confucianism, 50, 640
neurotransmitters, 898–899, 902
new frame (*xinjia*), 11–12, 24, 26, 97–98, 314, 317, 374, 457, 459–460, 463–464, 483, 543 573, 708, 573, 833
New Method of Self-Study in Taijiquan, 213, 699
New York, 14–15, 20, 123–127, 150, 161, 162 note 1, 163 note 5, 165, 172–174, 176, 184 note 26, 214–215, 243, 322, 465, 691 note 2, 718–719, 730 note 13, 797, 804, 812
no tension (*song*), 78–79, 397, 401, 474, 478

O
old frame (*laojia*), 24, 26, 93, 95–98, 314, 317, 454, 457, 459–460, 462–464, 473–474, 542–543, 551, 573, 700, 703, 865–866, 880
Opium War, 756–757
outer elixir school (*waidan*), 48, 265, 348–351, 643

P
Paris, 127, 172–173, 373, 718
patience, 61, 78, 89, 118, 153, 242, 322, 347, 386, 393, 432, 543, 548, 916
Peng, Tingjun, 673–674
pill of immortality, 341, 348–349
Po, Bingru, 407
posture, 9, 63, 79, 95, 119–121, 269, 284–285, 324–325, 329, 351, 363, 386, 389, 392, 574, 576–579, 599–603, 609, 717, 833–834, 843, 846
prenatal qi, 671, 677, 682, 684–685
press (*ji*), 144–145, 247, 292, 476–477, 509, 736

945

primordial taijiquan (*xiantian taijiquan*), 656
push (*an*), 135, 145, 247, 433
push-hands (*tuishou*), 7, 62–64, 79, 85, 89–90, 97, 99, 117–119, 122, 125–127, 132, 137–138, 156–158, 160, 199, 201–203, 208, 246–249, 255 note 16, 277, 280, 283, 290–291, 309, 316, 320, 326, 337–338, 362–363, 387, 408, 417, 422–426, 431, 433–436, 438, 440–442, 457, 459–460, 464, 489, 507, 509, 526, 547, 551

Q

qi, 41–45, 47, 49, 53 note 38, 63, 67, 73–74, 95–96, 98–99, 139, 153, 159, 175, 183 note 15, 186 note 56, 193–194, 206, 208, 211–213, 215–216, 219–221, 227, 233 note 17, 248–249, 255 note 15, 262, 265–270, 272–273, 279, 307, 318, 320, 322, 324–325, 327–331, 333, 335–337, 348, 350–354, 356 note 8, 373, 422, 548–549, 557, 571–574, 607–608, 610–611, 638, 643–646, 658, 671, 679–680, 686–688, 692 note 6, 836–837, 866, 922–923
Qi, Jiguang, 8, 313, 508, 581, 645, 648–649, 654, 698–699, 866
Qian, Mingshan, 169, 183 note 19
qigong, 41–42, 45, 47–51, 52 note 13, 54 note 43, 90, 96, 98, 134, 220, 255 note 20, 231 note 7, 249, 265, 283, 315, 318, 320, 322, 341, 348–349, 351–352, 373, 383, 423, 428, 430, 434–438, 440–441, 451, 459, 627, 637, 643, 646, 651, 671–688, 865–884, 886–903
Qin Shi Huangdi, 344
Qin Xu, 673
Qing Dynasty, 6, 10, 13, 23, 26–27, 167, 177, 253 note 2, 278, 312, 376, 412, 418–419, 560, 582, 585, 606, 625, 630–631, 640–641, 649, 655, 702, 711, 756–757, 760, 772
qinna (see locking techniques)
Questions and Answers on Taiji Boxing, 120, 215, 239, 279, 285

R

receiving energy (*jiejing*), 204, 281
relaxation (*song*), 89, 96, 120, 132, 215, 227, 320, 323, 328, 338, 397, 401, 474, 478, 716, 814
relaxation exercise, 89, 107, 110, 220
Ren, Changchun, 653
Ren, Guangyi, 312, 314–315, 318–319, 323, 326, 337–338, 832–833, 837–838
renmai meridian, 884
Republic of China Cultural Renaissance, 174, 718
ROC Chinese Boxing Association, 717
rollback, 68, 70, 135, 137, 144, 148, 246–247, 291, 294–295, 477, 491, 614, 736, 740–741, 848, 852–853
rooster stands on one leg, 9, 212, 277, 303, 313, 572, 767
root, 117, 133, 319, 337, 361, 397–404, 469–471, 515, 556, 571, 582, 621, 719, 799, 843

S

San Francisco, 11, 15, 23, 239, 673, 800, 804
sanshou (see dispersing hands), 83, 89–90, 137, 199, 290–291, 388, 605–615, 763, 771, 773
scholar tree, 696–697
Scripture of the Yellow Court, 634
sealing accupoints, 206
second routine (*erlu, paochui*), 8, 93, 97–98, 313, 316–318, 325, 424–425, 438–439, 484–485, 489, 544, 573, 698, 700, 770, 865, 883
Secret Transmissions on Taiji Elixir Cultivation, 628, 653, 659
Secrets of Shaolin Boxing, 639
self-cultivation, 3, 42, 49, 177, 198, 363, 507, 638, 642–644, 647, 685, 812
Self-defense Applications of Taijiquan, 631
sensitivity (*tingjing*), 79, 133, 137, 200, 202, 207–208, 319, 321–322, 325–328, 347, 388, 441, 486, 489–491, 557–558, 575, 577, 607, 622–623, 648, 680–681, 700, 735, 843, 846, 848–854, 858
sexual cultivation, 47, 213, 234 note 22
Shaanxi Province, 2, 6, 463, 630, 702
Shandong Province, 10, 15, 151, 154, 157, 168–169, 312–313, 459–460, 582, 700, 702
Shanghai city, 14, 117, 182 note 10, 183 note 16, 194, 277–279, 285, 287 notes 1 and 2, 359, 406, 424, 426–428, 433, 439, 475, 585–586, 588–589, 713–714, 729 note 7, 755, 761
Shanghai School of Fine Arts, 255 note 11, 713
Shanxi Province, 6, 116–117, 119, 122, 124, 169, 481, 634, 648, 654, 660, 673, 678, 696–697, 702

Shaolin boxing, 52 note 24, 78, 83, 183 note 15, 220–221, 226, 232 note 10, 253 note 2, 313, 361, 363, 505, 626, 628, 630, 639, 642, 651, 691 note 2, 733, 754, 757, 760–761, 763, 933
Shaolin Temple, 3, 6, 98, 220, 417, 423, 463, 695, 698, 709, 933
Shen, Xianglin, 587
Shi, Diaomei, 763
Shi, Shufang, 153, 221, 232 note 10
Shizhong (Shr Jung, Shih Chung), 165, 171–173, 176, 184 note 22, 717–720, 724, 727, 730 notes 13 and 16, 797, 800, 804, 806, 809, 812, 817–819
short energy, 122, 487,
Short Introduction to Taijiquan, 630
shoulder stroke (*kao*), 70, 246, 317, 364, 719, 734
Sichuan Province, 2, 20, 46, 124, 169, 285, 359, 642, 655, 672, 716
silk reeling (*changsijing, chansigong*), 315–316, 319–320, 322–323, 325–328, 331–338, 360–361, 422–423, 434–438, 440–442, 444, 451, 456, 458, 464, 527, 529, 532–534, 544, 553, 831, 835–836, 866–876, 882–883
Singapore, 14, 83–84, 87–88, 119, 176, 588, 719
single whip, 38–39, 284, 286, 318, 323, 460, 478, 529, 532–533, 549, 552, 574, 649, 715, 720
Sino-French War, 757
Sino-Japanese War, 714–716, 757, 817
six seal, four close, 368, 551, 840
slow-twitch muscle, 895–898, 902, 904 notes 7 and 8
small frame (*xiaojia*), 8, 299 note 1, 314, 360, 474, 482, 564, 566, 703
Smith, Robert W., 81, 156–157, 171, 244, 292–296, 356 note 5, 717, 721, 729 note 4, 729 notes 8 and 10, 730 note 14, 813, 823, 925–926
solo practice, 556–558
Song, Jianzhi, 638
Song, Shuming, 287 note 1, 630, 632–633, 637, 650
Song, You'an, 168, 714
Song, Zhijian, 633
Song, Zijian, 79–80, 84
South China Sports Association, 586
spear (*qiang*), 26, 93, 97, 313, 456, 501, 506, 576, 579, 581
spirit (*shen*), 74, 213, 265–268, 27–273, 350–352, 548, 638, 646, 684
splitting energy, 70, 576
stability, 104, 134, 404, 438, 531, 574
standard meridians, 867, 869–871
standing post (*zhanzhuang*), 315, 319, 322, 329–331, 397, 399, 458, 570, 678, 831, 841, 867–868, 872–874
Steel, Kelvin, 590
sticking energy (*nianjing, zhan*), 73, 199–200, 282, 576, 613–615, 631, 639, 736, 777–796, 814, 848, 851, 925–926, 934, 936
stimulated energy (*jing*), 73, 197, 267–270, 272–273, 350–351, 374, 574, 576, 646, 684, 687
straight sword (*jian*), 79, 90, 244, 279, 313, 385–388, 390, 496, 576, 579–580, 590, 606, 651, 655–656, 661, 690 note 1, 722, 797, 812, 855
Studies on Wudang Boxing, 652–653
Study of Taijiquan, 630, 633, 643, 734
Su, Jianyun, 427, 644, 733–734, 738
Summary of Zhang Sanfeng's Inner Elixir Theory, 656
Sun, Lutang, 11–12, 122, 193, 195, 278–279, 299, 314, 630, 637, 642–644, 691 note 3, 733–734, 736, 738–739, 751, 762
Sutton, Nigel, 115–116, 120–121, 123–127, 130 notes 12 and 13

T

Tai Chi and Mind-Body Research Program/Harvard Medical School, 901
Taiji: A Scientific Approach, 817
Taiji as philosophic term, 66–67, 248, 261–263, 306, 324–325
Taiji Classics, 65, 110, 140, 238–240, 245, 253 notes 5 and 6, 262–264, 268–269, 272– 273, 291, 351–352, 355, 467, 507, 549, 554
Taijiquan Academic Research Committee, 717
T'ai Chi Ch'uan for Health and Self-Defense, 66
Taijiquan for Health and Self-Defense, 171
Taijiquan Practical Methods, 606
Taijiquan Sticky Thirteen Spear, 631
Taiping Jing, 43, 46, 49
Taiping Rebellion, 539, 606, 701, 756

Tan, Chingngee, 87
Tan, Desmond, 199
Tang, Dianqing, 761
Tang Hao, 66, 312, 372, 581, 625, 634–636, 639, 648–649, 652, 660
Taoist Restoration Society, 412, 635
Tay, Guanleong, 90
teacher-student relationship, 173, 391, 773, *Ten Essential Points of Taijiquan*, 143
tensegrity, 828–839
Thirteen Chapters on Taijiquan, 90, 119, 285, 291, 372, 632, 659
thirteen postures, 6, 71, 291, 466–467, 612, 735–736
thirteen stances, 65, 68, 71–73, 75
Thirty-Eight Style, 97–99, 317–318
three heights, 135
Three Important Points on Partner Practice, 564
three powers posture (*santi*), 265–266, 738
three treasures (*jing, qi, shen*), 265–266, 350–351, 684
Tian, Xiuchen, 11
Tian, Zhaolin, 359
Tien, Moer, 696
Traditional Shaolin and Secret Transmissions of Shaolin Boxing, 639
thrusting hand, 146, 148, 579, 926
toes, 12, 106, 114, 330–332, 334, 397, 398–401, 531
training, learning process, 57–64, 254 note 9, 428, 429–442, 563–564, 569–584, 729 note 9, 754, 811, 855–864, 913
Treatise on Taijiquan, 654
Treatise on the Origins and Branches of Taijiquan, 630, 632
The True Essence of the Martial Arts, 643
Tu, Zongren, 24, 28–29, 57
tuberculosis, 20, 79, 168, 212, 220, 241, 277, 315, 713–714
tuishou (see push-hands)
two-person practices, 83, 89, 136–137, 326, 386–388, 435, 507, 525, 575, 606, 763, 771, 848
Twelve Continuous Fists, 562

U

Ueshiba, Morihei, 356 note 8
United Nations, 14, 171–172
uprooting, 202–203, 211, 319, 719, 799, 851, 915–916, 926

V

vertical dantian rotation, 877
vital energy (see *qi*)
vital points, 90, 154, 160, 162 note 1, 374, 474, 578, 646

W

waist, 9, 72, 110–111, 122, 143, 147–148, 159, 240, 263, 303, 317, 327, 332–334, 336–338, 360, 362, 487, 519, 609, 610–611
Waley, Arthur, 42, 45
Wan Chun, 561
Wan, Laiping, 653
Wan, Laisheng, 116–117, 156, 163 note 3, 216, 653
Wanchai District, 586, 594 note 2
Wang, Haijun, 543, 554
Wang, Jiaxiang, 10, 23–24, 27–28, 30–31
Wang, Juexin, 636
Wang, Lanting, 14, 282, 561–563
Wang, Peisheng, 359, 427, 934
Wang, Xi'an, 481, 484, 486, 489, 496, 704, 706
Wang, Xianggen, 198, 359, 363
Wang, Xiling, 655
Wang, Xiuai, 151
Wang, Yangming, 180, 647
Wang, Yannian, 116–118, 128 note 2, 158, 227, 288 note 11, 717, 721, 798
Wang, Yongfu, 673
Wang, Zongyue, 6–8, 14, 65–66, 122, 146, 241, 253 notes 2 and 5, 375, 403, 612, 630–631, 633, 636, 648, 659–660
ward off (*peng*), 70, 126, 143–144, 477, 510, 516, 521, 736, 834, 840, 847, 925–926
Warlord Period, 585, 634, 702, 757–758, 816
water image, 44, 58, 69–70, 103–104, 197, 259–274, 485, 549, 778
Waterside Pavilion, Beijing, 713
Wave Hands Like Clouds, 258, 403, 862
wei-so garrison units, 7, 384, 606, 649, 698, 759, 761
Wenzhou, 83, 167, 182 note 5, 712
White Cloud Monastery, 2, 351, 394
White Crane, 83, 442, 594 note 4, 691 note 2, 833, 862
White Lotus Society, 50, 756
World Health Organization/health guidelines, 384
women, 172, 177, 179, 406

Wu-Chan fight, 588
Wu, Chaojie, 590
Wu, Dakui, 586–588, 590–591, 594 note 2
Wu, Daqi, 587, 590
Wu, Gongyi, 585–588, 590–591, 594 note 4
Wu, Gongzao, 119, 585, 588–590, 594 note 3, 633, 640
Wu, Guozhong, 80–82, 84–88, 91 note 6, 118–119, 123, 130 note 10, 255 note 20
Wu, Hoqing, 14
Wu, Jianquan, 14, 119, 123, 130 note 9, 240, 287 notes 1 and 2, 314, 407, 508, 568 notes 2 and 8, 585–588, 590, 592, 594 notes 1 and 4, 631, 633, 637, 762
Wu, Kangnian, 588, 590
Wu, Mengxia, 156, 163
Wu, Quanyou, 14, 123, 130 note 9, 561, 590, 691 note 3, 934
Wu, Ruqing, 560
Wu style, 12, 14, 240, 253 note 5, 255 note 16, 287 note 2, 314, 359–360, 407, 427, 509, 525, 568, note 8, 585, 592, 691 note 3
Wu, Tunan, 122, 240, 375, 560, 633, 637, 659, 676, 817
Wu, Wenbiao, 590
Wu, Yanxia, 587, 590
Wu, Yinghua, 589
Wu, Yuxiang, 11–12, 14, 120, 122, 241, 253 notes 5 and 6, 299 note 1, 509, 568 note 1, 630–631, 641, 654, 659, 701, 734
Wu, Xiubao, 423
Wu, Zhiqing, 630, 636
Wudang Martial Arts Research Association, 652–653
Wudang Mountain, 2–3, 238, 252, 279, 344, 625, 627, 635–636, 648, 651–652, 695
Wudang Taijiquan, 653
Wudang sword, 359
wuji, 66–69, 75, 263, 324–325, 377–378, 402, 425, 570, 737–738, 745, 830–831, 833–835, 830, 840–841
Wuqing Taijiquan, 562
wuwei (non-action), 258, 274, 309, 346, 415, 639

X

Xia Tao, 132, 207, 272
Xi'an city, 2, 341, 360, 374, 387, 423, 463, 481, 579
Xiao, Huilong, 592

xingyiquan, 157, 194–195, 216, 248, 278–279, 314, 629–630, 639, 644, 657, 677–678, 691 notes 2 and 3, 733–736, 638–639, 777–778, 788–791
xinjia (see new frame)
xinyiquan, 359–360, 413, 416–417, 562, 673, 691 note 4
Xiong, Yanghe, 717, 752 –753, 760–773, 776
Xu, Chongming, 721
Xu, Tingsen, 406–407
Xu, Yizhong, 151, 156, 184 note 22, 717, 719
Xu, Yusheng, 11, 177, 283, 285, 287 note 1, 630, 632, 637
Xu, Yuxiang, 299 note 1, 568 note 1, 630–631, 641, 654, 659, 701, 734
Xu, Zhengmei, 797, 816–819
Xuanwu (god of war), 628, 642, 651, 661, 675

Y

Yang, Banhou, 13–15, 119, 121, 123, 130 note 9, 136, 195, 199, 238, 255 note 16, 280–282, 287 notes 2 and 4, 299 note 1, 359, 474, 561–562, 606, 633, 646, 730 notes 10 and 11, 755, 759–760
Yang, Chengfu, 15, 20, 77–79, 115–124, 128 note 2, 143, 157–158, 160, 163 note 4, 169–170, 177, 179, 183 notes 17, 314, 359–360, 385, 407, 473–475, 478–480, 606, 631–632, 635–637, 639, 653, 714–716, 729 notes 6, 7, 8, and 9, 730 note 10, 755, 759–760, 762–763, 773, 797, 807, 925
Yang, Hongling, 656
Yang, Jianhou, 13–15, 116, 121–122, 195, 238, 280, 282, 287 note 1, 359, 473–475, 606, 729 note 9, 755, 763, 771
Yang, Jwing-Ming, 417, 509, 525
Yang, Luchan, 9, 12–15, 116, 121–122, 177, 185 note 47, 192–193, 195, 198–199, 204, 206, 238, 240–241, 248–249, 252–253 notes 2 and 5, 254 note 7, 255 note 16, 278–282, 287 note 7, 359, 375, 385, 454–455, 457, 474–475, 537, 560–563, 565–566, 568 notes 1 and 3, 583, 606, 615, 630, 634–636, 649, 654, 660, 691 note 3, 701, 709, 752–756, 759, 760, 772–773, 934
Yang, Qingyu, 57, 383, 764
Yang, Sau Chung, 480
Yang, Shaohou, 15, 122, 193, 279–280, 287 notes 1 and 4, 631, 730, 755, 759–760, 762

Yang, Zhengduo, 427
Yang, Zhenduo, 288 note 10, 401, 474–475
Yao, Hanchen, 314
Ye, Shuliang, 591–592
Yellow Emperor (Huangdi), 46, 50, 52 note 13, 344–345, 354, 355 note 1, 356 note 11, 344–345, 354, 355 note 1, 356 note 11, 630, 632
Yijing (see Book of Changes)
Yin, Wanbang, 761
Yip Man, 586
Yongnian, 15, 560, 568 note 1, 635, 754
yongquan acupoint, 329, 397, 881
Yuan, Shikai, 10, 759
Yuan, Shiming, 423–424
Yuan, Weiming, 727, 797, 799 note 1, 808–815
Yue Fei (General), 630, 655, 658, 691 note 4
Yue, Shuting, 82–86, 88–89, 124 note 11
Yuwen University, 168, 255, 713

Z

Zhan, Deshen, 721
Zhang, Daoling, 46
Zhang, Fengqi, 560–561
Zhang, Guan, 167, 182 note 10
Zhang, Qinlin, 116–117, 119, 124, 158, 169, 231 note 7, 255 note 20, 287 note 3, 288 note 11, 730
Zhang, Qingling, 78–79
Zhang, Sanfeng, 2–3, 5–6, 8, 87, 147, 238, 240–241, 252 note 2, 253 note 5, 254 note 7, 258, 279, 287 note 5 343–344, 354, 397, 399, 412, 587, 590–591, 625, 627–637, 639–642, 647–661, 672, 725
Zhang Sanfeng Classic, 147
Zhang, Shaotang, 560
Zhang, Wansheng, 563
Zhang, Xitang, 423, 427
Zhang, Youquan, 358–360, 360
Zhang, Zhigang, 20
Zhao, Kuangyin, 672
Zhao, Youbin, 635, 659
Zhao, Zhongdao, 672–674, 676–678, 682–685, 691 note 2, 692 note 5
Zhaobao, 11, 630, 634, 650–651, 653–654, 702, 791, 794
Zheng, Manqing, 15, 20, 77, 80–81, 84, 88, 91 note 11, 115–118, 121–124, 126–127, 128 notes 1 and 2, 129 note 4, 150–152, 154–156, 158, 161–162, 164 notes 6 and 8, 165–171, 173–174, 175–181, 181 note 2, 183 notes 14 and 17, 184 note 28, 185 note 37, 202, 204, 211–212, 215–216, 220, 229 note 4, 231 notes 7, 8 and 9, 232 note 11, 235 note 28, 277–288, 291, 297, 299, 346, 372, 507–509, 524, 607, 611, 623–624, 631–633, 636–638, 641, 646, 711–731, 763, 797–798, 800–802, 806–807, 809–811, 817–818, 821–822, 850, 916, 918, 925 note 19
thirty-seven-posture form, 78, 120, 122, 169–170, 179, 239
Zheng Manqing Memorial Hall, 720–721, 725, 731 note
Zheng, Patrick, 160–163, 164 note 8, 244
Zhong, Yueping, 587–588, 594 note 1
Zhongshan Hall, 716, 801–802, 807, 817
Zhou, Dunyi, 380 note 12
Zhou, Jiannan, 636
Zhu, Tiancai, 548, 704
Zhu, Yuanzhang, 696, 698
Zhu Xi, 42, 262, 350, 378, 637
Zhuang Shen, 636
Zhuangzi, 44, 219, 233 note 16, 260, 273, 308, 343, 377, 415, 626, 637, 642, 662, 812
Zuo, Laipeng, 78, 80, 84, 116–119, 124, 249, 255 note 20

Other Titles by Via Media Publishing

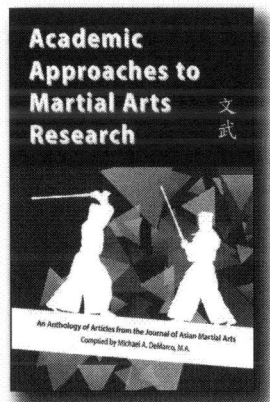

Academic Approaches
to Martial Art Research

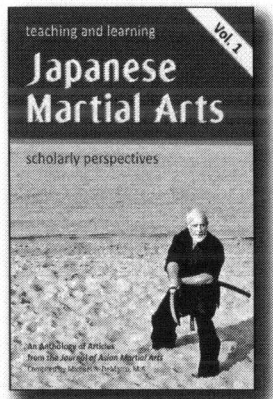

Teaching and Learning Japanese Martial Art Arts
Volume I and Volume II

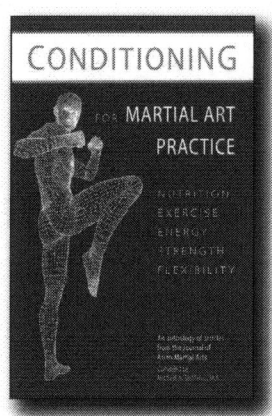

Conditioning for
Martial Art Practice

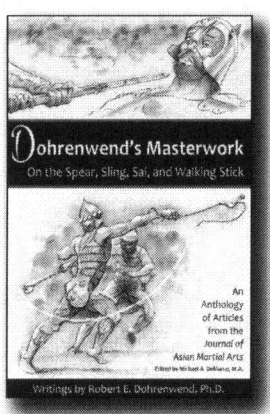

Dohrenwend's Masterwork
spear, sling, sai, walking stick

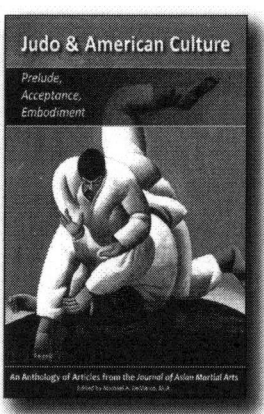

Judo and
American Culture

Fiction

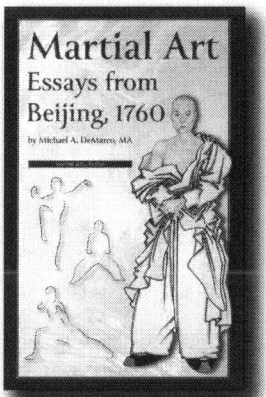

Wuxia America - Emergence
of a Chinese American Hero

Martial Art Essays
from Beijing, 1760

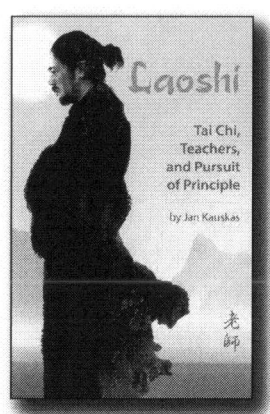

Laoshi: Tai Chi, Teachers,
and Pursuit of Principle

Printed in Great Britain
by Amazon

50021a49-1742-483d-b0d9-25b8adebca78R01